Colposcopy

PRINCIPLES AND PRACTICE

An Integrated Textbook and Atlas

Colposcopy

PRINCIPLES AND PRACTICE

An Integrated Textbook and Atlas

BARBARA S. APGAR, MD, MS
Clinical Professor
Department of Family Medicine
University of Michigan Medical School
Ann Arbor, Michigan

GREGORY L. BROTZMAN, MD
Professor
Department of Family and Community Medicine
Medical College of Wisconsin
Milwaukee, Wisconsin

MARK SPITZER, MD
Professor of Clinical Obstetrics and Gynecology
New York University School of Medicine
Department of Obstetrics and Gynecology
North Shore University Hospital
Manhasset, New York

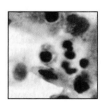

W.B. SAUNDERS COMPANY
An Imprint of Elsevier Science
Philadelphia   London   New York   St. Louis   Sydney   Toronto

W.B. SAUNDERS COMPANY
An Imprint of Elsevier Science

The Curtis Center
Independence Square West
Philadelphia, Pennsylvania 19106

Library of Congress Cataloging-in-Publication Data

Colposcopy, principles & practice: an integrated textbook and atlas / [edited by] Barbara S. Apgar, Mark Spitzer, Gregory L. Brotzman.

   p.; cm.

   ISBN 0–7216–8494–7

   1. Colposcopy—atlases. I. Title: Colposcopy, principles and practice. II. Apgar, Barbara S.
III. Spitzer, Mark. IV. Brotzman, Gregory L.
   [DNLM: 1. Colposcopy—methods. 2. Colposcopy—atlases. WP 250 C721 2002]

RG107.5.C6 C65 2002

618.1′075—dc21   2001057596

Executive Editor: Raymond Kersey
Developmental Editor: Denise LeMelledo
Project Manager: Agnes Byrne
Manuscript Editor: Jennifer Ehlers
Senior Production Manager: Peter Faber
Illustration Specialist: Lisa Lambert
Designer: Karen O'Keefe-Owens
Illustrator: Esteban Cabrera
Indexer: Dennis Dolan

COLPOSCOPY PRINCIPLES & PRACTICE:
AN INTEGRATED TEXTBOOK AND ATLAS   ISBN 0–7216–8494–7

Printed in the United States of America

Last digit is the print number: 9   8   7   6   5   4   3   2   1

To my beloved teachers, Virginia and Gloria, whose spirits continue to enrich my life; to Larisa for teaching me about rainbows; and to my caring and energetic residents, who have given me a wealth of fond memories over the years.

B.A.

To my wife Cindy and my children, Ethan, Isaac, and Elyse, who have supported me, loved me, and put up with the long hours of work on this book.

G.B.

To my beloved mother, Miriam Spitzer, and my late father, Sam Spitzer, of blessed memory, who sacrificed everything for their children's happiness and success; to my wonderful daughters, Gila, Ayelet, and Elkie; and, most of all, to my beloved wife and partner through life, Peri, without whose love and understanding this book could not have happened.

M.S.

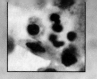

Contributors

BARBARA S. APGAR, MD, MS
Clinical Professor, Department of Family Medicine, University of Michigan Medical School, Ann Arbor, Michigan
Principles and Technique of the Colposcopic Examination; Glossary; Abnormal Transformation Zone; High-Grade Squamous Intraepithelial Lesion; Practical Therapeutic Options for Treatment of Cervical Intraepithelial Neoplasia

DOROTHY M. BARBO, MD
Professor Emerita, Department of Obstetrics and Gynecology, University of New Mexico, Albuquerque, New Mexico
Colposcopic Assessment System: Rubin and Barbo Colposcopic Assessment System

ROBERT E. BRISTOW, MD
Assistant Professor, Departments of Obstetrics & Gynecology and Oncology, The Johns Hopkins University School of Medicine, Baltimore, Maryland; Surgeon, The Kelly Gynecologic Oncology Service, The Johns Hopkins Hospital and Medical Institutions, Baltimore, Maryland
Management Scenarios: Management of Positive Margins and Positive Endocervical Curettage

GREGORY L. BROTZMAN, MD
Professor, Department of Family and Community Medicine, Medical College of Wisconsin, Milwaukee, Wisconsin; Assistant Director, Columbia Hospital Family Practice Residency Program, Milwaukee, Wisconsin
Adjunctive Testing: Cervicography; Principles and Technique of the Colposcopic Examination; Glossary; Abnormal Transformation Zone; High-Grade Squamous Intraepithelial Lesion, Psychosocial Aspects of Colposcopy; Practical Therapeutic Options for Treatment of Cervical Intraepithelial Neoplasia

DENNIS J. BUTLER, PhD
Associate Professor, Department of Family and Community Medicine, Medical College of Wisconsin, Milwaukee, Wisconsin; Director of Behavioral Science, Columbia Hospital Family Practice Program, Milwaukee, Wisconsin
Psychosocial Aspects of Colposcopy

GORDON DAVIS, MD
Director, Arizona Vulva Clinic, Phoenix, Arizona
Vulvar Intraepithelial Neoplasia: Clinical Manifestations

JUAN FELIX, MD
Associate Professor of Pathology and Obstetrics & Gynecology, Keck School of Medicine, University of Southern California, Los Angeles, California; Director of Surgical Pathology, Los Angeles County Women's and Children's Hospital, Los Angeles, California
The Papanicolaou Smear: Liquid-Based, Thin-Layer Cytology

ALEX FERENCZY, MD
Professor of Pathology and Obstetrics & Gynecology, McGill University, Montreal, Quebec, Canada; Physician, SMBD-Jewish General Hospital, Department of Pathology, Montreal, Quebec, Canada
Vulvar Intraepithelial Neoplasia

FRANK GIRARDI, MD
Professor, Department of Obstetrics and Gynecology, University of Graz, Graz, Austria; Chairman, Department of Obstetrics and Gynecology, General Hospital, Badeu/Vienna, Austria
Colposcopic Assessment System: Burghardt's System

MITCHELL D. GREENBERG, MD
Senior Vice President, Corporate Clinical Affairs, U.S. HealthConnect, Philadelphia, Pennsylvania
Colposcopic Assessment System: Reid's Colposcopic Index

MARY K. HOWETT, PhD
Professor of Microbiology and Immunology, Pennsylvania State University College of Medicine, Hershey, Pennsylvania
Human Papillomaviruses: Molecular Aspects of the Viral Life Cycle and Pathogenesis

CYNDA JOHNSON, MD, MBA
Professor and Head, Department of Family Medicine, University of Iowa College of Medicine, Iowa City, Iowa
The Papanicolaou Smear: Terminology in Cervical Cytology: The Bethesda System; The Papanicolaou Smear: Conventional Cytology

RAYMOND H. KAUFMAN, MD
Professor, Departments of Obstetrics & Gynecology and Pathology, Baylor College of Medicine, Houston, Texas
Lower Genital Tract Changes Associated with in Utero Exposure to Diethylstilbestrol

BURTON A. KRUMHOLZ, MD
Professor of Obstetrics, Gynecology, and Women's Health Care, Albert Einstein College of Medicine, The Yeshiva University, New York, New York; Attending Physician, Obstetrics and Gynecology, Long Island Jewish Medical Center, New Hyde Park, New York
Vagina: Normal, Premalignant, and Malignant

NEAL M. LONKY, MD, MPH
Clinical Professor, Department of Obstetrics and Gynecology, University of California, Irvine School of Medicine, Irvine, California; Assistant Chief of Obstetrics and Gynecology, Area Research and Education Chairman, Director of Colposcopic Services, Kaiser Permanente, Anaheim, California
Adjunctive Testing: Cervical Screening with in Vivo and in Vitro Modalities: Speculoscopy Combined with Cytology

ATTILA T. LORINCZ, PhD
Senior Vice President and Chief Scientific Officer, Digene Corporation, Gaithersburg, Maryland
Adjunctive Testing: Human Papillomavirus Testing

KELLY J. MANAHAN, MD
Assistant Professor, Division of Gynecologic Oncology, University of Iowa, Iowa City, Iowa
Squamous Cervical Cancer: Invasion and Microinvasion

LYNETTE MARGESSON, MD
Assistant Professor of Obstetrics and Gynecology, Dartmouth Medical School, Hanover, New Hampshire
Non-neoplastic Epithelial Lesions of the Vulva

F. J. MONTZ, MD
Professor, Departments of Obstetrics & Gynecology and Oncology, The Johns Hopkins University School of Medicine, Baltimore, Maryland; Director and Surgeon, The Kelly Gynecologic Oncology Service, The Johns Hopkins Hospital and Medical Institutions, Baltimore, Maryland
Management Scenarios: Management of Positive Margins and Positive Endocervical Curettage

DENNIS M. O'CONNOR, MD
Associate Clinical Professor, Department of Obstetrics & Gynecology and Department of Pathology & Laboratory Medicine, University of Louisville School of Medicine, Louisville, Kentucky; Pathologist, Clinical Associates, PSC, Norton Suburban Hospital, Louisville, Kentucky
Glossary; Normal Transformation Zone

BRUCE PATSNER, MD, MBA
Womens Cancer Center, Palo Alto, California
Colposcopy of External Genital Condyloma

JOHN L. PFENNINGER, MD
President and Medical Director, The National Procedures Institute, Midland, Michigan; Medical Director, The Medical Procedures Center P.C., Midland, Michigan
Androscopy: Examination of the Male Partner

ANIL B.M. PINTO, MD
Clinical Instructor, Washington University School of Medicine, St. Louis, Missouri
Lower Genital Tract Intraepithelial Neoplasia in the Immunocompromised Woman

SWEE CHONG QUEK, MBBCh, MRCOG
Obstetrician and Gynecologist, Gynecologic Oncology Unit, KK Women's and Children's Hospital, Singapore
Adjunctive Testing: The Polarprobe

R. KEVIN REYNOLDS, MD
Associate Professor, Chief, Division of Gynecologic Oncology, University of Michigan, Ann Arbor, Michigan
Squamous Cervical Cancer: Invasion and Microinvasion

MARY M. RUBIN, RNC, PhD
Associate Clinical Professor, University of California–San Francisco, San Francisco, California; Director of Clinical Education and Director of Colposcopy Education Programs, California Family Health Council, Campbell, California
Principles and Technique of the Colposcopic Examination; Colposcopic Assessment System: Rubin and Barbo Colposcopic Assessment System

BETHANEE J. SCHLOSSER, BS
Graduate Assistant, Pennsylvania State University College of Medicine, Hershey, Pennsylvania
Human Papillomaviruses: Molecular Aspects of the Viral Life Cycle and Pathogenesis

ALBERT SINGER, PhD, DPhil
Professor and Consultant Gynecologist, Department of Women's and Children's Health, Whitlington Hospital, London, England
Adjunctive Testing: The Polarprobe

MARK SPITZER, MD
Professor of Clinical Obstetrics and Gynecology, New York University School of Medicine, Department of Obstetrics and Gynecology, North Shore University Hospital, Manhasset, New York
The Papanicolaou Smear: Terminology in Cervical Cytology: The Bethesda System; Adjunctive Testing: Cervicography; Lower Genital Tract Intraepithelial Neoplasia in the Immunocompromised Woman; Practical Therapeutic Options for Treatment of Cervical Intraepithelial Neoplasia; Management Scenarios: Guidelines for the Management of Colposcopic Findings; Management Scenarios: Management of Positive Margins and Positive Endocervical Curettage

ADOLF STAFL, MD, PhD
Professor of Obstetrics and Gynecology, Charles University, Prague, Czech Republic
Angiogenesis of Cervical Neoplasia

MARK H. STOLER, MD
Professor of Pathology and Gynecology, University of Virginia Health System, Charlottesville, Virginia; Associate Director of Surgical and Cytopathology, University of Virginia Health System, Charlottesville, Virginia
Management Scenarios: Management of Atypical Squamous Cells of Undetermined Significance and Low-Grade Squamous Abnormalities of the Uterine Cervix

KARL TAMUSSINO, MD
Professor, Department of Obstetrics and Gynecology, University of Graz, Graz, Austria
Colposcopic Assessment System: Burghardt's System

RAPHAEL P. VISCIDI, MD
Associate Professor of Pediatrics, Johns Hopkins Univer-

sity School of Medicine, Baltimore, Maryland
Epidemiology of Genital Tract Human Papillomavirus Infections

ALAN G. WAXMAN, MD
Associate Professor, Department of Obstetrics and Gynecology, University of New Mexico School of Medicine, Albuquerque, New Mexico
Low-Grade Squamous Intraepithelial Lesion

DAVID G. WEISMILLER, MD, ScM
Assistant Professor of Family Medicine, Director of Women's Health, The Brody School of Medicine at East Carolina University, Greenville, North Carolina; Physician, Pitt County Memorial Hospital, Greenville, North Carolina
Triage of the Abnormal Papanicolaou Smear and Colposcopy in Pregnancy

EDWARD J. WILKINSON, MD
Professor and Vice Chairman, Department of Pathology and Laboratory Medicine, and Director, Division of Anatomic Pathology, University of Florida College of Medicine, Gainesville, Florida; Medical Director, Cytopathology and Histology Laboratories, Shands Hospital at the University of Florida, Gainesville, Florida; Medical Director, University of Florida Diagnostic Referral Laboratories, Shands Hospital at the University of Florida, Gainesville, Florida
The Papanicolaou Smear: Clinical Laboratories Improvement Act

V. CECIL WRIGHT, MD
Professor, Department of Obstetrics and Gynaecology, University of Western Ontario, London, Ontario, Canada
Colposcopic Features of Cervical Adenocarcinoma in Situ and Adenocarcinoma and Management of Preinvasive Disease

Preface

Colposcopy is an accepted and widely used procedure for examination of the lower genital tract. Since the early 1990s, the practice of colposcopy has evolved. New knowledge about the human papillomavirus has emerged. The triage guidelines for evaluation of abnormal cervical cytology have been revised, creating further interest in the role of colposcopy in evaluating preinvasive and invasive disease. Practitioners from various disciplines have been trained in colposcopy and have begun to include it among the services they offer in their practice. This integrated textbook and atlas provides a modern framework for all students and practitioners of colposcopy. Colposcopic practice is truly integrated now, and this book is written for all our colleagues.

A comprehensive textbook and atlas is not possible without the help of countless individuals. Our editors at W.B. Saunders especially Raymond Kersey and Denise LeMelledo, provided us with everything we needed to complete the project, and their encouragement kept us focused on the goal. Through their research and clinical practice initiatives, our international group of authors has helped define modern colposcopic practice, and we are grateful that they shared their work in this book. We would also like to honor the memory of Thomas L. Sedlacek, MD, who, before his untimely death, was involved in the initial planning of the book design.

One of the stumbling blocks in writing a colposcopy textbook is the large number of high-quality images needed to illustrate each clinical condition. Without the awesome and superb assistance of Mr. Fred Kostecki, president of National Testing Laboratories (NTL), we would not have been able to publish this book. Fred spent innumerable hours selecting the best Cervigrams from NTL's extensive collection. His extraordinary generosity enabled Greg to successfully digitalize and format the images in the book.

In addition to Mr. Kostecki, we want to gratefully thank our colleagues, Federico M. di Paola, MD, Chief, Laser Unit, Centro Medico de la Mujer in Buenos Aires, Argentina, and Vesna Kesic, MD, PhD, Associate Professor, Institute of Obstetrics and Gynecology, University Clinical Center, Beograd, Yugoslavia, for allowing us to use their Cervigrams. They provided invaluable assistance. Mr. John R. Voelz, Audiovisual Specialist at Colum-

bia–St. Mary's Hospital, Milwaukee, Wisconsin, helped in obtaining images of procedures and photofinishing pathology sections.

Two pathologists provided immeasurable help in selecting and labeling cytologic and histologic images. We would like to thank Edward J. Wilkinson, MD, Professor of Pathology and Laboratory Medicine at the University of Florida, Gainesville, Florida, and David J. Ferguson, MD, Staff Pathologist, Waukesha Memorial Hospital, Waukesha, Wisconsin, who selected the appropriate pathology material for the book.

From our own personal perspective, each of us has special thanks to render.

I would like to especially thank the individuals who taught and mentored me in my colposcopic practice. Very special thanks go to my chairman, Thomas L. Schwenk, MD, who has supported me throughout many endeavors but especially during the writing of this book. Most of all, I want to acknowledge the extraordinary efforts of my coeditors, Greg and Mark. Special and heartfelt thanks go to Greg for his uncanny and masterful ability to process the images and to Mark for his precise and brilliant editing and always sage advice. B.A.

A special thanks to my colleagues at the Medical College of Wisconsin–Columbia Family Practice Residency Program, who helped and supported me through this project, and to my editorial partners, Barbara and Mark, who helped make this book a reality. G.B.

In life, the difference between success and failure is often the presence of others who assist or enable an individual to reach goals. I would like to thank Burton A. Krumholz, MD, who has been my colposcopy mentor, and Vicki L. Seltzer, MD, who has been enormously supportive and enabled me to achieve my career goals. Finally, I would like to thank Barbara and Greg for allowing me to join them in this wonderful endeavor. M.S.

Our goal has been to provide a comprehensive and practical guide to colposcopic practice. We are deeply appreciative of all those who helped make the book a reality.

BARBARA S. APGAR, MD, MS
GREGORY L. BROTZMAN, MD
MARK SPITZER, MD

Contents

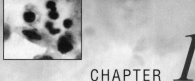

• Raphael P. Viscidi

CHAPTER *1*

Epidemiology of Genital Tract Human Papillomavirus Infections

Papillomaviruses are a class of viruses that cause warts (papillomas) in many vertebrate species, including humans. Warts are the clinical manifestation of the proliferation of squamous epithelial cells. They may appear as well-circumscribed, elevated lesions or as flat lesions, or they may be recognizable only by their characteristic histologic features. Warts have been identified at many different sites in humans, including the genital tract, oral cavity, respiratory tract, and skin. Most warts are benign, but they may rarely undergo malignant transformation, a process intimately linked to their viral etiology.

VIRAL ETIOLOGY OF WARTS

HPV infections of the female genital tract are very common, and the vast majority of them are clinically inapparent.

The viral etiology of common skin warts was established in 1907 by Ciuffo, who demonstrated that warts could be induced by transmission of a cell-free filtrate from person to person.[1] Subsequently, similar transmission studies showed that warts at other sites in humans, including the genital tract, were also of viral origin.[2, 3] In 1949, the responsible agent—the papillomavirus—was first visualized with the electron microscope in material taken from a common skin wart.[4, 5] The presence of particles resembling papillomaviruses in genital warts was not definitively established until 1970.[6] Further progress in characterization of papillomaviruses was greatly slowed by the inability to propagate the virus in a tissue culture system. The cloning of human and animal papillomavirus genomes in the 1970s opened up a new era in papillomavirus virology. The genomic organization of papillomaviruses was determined, and considerable progress was made in elucidating the function of several papillomavirus genes. The partial sequencing of multiple human papillomavirus (HPV) genomes led to an appreciation of the tremendous heterogeneity of the species. More than 100 HPV types have now been identified, and specific clinical lesions have been associated with different types. For epidemiologic studies, the chief benefit from the application of molecular biologic techniques to HPV is the development of molecular diagnostic tools. These developments culminated in 1989 with the introduction of diagnostic methods based on the polymerase chain reaction (PCR).[7] These methods are now the "gold standard" for detection of HPV in biologic specimens. Their use in epidemiologic studies has provided estimates of the prevalence of HPV infection in various populations. It is clear from these studies that HPV infections of the female genital tract are very common and that the vast majority of these infections are clinically inapparent.

WARTS AND CANCER

The etiologic relationship of HPVs to cervical cancer, as well as to cancers at several other sites, is firmly established.

The work of Shope in 1933 first established a connection between papillomaviruses and cancer.[8] He showed that viruses recovered from naturally occurring papillomas in cottontail rabbits produced warts in domestic rabbits that progressed to carcinoma. A possible connection between cervical cancer and a venereally transmitted infectious agent had long been suspected. In 1842, a relationship between cervical cancer and sexual activity was described by Rigoni-Stern, who observed that cervical cancer is almost never seen in virgins and is most common in prostitutes.[9] In the modern era, epidemiologic studies have shown that the risk of cervical cancer is increased among women who begin having sexual intercourse at earlier ages and who have greater numbers of sexual partners. In 1976, zur Hausen suggested that HPV might be etiologically related to anogenital cancers.[10] His argument was based on the mode of venereal transmission of HPV, the anecdotal reports of malignant transformation of genital warts, and the known oncogenic potential of papillomaviruses. In the same year, Meisels and Fortin noted that the cytologic features of condylomatous genital warts resemble those of mild cervical intraepithelial neoplasia (CIN), suggesting a link between the two pathologic processes.[11] In 1983, Durst, working in zur

Hausen's laboratory, discovered a new HPV genotype, type 16 (HPV 16), in a biopsy sample from an invasive cervical cancer.[12] Using a cloned portion of the genome as a probe, he demonstrated the presence of HPV 16 DNA in more than 60% of cervical cancer biopsy specimens from German patients. Today, the epidemiologic evidence from case-control and cohort studies for an association between HPV and cervical cancer is overwhelming. In addition, laboratory studies detailing the transforming properties of HPV oncoproteins provide support for a plausible mechanism of HPV-induced carcinogenesis. Now that the etiologic relationship of HPVs to cervical cancer, as well as to cancers at several other sites, is firmly established, the focus of epidemiologic studies has turned to determining why only a small number of persons infected with HPV go on to develop cancer.

OVERVIEW OF BIOLOGY AND PATHOGENESIS OF PAPILLOMAVIRUSES

A detailed treatment of the molecular biology and pathogenesis of HPV is provided in Chapter 2.

Biology of Papillomaviruses

Papillomaviruses are small, nonenveloped DNA viruses. The genome is a double-stranded circular DNA molecule of approximately 8000 base pairs that is contained within a spherical protein coat or capsid. The capsid consists of two structural proteins: the major capsid protein (L1), which constitutes 80% of the total protein, and the minor capsid protein (L2). All papillomaviruses have a similar genetic organization. The viral genome is divided into an early region, which encodes the genes required for viral transcription and replication and for cellular transformation; a late region, which encodes for the viral capsid proteins; and a noncoding regulatory region, also referred to as the long control region, that contains the control elements for transcription and replication and the viral origin of replication.

> **The current list of cancer-associated HPVs includes four high-risk types (types 16, 18, 31, and 45) and nine intermediate risk types (types 33, 35, 39, 51, 52, 56, 58, 59, and 68). Seventy-five percent of cervical cancers are infected with type 16, 18, 31, or 45.**

Papillomaviruses are classified on the basis of the species they infect and on the degree of genetic relationship with other papillomaviruses of the same species. Presently, 34 animal papillomavirus types and more than 115 different HPV types have been described (HPV sequence database; www.hpv-web.lanl.gov). On the basis of criteria adopted by the Papillomavirus Nomenclature Committee, the combined nucleotide sequence of the E6, E7, and L1 open reading frame (~2.4 kb, or roughly one third of the genome) of a new type should differ by more than 10% from the corresponding sequence of other known HPV types.[13] The investigator who discovers the papillomavirus usually names the type, and a nomenclature committee later assigns a number. Isolates within the same type differing by 0% to 2% in their nucleotide sequence from a reference sequence are considered variants. HPVs are also commonly grouped on the basis of site of infection into cutaneous and mucosal types or, on the basis of the strength of their association with cancer, into high-risk and low-risk types. The current list of cancer-associated HPVs includes four high-risk types (types 16, 18, 31, and 45) and nine intermediate-risk types (types 33, 35, 39, 51, 52, 56, 58, 59, and 68). Seventy-five percent of cervical cancers are infected with type 16, 18, 31, or 45. In general, different types are associated with different clinical entities. However, extensive analyses have not always been carried out to establish the specificity of these associations. All the types can cause subclinical infection, the most common manifestation of HPV infection. More than 35 types have been recovered from the female lower genital tract, which is the main reservoir for the mucosal types.

Pathogenesis of Papillomavirus Infection

> **HPV infections are initiated when the virus gains access to basal cells of a squamous epithelial surface either through minor traumas such as skin abrasion or during sexual intercourse.**

Papillomaviruses have a specific tropism for surface epithelial cells of the skin or the mucosa. Infection is entirely confined to the epithelium, and consequently viremia does not occur during the course of infection. HPV infections are initiated when the virus gains access to basal cells of a squamous epithelial surface either through minor traumas such as skin abrasion or during sexual intercourse. The life cycle of the papillomavirus within infected cells can be divided into an early stage and a late stage. The stages are linked to the differentiation state of the epithelial cell. In the early stage, a low level of viral replication is maintained in the basal cell, and only the early genes are transcribed. The late stage occurs in terminally differentiated squamous epithelial cells and is associated with late gene expression, synthesis of capsid proteins, vegetative viral DNA synthesis, and formation of viral particles. Common histologic features of HPV infection are localized hyperplasia of basal cells, thickening or keratosis of the superficial cell layer, and a degenerative cellular process known as koilocytosis. Koilocytes are characterized by perinuclear cytoplasmic vacuolization, nuclear enlargement, and hyperchromasia. The nuclear changes reflect the fact that papillomaviruses multiply in the nucleus.

Clinical Manifestations of HPV Infection of the Female Genital Tract

The most commonly recognized visible clinical lesions associated with HPV infection of the female lower genital tract are genital or venereal warts (condylomata acuminata). The lesions are typically multiple, well-circumscribed, papillomatous growths that may involve the vaginal introitus, the vulva, the perineum, the anus, and, rarely, the cervix. Most HPV infections of the genital tract are subclinical, but in many cases they can be diagnosed cytologically. Cervical cytology is the most frequently used method of assessing women for cytologic evidence of HPV infection and of HPV-associated neoplasia. The cytologic effects of HPV infection include a spectrum of abnormalities. The mildest abnormalities are usually called condylomatous atypia or koilocytotic atypia. The more severe abnormalities correspond to the traditional classification of precursor lesions of invasive cervical cancer—namely, mild, moderate, or severe dysplasia (CIN 1, CIN 2, or CIN 3, respectively). The observation initially made by Meisels and colleagues that condylomatous atypia is nearly indistinguishable from CIN 1 led to the development of the Bethesda System of cytopathology, in which these two diagnoses are combined as low-grade squamous intraepithelial lesions (LSIL), whereas CIN 2 and CIN 3 are combined as high-grade squamous intraepithelial lesions (HSIL).

PREVALENCE AND INCIDENCE OF HPV INFECTION OF THE FEMALE GENITAL TRACT

Estimates of the prevalence of cervical HPV infection vary greatly depending on the method of diagnosis and the demographic and behavioral characteristics of the study population. Infection can be diagnosed clinically (observation of genital warts), cytologically (Papanicolaou [Pap] smear), or virologically (DNA detection). The most sensitive virologic techniques for detection of HPV infection are polymerase chain reaction (PCR)-based. These methods can also provide information on type-specific prevalence, which is important because of differences in the oncogenic potential of HPV types. In the following discussion, reliance is placed largely on studies in which PCR-based methods were used to detect HPV DNA.

Prevalence of HPV in Women with Cytomorphologically Normal Cervices

The most prevalent HPV type was HPV 16; from approximately 3% to 9% of women were infected with HPV 16. The next most common type usually had a prevalence of about half that of HPV 16.

Multiple infections were common, with prevalence ranging from 2% to 20% of women.

The results from several studies reporting the prevalence of type-specific HPV cervical infection in cytologically normal women are summarized in Table 1–1.[14–18] In these studies, the prevalence of cervical HPV infection varied from 14% to 35%. It is clear from these and many other studies that HPV infection is very common in young, sexually active women. With the exception of the Costa Rican study, the studies' most prevalent HPV type was HPV 16; approximately 3% to 9% of women were infected with HPV 16. The next most common type usually had a prevalence of about half that of HPV 16, and most types were detected much less frequently than was HPV 16. Although type-specific prevalence differed

among studies, other common types included 6 and 11, 18, 31, 33, 45, 51, 52, 53, 58, 59, and 66. In most studies, a relatively high proportion (6% to 13%) of women were infected with nontypable or unidentified types. However, in more recent studies from Brazil and Costa Rica that used assays capable of detecting more types, only 1% to 2% of women harbored nontypable viruses, suggesting that most types capable of infecting the female genital tract have now been identified. Although there was a wide variation among studies, multiple infections were common, with prevalence rates ranging from 2% to 20%. The distribution of types in women from Brazil and Costa Rica was similar to that in women from the United States, suggesting that there may not be major differences in type-specific HPV prevalence worldwide. However, too few surveys have been done to exclude regional differences. Furthermore, there are geographic differences in the type-specific prevalence of HPV in invasive cancers, and it is tempting to attribute this to differences in exposure to HPV types. The proportions of HPV types classified as high-risk, intermediate-risk, or low-risk/untyped were similar in the six studies. Collectively, the low-risk/untyped group composed approximately 40% of HPV types identified in these studies; from about a fifth to a third of the types fell into the high-risk group, and a similar proportion into the intermediate-risk group.

Cumulative Prevalence of Cervical HPV Infection

Within individuals, the detection of HPV DNA was highly variable, indicating the limitations of single-point measurements of cervical HPV infection for calculating prevalence.

The estimates in the studies referenced previously are point prevalences. Studies in which women have been sampled repeatedly suggest that exposure to genital HPVs is much higher than is indicated by point prevalence studies.[19–21] In a study of 608 female students with an average age of 20 years, recruited from a state university in New Brunswick, New Jersey and followed up at 6-month intervals for an average of 2.2 years, the prevalence of HPV infection at baseline was 26%.[17] However, about 60% of the women were infected with HPV at some time during the 3-year period of study. The baseline prevalence and cumulative prevalence for HPV 16 were 3.8% and 10%, respectively. In a smaller study with more frequent sampling, 72 college women were followed over 10 weeks.[19] The weekly point prevalences of cervical HPV infection detected by PCR ranged from 20.8% to 47.2%, and the cumulative HPV prevalence was 59.3%. Within individuals, the detection of HPV DNA was highly variable, indicating the limitations of single-point measurements of cervical HPV infection for calculating prevalence. In studies for which the intervals between samplings were longer, the reported cumulative HPV prevalence was lower. In a study of predominantly white, middle-class women of a median age of 26 years with normal cervical cytologic findings, 36% of the women were HPV DNA positive by PCR at either of two visits a

▼ Table 1–1

Prevalence of Human Papillomavirus (HPV) Types Determined by Polymerase Chain Reaction Among Women Who Are Cytologically Normal

Population (Reference)	University health service[1] (14)	University health service (15)	University students[2] (17)	Kaiser Permanente HMO[3] (18)	Low-income urban (16)	Low-income rural[4]
Location	Berkeley, California	College Park, Maryland	New Brunswick, New Jersey	Portland, Oregon	Sao Paulo, Brazil	Guanacaste Province, Costa Rica
Number	462	414	604	1030	1425	305
Mean Age (yr)	22.9	22.5	20	35[5]	33	NA[6]
HPV Type	N (%)	N (%)	N (%)	N (%)	N (%)	N (%)
High Cancer Risk						
16	40 (8.7)	32 (7.7)	23 (3.8)	57 (5.9)	38 (2.7)	3 (1)
18	24 (5.2)	8 (1.9)	12 (2)	18 (1.8)	11 (0.8)	3 (1)
31	21 (4.5)	8 (1.9)	(≤ 1)	27 (2.7)	15 (1.1)	1 (0.3)
45	5 (1.1)	15 (3.6)	8 (1.3)	16 (1.6)	7 (0.5)	0 (0)
Intermediate Cancer Risk						
33	12 (2.6)	1 (0.2)	(≤ 1)	8 (0.8)	6 (0.4)	2 (0.7)
35	2 (0.4)	3 (0.7)	(≤ 1)	14 (1.4)	3 (0.2)	1 (0.3)
39	15 (3.3)	4 (1)	9 (1.5)	13 (1.3)	1 (0.1)	2 (0.7)
51	12 (2.6)	17 (4.1)	9 (1.5)	31 (3.1)	10 (0.7)	1 (0.3)
52	20 (4.3)	7 (1.7)	(≤ 1)	19 (1.9)	9 (0.6)	3 (1)
56	ND[7]	5 (1.2)	(≤ 1)	23 (2.3)	8 (0.6)	0 (0)
58	11 (2.4)	7 (1.7)	8 (1.3)	20 (2)	17 (1.2)	5 (1.6)
59	ND	8 (1.9)	10 (1.7)	12 (1.2)	1 (0.1)	0 (0)
W13B	ND	4 (1)	ND	3 (0.3)	1 (0.1)	ND
Low Cancer Risk						
6,11	16 (3.5)	13 (3.1)	(≤ 1)	28 (2.7)	14 (1)	2 (0.7)
53	ND	9 (2.2)	14 (2.3)	35 (3.5)	20 (1.4)	3 (1)
54	ND	4 (1)	(≤ 1)	23 (2.3)	1 (0.1)	3 (1)
66	21 (4.5)	8 (1.9)	8 (1.3)	8 (0.8)	0 (0)	0 (0)
PAP155	16 (3.5)	8 (1.9)	11 (1.8)	13 (1.3)	7 (0.5)	1 (0.3)
PAP291	ND	2 (0.5)	(≤ 1)	12 (1.2)	2 (0.1)	0 (0)
Other or Nontypable	61 (13.2)	36 (8.7)	46 (7.6)[8] 33 (5.5)	67 (6.5)	45 (3.2)[9] 11 (0.8)	33 (10.8)[10] 6 (2)
Any HPV Type	208 (45)[11]	145 (35)	168 (27.8)[12]	80 (17.7)[13]	196 (13.8)	45 (14.8)
Multiple Types	60 (13)	33 (8)	34 (5.6)	~20%[12]	31 (2.2)	13 (4.3)

[1] In this study, the vulva and cervix were sampled; data for combined prevalence from both sites are presented. Five women with mild cervical dysplasia are excluded.

[2] Women were recruited by advertisement. Eleven (1.9%) women with squamous epithelial lesions are included in the total number.

[3] Health maintenance organization.

[4] Unpublished data.

[5] Median age.

[6] Not available.

[7] Not done.

[8] Other HPV types include those in the table with prevalence ≤ 1 and HPV types 26, 32, 40, 55, 68, and 70.

[9] Other HPV types include 26, 32, 34, 40, 55, 61, 62, 68, 70, 72, and 73 and three types that have not been assigned numbers.

[10] Other HPV types include 26, 32, 40, 55, 67, 68, 70, and 72 and several types that have not been assigned numbers.

[11] Prevalence at cervix was 32% (n = 149).

[12] Prevalence among 124 subjects with specific HPV types detected by polymerase chain reaction; 33 subjects with an uncharacterized HPV type are excluded.

[13] Prevalence based on a subset of 453 women (72).

mean of 14.9 months apart.[22] In a population-based survey of young Swedish women, the cumulative prevalence of HPV DNA was 25% after two examinations an average of 24 months apart.[23] The acquisition of cervical HPV infection was examined in a large, longitudinal study of 1425 low-income women from Brazil with a median age of 33 years who provided an average of 3.4 specimens over a mean follow-up period of 10 months (range, 4 to 36 months).[16] The overall prevalence of HPV infection at enrollment was 13.8%, and the cumulative prevalence was 25.1%. HPV 16 was the most common type identified, with a cumulative prevalence of 4.2%. The cumulative prevalence of HPV (range, 25% to 60%) in these studies varies probably due largely to differences in the ages of the women and in their sexual behavior risk factors. The HPV detection methods used in the studies may also have differed in their efficiency of detection of HPV DNA.

Incidence of Cervical HPV Infection

For a variety of reasons, the incidence of genital HPV infection (the rate of newly acquired infections) is still poorly defined. The longitudinal studies required to derive an estimate are costly and difficult to conduct. Given the short-term fluctuations in the detection of HPV DNA, it is unclear how frequently women should be sampled. Additionally, among women past their onset of sexual activity, it is impossible with current molecular techniques to distinguish a new infection from a recurrence or reactivation of a previously latent infection. The best estimates of incident infection are provided by the previously mentioned studies conducted in New Brunswick, New Jersey and in Brazil.[16, 17] In these studies, estimates of incident HPV infection were similar—1.2% and 1.3% new infections per month, respectively. In both studies, the incidence rates were generally higher for younger women. In both studies, the incidence of HPV 16 was among the highest of the types that were surveyed— 0.14% and 0.29% new infections per month in the Brazil and the U.S. studies, respectively. It is therefore clear that a very high proportion of women will become infected with HPV in their lifetime, and a substantial proportion will become infected with HPV 16, the principal oncogenic HPV type.

Prevalence of HPV in Women with Cervical Disease

> **Most HPV types cause mild cervical cytologic abnormalities.**

The pattern of HPV type distribution among women with cervical disease is different from that among cytologically normal women. The results from studies reporting the prevalence of type-specific HPV cervical infection in women with low-grade cervical dysplasia, high-grade cervical dysplasia, or invasive cervical cancer are summarized in Table 1−2.[18, 24, 25] As compared with the prevalence of cervical HPV infection in cytologically normal women (14% to 35%), the prevalence in women with cervical disease is much higher, ranging from 70% to 80% in women with low-grade cervical dysplasia to approximately 90% in women with high-grade cervical dysplasia or invasive cervical cancer. In the Portland, Oregon and Costa Rica studies of women with low-grade cervical dysplasia, the HPV types identified were distributed nearly equally among the high-risk (18% to 32%), intermediate-risk (36% to 38%) or low-risk/untyped (31% to 44%) groups. The distribution of types is similar to that seen in cytologically normal women and suggests that most HPV types can cause mild cervical cytologic abnormalities. In the study from the Netherlands, a greater proportion of the HPV types were in the high-risk or intermediate-risk groups (74%), perhaps owing to the in-

clusion of more women with CIN 1 and fewer women with condylomatous atypia. Among women with high-grade dysplasia or invasive cervical cancer, the majority of HPV types identified were high-risk types (54% to 80%); only 5% to 11% of HPV types were in the low-risk/untyped group. In the study from the Netherlands, the prevalence of HPV types 16, 18, 31, and 45 increased with increasing grade of cervical dysplasia, supporting the proposed higher oncogenic potential of these types as compared with the intermediate-risk and low-risk types. This study also clearly documented a decrease in HPV heterogeneity with increasing severity of dysplasia. Six HPV types (39, 56, 40, 42, 5, and 66) detected in women with low-grade cervical dysplasia were not found in any women with high-grade dysplasia. Other investigators have also noted the homogeneity with regard to associated HPV types in CIN 2 and CIN 3 lesions as compared with the heterogeneity in CIN 1 lesions.[26]

> **The geographic differences in HPV types associated with cervical neoplasia may be due to differences in exposure, in sampling, or in oncogenic potential of HPV types in different host populations.**

> **HPV 16 or related viruses accounted for 68% of the viral types found in squamous cell tumors; HPV 18 or related types accounted for 71% of the viral types found in adenocarcinomas.**

The International Biological Study on Cervical Cancer (IBSCC), an international survey of invasive cervical cancer, showed that HPV 16 was the predominant type in cancers from all geographic regions (43% to 65% of all cancers).[25] HPV 18 and its related virus, HPV 45, were frequently detected in cancers from Africa (30%), North America (29.8%), and southeast Asia (40%) but were less commonly detected in those from Europe (10.4%) and Central and South America (16.8%). Despite regional similarities, the distribution of HPV types varied in some countries. HPV 18 accounted for more than 50% of cancers in Indonesia; HPV 45 was highly prevalent in Mali (western Africa); and HPV 39 and HPV 59 were found predominantly in Central and South America. The geographic differences in HPV types associated with cervical neoplasia may be due to differences in exposure, in sampling, or in oncogenic potential of HPV types in different host populations. Although two thirds to three fourths of cancers were associated with either HPV 16 or HPV 18, 21 different viruses and several variants were detected at least once each in the cancer survey. Only one novel type was detected, indicating that most HPV types associated with cancer have been identified. HPV 16 or related viruses accounted for 68% of the viral types found in squamous cell tumors; HPV 18 or related types accounted for 71% of the viral types found in adenocarcinomas. The association of HPV 16 and HPV 18 with these histologic types of cervical cancer has been reported previously, but the biologic basis for the different associations is unknown.[27, 28] In most studies, HPV prevalence has not been 100% in women with cytologic abnormalities, including those with invasive cervical cancer. The most

▼ Table 1–2

Prevalence of Human Papillomavirus (HPV) Types Determined by Polymerase Chain Reaction Among Women with Low-Grade Cervical Dysplasia, High-Grade Cervical Dysplasia, or Invasive Cervical Cancer

Cervical Disease	Low-grade cervical dysplasia			High-grade cervical dysplasia or invasive cervical cancer		
Population (Reference)	Kaiser Permanente HMO[1] (18)	Low-income rural[2]	Outpatient clinic (24)	Outpatient clinic (24)	Low-income rural[2]	Hospital patients (25)
Location	Portland, Oregon	Guanacaste Province, Costa Rica	Netherlands	Netherlands	Guanacaste Province, Costa Rica	22 countries
Number	426	325	971	402	159[3]	932
HPV Type	N (%)	N (%)	N (%)	N (%)	N (%)	N (%)
High Cancer Risk						
16	101 (23.7)	35 (10.8)	240 (24.7)	202 (50)	72 (45.3)	465 (49.9)
18	38 (8.9)	12 (3.7)	52 (5.4)	36 (8.9)	12 (5.3)	128 (13.7)
31	37 (8.7)	15 (4.6)	67 (6.9)	32 (7.9)	10 (6.3)	49 (5.3)
45	20 (4.7)	10 (3.1)	8 (0.8)	5 (1.2)	3 (1.9)	78 (8.4)
Intermediate Cancer Risk						
33	19 (4.5)	3 (0.9)	37 (3.8)	15 (3.7)	7 (4.4)	26 (2.8)
35	27 (6.3)	8 (2.5)	6 (0.6)	1 (0.2)	5 (3.1)	16 (1.7)
39	30 (7)	17 (5.2)	1 (0.1)	0 (0)	4 (2.5)	14 (1.5)
51	24 (5.6)	22 (6.8)	11 (1.1)	3 (0.7)	10 (6.3)	7 (0.8)
52	25 (5.9)	19 (5.9)	16 (1.6)	5 (1.2)	9 (5.7)	25 (2.7)
56	49 (11.5)	23 (7.1)	2 (0.2)	0 (0)	5 (3.1)	16 (1.7)
58	13 (3.1)	27 (8.3)	18 (1.9)	3 (0.7)	17 (10.7)	19 (2.0)
59	13 (3.1)	6 (1.9)	3 (0.3)	4 (0.1)	2 (1.3)	15 (1.6)
Low Cancer Risk						
6,11	26 (6.1)	24 (7.4)	24 (2.5)	5 (1.2)	5 (3.1)	2 (0.2)
40	4 (0.9)	3 (0.9)	1 (0.1)	0 (0)	0 (0)	0 (0)
42	7 (1.6)	ND[4]	3 (0.3)	0 (0)	ND	0 (0)
53	20 (4.7)	26 (8)	0 (0)	0 (0)	5 (3.1)	0 (0)
54	11 (2.6)	4 (1.2)	3 (0.3)	2 (0.5)	3 (1.9)	0 (0)
55	5 (1.2)	4 (1.2)	1 (0.1)	0 (0)	1 (0.6)	2 (0.2)
66	33 (7.8)	13 (4)	10 (1)	0 (0)	1 (0.6)	0 (0)
PAP155	17 (4)	9 (2.8)	ND	ND	0 (0)	0 (0)
PAP291	22 (5.2)	4 (1.2)	ND	ND	3 (1.9)	1 (0.1)
Other or Nontypable	63 (14.8)	94 (28.9) 23 (7.1)	119 (12.3)	27 (6.7)	30 (18.9) 7 (4.4)	39 (4.2)
Any HPV Type	338 (80.1)[5]	226 (69.5)	695 (71.6)	359 (88.9)	141 (88.7)	866 (92.9)
Multiple Types	134 (28.4)[6]	88 (27.1)	66 (6.8)[7]	19 (4.7)[7]	49 (30.8)	36 (3.9)

[1] Health maintenance organization.
[2] Unpublished data.
[3] Includes 34 cases of invasive cervical cancer.
[4] Not done.
[5] Denominator for this calculation was 422 cases (37).
[6] Value is based on 472 cases, including 50 with high-grade cervical dysplasia (37).
[7] Multiple infections containing HPV types 6, 11, 16, 18, 31, or 33 and one of the other types listed would not be detected with the protocol used.

likely reasons for the failure to detect HPV are inadequate specimen collection, cytopathologic misclassification, presence of unrecognized types or of types not amplified by the primer sets used, low copy number of target DNA, and disruption of the genomic segment targeted by PCR. In a reanalysis of the HPV-negative tumors from the IBSCC study, using PCR assays for multiple regions of the HPV genome and rigorous evaluations of specimen adequacy, HPV DNA was detected in all but two of the tumors from which adequate tissue samples were available, giving an overall HPV prevalence of 99.7%.[29]

Epidemiologic Evidence for the Association of HPV with Cervical Neoplasia

The odds ratios for the presence of HPV DNA ranged from about 15 to 120, and the odds ratios for HPV 16 DNA ranged from about 12 to 300.

> A number of studies have shown a twofold to sevenfold increased risk for cervical dysplasia in women infected with multiple HPV types as compared with those infected with a single type.

Numerous studies have examined the prevalence of HPV in cases and controls to determine the association of HPV infection with invasive cervical cancer. The results of several studies that used PCR for HPV diagnosis are summarized in Table 1–3.[30-35] The odds ratios for the presence of HPV DNA ranged from about 15 to 120, and the odds ratios for HPV 16 DNA ranged from about 12 to 300. The causal role of the virus in carcinogenesis of cervical cancer is supported from an epidemiologic perspective by the very strong and consistent association of HPV with invasive cervical cancer and carcinoma in situ. The majority of these studies have also examined previously established risk factors for cervical cancer in relation to the detection of HPV DNA. In most studies, HPV infection was shown to explain the sexual risk factors for cervical dysplasia (for example, increasing lifetime number of sexual partners) as well as other behavioral and demographic determinants (low family income, low educational level, smoking, use of oral contraceptives, and age at first sexual intercourse). A number of studies have shown a twofold to sevenfold increased risk for cervical dysplasia in women infected with multiple HPV types as compared with those infected with a single type.[34-37] Further studies are needed to confirm these observations and to investigate a biologic basis for interaction between HPV types. For example, it is not known whether infection with particular HPV types can promote infection with other HPV types or influence the oncogenic potential of an HPV type. The occurrence of infection with multiple HPV types does not appear to be simply a chance event. In a large survey of type-specific infection, certain combinations of HPV types were observed to occur as joint infections far more frequently than could be attributed to chance.[16]

PREVALENCE AND INCIDENCE OF GENITAL WARTS

> In the annual survey of the Centers for Disease Control and Prevention, between 1966 and 1987, the number of consultations for genital warts increased from 70,000 to 360,000, but by 1997 the number had declined to 150,000.

The most common clinical manifestation of an HPV infection is genital warts. Unlike some other sexually transmitted diseases, the true prevalence and incidence of genital warts in the United States is unknown because genital warts are not a reportable disease. In addition, because contact tracing is not carried out, many cases may go undiagnosed. However, the occurrence of genital warts can be measured indirectly by surveys of first office visits to physicians as compiled annually by the Centers for Disease Control and Prevention (CDC) (www.cdc.gov). Between 1966 and 1987, the number of consultations for genital warts increased from about 70,000 to 360,000. Declines in the number of visits have occurred since 1987. In 1997, the most recently available year, there were about 150,000 visits. The number of comparable consultations for genital herpes in 1997 was 175,000. Similar temporal trends in the prevalence of

▼ Table 1–3

Risk of Cervical Dysplasia and Invasive Cervical Cancer Associated with HPV Infection As Determined by PCR

Location	Cervical Diagnosis	Cervical HPV DNA			Cervical HPV 16 DNA			Reference
		No. Cases (% Pos)	No. Controls (% Pos)	OR (95% CI)	No. Cases (% Pos)	No. Controls (% Pos)	OR (95% CI)	
Colombia	Invasive cancer	87 (72.4)	98 (13.3)	15.6 (7–35)	229 (47.6)	228 (5.7)	29.7 (15–57)	30
Spain	Invasive cancer	142 (69)	130 (4.6)	46.2 (19–115)				
Brazil	Invasive cancer	186 (84.4)	190 (16.8)	37.1 (20–70)	186 (53.8)	10 (5.3)	74.9 (33–173)	31
Taiwan	CIN 2–3; invasive cancer	48 (91.7)	260 (9.2)	122.3 (39–389)	48 (58.3)*	260 (0.8)	1280 (185–8830)	35
Colombia	CIN 3	125 (63.2)	181 (10.5)	15.5 (8–29)	125 (32.8)	181 (3.3)	27.1 (11–70)	32
Spain	CIN 3	157 (70.7)	193 (4.7)	56.9 (25–131)	157 (49)	193 (0.5)	295.5 (45–1946)	32
Norway	CIN 2–3	98 (90.8)	221 (15.4)	67.2 (29–158)	98 (65.3)	221 (6.3)	123.9 (47–329)	33
New Mexico	CIN 2–3	176 (93.8)	311 (42)	20.6 (11–40)	187 (52.4)	325 (8.6)	11.7 (7–19)	34
Taiwan	CIN 1	37 (54)	260 (9.2)	14 (6–32)	6 (16.2)	260 (9.2)	54.8 (9–333)	35

* Includes HPV types 16, 18, 31, and 45.
CI, confidence interval; CIN, cervical intraepithelial neoplasia; HPV, human papillomavirus; OR, odds ratio; PCR, polymerase chain reaction.

genital warts have been observed in England and Wales.[38] Rates of doctor visits for genital warts increased dramatically between 1980 and 1986. The rate leveled off from 1986 to 1991, but since 1992 it has risen by 15%. In addition to the summary data from the CDC, estimates of the prevalence of genital warts in the United States have been made by surveys of selected populations. A survey of 750 women consecutively attending a university student health clinic between 1984 and 1987 found that 1.5% of the women had genital warts.[39] Among women seen for annual gynecologic examinations at a health maintenance organization between 1984 and 1987, the prevalence of genital warts was 0.8% for women between the ages of 21 and 29 years and 0.6% for women between 29 and 39 years of age.[39] The prevalence of genital warts is higher in persons visiting sexually transmitted disease clinics. In a study of patients seen at the Kings County Clinic, Seattle, Washington, in 1986, 13% of men and 9% of women had genital warts.[39]

The actual incidence of genital warts was measured in a study conducted by the Mayo Clinic in Rochester, Minnesota from 1950 to 1978.[40] The incidence increased about eightfold, from 13 per 100,000 between 1950 and 1954 to 106 per 100,000 between 1975 and 1978. The highest recorded incidence was for women between the ages of 20 and 24 years (619 per 1000 in 1975–1978). More recently, the incidence of genital warts during a 2-year period, 1989 through 1990, in a middle-sized urban area in Sweden was determined.[41] The overall incidence was 240 per 100,000, more than twice the rate in Minnesota a little more than a decade earlier. As in Minnesota, the highest age-specific incidence occurred in the 20- to 24-year age group, 1200 per 100,000.

> **Several HPV types have been associated with genital warts, but HPV 6 is the most commonly identified type.**

Several HPV types have been associated with genital warts, but HPV 6 is the most commonly identified type. In a study using PCR and type-specific oligonucleotide probes, the distribution of HPV types was determined in 37 patients with genital warts.[42] The types most commonly found were HPV 6 (94%), HPV 11 (8%), HPV 54 (8%), and HPV 58 (8%). Eight patients (21.6%) had multiple HPV types detected. In previous studies using Southern blot hybridization, HPV 6 DNA was detected in 62% to 70% of genital warts, and HPV 11 DNA was detected in 12% to 30% of lesions.[43, 44]

PREVALENCE OF HPV-ASSOCIATED CYTOLOGIC ABNORMALITIES

> **From the National Breast and Cervical Cancer Early Detection Program, the overall rate of abnormal Pap tests was 3.8%. The rates for low-grade squamous lesions, high-grade lesions, and squamous cancer were 2.9%, 0.8%, and less than 0.1%, respectively.**

All HPV types that infect the female genital tract can induce low-grade squamous intraepithelial lesions, which are the morphologic correlate of a productive infection. Rarely, HPV induces a proliferative epithelial lesion that pathologists recognize as a high-grade squamous intraepithelial lesion. Because these lesions are known to be cytohistologic precursors of invasive cervical cancer, cervical cytology screening has been used widely for many years to identify women at risk for invasive cancer. Data from screening programs provide a crude estimate of the prevalence of HPV infections associated with cytohistologic abnormalities. However, limitations of the data include the selective nature of screened populations, the interobserver and intraobserver variations in interpretation of cytologic abnormalities, and the potential lack of correlation between smears and underlying pathology. In addition, studies that have used the Bethesda System in reporting test results are difficult to compare with studies for which other nomenclatures were used. Numerous studies have reported the prevalence of cytologic abnormalities in various populations. The most recently available data for U.S. women come from the National Breast and Cervical Cancer Early Detection Program.[45] Between October 1991 and June 1995, 312,858 women participating in this program were screened by Pap tests. About one fourth of the women were younger than 30 years, and more than half were 40 years or older. The ethnicity of slightly less than half of the women was black or Hispanic. Results were reported using the Bethesda System categories. The overall rate of abnormal Pap tests was 3.8%. The rates for low-grade squamous lesions, high-grade lesions, and squamous cancer were 2.9%, 0.8%, and less than 0.1%, respectively. Rates in the United States are higher than those in other developed countries. In cancer screening programs conducted in Australia, the Netherlands, and Norway during the late 1980s or early 1990s, the rates of mild, moderate, and severe cervical dysplasia were 1.8%, 1.4%, and 1.6%, respectively.[46–48]

> **Subclinical HPV infections may be 10 to 30 times more common than cytologically apparent infections.**

The overall U.S. prevalence of 3.8% for HPV-associated cytologic abnormalities is from fourfold to ninefold lower than the point prevalence estimates for HPV infection determined by PCR (14% to 35%; see Table 1–1). The true ratio of subclinical to clinical HPV infection may be even higher. In three studies of unselected college-aged women who were evaluated by both Pap smears and HPV DNA detection by PCR, the prevalence of cytologic abnormalities ranged from 1% to 3.6%, whereas the prevalence of cervical HPV DNA ranged from 28% to 35%, indicating that subclinical HPV infections may be 10 to 30 times more common than cytologically apparent infections.[14, 15, 49] In most case series of abnormal Pap smears, the rates of low-grade cytologic abnormalities are higher among younger women, and the rates of invasive cancer are higher among older women. For example, among 796,337 smears obtained from

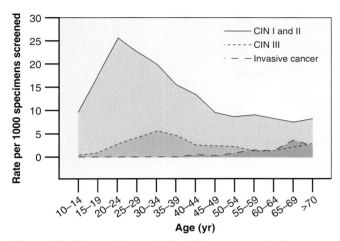

Figure 1–1. Rates of abnormal Papanicolaou smears in 5-year age groups of approximately 800,000 U.S. women screened in 1981. (Data from Sadeghi SB, Hsieh EW, Gunn S: Prevalence of cervical intraepithelial neoplasia in sexually active teenagers and young adults. Results of data analysis of mass Papanicolaou screening of 796,337 women in the United States in 1981. Am J Obstet Gynecol 1984;148:726.)

women of all ages during 1981, the prevalence of mild to moderate dysplasia was highest between ages 20 and 24 years, the prevalence of severe dysplasia was highest between ages 30 and 34 years, and the prevalence of invasive carcinoma was highest between ages 65 and 69 years (Fig. 1–1).[50]

PREVALENCE OF INVASIVE CERVICAL CANCER

Cervical cancer is one of the most common neoplastic diseases affecting women, with a combined worldwide incidence exceeded only by breast cancer and colorectal cancer.

Cervical cancer is one of the most common neoplastic diseases affecting women, with a combined worldwide incidence exceeded only by breast cancer and colorectal cancer (Fig. 1–2) (Web site of the International Agency for Research on Cancer; www-dep.iarc.fr). Approximately 370,000 new cases of invasive cervical cancer occurred worldwide in 1990, and the estimated age-standardized rate was approximately 15 per 100,000 women. The estimated number of deaths from invasive cervical cancer in 1990 was 190,000, making it the fifth leading cause of cancer-related deaths worldwide. The highest-risk areas are Latin America, the Caribbean, Africa, and southern Asia. In Central America the estimated age-standardized rate is 44 per 100,000, and in Africa rates range from 26 to 40 per 100,000 in various regions of the continent. In 1990, the highest incidence of cervical cancer was recorded in Haiti (92 per 100,000). The rate in less developed regions of the world is about 1.6 times that in more developed regions (18 versus 11 per 100,000). Cervical cancer is the second most common malignancy in women in less developed regions of the world, accounting for 15% of all cancers. In comparison, cervical cancer is the

fifth most common malignancy in women in more developed regions of the world and constitutes 5% of all cancers.

The projected number of new cases of invasive cervical cancer for 1999 in the United States is 12,800, and the estimated number of deaths that will occur because of this disease is 4800. The lifetime risk for U.S. women of being diagnosed with cervical cancer and the lifetime risk of dying from cervical cancer are 0.78% and 0.26%, respectively.

In the United States, cervical cancer is the eighth most common malignancy in women, with an estimated age-adjusted incidence for the period from 1990 to 1996 of 9 per 100,000 (Web site of the Surveillance, Epidemiology and End Results program of the National Cancer Institute; www-seer.ims.nci.nih.gov). The projected number of new cases of invasive cervical cancer for 1999 in the United States is 12,800, and the estimated number of deaths that will occur because of this disease is 4800. The lifetime risk for U.S. women of being diagnosed with cervical cancer and the lifetime risk of dying from cervical cancer are 0.78% and 0.26%, respectively. The incidence and mortality rates for cervical cancer in U.S. women differ significantly based on race and ethnicity (Table 1–4). In the period from 1990 to 1996, the highest incidence was observed among Hispanic women, who experienced a rate of more than twice that of white, non-Hispanic women. For black women, the comparable rate was more than 1.5 times that of white women. The incidence and mortality of cervical cancer have declined almost 50% since the early 1970s (Fig. 1–3). Rates for white women have

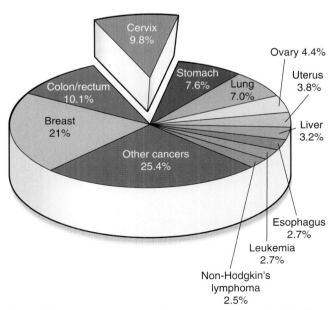

Figure 1–2. Incidence of cancer by sites in women worldwide. (Data from the Web site of the International Agency for Research on Cancer; www-dep.iarc.fr)

▼ Table 1–4

United States Age-Adjusted SEER* Incidence and Mortality Rates for Invasive Cervical Cancer

Race/Ethnicity	Incidence Rate 1990–1996 (Rate per 100,000 Persons)	Mortality Rate 1990–1996 (Rate per 100,000 Persons)
White non-Hispanic	7.1	2.4
White Hispanic	16.7	3.7
Black	11.8	6
Asian/Pacific Islander	10.3	2.8
American Indian	6	3.6
Hispanic	15.8	3.5

*Surveillance, Epidemiology and End Results (SEER) program. The program collects data from population-based tumor registries in five states (Connecticut, Hawaii, Iowa, New Mexico, and Utah) and six metropolitan areas (Atlanta, Detroit, Los Angeles, San Francisco–Oakland, San Jose–Monterey, and Seattle–Puget Sound), representing 14% of the U.S. population.

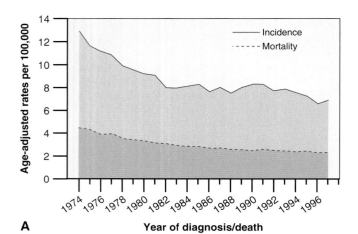

A   Year of diagnosis/death

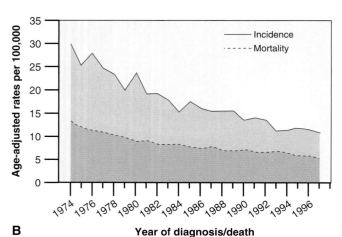

B   Year of diagnosis/death

Figure 1–3. U.S. incidence and mortality rates for invasive cervical cancer in white *(A)* and black *(B)* women from 1973 to 1996. (Data from the Web site of the Surveillance, Epidemiology and End Results [SEER] program of the National Cancer Institute; www-seer.ims.nci.nih.gov)

been level or gradually declining since the early 1980s, whereas the rates for black women fell steadily from the early 1970s to the early 1990s and have now leveled off. Cervical cancer is typically diagnosed at a relatively young median age compared with other cancers—at 46 years for white women and at 48 years for black women. By comparison, the median age of diagnosis for breast cancer is 63 years for all women, and the median age for all cancer sites in women is 68 years. The 5-year relative survival rate for the most recently available period (1989 to 1995) was about 70% for white women and 60% for black women.

DETERMINANTS OF CERVICAL HPV INFECTION

Sexual Transmission of HPV

That warts can be transmitted from one person to another was suspected long before the viral etiology of warts was established. Sir Astley Cooper, in his lectures on the principles and practice of surgery, published in 1835, stated that warts "frequently secrete a matter which is able to produce a similar disease in others."[51] Cervical HPV infections are usually sexually acquired. Genital HPV infections are rare in populations that are not sexually active and, conversely, the highest prevalence is recorded in the age group presumed to be the most sexually active. Additionally, sexual partners are commonly concordant for HPV infection. Finally, epidemiologic studies have identified sexual behavior as the major risk factor for genital HPV infection.

HPV Infection in Virgins and Neonates

Genital HPV infection is rare among virgins.

Genital HPV infection is rare among virgins. In a study of 130 women who had not experienced sexual intercourse, only two samples of epithelial cells collected from the vagina were HPV positive by PCR.[52] HPV 6 was detected in both samples. In another study, none of 55 virginal women had HPV DNA detectable by PCR in vaginal cells.[53] In a study of university women from Berkeley, California, none of 12 virgins had detectable HPV DNA by PCR in vaginal or cervical specimens.[14] In contrast, the prevalence of HPV infection in sexually active women was 46% in the Berkeley study. A carefully conducted, longitudinal study from Sweden provides the most convincing evidence for the absence of HPV cervical infection in virginal girls.[54] In this study, 98 adolescent girls were followed for 2 years with repeated cervical specimens and had structured interviews regarding sexuality every 6 months. None of the sexually inexperienced girls had HPV DNA in the cervix.

Genital HPV types appear to be uncommonly transmitted in the neonatal period. The presence of HPV DNA in newborn samples might simply indicate contamination with infected maternal cells rather than signify infection.

Genital HPV types appear to be uncommonly transmitted in the neonatal period, although published studies are conflicting. A study from Seattle, Washington included 151 subjects, the largest series of infants yet reported.[55] The pregnant women enrolled in the study had a high prevalence of genital HPV infection (41% HPV DNA positivity by PCR), and the women had many of the risk factors associated with perinatal transmission of HPV, including nulliparity, young age, and low cesarean section rate.[56] Cervical swab samples were obtained from the women during the first or second trimester, at 34 weeks' gestation, and at 6 weeks and 1 year post partum. Infants had samples collected from the oral cavity, the external genitalia, and the perianal region on multiple occasions after birth, beginning at age 6 weeks. At 579 infant visits, HPV DNA was detected by PCR from only 5 (1.5%) of the 335 genital, 4 (1.2%) of the 324 anal, and 0 of the 372 oral specimens. Perinatal transmission seems unlikely because the HPV DNA detection in the infants was not associated with maternal genital HPV DNA detection during pregnancy, and the HPV types detected in the infants were not the common genital types. These results were confirmed in another study of neonates that found HPV DNA in oral or genital specimens from 1 (4%) of 25 infants born to mothers with detectable HPV DNA in the genital tract and 1 (0.6%) of 178 infants born to mothers without detectable HPV DNA.[57] In contrast, several studies have reported HPV DNA prevalence in neonates and young children ranging from 32% to 72% in children born to women with HPV infection and from 5% to 29% in children born to women without HPV infection.[58-62] The widely varying estimates of prevalence are difficult to explain but may be due to differences in populations, in sampling methods, or in the specificity of laboratory assays. An additional consideration is that the presence of HPV DNA in newborn samples might simply indicate contamination with infected maternal cells rather than signify infection. Confirmation of infection would require additional evidence, preferably detection of viral messenger RNA or immune response to HPV proteins.

HPV Infection in Sex Partners

As many as two thirds to three fourths of persons sexually exposed to genital warts have been reported to develop genital warts subsequently. The observation of a concordant infection with the same HPV type or variant in one third to one half of regular sex partners suggests that the virus is transmitted sexually with modest efficiency.

As many as two thirds to three fourths of persons sexually exposed to genital warts have been reported to develop genital warts subsequently.[63, 64] In one study, more than one third of women who were sexual consorts of men with genital warts had concurrent cervical cytologic abnormalities.[64] Conversely, men who are sexual partners of women with cervical dysplasia are at risk of subclinical penile HPV infection. Among 25 men whose female sexual partners had CIN 3, 23 had histologic evidence of HPV infection, and 4 had severe penile dyspla-

sia or carcinoma in situ.[65] The development of highly sensitive, type-specific PCR assays for detection of HPV DNA in the genital tract has permitted studies of the transmission of subclinical genital HPV infection. In a study of 53 married couples, an HPV 16 infection was diagnosed in 26 couples.[66] In 9 (35%) of these 26 couples, both partners were infected. In a comparable study involving clients of a sexually transmitted disease clinic, an HPV infection was diagnosed in 41 of 45 couples.[67] Concordance for HPV infection was observed in 20 couples, and the same HPV type was found in 13 of the 20 couples. In a study of HPV 16 variants from genital lesions of married couples, the virus was detected in both husband and wife in eight couples.[68] In four couples, the husband and wife harbored the same HPV 16 variants, and in the other four couples, different HPV 16 variants were detected in the partners. The observation of a concordant infection with the same HPV type or variant in one third to one half of regular sex partners suggests that the virus is transmitted sexually with modest efficiency. Similar estimates of the sexual transmissibility of HPV have been recorded in the setting of sexual abuse. Among 15 girls with confirmed sexual abuse, HPV DNA was detected in 5 girls (33%) by using the Southern transfer hybridization technique.[69]

Risk Factors for Genital HPV Infection

The predominant risk factor for a genital HPV infection is the number of lifetime sexual partners. The other risk factor identified in most studies of HPV infection is young age.

PCR assays have made it possible to investigate risk factors for HPV infection independent of the correlated risk factors for development of cytologic abnormalities and cervical neoplasia. Several studies of cytologically normal women have shown that the predominant risk factor for a genital HPV infection is the number of lifetime sexual partners.[49, 70-75] In most studies, this factor alone has explained most or all the other putative risk factors identified by univariate analysis. The consistency with which this association has been observed in different populations provides strong epidemiologic support for a sexual route of transmission of genital HPV types. The other risk factor identified in most studies of HPV infection is young age. In a study of 5857 women age 15 to 55 years, excluding women with cytologic abnormalities on Pap smears, HPV prevalence by PCR was age dependent (Fig. 1–4).[76] The maximum prevalence occurred between 20 and 24 years of age (21%), followed by a decrease until age 35 years. The prevalence remained stable through age 50 years and then gradually declined again. The prevalence of HPV 16 and HPV 18 also peaked in the 20- to 24-year age group (6.6%) and declined gradually thereafter. The age trend is consistent with an epidemic curve of a sexually acquired infectious disease.[77] The prevalence rises as newly sexually active young women are exposed for the first time and then declines among older women because of decreased exposure or acquisition of protective immunity. Alternatively,

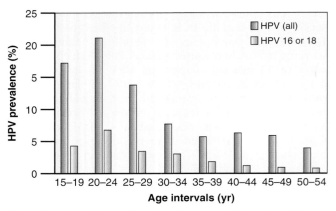

Figure 1-4. Prevalence of cervical human papillomavirus DNA by polymerase chain reaction assay in relation to age. (Data from Melkert PW, Hopman E, van den Brule AJ, et al: Prevalence of HPV in cyto-morphologically normal cervical smears, as determined by the polymerase chain reaction, is age-dependent. Int J Cancer 1993;53:919.)

the trend of decreasing prevalence of HPV with age could be explained as a cohort effect, owing to a higher risk of HPV infection among young women today than in the past, perhaps as a result of changes in sexual behavior since the 1960s.

In studies of cytologically normal women with HPV infection detected by PCR, age and sexual activity cannot explain some risk factors. However, these risk factors are not consistent across studies. Risk factors identified in some, but not all, studies include current or past pregnancies, black or Hispanic ethnicity, and use of oral contraceptives. Ethnicity may influence the prevalence of HPV infection owing to differences in genetic predisposition for acquisition or persistence of HPV infection. One possible mechanism might be differences in human leukocyte antigen haplotype among ethnic groups. These differences could influence host immune responses to HPV infection. Another mechanism invoked to explain ethnic differences in HPV prevalence is that different levels of endemic HPV infection may exist in given groups, thus increasing the risk of exposure to a group member.[78] The mechanism whereby pregnancy or oral contraceptive use might increase the prevalence of HPV infection is speculative. Hormonal perturbations of the immune response, steroid hormone–induced reactivation of latent infection, and hormone-induced upregulation of viral gene expression are potential mechanisms for which there is some support from in vitro studies.[79-81]

Male sexual behaviors have been shown to be an independent risk factor for infection in women.

Consistent with a sexual mode of transmission of genital HPV, male sexual behaviors have been shown to be an independent risk factor for infection in women. In a study of male partners of college women, the behaviors of the male partner that were associated with an increased risk included increasing number of lifetime sex partners, short-term relationship, lack of enrollment in college, age older than 20 years, and black or Hispanic ethnicity.[49]

These characteristics suggest that the male partners of HPV-infected women tend to be more sexually promiscuous. Similarly, in a case-control study of cervical cancer in Spain, a woman's risk of cervical cancer was strongly related to her husband's number of extramarital partners.[82] Most studies of risk factors for HPV DNA detection have not distinguished among HPV types. However, one study noted differences in the risk factors for high-risk oncogenic HPV types and low-risk nononcogenic HPV types.[75] The main risk factors for high-risk types were younger age and measures of lifetime sexual activity, such as number of partners. In contrast, the most important determinants for nononcogenic types were contraceptive variables related to the physical protection of the cervix, such as use of condoms or a diaphragm, and number of partners in the last 4 to 12 months. One explanation for this difference is that infections with low-risk HPV types are transient and thus correlate with recent sexual behavior, whereas infections with oncogenic types are more persistent and therefore correlate with measures of lifetime sexual exposure.

NATURAL HISTORY OF CERVICAL HPV INFECTION

Transient Cervical HPV Infection

Most cervical HPV infections diagnosed by PCR and other nucleic acid detection methods appear to be transient. The proportion of women who cleared their infection increased with younger age, longer interval between samplings, and infection with low-risk rather than high-risk HPV types.

Most cervical HPV infections diagnosed by PCR and other nucleic acid detection methods appear to be transient. In a number of studies, women have been sampled at intervals months apart to determine how frequently a cervical HPV infection is cleared or at least becomes undetectable using very sensitive assays such as PCR. For example, in a study of 393 cytologically normal women recruited from Kaiser Permanente clinics in Portland, Oregon, 51 (59.3%) of 86 women with a cervical HPV infection at enrollment did not have the same HPV type detectable at their second visit, an average of 14.9 months later.[22] The proportion of women who cleared their infection increased with younger age, longer interval between samplings, and infection with low-risk rather than high-risk HPV types. Only one third of women older than 30 years cleared their infection, compared with two thirds of those younger than 24 years. Slightly more than half of the initially infected women who had a follow-up visit within 12 months had lost the HPV type detected at entry, and nearly 75% of those who returned after more than 18 months had resolved their initial infection. Three fourths of the women infected with low-risk HPV types at entry no longer harbored the initial HPV type in their genital tract at the second visit. In contrast, among women infected with high-risk HPV types, only half had cleared their infection by the second visit. In other studies, the proportion of women with a transient cervical

HPV infection has been even higher. In a population-based study of young Swedish women, 57 (97%) of 59 women with cytomorphologically normal cervices presenting with an HPV infection were reported to clear their infection during a 2-year interval.[23]

Duration of Cervical HPV Infection

The time interval required for 50% of prevalent cases to become HPV DNA negative was 4.8 months for nononcogenic types and 8.1 months for oncogenic types.

Two studies in which women were followed with repeated measures of HPV DNA confirmed the transient nature of most cervical HPV infections and allowed estimates of the duration of infection. In the Brazil study cited previously, the time interval required for 50% of prevalent cases to become HPV DNA negative for the HPV type detected at enrollment was 4.8 months for nononcogenic types and 8.1 months for oncogenic types.[16] This is not a true measure of the duration of infections, because it is unknown how long the women had been infected by the time they were found to be positive at enrollment. In the New Brunswick, New Jersey study, the duration of infection was determined for incident infection.[17] The median duration of HPV infection was 8 months. The five HPV types with the longest median duration of infection were AE7 (16 months), 61 (15 months), 18 (12 months), 16 (11 months), and 71 (11 months). These HPV types include both low-risk and high-risk types. Larger studies are needed to determine whether the duration of infection differs significantly among HPV types and between nononcogenic and oncogenic types.

Incident Low-Grade Cytologic Abnormalities

The transient nature of most HPV cervical infections and the 3- to 10-fold lower prevalence of HPV-associated cytologic abnormalities compared with HPV DNA positivity suggest that only a small proportion of HPV-infected women are likely to develop cytologic abnormalities. However, estimates of incident low-grade cytologic abnormalities among HPV DNA–positive women have been quite high in some studies. In a cohort of young, sexually active women from the University of Maryland, the incidence of LSIL in HPV DNA–positive women was 9% over a 16-month observation period.[15] In a study that recruited young women from a family planning clinic and a university health clinic in San Francisco, California, the cumulative incidence of LSIL among 522 HPV DNA–positive, cytologically normal women was 25.5% after 40 months of follow-up (mean of 24 ± 15 months).[83] In the New Brunswick study, the cumulative percentage of HPV-infected women with squamous intraepithelial lesions (SIL) was 11% during a 24-month period.[17] In contrast, among 59 young Swedish women who were HPV DNA–positive and had normal cytology, only 1 woman (1.7%) had an atypical Pap smear at a median follow-up of 24 months.[23] These numbers may overesti-

mate the true risk of SIL because the subjects in the studies had a prevalent HPV infection and thus may have represented a high-risk subset of HPV-infected women. On the other hand, cytologic misclassification may lead to an underestimation of the risk of SIL. Because the koilocytotic cell is the production and assembly site of virions, some of these cells must be present in the genital tract for a DNA assay to be positive. The inability to detect them in every HPV infection probably reflects the inadequacy of sampling techniques.

Incident High-Grade Cytologic Abnormalities

In young women without a cytologic abnormality at the time the infection is diagnosed, high-grade squamous intraepithelial lesions are an uncommon outcome of HPV infection, even with high-risk HPV types.

In contrast to LSIL, which may be viewed as the cytopathologic manifestation of HPV infection, HSIL is uncommon and represents a truly premalignant lesion. With one exception, most studies have shown that HSIL is uncommon after an HPV infection. In a cohort of 241 women who presented to a sexually transmitted disease clinic in Seattle, Washington and had negative cervical cytologic tests, the cumulative incidence of moderate to severe CIN at 2 years was 28% among women with a positive test for HPV DNA at entry.[84] In contrast, a much lower incidence of severe cytologic abnormalities was observed in the Maryland and San Francisco studies. Among 522 women from a family planning clinic and a university health clinic in San Francisco, 11 (2.1%) developed HSIL over a mean follow-up interval of 21.8 months.[83] In addition, 44 (88%) of 50 women who were consistently positive for a high-risk HPV type for 1 year or longer did not develop HSIL over a 2-year period. Thus, in young women without a cytologic abnormality at the time the infection is diagnosed, HSIL is an uncommon outcome of HPV infection, even with high-risk HPV types. In the Maryland cohort, the incidence of HSIL after 16 months of observation was 5%.[15] In the New Brunswick study during an average of 2.2 years of follow-up (maximum 3.6 years), two cases of HSIL were observed among 443 women who had normal Pap smears at baseline.[17] There are several possible reasons for the discrepancy between the Seattle study and the other studies. The women from the sexually transmitted disease clinics were older than those from the family planning and student health clinics (26 years versus approximately 20 to 22 years). The women from the family planning and university health clinics had a relatively low prevalence of sexually transmitted diseases, which may be important cofactors for development of cytologic abnormalities. In the sexually transmitted disease clinic study, a less sensitive method was used to detect HPV DNA. As a result, only infections with a high viral load may have been identified, and these are more likely to induce cervical cytopathology. Differences among studies using cytology as an end point may also be due to interobserver variation in the interpretation of smears.

NATURAL HISTORY OF HPV-ASSOCIATED CYTOLOGIC ABNORMALITIES

Women with borderline and low-grade abnormalities on cervical cytology have a risk of progression to invasive cervical cancer over 24 months of 1 to 2 per 1000 women without treatment.

There have been numerous observational studies of the course of untreated cervical cytologic abnormalities. However, the interpretation of this literature is problematic for a number of reasons that have been discussed in several excellent review articles.[85, 86] Many of the controversies concern diagnostic criteria, because cytology is not always an accurate indicator of underlying pathology, and there is not uniform agreement on the cytologic definition of dysplasia. Even when biopsy is used for diagnosis, because lesions may be multifocal and histologically heterogeneous, the lesion may be missed, resulting in misclassification of disease status. Furthermore, it has been suggested that biopsy even for diagnostic purposes may influence the natural history of the disease. Because dysplasia is an asymptomatic condition, detection of disease depends on type, interval, and duration of follow-up. When changes in disease status occur over a short period of time, there is a greater likelihood that misclassification owing to sampling error is misinterpreted as true progression. In addition, comparisons of studies are difficult because rates of regression and progression of cytologic abnormalities may be influenced by demographic and clinical features of study subjects. A meta-analysis was applied to studies of the natural history of cervical squamous abnormalities.[87] Studies of women whose cervical smears showed squamous atypia or worse were identified by a search of the English-language medical literature for the years from 1966 to 1996. To be eligible for analysis, studies had to report a minimum of 6 months' follow-up without treatment; relate entry cytologic findings to outcomes; and report entry cytologic findings so that the study population could be stratified into categories of atypical cells of undetermined significance (ASCUS), LSIL, or HSIL. Fifteen of 81 studies that were reviewed, representing a total of 27,929 patients, were judged eligible for data analysis. The pooled rates for regression to normal, progression over time, and invasive cervical cancer are shown in Figure 1–5. The average rate of regression to normal of ASCUS was 68%. The corresponding rates for LSIL and HSIL were 47% and 35%, respectively. The rates of regression to normal did not vary significantly with the length of follow-up. The rate of progression of ASCUS was 2% at 6 months and 7% at 24 months. The rate of progression of LSIL was 6.5% at 6 months and 21% at 24 months. HSIL progressed at rates comparable to those of low-grade lesions—6.8% at 6 months and 23% at 24 months. The calculated rates for invasive cancer were as follows: ASCUS and LSIL combined at 6 and 24 months were 0.04% and 0.15%, respectively; HSIL at 6 months was 0.15%, and HSIL at 24 months was 1.44%. The findings from this analysis suggest that women with borderline and low-grade abnormalities on cervical cytology have a risk of progression to

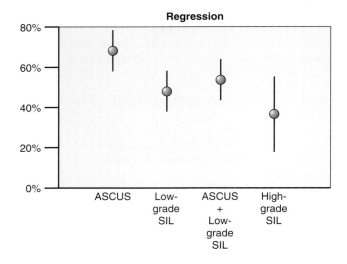

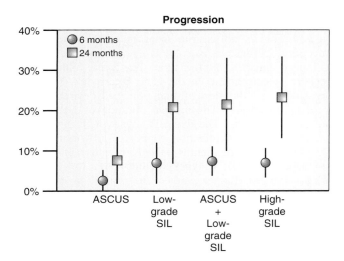

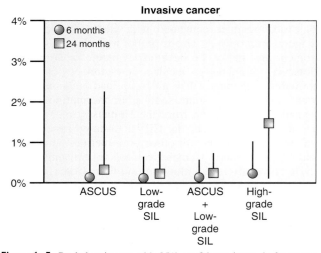

Figure 1–5. Pooled estimates with 95% confidence intervals for regression of cervical cytologic abnormalities to normal, progression over time to high-grade squamous epithelial lesions, and rates of invasive cervical cancer over time. (From Melnikow J, Nuovo J, Willan AR, et al: Natural history of cervical squamous intraepithelial lesions: A meta-analysis. Obstet Gynecol 1998;92:727.)

invasive cervical cancer over 24 months of 1 to 2 per 1000 women without treatment. The risk is small but not insignificant, and thus there continues to be controversy about how best to evaluate and manage these women.

RISK FACTORS FOR DEVELOPMENT OF CERVICAL NEOPLASIA

Although HPV infection is necessary for the development of HSIL and invasive cancer, it is not a sufficient cause.

From the extensive literature on the prevalence and natural history of cervical HPV infection that has appeared since the early 1990s, the picture that emerges is one of a viral infection that is nearly ubiquitous, is usually self-limited, and is uncommonly associated with disease. A question that still needs to be answered, however, is whether cervical HPV infections entirely resolve or simply persist at a level below the detection limit of current assays. Although HPV infection is necessary for the development of HSIL and invasive cancer, it is not a sufficient cause. Therefore, it is important to identify the additional risk factors for progression to disease. The kinds of risk factors postulated to influence the risk of progression to HSIL and invasive cervical cancer are viral factors, host factors, and environmental cofactors.

Viral Factors in the Development of Cervical Cancer

HPV Type and Viral Load

High viral load may marginally (odds ratio, 1.8) increase the risk for high-grade cytologic abnormalities.

Numerous studies have clearly demonstrated that HPV infection is a highly significant risk determinant of cervical neoplasia (see Epidemiologic Evidence for the Association of HPV with Cervical Neoplasia). Furthermore, the HPV types that are collectively referred to as the oncogenic or high-risk types exhibit the strongest association with cervical cancer.[88] High viral load may be another risk factor for high-grade cytologic abnormalities. Among patients referred for colposcopy because of a dysplastic cervical smear, underlying CIN 3 disease was diagnosed in 90% of women who had an intermediate or high amount of HPV 16 DNA detected in cervical cells by PCR.[89] In another study, women with a high viral load defined as detection of HPV DNA by both PCR and the less sensitive Southern blot method had a 13-fold increased risk of CIN compared with women who were HPV DNA positive by PCR only.[90] However, the influence of viral load on risk of CIN was less apparent after HPV type was taken into account. When a woman was infected with an oncogenic HPV type, a high viral load only marginally increased her risk for CIN (odds ratio, 1.8). In addition, among women with different grades of CIN, a high viral load was not associated with high-grade

lesions after controlling for other risk factors.[91] A potential limitation of studies reporting an association of high viral load with advanced cervical disease is the use of semiquantitative methods. A quantitative PCR-based fluorescent assay was used to measure viral DNA copy numbers for HPV types 16, 18, 31, and 45 in cervical cytobrush specimens from 149 women with CIN 2 or CIN 3, 176 women with CIN 1, and 270 women with normal cytology.[92] In this study, the amount of HPV DNA and the correlation of viral load with disease differed among the HPV types. Patients with CIN 2 or CIN 3 who were HPV 16 positive had 4000 to 6000 times as many copies of HPV DNA as had patients with the same disease infected with HPV 18, HPV 31, or HPV 45. The amount of HPV DNA for HPV 16 increased with increasing dysplasia, but there was no correlation of viral load and cervical disease for HPV types 18, 31, or 45. Furthermore, the range of HPV 16 DNA copies in women with cervical disease was very broad, making it difficult to establish a cutoff value that would predict high-grade disease. An additional observation from this study that may explain the association of CIN with viral load seen in some other studies is that the amount of cellular DNA in samples increased significantly with increasing disease.

Persistent HPV Infection

Longitudinal studies have also shown that persistent HPV infection is a risk factor for persistent or progressive cervical dysplasia.

The initial studies designed to investigate the role of HPV in cervical cancer were cross-sectional, case-control studies. More recently, prospective studies have examined the temporal association of HPV infection with the development of high-grade CIN. These studies have confirmed the association of HPV DNA positivity, and especially positivity for high-risk HPV types, with progressive cervical disease.[83, 93–97] Longitudinal studies have also shown that persistent HPV infection is a risk factor for persistent or progressive cervical dysplasia. The largest prospective study with the longest follow-up was conducted in the Netherlands.[94] Three hundred and fifty-three women referred to gynecologists with abnormal Pap smears were monitored every 3 to 4 months by cytology, colposcopy, and testing for high-risk HPV types. The median follow-up time was 33 months. Thirty-three women developed clinical progression, defined as a colposcopic impression of CIN 3 covering three or more cervical quadrants or a cervical smear showing suspected microinvasive disease. All 33 women had persistent infection with high-risk HPV types, although the same type may not have been detected at each visit. No clinical progression was seen in women negative for high-risk HPV types. The yearly incidence of clinical progression for women who remained positive for high-risk HPV types was 8% per year. At the last visit, all women had a colposcopically directed biopsy. One hundred and three women had an end histology diagnosis of CIN 3. At baseline, 100 (97.1%) of these women tested positive for high-risk HPV types, and infection was persistent in 98 women. In contrast, among women with negative results for high-risk HPV types at baseline, only three developed CIN 3. Women with persistent infection with high-risk HPV types from baseline until their last visit had a 327-fold greater risk of an end histologic diagnosis of CIN 3 than did women who had negative results throughout the study. Risk factors previously reported to contribute to the development of CIN 3, such as age, smoking, age at first intercourse, and number of sexual partners, were not found to be significant associations in this study.

The risk of incident cytologic abnormalities and invasive cervical cancer in relation to HPV infection among women with normal Pap smears at baseline has been evaluated in two studies. Among 17,654 women receiving routine cytologic screening at a health maintenance organization in Portland, Oregon and followed up for development of incident cytologic abnormalities, 380 incident cases were identified among initially cytologically normal women.[98] Cervical lavages collected at enrollment from the case women and lavages collected from matched control subjects were tested for HPV DNA by PCR. Women who tested positive for HPV DNA at enrollment were 3.8 times more likely to have LSIL subsequently diagnosed for the first time during follow-up and 12.7 times more likely to develop HSIL. In a study examining the risk of invasive cervical cancer in relation to HPV infection, the rate of detection of HPV in cytologically normal Pap smears of 118 women in whom cervical cancer subsequently developed was compared with that in the Pap smears of 118 age-matched women who did not have cancer.[99] Pap smears were obtained from the case women an average of 5.6 years before the time of diagnosis of cancer. HPV DNA was detected in the baseline Pap smears of 30% of the women with cervical cancer. In contrast, HPV was detected in only 3% of the baseline Pap smears of the control women. The study likely underestimates the true prevalence of HPV and the associated risk for cervical cancer, because detection of HPV DNA in archival specimens is suboptimal. Among women with cancer for whom tissue samples were available, 80 (77%) women were positive for HPV DNA, and in every case the HPV type was the same in the baseline smear and in the biopsy, supporting the hypothesis of viral persistence in the development of cervical cancer. When the baseline smears from the 118 women with cancer were re-examined at the time of the study, cytologic abnormalities were found to be present in 53 of the smears. Because of the cytologic misclassification of women at baseline, the true risk of cervical cancer for women with an HPV infection and a normal Pap smear is overestimated in this study.

Genetic Predisposition to Invasive Cervical Cancer

Individuals may possess a genetic susceptibility to cervical cancer, but the relative risks are small, and familial clustering would also be consistent with the known differences in cervical cancer risk associated with different socioeconomic groups.

Familial clustering has been observed for some human cancers, such as cancers of the breast, colon, prostate, lung, and stomach.[100, 101] The possibility of a genetic disposition to cervical cancer is suggested by occasional reports in the literature describing families in which several members have been affected by cervical cancer.[102–105] Furgyik and colleagues conducted the first prospective study of familial risk of cervical cancer.[106] They found that cervical cancer was diagnosed significantly more often in mothers and sisters of patients with cervical cancer (15.6%) than in female family members of male consorts (1%). Twin studies have also suggested that individuals may possess a genetic susceptibility to cervical cancer. Ahlbom and colleagues identified twin pairs in which one or both members had in situ cervical cancer by linking the Swedish Twin Registry to the Swedish Cancer Registry.[107] Monozygotic twins had a twofold greater risk of cervical cancer than did dizygotic twin pairs, suggesting a genetic effect as opposed to an environmental familial factor. In one study, the Swedish Cancer Registry was used to identify relatives of patients with cervical cancer and randomly selected age-matched controls.[108] Biologic mothers and full sisters of cases had a nearly twofold greater risk of developing cervical cancer compared with adoptive relatives of cases. In addition, familial cases with cervical cancer had a significantly lower age at diagnosis than did sporadic cases, consistent with the typically earlier age of onset of familial cancers. There was no difference in the risk for half-sisters of cases having a father or mother in common, suggesting that the clustering cannot be explained by vertical transmission of HPV from mother to child. An environmental, as opposed to a genetic, explanation for the familial clustering seems less likely because the risk for siblings who share an environment during the same time and age period was similar to that for mother-daughter relationships. The studies provide epidemiologic evidence for a genetic predisposition to cervical cancer. However, the relative risks are small, and familial clustering would also be consistent with the known differences in cervical cancer risk associated with different socioeconomic groups.[109]

Host and Environmental Factors in the Development of Cervical Cancer

Most of the sociodemographic, sexual, and obstetric factors traditionally associated with cervical cancer are now known to be largely correlates of HPV infection.

Most of the sociodemographic, sexual, and obstetric factors traditionally associated with cervical cancer are now known to be largely correlates of HPV infection. In most studies using PCR-based diagnostic methods, associations of cervical cancer with lower social class, fewer years of education, more lifetime sex partners, lower age at commencement of sexual intercourse, pregnancy, and parity have disappeared or been greatly weakened after HPV infection is taken into account.[31, 110–112] However, controversies continue regarding the role in cervical cancer risk of cigarette smoking, oral contraceptive use, chlamydia infection, and dietary factors.

Smoking, Oral Contraceptives, and Other Sexually Transmitted Infectious Agents

> **High concentrations of carcinogenic, tobacco-specific N-nitrosamines have been demonstrated in cervical mucus of smokers. However, many carefully conducted case-control studies have failed to find any association between cigarette smoking and cervical dysplasia or invasive cervical cancer after adjusting for HPV infection.**

Cigarette smoking has been linked to the etiology of HSIL or invasive cervical cancer in four case-control studies that used PCR methods to detect HPV infection.[91, 110, 113, 114] In these studies, relative risks ranged from 1.7 to 11.2. In support of an etiologic role for smoking, high concentrations of carcinogenic, tobacco-specific N-nitrosamines have been demonstrated in cervical mucus of smokers.[115] However, many carefully conducted case-control studies have failed to find any association between cigarette smoking and cervical dysplasia or invasive cervical cancer after adjusting for HPV infection.[31, 33, 35, 37, 111, 116]

Before the availability of PCR-based methods for detection of HPV infection, most epidemiologic studies demonstrated an increased risk of invasive cervical cancer associated with use of oral contraceptives.[117, 118] One study using PCR to detect HPV infection found a significantly elevated risk of cervical cancer among women who used oral contraceptives.[111] However, many comparable studies have failed to support this association.[31, 33, 35, 37, 110, 116, 119] In one study, oral contraceptive use was actually protective for high-grade cervical dysplasia.[120]

> **Seropositivity for antibodies against Chlamydia trachomatis and Neisseria gonorrhoeae is probably a surrogate marker for HPV infection, but it is possible that these infections may enhance the risk for cervical cancer.**

The recognition that the risk of cervical cancer is strongly influenced by sexual activity prompted the search for a sexually transmitted agent as an etiologic factor in cervical cancer and led to the discovery of the role of HPV infection. Several other sexually transmitted agents have also been associated with cervical cancer, but the significance of these associations is unclear. Early studies did not adjust for HPV status or used HPV assays that are not highly sensitive. However, in case-control studies of CIN 3 and invasive cervical cancer carried out in Spain and Colombia, exposure to other sexually transmitted agents was measured serologically in women who were examined for HPV using a PCR assay.[121] The presence and levels of antibody to cytomegalovirus, Treponema pallidum, and herpes simplex virus type 2 were not related to CIN 3 or to invasive cervical cancer. After adjustment for HPV DNA, women with antibodies against C. trachomatis were at moderate risk for CIN 3, and those in Spain with high antibody titers were at high risk for invasive cervical cancer. Spanish women with antibodies to N. gonorrhoeae were also at a significantly increased risk for invasive cervical cancer. In a prospective seroepidemiologic study of women from the Nordic countries, serum antibodies to C. trachomatis were associated with a 2.2-fold increased risk for squamous cell carcinoma after adjustment of HPV seropositivity.[122] The results of these studies most likely indicate that seropositivity to these agents is a surrogate marker for HPV infection. However, the possibility that infection with C. trachomatis or N. gonorrhoeae enhances the risk of cervical cancer cannot be excluded.

Dietary Factors

> **Low intakes of vitamin C, carotenoids, and possibly vitamin E and folate may increase the risk of cervical neoplasia, whereas vitamin A has little or no effect on cervical cancer risk.**

Potischman and Brinton reviewed the epidemiologic evidence for a relationship between nutrition and cervical cancer and concluded that low intakes of vitamin C, carotenoids, and possibly vitamin E and folate may increase the risk of cervical neoplasia, whereas vitamin A has little or no effect on cervical cancer risk.[123] However, the authors noted that a limitation in nearly all the studies examining the relationship of nutritional factors to cervical neoplasia was the absence of information on HPV status. Three case-control studies have examined the association of plasma micronutrients, particularly antioxidants, with the risk of cervical SIL in women whose HPV status was determined by sensitive and specific nucleic acid detection techniques. In a study of 123 low-income Hispanic women, the concentrations of serum carotenoids (betacarotene, β-cryptoxanthin, and lutein) and α-tocopherol and γ-tocopherol (vitamin E) were, on average, 24% lower among women with persistent HPV infection after 3 months of follow-up, compared with women with transient HPV infection or no infection.[124] In addition, serum α-tocopherol was significantly associated with grade of cervical dysplasia after adjustment for potential confounding sociodemographic factors and HPV infection. Plasma ascorbate concentration (vitamin C) was not associated with HPV status. In a study of 147 Hawaiian women with cervical SIL, plasma concentrations of carotenoids (lycopene and α-cryptoxanthin) were lower in cases than in clinic controls with negative cytologic smears.[125] The plasma level of vitamin C was also lower in cases than in controls, but the difference was not statistically significant. There was a significant inverse dose-response of α-cryptoxanthin and α-tocopherol to the risk of cervical SIL. In a third study, plasma micronutrients were measured in 378 CIN cases and 366 controls without a history of abnormal Pap smears.[90] After adjusting for HPV positivity and demographic factors, there was an inverse correlation between plasma α-tocopherol and CIN. Reduced ascorbic acid (vitamin C) showed a marginal inverse correlation with CIN. A plausible biologic mechanism for a protective effect of carotenoids, tocopherols, and vitamin C may be their function as antioxidants.[126–129] By scavenging the free oxygen radicals generated by many different intracellular reactions, antioxidants protect biologic macromolecules from oxidative damage. Antioxidants are particularly important for function of the immune system, which is essential for prevention and control of infectious diseases including HPV infection.[130] An additional biologic mechanism for the protective effect of betacarotene may derive from its conversion to retinoic acid.[131] Retinoic acid is a potent modulator of epithelial growth and differentiation and has been shown to have antiviral effects on HPV.[132, 133]

> **It is not clear whether women with low vitamin levels are at increased risk for cervical disease or whether persistent HPV infection results in lower concentrations of these nutrients.**

Whether nutrients influence HPV infection, persistence, or progression of cervical disease is unknown. In a randomized trial of betacarotene supplementation in women with moderate cervical dysplasia, there was no difference between the betacarotene group and the placebo group in the risk for having CIN at 9 months, suggesting that the vitamin had no effect on resolution of HPV infection once HPV-induced disease had developed.[134] In a prospective study that used a questionnaire to estimate nutrient intake, the risk of incident SIL among women infected with high-risk HPV types was similar in women who reported high vitamin A, C, or E intake and in women who reported low vitamin intake, suggesting that in the presence of an HPV infection the vitamins are not important protective cofactors against development of LSIL.[135] Although plasma micronutrients do not appear to influence the initial course of an HPV infection or the persistence of cytologic abnormalities, they may nevertheless have an effect on progression of LSIL lesions to HSIL or invasive cervical cancer. To date, studies have not been conducted to test this hypothesis. One difficulty with the interpretation of observational studies of nutrient intake is that it is not clear whether women with low vitamin levels are at increased risk for cervical disease or whether persistent HPV infection results in lower concentrations of these nutrients. In conclusion, the published studies indicate that low plasma levels of antioxidants are associated with HPV-related cervical disease; however, establishing a causal role for plasma micronutrients in cervical cancer will require prospective studies and possibly intervention trials with vitamin supplementation.

CONCLUSIONS

Although HPV infection explains many of the classic risk factors for cervical neoplasia, particularly its relationship to sexual activity, our knowledge of potential cofactors is still limited. Environmental factors such as smoking, diet, and exposure to other sexually transmitted diseases; protective and susceptibility genetic determinants; and viral characteristics of infection such as HPV type, viral load, and mixed cervical infection appear to contribute to cancer risk. However, a coherent picture of the natural history of HPV-induced cervical carcinogenesis is lacking, and putting the various pieces together is the principal challenge for future epidemiologic studies of HPV. The largest gap in our knowledge of HPV infection is in the area of immune responses, particularly as they relate to

susceptibility to HPV infection and progression to cervical disease. Filling this gap will likely be a major focus of future epidemiologic studies.

Acknowledgments

This work was supported by grant AI-42058 (R.P.V.) from the National Institutes of Health. The author thanks Keerti Shah for reading the manuscript and providing helpful comments.

SUMMARY OF KEY POINTS

- The etiologic relationship of HPV to cervical cancer, as well as to cancers at several other sites, is firmly established.

- The current list of cancer-associated HPV types includes four high-risk types (types 16, 18, 31, and 45) and nine intermediate-risk types (types 33, 35, 39, 51, 52, 56, 58, 59, and 68). Seventy-five percent of cervical cancers are infected with type 16, 18, 31, or 45.

- HPV infections are initiated when the virus gains access to basal cells of a squamous epithelial surface through minor traumas such as skin abrasion or during sexual intercourse.

- The most prevalent HPV type is HPV 16. HPV 16 is the predominant type in squamous cancers. HPV 18 is the predominant type in adenocarcinomas. Multiple infections are common, with prevalence ranging from 2% to 20% of women.

- Within individuals, the detection of HPV DNA is highly variable, indicating the limitations of single-point measurements of cervical HPV infection for calculating prevalence.

- The odds ratios for developing cervical dysplasia in the presence of HPV DNA range from about 15 to 120 compared with controls and from about 12 to 300 in the presence of HPV 16 DNA.

- A number of studies have shown a twofold to sevenfold increased risk for cervical dysplasia in women infected with multiple HPV types as compared with those infected with a single type.

- Several HPV types have been associated with genital warts, but HPV 6 is the most commonly identified type.

- From the National Breast and Cervical Cancer Early Detection Program, the overall rate of abnormal Pap tests was 3.8%. The rates for low-grade squamous lesions, high-grade lesions, and squamous cancer were 2.9%, 0.8%, and less than 0.1%, respectively.

- Subclinical HPV infections may be 10 to 30 times more common than cytologically apparent infections.

- Cervical cancer is one of the most common neoplastic diseases affecting women, with a combined worldwide incidence exceeded only by breast cancer and colorectal cancer.

- In the United States, cervical cancer is the eighth most common malignancy in women.

- In the United States, the projected number of new cases of invasive cervical cancer for 1999 is 12,800, and the estimated number of deaths that will occur from this disease is 4800. The lifetime risk for U.S. women of being diagnosed with cervical cancer and the lifetime risk of dying from cervical cancer are 0.78% and 0.26%, respectively.

- Neonatal transmission of genital HPV appears to be uncommon.

- The presence of HPV DNA in newborn samples might simply indicate contamination with infected maternal cells rather than infection.

- HPV is transmitted sexually with modest efficiency. As many as two thirds to three fourths of persons sexually exposed to genital warts have been reported to develop genital warts subsequently.

- The predominant risk factor for a genital HPV infection is the number of lifetime sexual partners, with male sexual behavior being an independent risk factor for infection in women.

- Most cervical HPV infections diagnosed by PCR and other nucleic acid detection methods appear to be transient. The proportion of women who cleared their infection increased with younger age, longer interval between samplings, and infection with low-risk as opposed to high-risk HPV types.

- The time interval required for 50% of prevalent cases to become HPV DNA negative was 4.8 months for nononcogenic types and 8.1 months for oncogenic types.

- In young women without a cytologic abnormality at the time the infection is diagnosed, HSIL is an uncommon outcome of HPV infection, even with high-risk HPV types.

- Women with borderline and low-grade abnormalities on cervical cytology have a risk for progression to invasive cervical cancer over 24 months of 1 to 2 per 1000 women without treatment. High viral load and persistent HPV infection may be risk factors for high-grade cytologic abnormalities.

- Although HPV infection is necessary for the development of HSIL and invasive cancer, it is not a sufficient cause.

References

1. Ciuffo G: Innesto positivo con filtrate di verruca volgare. Giorn Ital Mal Venereol 1907;48:12.

2. Waelsch L: Ubertragungsversuche mit Spitzen Kondylome. Arch Dermatol Syphilis 1917;124:625.

3. Serra, A: Richerche istologiche e sperimentali sul condiloma acuminato: I papillomi del capo e la verruca volgare. Contributo all'etiologia, patogenesi, filtrabilita. Giorn Ital Mal Venereol 1908; 49:11.

4. Strauss MJ, Shaw EW, Bunting H, Melnick JJ: Crystalline virus-like particles from skin papillomas characterized by intranuclear inclusion bodies. Proc Soc Exptl Biol Med 1949;72:46.

5. Bunting H: Close-packed array of virus particles in human genital warts. Proc Soc Exptl Biol Med 1953;84:327.

6. Oriel JD, Almeida JD: Demonstration of virus particles in human genital warts. Br J Vener Dis 1970;46:37.

7. Manos MM, Ting Y, Wright DK, et al: Use of polymerase chain reaction amplification for the detection of genital human papillomaviruses. In Furth M, Greaves M (eds): Cancer Cells 7, Molecular Diagnostics of Human Cancer. New York, Cold Spring Harbor Laboratory Press, 1989, pp 209–214.

8. Shope R: Infectious papillomatosis of rabbits. J Exp Med 1933;58: 607.

9. Rigoni-Stern D: Fatti statistici relativi alle malatia cancerose. G Serv Prog Pathol Therap 1842;2:507.

10. zur Hausen H: Condylomata acuminata and human genital cancer. Cancer Res 1976;36:794.

11. Meisels A, Fortin R: Condylomatous lesions of the cervix and vagina. I. Cytologic patterns. Acta Cytol 1976;20:505.

12. Durst M, Gissmann L, Ikenberg H, zur Hausen H: A papillomavirus DNA from a cervical carcinoma and its prevalence in cancer biopsy samples from different geographic regions. Proc Natl Acad Sci USA 1983;80:3812.

13. deVilliers EM: Human pathogenic papillomavirus types: An update. Curr Top Microbiol Immunol 1994;186:1.

14. Bauer HM, Ting Y, Greer CE, et al: Genital human papillomavirus infection in female university students as determined by a PCR-based method. JAMA 1991;265:472.

15. Kotloff KL, Wasserman SS, Russ K, et al: Detection of genital human papillomavirus and associated cytological abnormalities among college women. Sex Transm Dis 1998;25:243.

16. Franco EL, Villa LL, Sobrinho JP, et al: Epidemiology of acquisition and clearance of cervical human papillomavirus infection in women from a high-risk area for cervical cancer. J Infect Dis 1999;180:1415.

17. Ho GY, Bierman R, Beardsley L, et al: Natural history of cervicovaginal papillomavirus infection in young women. N Engl J Med 1998;338:423.

18. Wheeler CM: Human papillomavirus type-specific prevalence. In Myers G, Baker C, Wheeler CM, et al (eds): Human Papillomaviruses 1996: A Compilation and Analysis of Nucleic Acid and Amino Acid Sequences. Los Alamos, NM, Los Alamos National Laboratory, 1996, pp III112–III124.

19. Wheeler CM, Greer CE, Becker TM, et al: Short-term fluctuations in the detection of cervical human papillomavirus DNA. Obstet Gynecol 1996;88:261.

20. Schneider A, Kirchhoff T, Meinhardt G, Gissmann L: Repeated evaluation of human papillomavirus 16 status in cervical swabs of young women with a history of normal Papanicolaou smears. Obstet Gynecol 1992;79:683.

21. Moscicki AB, Palefsky J, Smith G, et al: Variability of human papillomavirus DNA testing in a longitudinal cohort of young women. Obstet Gynecol 1993;82:578.

22. Hildesheim A, Schiffman MH, Gravitt PE, et al: Persistence of type-specific human papillomavirus infection among cytologically normal women. J Infect Dis 1994;169:235.

23. Evander M, Edlund K, Gustafsson A, et al: Human papillomavirus infection is transient in young women: A population-based cohort study. J Infect Dis 1995;171:1026.

24. deRoda H, Walboomers JM, Meijer CJ, et al: Analysis of cytomorphologically abnormal cervical scrapes for the presence of 27 mucosotropic human papillomavirus genotypes, using polymerase chain reaction. Int J Cancer 1994;56:802.

25. Bosch FX, Manos MM, Munoz N, et al: Prevalence of human papillomavirus in cervical cancer: A worldwide perspective. International biological study on cervical cancer (IBSCC) study group. J Natl Cancer Inst 1995;87:796.

26. Lungu O, Sun XW, Felix J, et al: Relationship of human papillomavirus type to grade of cervical intraepithelial neoplasia. JAMA 1992;267:2493.

27. Tase T, Okagaki T, Clark BA, et al: Human papillomavirus types and localization in adenocarcinoma and adenosquamous carcinoma of the uterine cervix: A study by in situ DNA hybridization. Cancer Res 1988;48:993.

28. Wilczynski SP, Bergen S, Walker J, et al: Human papillomaviruses and cervical cancer: Analysis of histopathologic features associated with different viral types. Hum Pathol 1988;19:697.

29. Walboomers JM, Jacobs MV, Manos MM, et al: Human papillomavirus is a necessary cause of invasive cervical cancer worldwide. J Pathol 1999;189:12.

30. Munoz N, Bosch FX, deSanjose S, et al: The causal link between human papillomavirus and invasive cervical cancer: A population-based case-control study in Colombia and Spain. Int J Cancer 1992;52:743.

31. Eluf-Neto J, Booth M, Munoz N, et al: Human papillomavirus and invasive cervical cancer in Brazil. Br J Cancer 1994;69:114.

32. Bosch FX, Munoz N, deSanjose S, et al: Human papillomavirus and cervical intraepithelial neoplasia grade III/carcinoma in situ: A case-control study in Spain and Colombia. Cancer Epidemiol Biomarkers Prev 1993;2:415.

33. Olsen AO, Gjoen K, Sauer T, et al: Human papillomavirus and cervical intraepithelial neoplasia grade II–III: A population-based case-control study. Int J Cancer 1995;61:312.

34. Becker TM, Wheeler CM, McGough NS, et al: Sexually transmitted diseases and other risk factors for cervical dysplasia among southwestern Hispanic and non-Hispanic white women. JAMA 1994;271:1181.

35. Liaw KL, Hsing AW, Chen CJ, et al: Human papillomavirus and cervical neoplasia: A case-control study in Taiwan. Int J Cancer 1995;62:565.

36. Morrison EA, Ho GY, Vermund SH, et al: Human papillomavirus infection and other risk factors for cervical neoplasia: A case-control study. Int J Cancer 1991;49:6.

37. Schiffman MH, Bauer HM, Hoover RN, et al: Epidemiologic evidence showing that human papillomavirus infection causes most cervical intraepithelial neoplasia. J Natl Cancer Inst 1993;85:958.

38. Simms I, Fairley CK: Epidemiology of genital warts in England and Wales: 1971 to 1994. Genitourin Med 1997;73:365.

39. Koutsky LA, Galloway DA, Holmes, KK: Epidemiology of genital human papillomavirus infection. Epidemiol Rev 1988;10:122.

40. Chuang TY, Perry HO, Kurland LT, Ilstrup DM: Condyloma acuminatum in Rochester, Minn., 1950–1978. I. Epidemiology and clinical features. Arch Dermatol 1984;120:469.

41. Persson G, Andersson K, Krantz I: Symptomatic genital papillomavirus infection in a community. Incidence and clinical picture. Acta Obstet Gynecol Scand 1996;75:287.

42. Greer CE, Wheeler CM, Ladner MB, et al: Human papillomavirus (HPV) type distribution and serological response to HPV type 6 virus-like particles in patients with genital warts. J Clin Microbiol 1995;33:2058.

43. Sugase M, Moriyama S, Matsukura T: Human papillomavirus in exophytic condylomatous lesions on different female genital regions. J Med Virol 1991;34:1.

44. Langenberg A, Cone RW, McDougall J, et al: Dual infection with human papillomavirus in a population with overt genital condylomas. J Am Acad Dermatol 1993;28:434.

45. Lawson HW, Lee NC, Thames SF, et al: Cervical cancer screening among low-income women: Results of a national screening program, 1991–1995. Obstet Gynecol 1998;92:745.

46. Mitchell H, Medley G: Age and time trends in the prevalence of cervical intraepithelial neoplasia on Papanicolaou smear tests, 1970–1988. Med J Aust 1990;152:252.

47. Kreuger FA, Beerman H, Nijs HG, van Ballegooijen, M: Positive diagnostic values and histological detection ratios from the Rotterdam cervical cancer screening programme. Int J Epidemiol 1998;27:377.

48. Bjorge T, Gunbjorud AB, Langmark F, et al: Cervical mass screening in Norway—510,000 smears a year. Cancer Detect Prev 1994;18:463.

49. Burk RD, Ho GY, Beardsley L, et al: Sexual behavior and partner characteristics are the predominant risk factors for genital human papillomavirus infection in young women. J Infect Dis 1996;174:679.

50. Sadeghi SB, Hsieh EW, Gunn SW: Prevalence of cervical intraepithelial neoplasia in sexually active teenagers and young adults. Results of data analysis of mass Papanicolaou screening of 796,337 women in the United States in 1981. Am J Obstet Gynecol 1984;148:726.

51. Cooper A: Lectures on the Principles and Practice of Surgery, 8th ed. London, Cox and Portwine, 1835.

52. Rylander E, Ruusuvaara L, Almstromer MW, et al: The absence of vaginal human papillomavirus 16 DNA in women who have not experienced sexual intercourse. Obstet Gynecol 1994;83:735.

53. Fairley CK, Chen S, Tabrizi SN, et al: The absence of genital human papillomavirus DNA in virginal women. Int J STD AIDS 1992;3:414.

54. Andersson-Ellstrom A, Hagmar BM, Johansson B, et al: Human papillomavirus deoxyribonucleic acid in cervix only detected in girls after coitus. Int J STD AIDS 1996;7:333.

55. Watts DH, Koutsky LA, Holmes KK, et al: Low risk of perinatal transmission of human papillomavirus: Results from a prospective cohort study. Am J Obstet Gynecol 1998;178:365.

56. Kashima HK, Shah F, Lyles A, et al: A comparison of risk factors in juvenile-onset and adult-onset recurrent respiratory papillomatosis. Laryngoscope 1992;102:9.

57. Smith EM, Johnson SR, Cripe T, et al: Perinatal transmission and maternal risks of human papillomavirus infection. Cancer Detect Prev 1995;19:196.

58. Pakarian F, Kaye J, Cason J, et al: Cancer associated human papillomaviruses: Perinatal transmission and persistence. Br J Obstet Gynaecol 1994;101:514.

59. Cason J, Kaye JN, Jewers RJ, et al: Perinatal infection and persistence of human papillomavirus types 16 and 18 in infants. J Med Virol 1995;47:209.

60. Puranen M, Yliskoski M, Saarikoski S, et al: Vertical transmission of human papillomavirus from infected mothers to their newborn babies and persistence of the virus in childhood. Am J Obstet Gynecol 1996;174:694.

61. Fredericks BD, Balkin A, Daniel HW, et al: Transmission of human papillomaviruses from mother to child. Aust N Z J Obstet Gynaecol 1993;33:30.

62. Tenti P, Zappatore R, Migliora P, et al: Perinatal transmission of human papillomavirus from gravidas with latent infections. Obstet Gynecol 1999;93:475.

63. Oriel JD: Natural history of genital warts. Br J Vener Dis 1971;47:1.

64. Campion MJ, Singer A, Clarkson PK, McCance DJ: Increased risk of cervical neoplasia in consorts of men with penile condylomata acuminata. Lancet 1985;1:943.

65. Campion MJ, McCance DJ, Mitchell HS, et al: Subclinical penile human papillomavirus infection and dysplasia in consorts of women with cervical neoplasia. Genitourin Med 1988;64:90.

66. Kyo S, Inoue M, Koyama M, et al: Detection of high-risk human papillomavirus in the cervix and semen of sex partners. J Infect Dis 1994;170:682.

67. Baken LA, Koutsky LA, Kuypers J, et al: Genital human papillomavirus infection among male and female sex partners: Prevalence and type-specific concordance. J Infect Dis 1995;171:429.

68. Ho L, Tay SK, Chan SY, Bernard HU: Sequence variants of human papillomavirus type 16 from couples suggest sexual transmission with low infectivity and polyclonality in genital neoplasia. J Infect Dis 1993;168:803.

69. Gutman LT, St Claire K, Herman-Giddens ME, et al: Evaluation of sexually abused and nonabused young girls for intravaginal human papillomavirus infection. Am J Dis Child 1992;146:694.

70. Ley C, Bauer HM, Reingold A, et al: Determinants of genital human papillomavirus infection in young women. J Natl Cancer Inst 1991;83:997.

71. Hildesheim A, Gravitt P, Schiffman MH, et al: Determinants of genital human papillomavirus infection in low-income women in Washington, D.C. Sex Transm Dis 1993;20:279.

72. Bauer HM, Hildesheim A, Schiffman MH, et al: Determinants of genital human papillomavirus infection in low-risk women in Portland, Oregon. Sex Transm Dis 1993;20:274.

73. Wheeler CM, Parmenter CA, Hunt WC, et al: Determinants of genital human papillomavirus infection among cytologically normal women attending the University of New Mexico student health center. Sex Transm Dis 1993;20:286.

74. Karlsson R, Jonsson M, Edlund K, et al: Lifetime number of partners as the only independent risk factor for human papillomavirus infection: A population-based study. Sex Transm Dis 1995;22:119.

75. Kjaer SK, van den Brule AJ, Bock JE, et al: Determinants for genital human papillomavirus (HPV) infection in 1000 randomly chosen young Danish women with normal Pap smear: Are there different risk profiles for oncogenic and nononcogenic HPV types? Cancer Epidemiol Biomarkers Prev 1997;6:799.

76. Melkert PW, Hopman E, van den Brule AJ, et al: Prevalence of HPV in cytomorphologically normal cervical smears, as determined by the polymerase chain reaction, is age-dependent. Int J Cancer 1993;53:919.

77. Schiffman MH: Epidemiology of cervical human papillomavirus infections. Curr Top Microbiol Immunol 1994;186:55.

78. Bosch FX, Munoz N, deSanjose S, et al: Importance of human papillomavirus endemicity in the incidence of cervical cancer: An extension of the hypothesis on sexual behavior. Cancer Epidemiol Biomarkers Prev 1994;3:375.

79. Gloss B, Bernard HU, Seedorf K, Klock G: The upstream regulatory region of the human papilloma virus-16 contains an e2 protein-independent enhancer which is specific for cervical carcinoma cells and regulated by glucocorticoid hormones. EMBO J 1987;6:3735.

80. Mittal R, Tsutsumi K, Pater A, Pater MM: Human papillomavirus type 16 expression in cervical keratinocytes: Role of progesterone and glucocorticoid hormones. Obstet Gynecol 1993;81:5.

81. Pater MM, Hughes GA, Hyslop DE, et al: Glucocorticoid-dependent oncogenic transformation by type 16 but not type 11 human papilloma virus DNA. Nature 1988;335:832.

82. Bosch FX, Castellsague X, Munoz N, et al: Male sexual behavior and human papillomavirus DNA: Key risk factors for cervical cancer in Spain. J Natl Cancer Inst 1996;88:1060.

83. Moscicki AB, Shiboski S, Broering J, et al: The natural history of human papillomavirus infection as measured by repeated DNA testing in adolescent and young women. J Pediatr 1998;132:277.

84. Koutsky LA, Holmes KK, Critchlow CW, et al: A cohort study of the risk of cervical intraepithelial neoplasia grade 2 or 3 in relation to papillomavirus infection. N Engl J Med 1992;327:1272.

85. Syrjanen KJ: Spontaneous evolution of intraepithelial lesions according to the grade and type of the implicated human papillomavirus (HPV). Eur J Obstet Gynecol Reprod Biol 1996;65:45.

86. Ostor AG: Natural history of cervical intraepithelial neoplasia: A critical review. Int J Gynecol Pathol 1993;12:186.

87. Melnikow J, Nuovo J, Willan AR, et al: Natural history of cervical squamous intraepithelial lesions: A meta-analysis. Obstet Gynecol 1998;92:727.

88. Lorincz AT, Reid R, Jenson AB, et al: Human papillomavirus infection of the cervix: Relative risk associations of 15 common anogenital types. Obstet Gynecol 1992;79:328.

89. Cuzick J, Terry G, Ho L, et al: Human papillomavirus type 16 in cervical smears as predictor of high-grade cervical intraepithelial neoplasia. Lancet 1992;339:959.

90. Ho GY, Palan PR, Basu J, et al: Viral characteristics of human papillomavirus infection and antioxidant levels as risk factors for cervical dysplasia. Int J Cancer 1998;78:594.

91. Ho GY, Kadish AS, Burk RD, et al: HPV 16 and cigarette smoking as risk factors for high-grade cervical intra-epithelial neoplasia. Int J Cancer 1998;78:281.

92. Swan DC, Tucker RA, Tortolero-Luna G, et al: Human papillomavirus (HPV) DNA copy number is dependent on grade of cervical disease and HPV type. J Clin Microbiol 1999;37:1030.

93. Woodman CB, Rollason T, Ellis J, et al: Human papillomavirus infection and risk of progression of epithelial abnormalities of the cervix. Br J Cancer 1996;73:553.

94. Nobbenhuis MA, Walboomers JM, Helmerhorst TJ, et al: Relation of human papillomavirus status to cervical lesions and consequences for cervical-cancer screening: A prospective study. Lancet 1999;354:20.

95. Remmink AJ, Walboomers JM, Helmerhorst TJ, et al: The presence of persistent high-risk HPV genotypes in dysplastic cervical lesions is associated with progressive disease: Natural history up to 36 months. Int J Cancer 1995;61:306.

96. Ho GY, Burk RD, Klein S, et al: Persistent genital human papillomavirus infection as a risk factor for persistent cervical dysplasia. J Natl Cancer Inst 1995;87:1365.

97. ter Harmsel B, Smedts F, Kuijpers J, et al: Relationship between human papillomavirus type 16 in the cervix and intraepithelial neoplasia. Obstet Gynecol 1999;93:46.

98. Liaw KL, Glass AG, Manos MM, et al: Detection of human papillomavirus DNA in cytologically normal women and subsequent cervical squamous intraepithelial lesions. J Natl Cancer Inst 1999;91:954.

99. Wallin KL, Wiklund F, Angstrom T, et al: Type-specific persistence of human papillomavirus DNA before the development of invasive cervical cancer. N Engl J Med 1999;341:1633.

100. Easton DF: The inherited component of cancer. Br Med Bull 1994;50:527.

101. Lynch HT, Fusaro RM, Lynch J: Hereditary cancer in adults. Cancer Detect Prev 1995;19:219.

102. Andrews FJ, Linehan JJ, Melcher DH: Cervical carcinoma in both mother and daughter. Acta Cytol 1981;25:3.

103. Way S: Letter: Carcinoma-in-situ of cervix in sisters. Br Med J 1976;1:834.

104. Way S, Hetherington J, Galloway, DC: Simultaneous cytological diagnosis of cervical cancer in three sisters. Lancet 1959;2:890.

105. Bender S: Carcinoma in-situ of cervix in sisters. Br Med J 1976;1:502.

106. Furgyik S, Grubb R, Kullander S, et al: Familial occurrence of cervical cancer, stages 0–IV. Acta Obstet Gynecol Scand 1986;65:223.

107. Ahlbom A, Lichtenstein P, Malmstrom H, et al: Cancer in twins: Genetic and nongenetic familial risk factors. J Natl Cancer Inst 1997;89:287.

108. Magnusson PK, Sparen P, Gyllensten UB: Genetic link to cervical tumours. Nature 1999;400:29.

109. Fasal E, Simmons ME, Kampert JB: Factors associated with high and low risk of cervical neoplasia. J Natl Cancer Inst 1981;66:631.

110. Ngelangel C, Munoz N, Bosch FX, et al: Causes of cervical cancer in the Philippines: A case-control study. J Natl Cancer Inst 1998;90:43.

111. Bosch FX, Munoz N, deSanjose S, et al: Risk factors for cervical cancer in Colombia and Spain. Int J Cancer 1992;52:750.

112. Peng HQ, Liu SL, Mann V, et al: Human papillomavirus types 16 and 33, herpes simplex virus type 2 and other risk factors for cervical cancer in Sichuan Province, China. Int J Cancer 1991;47:711.

113. Becker TM, Wheeler CM, McGough NS, et al: Cigarette smoking and other risk factors for cervical dysplasia in southwestern Hispanic and non-Hispanic white women. Cancer Epidemiol Biomarkers Prev 1994;3:113.

114. Kjaer SK, Engholm G, Dahl C, Bock JE: Case-control study of risk factors for cervical squamous cell neoplasia in Denmark. IV: Role of smoking habits. Eur J Cancer Prev 1996;5:359.

115. Prokopczyk B, Cox JE, Hoffmann D, Waggoner SE: Identification of tobacco-specific carcinogen in the cervical mucus of smokers and nonsmokers. J Natl Cancer Inst 1997;89:868.

116. Munoz N, Bosch FX, deSanjose S, et al: Risk factors for cervical intraepithelial neoplasia grade iii/carcinoma in situ in Spain and Colombia. Cancer Epidemiol Biomarkers Prev 1993;2:423.

117. Brinton LA: Oral contraceptives and cervical neoplasia. Contraception 1991;43:581.

118. Invasive squamous-cell cervical carcinoma and combined oral contraceptives: Results from a multinational study. WHO collaborative study of neoplasia and steroid contraceptives. Int J Cancer 1993;55:228.

119. Kjaer SK, van den Brule AJ, Bock JE, et al: Human papillomavirus—the most significant risk determinant of cervical intraepithelial neoplasia. Int J Cancer 1996;65:601.

120. Becker TM, Wheeler CM, McGough NS, et al: Contraceptive and reproductive risks for cervical dysplasia in southwestern Hispanic and non-Hispanic white women. Int J Epidemiol 1994;23:913.

121. deSanjose S, Munoz N, Bosch FX, et al: Sexually transmitted agents and cervical neoplasia in Colombia and Spain. Int J Cancer 1994;56:358.

122. Koskela P, Anttila T, Bjorge T, et al: Chlamydia trachomatis infection as a risk factor for invasive cervical cancer. Int J Cancer 2000;85:35.

123. Potischman N, Brinton LA: Nutrition and cervical neoplasia. Cancer Causes Control 1996;7:113.

124. Giuliano AR, Papenfuss M, Nour M, et al: Antioxidant nutrients: Associations with persistent human papillomavirus infection. Cancer Epidemiol Biomarkers Prev 1997;6:917.

125. Goodman MT, Kiviat N, McDuffie K, et al: The association of

plasma micronutrients with the risk of cervical dysplasia in Hawaii. Cancer Epidemiol Biomarkers Prev 1998;7:537.

126. Di Mascio P, Murphy ME, Sies H: Antioxidant defense systems: The role of carotenoids, tocopherols, and thiols. Am J Clin Nutr 1991;53(suppl 1):194S.

127. Burton GW: Antioxidant action of carotenoids. J Nutr 1989;119:109.

128. Burton GW, Ingold KU: Vitamin E as an in vitro and in vivo antioxidant. Ann NY Acad Sci 1989;570:7.

129. Niki E, Noguchi N, Tsuchihashi H, Gotoh N: Interaction among vitamin C, vitamin E, and beta-carotene. Am J Clin Nutr 1995; 62(suppl 6):1322S.

130. Bendich A: Carotenoids and the immune response. J Nutr 1989; 119:112.

131. Hebuterne X, Wang XD, Johnson EJ, et al: Intestinal absorption and metabolism of 9-cis-beta-carotene in vivo: Biosynthesis of 9-cis-retinoic acid. J Lipid Res 1995;36:1264.

132. Khan MA, Jenkins GR, Tolleson WH, et al: Retinoic acid inhibition of human papillomavirus type 16-mediated transformation of human keratinocytes. Cancer Res 1993;53:905.

133. Shindoh M, Sun Q, Pater A, Pater MM: Prevention of carcinoma in situ of human papillomavirus type 16-immortalized human endocervical cells by retinoic acid in organotypic raft culture. Obstet Gynecol 1995;85:721.

134. Romney SL, Ho GY, Palan PR, et al: Effects of beta-carotene and other factors on outcome of cervical dysplasia and human papillomavirus infection. Gynecol Oncol 1997;65:483.

135. Wideroff L, Potischman N, Glass AG, et al: A nested case-control study of dietary factors and the risk of incident cytological abnormalities of the cervix. Nutr Cancer 1998;30:130.

• Bethanee J. Schlosser
• Mary K. Howett

CHAPTER *2*

Human Papillomaviruses: Molecular Aspects of the Viral Life Cycle and Pathogenesis

All papillomaviruses infect epithelial tissues in a species-specific manner and induce epithelial proliferation.

Papillomaviruses (PVs) are ubiquitous microorganisms that cause productive and/or latent infections in a wide variety of species and tissues. To date, more than 90 types of human papillomavirus (HPV) have been catalogued, including those that preferentially infect cutaneous or mucosal stratified squamous epithelia.[1] Animal PVs also infect numerous species and include the well-studied Shope cottontail rabbit papillomavirus (CRPV) and bovine papillomavirus type 1 (BPV1). All PVs infect epithelial tissues in a species-specific manner and induce epithelial proliferation. All PVs, both animal and human, share a common genomic organizational structure, but sequence similarity among HPV types and between HPVs and animal PVs varies substantially.

Because it proficiently infects and transforms mono-layer cell cultures, BPV1 has often been used as the prototype for investigations of the PV life cycle. However, differences between the life cycles and the gene products of BPV1 and HPV do exist. The following discussion will therefore elaborate on investigations of HPV and, where information is lacking for HPV, will also include what is known for BPV1.

OVERVIEW OF THE PV LIFE CYCLE

The life cycle of PV is strictly linked to differentiation of the keratinocyte, the host cell for infection.

HPVs can bind to cells from a wide range of human tissues; however, greatest binding is observed with epithelial and mesenchymal cells. Approximately half the currently identified HPVs infect cutaneous epithelial surfaces, whereas the remainder preferentially target the mucosal epithelium of the anogenital tract.[2] The life cycle of PV is strictly linked to differentiation of the keratinocyte, the host cell for infection.[3] Investigations of the productive PV life cycle have been hindered by the requirement for differentiation and the lack of complete keratinocyte differentiation in cell culture in the absence of special manipulation. Fortunately, several in vivo and in vitro systems are now available that facilitate investigation of the entire virus life cycle.

Successful HPV infection requires access to actively dividing basal epithelial cells and is likely facilitated by epithelial microabrasions.

Current knowledge suggests that PV virions are shed from infected epithelial surfaces within the nuclei of highly keratinized, metabolically inert squames. Access to actively dividing basal epithelial cells is required for successful PV infection and is likely facilitated by epithelial microabrasions (Fig. 2–1).[4] Fibrinolysis, which occurs routinely during wound healing, may facilitate dissolution of the infected squame with subsequent deposition of free virus at the basal cell layer.[5]

It is postulated that PV enters target cells through one or more cell surface receptors.

The mechanism by which PVs enter target cells is largely unknown. Several studies have provided evidence for the presence of one or more PV cell surface receptors.[6] The α_6 integrin subunit[7] and heparan sulfate[8] are two cell surface molecules that may facilitate PV binding to host cells. Replication of PVs occurs entirely within the host cell nucleus. On viral entry to basal keratinocytes, expression of early viral genes is initiated. The host cell DNA replication machinery, in conjunction with the viral E1 and E2 proteins, then facilitates replication of the episomal viral genome to a low copy number (20 to 100 copies per cell). On mitotic division of the infected basal cell, approximately half the viral DNA episomes are par-

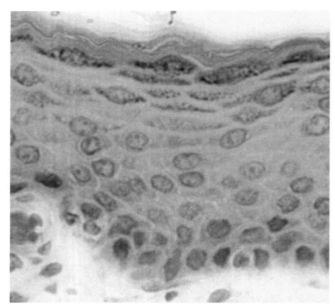

Epithelial Differentiation		
Cornified Layer	• Keratin cross-linking • Metabolically inert squames	• Virion assembly in nucleus • Release of infected squames
Granular Layer	• Keratohyalin granule formation • Reduced cell metabolism • Nuclear breakdown	• Expression of capsid proteins • PV DNA amplification
Spinous Layer	• Initiation of differentiation • High molecular weight keratin synthesis • Increased cell size	• PV DNA maintenance • Production of early proteins
Basal Layer	• Cell division & proliferation • Active cell DNA replication	• Low-copy PV DNA replication • Early gene expression

Figure 2–1. Stages of normal epithelial differentiation and papillomavirus infection. This photomicrograph shows a normal foreskin epithelium that has been stained with hematoxylin and eosin, demonstrating the multiple layers of differentiated epithelium. The biochemical and morphologic events that accompany differentiation are noted for each epithelial layer. In addition, events associated with papillomavirus infection are elucidated according to spatial localization.

titioned to the daughter cell that subsequently progresses to the spinous layer and begins to differentiate (see Fig. 2–1). The remaining genomes persist within the infected basal stem cell.

As differentiation continues, the episomal PV genome is further amplified to a high copy number (200 to 1000 copies per cell) in preparation for production of progeny virions.[9] Late viral gene transcription begins in the more differentiated suprabasal epithelial layers.[10] Viral capsid proteins, L1 and L2, are then produced and facilitate packaging of viral genomes. Ultimately, cornified virus-containing squames are formed.[11]

Benign HPV-induced lesions can progress to carcinoma, often coincident with integration of the PV genome into host DNA.

PV infections do not always result in the production of progeny virions. In some instances, HPV DNA, but not HPV RNA, can be detected, representing a state of apparent clinical latency. It is common, especially in some tissue types, such as genital epithelium, to find HPV DNA in the absence of infectious virus or histopathology.[12] Reactivation of these latent infections with subsequent virus production can occur. Mechanisms of HPV latency and reactivation are poorly understood. Benign HPV-induced lesions can progress to carcinoma, often coincident with integration of the PV genome into host DNA.

VIRION STRUCTURE

PVs are small, nonenveloped, icosahedral DNA viruses.

The PV genome is encapsulated in a proteinaceous capsid composed of L1 and L2, the major and minor structural proteins that are encoded by the late viral genes.

PVs are small, nonenveloped, icosahedral DNA viruses. Each virion is approximately 52 to 55 nm in diameter and contains a single copy of the double-stranded, circular, covalently closed viral DNA. The PV genome is 7200 to 8000 base pairs (bp) in size and is encapsulated in a spherical, 2-nm–thick proteinaceous capsid.

The PV capsid is composed of L1 and L2, the major and minor structural proteins, respectively, that are encoded by the late viral genes.[13] Because L2 is present in small quantities, it is believed that most of the PV capsid's pentameric capsomers contain five L1 molecules. The exact location of L2 within the virus capsid remains unclear. L2 expression is apparently not required for virus assembly because synthetically expressed L1 monomers spontaneously assemble into virus-like particles (VLPs) that are morphologically similar to authentic virions by electron microscopy.[14] However, coexpression of L2 increases the yield and stability of VLPs[15] and is required for efficient packaging of DNA.[16] Because the capsid is nonenveloped, PV virions are resistant to desiccation. PV stability may also be enhanced by the protection of virions within the nuclei of shed squames.

GENOME ORGANIZATION

One strand of PV DNA contains all the open reading frames or gene-encoding segments for all viral proteins.

Figure 2-2. Organization of the HPV 16 genome. The genome of HPV 16 consists of 7905 base pairs of circular, covalently closed, double-stranded DNA shown here in linearized form. The six early (E) and two late (L) open reading frames (ORFs) are depicted and are categorized by translational reading frame. The biologic functions associated with the products of the HPV 16 genes are also delineated. The upstream regulatory region (URR) is located between the L1 and E6 ORFs. Although the URR does not contain any ORFs, the promoter and enhancer elements found within the URR regulate the expression of all HPV genes. HPV, human papillomavirus.

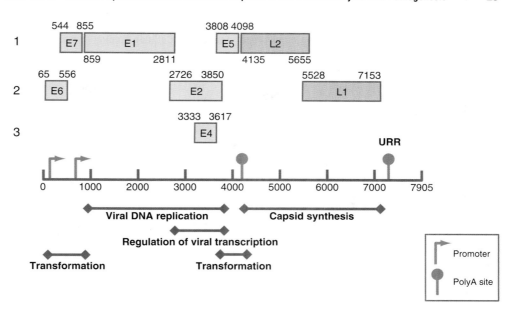

All PV genomes share a common pattern of organization (Fig. 2–2). One strand of the PV DNA contains all the open reading frames (ORFs) or gene-encoding segments (8 for HPV 16, 9 for HPV 11, and 10 for BPV 1).[17, 18] Through complex patterns of gene splicing, these ORFs encode all viral proteins. The early (E) region of the genome is transcribed before, as well as during, viral DNA synthesis. This region was originally identified as the specific fragment of the BPV1 genome sufficient for cellular transformation, and the analogous region in all PV genomes was subsequently termed the *early region*. The early gene products are detectable within proliferative areas of most HPV lesions.[19] The late (L) region of the genome contains the L1 and L2 ORFs, which, unlike the early genes, are expressed only in productive viral infections where their gene products are restricted to suprabasal differentiating epithelial cells. Overall, the size and location of most ORFs, as well as the functions of the viral proteins (Table 2–1), are conserved among PVs.[20]

The PV genome is divided into early (E) and late (L) regions corresponding to before and after DNA synthesis, respectively.

The L1 and E6 ORFs are separated by a 400- to 1000-bp region of DNA that does not encode any viral proteins but does contain the origin (ori) of viral DNA replication and many *cis*-acting promoter and enhancer elements (Fig. 2–3).[18] Binding of these sites by various cellular and viral proteins modulates viral transcription and DNA replication. This regulatory region has been called the noncoding region, the long control region, and the upstream regulatory region (URR). Numerous cellular factors positively or negatively influence HPV transcription by binding to the URR (see Fig. 2–3).[21] Viral gene expression is also regulated by posttranscriptional mechanisms such as alternative messenger RNA splicing,[22] variations in polyadenylation site usage,[23] and changes in messenger RNA stability.[24]

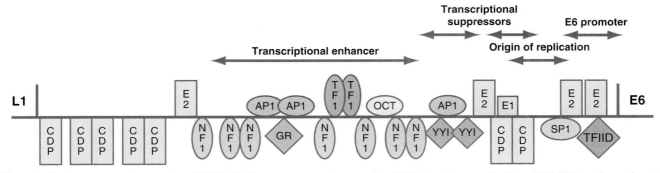

Figure 2-3. Upstream regulatory region of HPV 16. The upstream regulatory region (URR) lies between the L1 and E6 ORFs and contains *cis*-responsive enhancer elements to which numerous cellular proteins bind. The viral E1 and E2 proteins also bind to specific sequences within the URR. The binding of both cellular and viral proteins to the URR modulates the level of viral transcriptional activity. The URR also contains origin of replication sequences, which drive viral DNA replication. AP1, activator protein 1; CDP, CCAAT displacement protein; GR, glucocorticoid receptor; NF1, nuclear factor 1; OCT, octamer binding factor 1; ORF, open reading frame; TF1, transcription enhancer factor 1; TFIID, transcription factor IID; YY1, yin yang 1.

▼ Table 2-1

Viral Gene Products, Associated Biologic Functions, and Known Cellular Binding Partners

Viral Protein	Biologic Function	Interacting Cellular Molecules
E1	Initiates viral DNA replication Maintains episomal DNA copy number Regulates viral transcription Regulates viral transformation	Cyclin E DNA polymerase α/primase (p180, p70 subunits) Hsp40 chaperone protein hUBC9 Replication protein A (RPA70 subunit) 16E1-binding protein (16E1BP)
E2	Major viral transcription regulator Regulates viral DNA replication Activates and represses viral transcription Regulates viral transformation	Activation domain modulating factor (AMF-1) Replication protein A (RPA) Sp1 TATA box-binding protein (TBP) Transcription factor IIB (TFIIB)
E1^E4	May facilitate virion release	Cytokeratins
E5	Minor transforming oncoprotein Enhances mitogenic signaling pathways	Epidermal growth factor receptor (EGFR) Platelet-derived growth factor β receptor (PDGFβR) p125/α-adaptin 16-kD vacuolar H^+-ATPase subunit (16K)
E6	Major transforming oncoprotein Binds p53 and induces p53 degradation Alters cell cycle progression and genomic stability	p53 Bak CBP/p300 E6-associated protein (E6AP) E6-binding protein (E6BP) E6-targeted protein 1 (E6TP1) Multicopy maintenance protein 7 (mcm7) Paxillin TATA box-binding protein (TBP)
E7	Major transforming oncoprotein Sequesters pRb/p107 and releases E2F Alters cell cycle progression	Retinoblastoma family members (pRb, p107, p130) AP1 family members (c-jun, junB, junD, c-fos) cdk inhibitors (p21/Cip1, p27/Kip1) Cyclin A TATA box-binding protein (TBP)
L1	Major structural protein of virus capsid Essential for capsid formation and stability Facilitates initial binding to host cell surface May facilitate viral DNA entry to nucleus	α_6 integrin subunit Heparan sulfate Karyopherin $\alpha_2\beta_1$
L2	Minor structural protein of virus capsid Facilitates packaging of DNA to virions and VLPs	

AP, activator protein; ATPase, adenosine triphosphatase; cdk, cyclin-dependent kinase; E, early; L, late; pRb, retinoblastoma tumor suppressor protein; VLP, virus-like particle.

Classification or typing of HPVs is based on the degree of similarity present in select regions of the genome.

Significant genomic diversity exists among HPV types. Classification, or typing, of HPVs is based on the degree of similarity present in select regions of the genome. The first HPV typing scheme was based on the degree of overall nucleotide homology, as determined by liquid hybridization. HPV typing was then based on DNA sequence homology within the E6, E7, and L1 ORFs. Most recently, however, typing strategies have focused on sequence homology exclusively within the L1 gene, the most highly conserved HPV ORF.[25] HPV classification now requires that a novel virus type share less than 90%

DNA sequence homology in the L1 gene with existing types. Subtypes exhibit 90% to 98% sequence homology, whereas variants demonstrate more than 98% homology with currently catalogued HPV types.

VIRAL ATTACHMENT AND ENTRY

Productive PV infection occurs only in stratified squamous epithelial cells, and initial binding and attachment of virus to target cells require the L1 protein.

PVs bind to a wide variety of cell types from multiple species in a dose-dependent fashion. Internalization of PV virions also occurs in several cell types.[26] However, productive PV infection occurs only in stratified squamous epithelial tissue.[11] Initial binding and attachment of virus to the surface of target host cells require the L1 protein but do not appear to involve L2.[27]

PV binding to epithelial and other cell lines is specific and saturable.[27] Although pretreatment of target cells with trypsin significantly reduces the binding of PV capsids, pretreatment of cells with sialidase, N-glycosidase, or octyl-β-D-glycopyranoside has no effect on binding, suggesting that a cell surface protein mediates PV attachment.[28] Because HPV 16 VLPs competitively inhibit BPV1 binding and transformation of C127 cells,[6] the putative receptor may be used by different PVs. Virus entry into cells is believed to occur by endocytosis, and uptake of HPV 33 VLPs into smooth endocytic vesicles has been documented by immunoelectron microscopy.

Successful PV infection requires the import of the virus genome to the nucleus and the partial uncoating of the viral capsid.

Little is known about the intracellular events that immediately follow virus entry. Successful infection does, however, require import of the virus genome to the nucleus. As with other DNA viruses, nuclear import of the PV genome likely requires partial uncoating of the virus capsid. Intact L1 VLP capsids are unable to enter the nucleus.[2] Some neutralizing L1 antibodies do not block virus binding but still prevent infection; such antibodies may cross-link L1 capsomers and thereby prohibit viral uncoating.[29] How uncoated viral DNA accesses the host cell nucleus is presently unknown.

EARLY GENE EXPRESSION

The use of multiple promoters, alternative splicing, and differentiation-linked regulation of transcription complicates PV gene expression. Following successful entry, cellular factors bind to the URR and initiate transcription from the major early promoter located at the 5′ end of the E6 ORF.[10] Early transcripts that code for E6, E7, E1, E2, and E5 are polycistronic and terminate at a series of polyadenylation sites between the E5 and L2 ORFs.[30] Translation of internal ORFs within polycistronic transcripts appears to occur by reinitiation of translation rather than through internal ribosomal entry sites.

E6 and E7 are detected at low levels in basal cells and facilitate viral DNA replication by maintaining cell cycle progression.

E6 and E7 can be detected at low levels in basal cells and facilitate viral DNA replication by maintaining cell cycle progression.[21] The early viral genes encoding E1 and E2 are the next to be expressed. In HPV infections, the E2 protein then binds to multiple E2-binding sites (E2BSs) within the URR and blocks early gene transcription. At the same time, E2 facilitates specific binding of the E1 protein to the ori within the URR, which initiates

replication of the viral DNA genome. Early gene transcription increases with progression of cells to the intermediate epithelial layers concomitant with the onset of vegetative viral DNA replication. At this point in the infected epithelium, the most abundant viral transcript is the bicistronic E1^E4 messenger RNA initiated from a differentiation-dependent promoter within the E7 ORF.[31] Owing to its accumulation in the terminally differentiated layers of an infected epithelium, E1^E4 has been classified as a "late" viral product.

E1: The Replication Initiation Protein

The E1 ORF is a large and relatively conserved early gene that has an essential role in viral DNA replication and transcription.

The E1 ORF is a large and relatively conserved early gene. Full-length BPV1 E1 is expressed as a 68- to 72-kD nuclear phosphoprotein and exhibits structural similarity to SV40 T antigen. E1 contains a bipartite nuclear localization signal[32] and multiple phosphorylation sites.[33] The E1 protein binds specifically, yet weakly, to the relatively conserved E1-binding site (E1BS) within the ori[34] and significantly changes the conformation of the DNA.[35] In cell-free replication assays, high concentrations of BPV1 E1 alone support ori-independent DNA replication, likely owing to E1's strong and nonspecific affinity for DNA.[36] However, binding of E1 by E2 enhances the binding affinity of E1 for ori-containing DNA sequences and promotes ori-specific DNA replication.[37]

In addition to its essential role in viral DNA replication, E1 also regulates viral transcription. Demeret and colleagues[38] demonstrated that HPV 18 E1 activates transcription in the presence of the DNA-binding domain (DBD) of E2; therefore, like full-length E2, E1 may have intrinsic transactivation activity.

E2 Proteins: Modulation of Viral DNA Replication and Transcription

The E2 proteins are site-specific DNA-binding proteins that play important roles in viral DNA replication and transcription.

Owing to the use of multiple promoters and alternative messenger RNA splicing, BPV1 produces three E2 proteins: the full-length 48-kD E2TA, the 31-kD E2-TR, and the 28-kD E8/E2 fusion protein. Similarly, HPV 11 expresses full-length 40-kD E2, truncated E2C, and spliced E1M^E2C. In BPV1-transformed C127 cells, E2TA, E2-TR, and E8/E2 are present in a ratio of 1:10:3[39]; however, the relative abundance of E2 proteins does change with the cell cycle.[40] For all PVs, the full-length E2 protein consists of three structural and functional domains. The N-terminal transactivation domain (TAD), approximately 200 amino acids (aa) in length, is very highly conserved among PV types and accounts for E2's ability to transactivate transcription. The central region of full-length E2, known as the hinge region, exhibits flexible secondary structure as well as significant variability in length and sequence among PV types.[41] The C-terminus of the E2 protein consists of a DBD that also facilitates E2 protein homodimer and heterodimer formation.[42] All the PV E2 products possess the C-terminal DBD and the central hinge region but have different N-termini; E2C lacks the TAD completely.

The E2 proteins are site-specific DNA-binding proteins that play important roles in both viral DNA replication and transcription. E2 binds as a dimer to the palindromic consensus sequence, $ACCN_6GGT$, present multiple times throughout the URR.[43] Among genital HPV types, there are four highly conserved E2BSs upstream of the major early promoter, P_{97}, which flank a solitary and less conserved E1BS (Fig. 2–3); the distribution and location of these E2BSs are highly conserved.[44] E2 plays an important role in the initiation of ori-dependent DNA replication.[45] In fact, BPV1 DNA replication in vitro requires the presence of full-length E2 and at least one E2BS.[46] E2 directly binds to E1[47] and involves aa 18 to aa 41 of HPV 16 E2.[48]

The various forms of E2 affect transcription differently and may act as either activators or repressors.

The E2 proteins are important regulators of viral transcription. However, the various forms of E2 affect transcription differently, as either activators or repressors. Generally, full-length E2 activates viral transcription, whereas the truncated E2 proteins, which lack intact TADs, repress transcription. The relative abundance of the various forms of E2 and the context of bound E2BSs within the genome also affect the transcriptional activity of the PV genome. The full-length E2 proteins of mucosal HPVs, including HPV 11, HPV 16, and HPV 18, repress transcription from the major early, or E6, promoter.[49, 50] Variation in transcriptional activation by E2 also exists among HPV types, because the E2 proteins of oncogenic HPV types activate E2-responsive promoters more efficiently than do nononcogenic HPV type E2 proteins.[51]

It is widely believed that HPV E2 regulates cell growth indirectly by downregulating the expression of the E6 and E7 oncogenes from the major early promoter.

It is widely believed that HPV E2 regulates cell growth indirectly by downregulating the expression of the E6 and E7 oncogenes from the major early promoter. Exogenous expression of BPV1 E2TA suppresses growth and induces apoptosis of HPV 18–positive HeLa cells.[52, 53] BPV1 E2TA expression also inhibits growth of the HPV-negative cervical cancer cell line, HT-3, which must be independent of E6/E7 activity.[54] Overexpression of HPV 31 E2 in primary human keratinocytes induces S-phase cell cycle arrest followed by multiple rounds of DNA replication without mitotic division.[55] Therefore, E2 may play an important role in vegetative viral DNA amplification by altering cell cycle progression.

VIRAL GENOME REPLICATION

Following initial expression of E1 and E2 within the infected basal keratinocytes, the episomal genome is replicated to a low copy number by the cellular DNA replication machinery.

Following initial expression of E1 and E2 within infected basal keratinocytes, the episomal genome is replicated to a low copy number by the cellular DNA replication machinery. In vitro studies of stable episomal BPV1 genomes in transformed cells indicate that nonvegetative episomal viral DNA replication occurs in two phases, an establishment phase during which the viral genome is amplified from a low to a moderate copy number and a maintenance phase characterized by a constant episome copy number.[56]

Some viral episomes may replicate more than once, but overall the total number of genomes per cell in undifferentiated cells remains relatively constant.

The mechanism by which viral genome copy number is regulated is currently unknown. Replicated virus episomes were originally thought to be "marked" so as to prevent their re-entry into the replication pool. Evidence indicates that marking does not occur but that replication occurs on average once per genome per cell cycle; some virus episomes may replicate more than once, but overall the total number of genomes per cell remains relatively constant.[57]

A second and more robust phase of genome replication, termed *vegetative amplification,* occurs in the upper strata of differentiated epithelia and results in a high number of episomal genomes per cell.[11] The exact mechanism by which the infected host cell is triggered to switch from plasmid maintenance to vegetative DNA amplification is unclear. Because vegetative DNA amplification occurs only in terminally differentiating cells, induction of vegetative amplification may depend on the controlled and differentiation-dependent expression of cellular factors.

The exact mechanism by which the infected host cell is triggered to switch from plasmid maintenance to DNA amplification is unclear.

Although it is clear that PV DNA replication occurs in the nucleus, little is known about the mechanism and order of assembly of the necessary viral and cellular factors. Viral DNA replication is dependent on the specific binding of E1 and E2 to viral DNA sequences within the URR.[58] Efficient PV DNA replication also requires a myriad of host cell factors including DNA polymerases α/primase and δ, replication protein A, topoisomerases I and II, replication factor C, and proliferating-cell nuclear antigen.[59]

LATE GENE EXPRESSION

The signal for transition from the latent phase to the productive phase of PV infection is poorly understood. However, differentiation-dependent signals are crucial for the increased expression of the late gene products L1 and L2. Polycistronic transcripts coding for L1 and L2 are limited to the terminally differentiated epithelial layers in HPV 31–positive organotypic raft cultures.[60] L1 and/or L2, as well as E1^E4 and E5, are expressed from the bicistronic E1^E4, L1 and polycistronic E1^E4, E5, L2, L1 transcripts.[61, 62] These late messenger RNAs are transcribed from a differentiation-dependent promoter located within the E7 ORF.[31] Late gene transcription is regulated by putative differentiation-specific transcriptional enhancers, inhibitory late gene DNA sequences, and transcriptional repressor proteins.[63] However, the presence of L1/L2–containing transcripts in the absence of L1 and/or L2 protein suggests that posttranscriptional mechanisms also play a crucial role in spatially restricting late protein expression.[64]

L1 and L2: Structural Viral Proteins

Although late protein expression is confined to terminally differentiated keratinocytes, transcripts coding for L1 and L2 are found more widely throughout the strata of an infected epithelium. Although mucosal HPVs, such as HPV 6 and HPV 11, produce only a bicistronic messenger RNA (the E1^E4, L1 transcript) that codes for L1, the cutaneous HPVs (e.g., HPV 1, 2, 4) and BPV1 produce this bicistronic transcript as well as a monocistronic L1-encoding messenger RNA.[65] The L1 gene product is highly conserved among PVs, whereas L2 is less well conserved. Despite some variation between PVs and HPV types, the molecular weights of L1 and L2 are approximately 55 to 60 kD and 70 to 75 kD, respectively, as determined by sodium dodecyl sulfate–polyacrylamide gel electrophoresis (SDS-PAGE) analysis.[66, 67]

E1^E4: An Abundant Yet Enigmatic Viral Product

> **Closely related HPV types exhibit significant E1^E4 aa sequence homology and conserved physical traits in the protein.**

E4 is the most divergent ORF among HPV types, and the E1^E4 protein shows little conservation among HPV types. However, closely related HPV types (e.g., HPV 1, 2, 4) exhibit significant aa sequence homology and conserved physical traits.[68] Although the E4 ORF does contain a translation initiation codon in some, but not all, HPV genomes, a product derived solely from the E4 ORF has not been detected. E1^E4 is the most abundant product of both viral transcription, which constitutes approxi-

mately 90% of virus transcripts within genital condylomata, and viral translation.[65, 69]

> **E1^E4 is the most abundant product of both viral transcription, which constitutes approximately 90% of viral transcripts within genital condylomata, and viral translation.**

E1^E4 messenger RNA is initially detected in the parabasal layer but is expressed throughout the infected epithelium.[70] The E1^E4 protein is primarily encoded by two transcripts, the E1^E4, E5 and the E1^E4, L1 messenger RNAs.[61, 71] In experimental HPV 11–induced papillomas, the E1^E4 protein is detected as a 10-kD/11-kD doublet and represents approximately 8% of the total extractable protein within shed epithelial cells.[72] Although the total amount of E1^E4 protein within lesions varies among HPV types, E1^E4 may constitute up to 20% of total protein in naturally occurring HPV 1–induced warts. Because E1^E4 is produced in large quantities in productive infections, it has been suggested that the level of E1^E4 expression may correlate with the level of virion production.[73] However, E1^E4 is not found in progeny virions. Owing to its abundance in terminally differentiated layers of the infected epithelium, as well as to its cellular colocalization with L1, E1^E4 may be involved in virus maturation as a scaffold or transport protein.[74]

> **Sustained expression of HPV 16 E1^E4 specifically induces collapse of the cytokeratin network in cultured cells, potentially weakening cell-cell junctions.**

When expressed in cell culture systems, the E1^E4 protein of some HPVs (e.g., HPV 1, 16, 31b) displays a filamentous distribution within the cell cytoplasm that colocalizes with cytokeratin intermediate filaments.[64] Sustained expression of HPV 16 E1^E4 specifically induces collapse of the cytokeratin network.[75] By collapsing the cytokeratin network, and potentially weakening cell-cell junctions, E1^E4 may augment virus release during surface shedding of these more fragile squames.[75] It should be noted, however, that association of E1^E4 with cytokeratins has not been detected in naturally occurring HPV lesions.[76]

VIRION MORPHOGENESIS

The processes of genome packaging and virion assembly are still poorly understood. In addition, little is known about the conformational structures of the L1 and L2 proteins. However, evidence indicates that disulfide bonds between L1 molecules are important for capsid assembly and stability.[14] Prolonged incubation with reducing agents such as β-mercaptoethanol or dithiothreitol is sufficient and necessary for disassembly of HPV L1 VLPs or native HPV 1 virions to capsomers.[77] Reduction of intercapsomeric disulfide bonds abrogates the formation of L1 trimers that are essential for capsid assembly. Data suggest that the reducing environment of the host cell cytoplasm, in the context of physiologic ionic strength, may facilitate capsid disassembly and genome uncoating. Concomitantly, locally elevated ionic strength, owing to the presence of viral and cellular DNA, may facilitate capsid formation within infected cell nuclei.[77] Intercapsomeric disulfide bonds may form within the nucleus and/or upon virion release. Although not required for empty VLP assembly, L2 is required for encapsidation of the viral genome.[16]

MODEL SYSTEMS TO STUDY THE PATHOGENESIS OF PV

Human Tissue Xenografts

> Attempts to induce full, vegetative PV replication in traditional culture systems have been hindered by the strict requirement for differentiated tissue and the extreme host specificity of PVs.

For more than 50 years, attempts to induce full, vegetative PV replication in traditional culture systems have been hindered by the strict requirement for differentiated tissue and extreme host specificity of PVs. HPVs target human epithelium exclusively, and subsets of HPVs show specificity for epithelia of designated anatomic sites. For example, genital HPVs are restricted, with few exceptions, to growth in genital targets. Presumably, this high level of specificity is controlled by host cell factors present in permissive target cells. A review of the targets of individual HPV types can be found in the work of de Villiers.[78]

Original evidence that HPVs cause skin warts was obtained in human volunteers, an approach now considered unethical. Furthermore, the host restriction of HPVs precludes development of an animal model. The development of immunocompromised animals, however, has allowed extension of classic skin grafting and immunotransfer approaches to "xenografting" of a variety of tissues across species barriers. Xenografts have been routinely established in both athymic[79] and severe combined immunodeficient (SCID)[80] mice. These animals exhibit deficiencies of immune system components, most notably of the T cell lineage, that prevent rejection of grafted heterologous tissues. In the in vivo xenograft setting, a variety of growth factors are present, and angiogenesis establishes a blood supply to the tissue. A major advantage is that tissues grow in a fully differentiated, in vivo condition, allowing study of normal physiologic and biochemical tissue processes. Xenografted human tissues differentiate completely and allow recapitulation of the natural history of fastidious human pathogens. A wide variety of human tissues, both normal and neoplastic, have been successfully transplanted and maintained as xenografts over the life span of the host mouse.

> Xenografted human tissues offer a fully competent, susceptible target for HPV. Xenografts produce abundant virus. HPV-transformed grafts exhibit mild to moderate dysplasia.

Xenografted human tissues offer a fully competent, susceptible target for HPVs (Fig. 2–4). HPV-transformed grafts exhibit mild to moderate dysplasia. HPV 11 induces papillomas that show hyperproliferation of the epithelium and that closely resemble condylomata acuminata, characterized by koilocytosis, nuclear hyperchromasia, and binucleation. To date, five HPVs and several animal

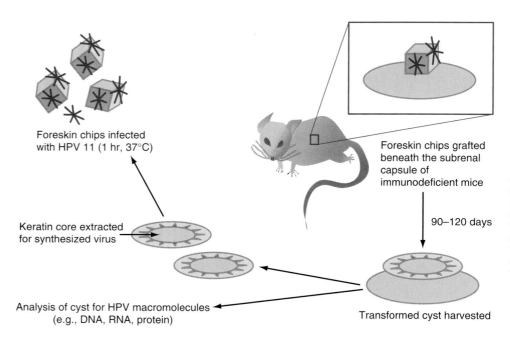

Foreskin chips infected with HPV 11 (1 hr, 37°C)

Keratin core extracted for synthesized virus

Analysis of cyst for HPV macromolecules (e.g., DNA, RNA, protein)

Foreskin chips grafted beneath the subrenal capsule of immunodeficient mice

90–120 days

Transformed cyst harvested

Figure 2–4. Schematic diagram of the human tissue xenograft system. Chips of human tissues, which have included foreskin, vagina, cervix and others, are infected in vitro with infectious stocks of PVs (e.g., HPV 11). The infected tissue chips are then transplanted to the subrenal capsule of immunocompromised mice. Following prolonged in vivo incubation, the tissue is morphologically transformed into a papillomatous cyst that contains PV macromolecules (i.e., DNA and RNA) as well as progeny virions. HPV, human papillomavirus; PV, papillomavirus.

▼ Table 2–2
Viruses Successfully Propagated Using the Xenograft System

Papillomaviruses
BPV1
BPV4
CRPV
HPV 1
HPV 2
HPV 11
HPV 40
LVX82/MM7
Poxviruses
Molluscum contagiosum
Herpesviruses
Herpes simplex virus 2
Varicella-zoster virus
Others
Vaccinia virus
Norwalk virus

BPV, bovine papillomavirus, CRPV, cottontail rabbit papillomavirus; HPV, human papillomavirus.

PVs have been successfully grown in xenografts (Table 2–2).

Keratinocyte Cell Culture Models

> **Parallel to the growth of PVs in xenografts, there have been remarkable advances in the ability to grow differentiated keratinocytes in culture.**

Parallel to the growth of PVs in xenografts, there have been remarkable advances in the ability to grow differentiated keratinocytes in culture. Cell culture medium has been adapted to favor keratinocyte differentiation. Specialized culture protocols, namely the organotypic raft culture system, have also been developed, in which epithelial cells are grown on top of a dermal equivalent, composed of fibroblasts in a collagen matrix, and then raised to the air-liquid interface to simulate the in vivo growth environment.

Meyers and colleagues[3] have used the low-grade cervical intraepithelial neoplasia–derived cell line, CIN-612,[81] to demonstrate complete HPV 31b vegetative replication in raft cultures. In raft cultures, full induction of virus production requires induction of epithelial differentiation by chronic and intermittent addition of 12-O-tetradecanoyl phorbol-13 acetate, a known activator of protein kinase C (PKC), to the medium. The molecular link between PKC activation and virion morphogenesis is not yet fully understood. The organotypic culture system has been used to study the natural history of HPV 31b infection, and a large number of virus-specific transcripts and regulatory regions have been mapped using this approach.[82] Additionally, HPV 18[83] and other HPV types have been grown using the organotypic raft culture system.

ASSOCIATION OF HPV WITH CANCER

Estimates indicate that up to 15% to 20% of all human cancers may be attributed to HPV infection. Dysplasia and squamous carcinoma of the cervix are unequivocally the most common forms of neoplastic disease associated with HPV infection. HPV DNA can be detected in more than 95% of cervical cancers worldwide. As a result, HPV types have been categorized according to their association with neoplastic progression.[84] "Low-risk" types, for which the genital types HPV 6 and HPV 11 serve as prototypes, typically produce benign hyperproliferative lesions that have a very low, yet detectable, frequency for progression to invasive cancer.[85] "High-risk" types, on the other hand, are associated with a significant tendency for lesion progression to cancer and include HPV types 16, 18, 31, 33, 35, and 45.[84]

> **HPV 16 is consistently the most frequent type associated with cervical cancer, accounting for approximately 50% to 60% of all HPV-positive cases.**

Altogether, high-risk types account for more than 90% of all HPV sequences detected in invasive cervical cancers.[86, 87] HPV 16 is consistently the most frequent type associated with cervical cancer, accounting for approximately 50% to 60% of all HPV-positive cases; HPV 18 DNA is detected in 10% to 20% of such cancers.[86, 87] Overall, however, there is a strong tendency for spontaneous regression of HPV-induced preinvasive cervical intraepithelial neoplasia even in the presence of high-risk HPV DNA. This is especially true in young women. Therefore, secondary cofactors, such as smoking, oral contraceptive use, HLA type, and immune status, contribute significantly to cervical carcinogenesis.[10] Chapter 1 addresses the association of HPV with cancer as well as the presence of specific HPV types in preneoplastic and neoplastic lesions.

CELLULAR TRANSFORMATION BY PVs

> **In HPV-induced condylomata and mild and moderate dysplasias, the HPV genome is generally episomal, whereas in highly dysplastic or cancerous HPV-positive lesions, the HPV DNA is frequently integrated into the host cell DNA.**

In HPV-induced condylomata, papillomas, and mild to moderate dysplasias, the HPV genome is generally episomal.[88] However, in highly dysplastic and cancerous HPV-positive lesions, the HPV DNA is frequently integrated into the host cell DNA.[89] Integration, however, is not advantageous for new virus production. Integration of HPV DNA necessarily disrupts one or more HPV genes and frequently occurs in the E1 and/or E2 ORFs, thereby abrogating expression of these proteins. Loss of E1 and E2 prevents replication of viral DNA and leads to dysregulated expression of other viral genes. E6 and E7 are transcribed predominantly from the major early promoter, the basal activity of which is repressed by E2, and loss of E2 results in uncontrolled, elevated expression of E6 and

E7. HPV-positive cervical cancers and tumor-derived cell lines continue to express E6 and E7, suggesting that these viral products are required for continued cell growth[90, 91] and maintenance of the transformed phenotype.[92]

> **Integration of HPV DNA disrupts one or more HPV genes and frequently occurs in the E1 or E2 ORFs, thereby abrogating expression of these proteins.**

> **Loss of E2 results in uncontrolled, elevated expression of E6 and E7. Cervical cancers continue to express E6 and E7, suggesting that these viral products are required for continued cell growth and maintenance of the transformed phenotype.**

The E6 and E7 proteins are relatively well conserved among HPV types and dramatically affect cell proliferation and genome stability through their effects on cellular molecules involved in cell cycle progression and apoptosis (Fig. 2–5). In vitro, E6 and E7 abrogate cell cycle checkpoints by binding cyclin/cyclin-dependent kinase (cdk) complexes and other regulatory proteins; not surprisingly, high-risk oncoproteins more effectively dysregulate the cell cycle than do low-risk E6 and E7.[87] In productive infections, E6/E7–induced cell cycle progression facilitates viral DNA replication in cells that have withdrawn from the cell cycle and would otherwise lack DNA replication capabilities.

In vivo effects of E6 and E7 have been examined using transgenic mouse models. Under the control of the human keratin 14 promoter, which targets transgene expression to basal epithelial cells, simultaneous expression of HPV 16 E6 and E7 in transgenic mice results in hyperplasia, papillomatosis, and dysplasia at epidermal and squamous mucosal tissues.[93] Data suggest that HPV 16 E7 predominantly induces benign tumor formation, whereas HPV 16 E6 dramatically enhances malignant progression of preexisting benign tumors.

> **It is suggested that HPV 16 E7 predominantly induces benign tumor formation, whereas HPV 16 E6 dramatically enhances malignant progression of preexisting benign tumors.**

E6: Degradation of p53

Full-length HPV E6 is approximately 150 aa in length. The E6 protein is highly variable but does contain several conserved motifs. Four highly conserved cysteine-containing motifs (CXXC) form two zinc-finger domains, characteristic of some transcriptional transactivator proteins. These zinc-finger domains enable HPV 16 and 18 E6 to bind zinc,[94, 95] and ablation of either renders E6 defective in transformation assays.[96] The E6 N-terminus is hydrophilic, whereas the central region separating the zinc-finger motifs is hydrophobic. E6 has a short C-terminus, which, for high-risk HPV E6 proteins, contains a PDZ

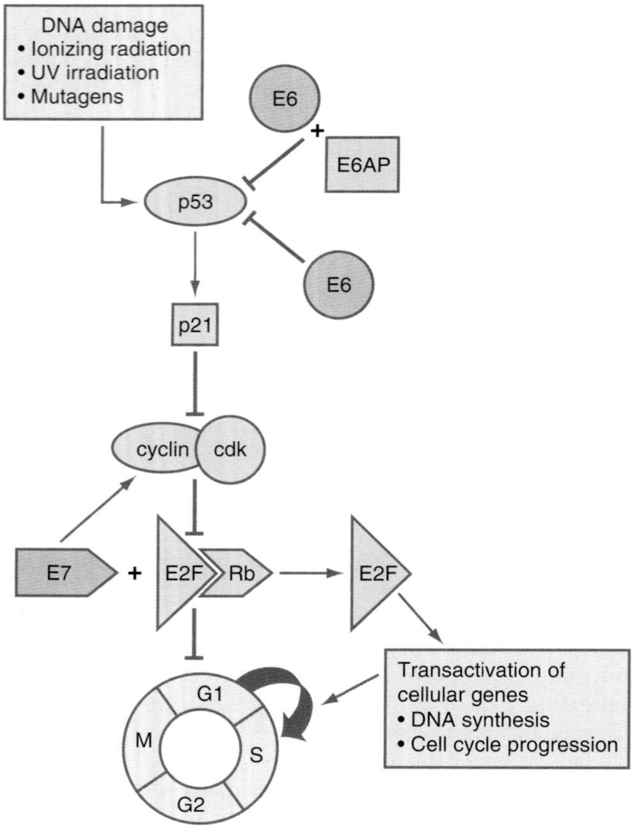

Figure 2–5. Alteration of the cell cycle by oncogenic E6 and E7. The normal cellular response to DNA-damaging agents includes activation of p53 and transcription of p53-responsive genes such as p21. p21 and other cyclin-dependent kinase (cdk) inhibitors block the activity of cyclin/cdk complexes and thereby prevent phosphorylation and inactivation of pRb. When active, pRb binds and sequesters the transcription factor E2F, preventing its ability to transactive cellular genes. High-risk E6 can bind to the C-terminus of p53 and prevent transactivation of p53-responsive genes. In combination with the cellular protein E6-associated protein (E6AP), E6 can also bind and target p53 for ubiquitin-mediated degradation. High-risk E7 binds to pRb and results in the release of active E2F. E2F induces the transcription of cellular genes involved in DNA synthesis and cell cycle progression. E7 also upregulates the level of cyclins and cdks, which phosphorylate and inactivate pRb, thereby releasing E2F. Overall, oncogenic E6 and E7 promote cell cycle progression and prevent p53- and pRb-mediated apoptosis and growth arrest, respectively. pRb, retinoblastoma protein.

(*PSD-95, Discs—large, ZO-1*)-binding motif that mediates protein-protein interactions.[97] The E6 protein is both nuclear and cytoplasmic and is present at low levels in transformed cells.

The most well-characterized E6 binding partner is the tumor suppressor protein p53.

The most well-characterized E6 binding partner is the tumor suppressor protein p53. HPV 16 and 18 E6 have been shown to interact with p53 in vitro.[98] High-risk E6 proteins have a higher binding affinity for p53 than do low-risk E6 proteins. Low-risk and high-risk E6 proteins interact with the C-terminus of p53, but only high-risk E6 proteins also bind p53's core DBD.[99] Interaction of E6 with the p53 DBD requires prior binding of E6 to E6-associated protein and results in ubiquitin-mediated degradation of p53.[99] By inducing degradation of p53, E6 effectively abrogates p53-mediated growth arrest and apoptosis in response to DNA-damaging agents (see Fig. 2–5). HPV 16 or 18 E6 expression in transformed cells disrupts the G1 cell cycle checkpoint,[100] and HPV 16 E6 expression in human foreskin keratinocytes inhibits the mitotic spindle checkpoint, resulting in an abnormally high cellular DNA content.[101] Several mutant high-risk E6 proteins bind p53 without inducing its degradation.[102] These E6 mutants are still able to transform established murine cells[103] and immortalize human embryonic cells.[104] E6/p53 complex formation, even in the absence of p53 degradation, prevents binding of p53 to DNA and inhibits p53-mediated transcriptional repression and activation.[105]

Intratypic HPV diversity within the E6 ORF results in the expression of E6 variants with differing capacities for p53 degradation and cellular transformation.

The overall prevalence of HPV E6 variants varies by geographic location and demographic population. HPV 16 E6 variants may be more prevalent in cervical carcinomas than the HPV 16 E6 prototype.

Intratypic HPV diversity within the E6 ORF results in the expression of E6 variants with differing capacities for p53 degradation and cellular transformation.[106] The clinical implications of such variants may be significant. Zehbe and colleagues[107] have detected the HPV 16 E6 prototype in 44% of high-grade cervical intraepithelial neoplasias but in less than 10% of invasive cervical cancers, and HPV 16 E6 variants may be more prevalent in cervical carcinomas than the E6 prototype. The overall prevalence of HPV E6 variants varies by geographic location and demographic population. Polymorphisms of p53 also exist among populations, the two most common of which have either proline or arginine at residue 72 (denoted p53Arg and p53Pro).[108] Although p53Pro is a stronger transactivator, p53Arg more effectively induces apoptosis and prevents immortalization of primary rodent

cells.[109] p53Arg is also more susceptible to HPV 18 E6–mediated degradation in vivo and is successfully targeted for degradation by HPV 11 E6.[110] The difference in susceptibility of these two p53 forms to E6-mediated degradation is echoed in the frequency of these p53 variants in cervical cancer. In some, but not all, studies, p53Arg is more frequently detected in cervical lesions than is p53Pro.[111, 112] The E6 protein may have evolved to more efficiently degrade the p53 variant that more effectively induces apoptosis and therefore poses the greatest risk to virus-induced cell proliferation. E6 has been shown to bind other cellular proteins, including c-myc, multicopy maintenance protein 7, Bak, E6-targeted protein 1, E6-binding protein (also known as ERC55), paxillin, and the human homolog of *Drosophila* discs—large protein.

In addition to the full-length E6 protein, high-risk mucosal HPV types produce a series of alternatively spliced transcripts, denoted E6*, that lack the E6 C-terminal domain.[113] Although E6* transcripts are highly abundant, E6* proteins (denoted E6* I to IV) are barely detectable in vivo. HPV 16 E6* I fails to immortalize primary human keratinocytes in culture.[114] However, HPV 18 E6* I has been shown to interact in vitro with both E6 and E6AP, but not p53, and it effectively blocks the association of E6 with p53.[115] By preventing the E6-p53 interaction, E6* prevents E6-mediated degradation of p53, resulting in increased activity of p53-responsive promoters and decreased proliferation of cells that contain both E6 and p53.[115] The ability of E6* to bind E6 dictates these antiproliferative and proapoptotic effects.

E7: Abrogation of Cell Cycle Regulation

The E7 ORF produces a small, acidic protein, approximately 100 aa in length, that localizes to both the nucleus and the cytoplasm. The C-terminus of E7 contains two CXXC motifs that form a zinc-finger domain that has been shown to bind zinc.[94] Phosphorylation of HPV 16 E7 by casein kinase II (CK II) is required for efficient cellular transformation by E7 but is not necessary for binding of E7 to the retinoblastoma tumor suppressor protein (pRb). Low-risk E7 proteins are phosphorylated by CK II less efficiently than are those of high-risk HPVs.

Generally, E7 proteins of low-risk types (HPV types 6 and 11) have a lower binding affinity for pRb than do high-risk E7s (HPV types 16, 18, and 33).

HPV 16 E7 has been shown to bind pRb, p107, and p130.[116, 117] Generally, E7 proteins of low-risk types (HPV 6, 11) have a lower binding affinity for pRb, both in vitro and in vivo, compared with high-risk E7s (HPV 16, 18, 33). As a result, low-risk E7 proteins cooperate very poorly with the activated *ras* oncogene in transformation assays.[118] E7 competes directly with the cellular transcription factor, E2F, for binding to pRb, resulting in elevated levels of free, active E2F (see Fig. 2–5).[119] Release of E2F results in transactivation of cellular target genes involved in DNA synthesis induction (e.g., thymidine kinase, dihydrofolate reductase, DNA polymerase α)

and cell cycle progression (e.g., cyclin A, D, E).[120] Active E2F promotes the progression from G1 to S phase, thereby stimulating quiescent cells to replicate DNA and proliferate. Interaction between E7 and pRb may also induce degradation of pRb via the ubiquitin-proteasome pathway. Other binding targets of E7 include the cdk2-cyclin A/cyclin E complex, TATA box-binding protein, the activator protein 1 transcription factors, and the cdk inhibitors p21/Cip1 and p27/Kip1.

> **Although efficient immortalization of primary human keratinocytes requires HPV 16 E6 and HPV 16 E7, HPV 16 E7 alone can immortalize these cells when present in high concentrations.**

Although efficient immortalization of primary human keratinocytes requires both HPV 16 E6 and HPV 16 E7, HPV 16 E7 can immortalize these cells when present at high concentrations.[121] High-risk E7 expression abrogates negative growth regulatory signals that include p53-mediated G1 arrest, transforming growth factor–mediated growth inhibition, and differentiation-induced quiescence. By circumventing p53-mediated G1 arrest, HPV 16 E7 successfully uncouples cell proliferation and differentiation. When overexpressed in primary human foreskin keratinocytes, HPV 16 E7, but not HPV 6 E7, invokes widespread alterations in cell cycle protein levels.[122] E7 expression results in increased levels of cyclins (most notably cyclin E), cdks, and the cdk inhibitors p21/Cip1 and p19, with overall elevations in cdk activity. Duration of the G1 phase is shortened in E7-expressing keratinocytes owing to premature activation of cyclin E–associated kinase activity.

E5: A Minor HPV-Transforming Protein

> **Unlike E6 and E7, E5 appears to alter cell growth by stimulating cellular growth signal transduction pathways.**

Although the genes encoding E6 and E7 are the main transforming genes of HPV, the E5 protein of several HPV types induces anchorage-independent growth and focus formation, and E5-expressing cells are tumorigenic in nude mice. Unlike E6 and E7, E5 appears to alter cell growth by stimulating cellular growth signal transduction pathways. Because E5 is the primary transforming protein of BPV 1, significant data have been collected on its functional aspects. Researchers have begun to characterize HPV E5 proteins as well.

Mucosal HPV types possess one (denoted E5) or two (denoted E5a and E5b) E5 ORFs located downstream of the E2 ORF. Little is known about the nature and function of E5b. The *E5/E5a* genes encode small, highly hydrophobic, membrane-associated proteins. In organotypic raft cultures of cervical intraepithelial neoplasia 612-9E cells, which contain episomal HPV 31b genomic DNA, E5a is detected primarily in the basal and granular cell layers. HPV E5 proteins bind platelet-derived growth factor β receptor and epidermal growth factor receptor (EGFR) and possess weak transforming activity. For example, HPV 16 E5 and HPV 6 E5a each cooperate with epidermal growth factor (EGF), the natural ligand of EGFR, to induce anchorage-independent growth of NIH3T3 cells and to stimulate DNA synthesis in primary human keratinocytes.[123] HPV 16 E5 also increases c-fos and c-jun expression in response to EGF.

It is clear that E5 expression induces, both directly and indirectly, increased mitogenic signaling via various growth factor receptors and other growth stimulatory pathways. By binding to the vacuolar H^+–adenosine triphosphatase 16-kD subunit, E5 inhibits cell-cell communication and may prevent optimal use of tumor suppressor signaling pathways. Although it is clear that the proliferative state induced by E5 is advantageous for viral DNA replication and virion production, a more direct role for E5 in the virus life cycle is under investigation.

PV VACCINE DEVELOPMENT

Prophylactic Vaccine Strategies

Animal models have demonstrated that injection of intact CRPV or BPV4 virions consistently protects immunized animals against experimental infection by the homologous virus type.[124] Furthermore, passive transfer of virion-induced antiserum to naive animals confers protection against subsequent virus challenge; such passive transfer does not, however, induce therapeutic regression of established lesions.[125, 126] Similar experiments using CRPV, BPV4, or canine oral PV VLPs demonstrate that VLP-based vaccines are successful prophylactic agents but offer little therapeutic benefit. Unlike intact virions and VLPs, disassembled virions or VLPs and denatured viral proteins fail to induce neutralizing antibodies or to consistently protect animals against viral challenge. Therefore, it is the immunodominant, conformational epitopes within intact virions and VLPs that confer protection against viral infection. VLP vaccines appear to facilitate predominantly type-specific immunity with little protection against closely related virus types. As such, the development of polyvalent VLP vaccines, which contain VLPs of numerous HPV types, is under investigation.

It is also clear, at least in animal models, that systemic immunization using VLP-based vaccines protects against virus infection at mucosal sites. Low-dose nasal immunization of mice with HPV 16 VLPs induces neutralizing systemic immunoglobulin G (IgG) and mucosal genital immunoglobulin A (IgA), the latter of which may be especially important in the prevention of HPV infection.[127] Nasal immunization of mice with attenuated *Salmonella typhimurium* expressing HPV 16 VLPs results in the detection of both IgG and IgA in cervical washes. Therefore, alternative, less-invasive methods of successful vaccine delivery may enhance the efficacy of vaccine programs by increasing the acceptability of vaccines to a broad patient population. Phase 1 clinical trials indicate that VLP-based vaccines composed of either HPV 11 L1 or HPV 16 L1 are well tolerated and effectively induce production of serologic neutralizing anti-HPV antibodies as measured in vitro.[128]

Therapeutic Vaccine Development

> **Because HPV proteins are not expressed on the surface of infected cells, it is unlikely that induction of an anti-HPV humoral response and associated antibody-dependent cytotoxicity would be therapeutically beneficial.**

Because the immunologic determinants associated with persistence or regression of viral infections remain poorly defined, the development of successful therapeutic vaccines has been slow. If developed, however, therapeutic vaccines could be used to treat cervical cancers and to reduce the significant disease burden of benign HPV-induced warts. Because HPV proteins are not expressed on the surface of infected cells, it is unlikely that induction of an anti-HPV humoral response and associated antibody-dependent cytotoxicity would be therapeutically beneficial. However, preliminary studies involving the induction of cytolytic T lymphocyte (CTL) responses show promise as a therapeutic strategy. The HPV antigen used in therapeutic vaccine studies varies with targeted disease state. For example, HPV E1 and E2 proteins are required for viral DNA replication and transcription and are therefore consistently present in benign hyperproliferative HPV lesions. Cervical cancers and high-grade dysplasias often exhibit integration of the HPV genome with disruption of the E1 and/or E2 ORFs but retain expression of HPV E6 and E7.

Stimulation of CTL responses can be achieved by introducing either naked HPV gene-encoding DNA or recombinant viral vectors to target cells with subsequent HPV gene expression. Human safety trials using recombinant vaccinia expressing HPV 16 or HPV 18 E6 and E7 demonstrate that recombinant vaccinia vaccines have no significant adverse effects at 21 months post vaccination.

Viral proteins and peptides may also induce therapeutic CTL responses. Immunization of mice with an HPV 16 CTL epitope-containing E7 peptide protects against subsequent challenge with HPV 16–transformed tumor cells in vivo.[129] Human studies also demonstrate that peptide epitopes of HPV 16 E7 can enhance CTL responses, resulting in the specific lysis of HPV 16–positive tumor cells in vitro.[130] In contrast to the variation observed with peptide immunizations, CTL responses are consistently induced by administration of particulate protein; therefore, VLPs may be an attractive delivery system for the induction of cell-mediated immune responses as well as humoral responses. Because L1 and L2 are absent in cervical carcinoma cells, L1 or L1/L2 VLPs alone will be ineffective in generating therapeutic CTLs in cervical cancer patients. However, chimeric VLPs that contain L1 or L1/L2 as well as other HPV gene products may augment the therapeutic utility of VLP vaccines. For example, immunization with HPV 16 L1/L2–E7 chimeric VLPs effectively protects mice against challenge with HPV 16 E7–positive tumor cells.

Acknowledgments

Research in the laboratory of Dr. Howett and Ms. Schlosser is funded in part by National Institutes of Health (NIH) grants 2 T32 CA60395-06 and 5 PO1 AI37829.

SUMMARY OF KEY POINTS

- PVs are ubiquitous microorganisms that cause productive and/or latent infections in a wide variety of species and tissues. All PVs infect epithelial tissues in a species-specific manner and induce epithelial proliferation. Although both animal and human PVs share a common genomic organizational structure, sequence similarity varies substantially.

- Approximately half of all currently identified HPVs infect cutaneous epithelial surfaces, whereas the remainder preferentially target the mucosal epithelium of the anogenital tract.

- In vivo and in vitro systems are now available that facilitate investigation of the entire PV life cycle. The life cycle of PV is strictly linked to differentiation of the keratinocyte, the host cell for infection. It is suggested that PV virions are shed from infected epithelial surfaces within the nuclei of highly keratinized, metabolically inert squames. Access to actively dividing basal epithelial cells is required for successful PV infection and is likely facilitated by epithelial microabrasions. Fibrinolysis that occurs during wound healing may facilitate dissolution of the infected squames with subsequent deposition of free virus at the basal cell layer.

- Replication of PVs occurs entirely within the host cell nucleus. On viral entry to basal keratinocytes, expression of early viral genes is initiated. The host cell DNA replication machinery, in conjunction with viral E1 and E2 proteins, facilitates replication of the episomal viral genome to a low copy number. As differentiation continues, the episomal PV genome is further amplified to a high copy number in preparation for production of progeny virions. Late viral gene transcription begins in the more differentiated suprabasal epithelial layers, and the viral capsid proteins, L1 and L2, facilitate packaging of viral genomes. Thus, cornified virus-containing squames are formed.

- PVs are small, nonenveloped, icosahedral DNA viruses. The PV genome is encapsulated in a proteinaceous capsid composed of L1 and L2, the major and minor structural proteins encoded by the late viral genes.

- All PV genomes share a common pattern of organization. Classification or typing of HPVs is based on the degree of similarity of various genomic regions. One strand of the PV DNA contains all

Continued on following page

the ORFs or gene-encoding segments. These ORFs encode all viral proteins. The early region of the genome is transcribed before and during viral DNA synthesis. The late region contains the L1 and L2 ORFs, which, unlike the early genes, are expressed only in productive viral infections. There is a section of the genome that is a noncoding region or URR. Binding to this site by various proteins modulates viral transcription and DNA replication.

- Successful PV infection requires import of the virus genome to the nucleus, which likely involves partial uncoating of the virus capsid. In HPV infections, the E2 protein binds to multiple sites and blocks early gene transcription. Early gene transcription increases with progression of cells to the intermediate epithelial layers. The various forms of E2 affect transcription differently, as either activators or repressors. It is believed that HPV E2 regulates cell growth indirectly by downregulating the expression of *E6* and *E7* oncogenes from the major early promoter. A robust phase of genome replication occurs in the upper epithelial layers and results in a high number of episomal genomes per cell.

- E1^E4 is the most abundant product of both viral transcription, which constitutes approximately 90% of virus transcripts within genital condylomata, and viral translation. Owing to its abundance in terminally differentiated layers of the infected epithelium, E1^E4 may be involved in virus maturation as a scaffold or a transport protein.

- Xenografted human tissues offer a fully competent, susceptible target for HPV. To date, five HPVs and several animal PVs have been successfully grown in xenografts.

- HPV 16 is the most frequent type associated with cervical cancer (50% to 60% of cases), whereas HPV 18 is detected in 10% to 20% of such cancers. In condylomata and mild and moderate dysplasia, the HPV genome is generally episomal. In highly dysplastic and cancerous lesions, the HPV DNA is frequently integrated into the host cell DNA. HPV-positive cervical cancers continue to express E6 and E7, suggesting that these viral products are required for continued cell growth and maintenance of the transformed phenotype. The most well-characterized E6 binding partner is the tumor suppressor protein p53.

- E6 and E7 are the main transforming genes of HPV. Cervical cancers and high-grade dysplasias exhibit integration of the HPV genome, with disruption of the E1 and/or E2 ORFs, but retain expression of HPV E6 and E7. Intratypic HPV diversity within the E6 ORF results in the expression of E6 variants with differing capacities for p53 degradation and cell transformation. The clinical implications of variants may be significant. The HPV 16 E6 prototype has been detected in 44% of high-grade cervical intraepithelial neoplasias but in less than 10% of invasive cervical cancers. HPV 16 E6 variants may be more prevalent in cervical carcinomas than the E6 prototype. The overall prevalence of HPV E6 variants varies by geographic location and demographic population. Although efficient immortalization of primary human keratinocytes requires both HPV 16 E6 and HPV 16 E7, HPV 16 E7 alone can immortalize these cells when it is present at high concentrations.

- Because the immunologic determinants associated with persistence or regression of viral infections remain poorly defined, the development of successful therapeutic vaccines has been slow. Because HPV proteins are not expressed on the surface of infected cells, it is unlikely that induction of an anti-HPV humoral response and associated antibody-dependent cytotoxicity would be therapeutically beneficial.

References

1. de Villiers EM: Papillomavirus and HPV typing. Clin Dermatol 1997;15:199.
2. Merle E, et al: Nuclear import of HPV11 L1 capsid protein is mediated by karyopherin alpha2beta1 heterodimers. J Cell Biochem 1999;74:628.
3. Meyers C, et al: Biosynthesis of human papillomavirus from a continuous cell line upon epithelial differentiation. Science 1992; 257:971.
4. Flores ER, et al: Establishment of the human papillomavirus type 16 (HPV-16) life cycle in an immortalized human foreskin keratinocyte cell line. Virology 1999;262:344.
5. Isom HC, Wigdahl B, Howett MK: Molecular pathology of human oncogenic viruses. In Sirica AE (ed): Cellular and Molecular Pathogenesis. Philadelphia, Lippincott-Raven, 1996, pp 341–387.
6. Muller M, et al: Papillomavirus capsid binding and uptake by cells from different tissues and species. J Virol 1995;69:948.
7. McMillan NA, et al: Expression of the alpha6 integrin confers papillomavirus binding upon receptor-negative B-cells. Virology 1999;261:271.
8. Joyce JG, et al: The L1 major capsid protein of human papillomavirus type 11 recombinant virus-like particles interacts with heparin and cell-surface glycosaminoglycans on human keratinocytes. J Biol Chem 1999;274:5810.
9. Frattini MG, Lim HB, Laimins LA: In vitro synthesis of oncogenic human papillomaviruses requires episomal genomes for differentiation-dependent late expression. Proc Natl Acad Sci USA 1996;93: 3062.
10. Syrjanen SM, Syrjanen KJ: New concepts on the role of human papillomaviruses in cell cycle regulation. Ann Med 1999;31:175.
11. Howley PM: Papillomavirinae: The viruses and their replication. In Fields BN, et al (eds): Fields Virology. Philadelphia, Lippincott-Raven, 1996, pp 2045–2076.
12. Pfister H: Biology and biochemistry of papillomaviruses. Rev Physiol Biochem Pharmacol 1984;99:111.
13. Larsen PM, Storgaard L, Fey SJ: Proteins present in bovine papillomavirus particles. J Virol 1987;61:3596.
14. Volpers C, et al: Assembly of the major and the minor capsid protein of human papillomavirus type 33 into virus-like particles and tubular structures in insect cells. Virology 1994;200:504.
15. Roden RB, et al: Papillomavirus L1 capsids agglutinate mouse erythrocytes through a proteinaceous receptor. J Virol 1995;69: 5147.
16. Roden RB, et al: In vitro generation and type-specific neutralization of a human papillomavirus type 16 virion pseudotype. J Virol 1996;70:5875.
17. Chen EY, et al: The primary structure and genetic organization of the bovine papillomavirus type 1 genome. Nature 1982;299:529.

18. Pfister H, Fuchs PG: Anatomy, taxonomy and evolution of papillomaviruses. Intervirology 1994;37:143.
19. Turek LP: The structure, function, and regulation of papillomaviral genes in infection and cervical cancer. Adv Virus Res 1994;44:305.
20. Bernard HU, Chan SY: Animal papillomaviruses. In Meyers G, et al (eds): Human Papillomaviruses: A Compilation and Analysis of Nucleic Acid and Amino Acid Sequences. Los Alamos, NM, Los Alamos National Laboratory, 1997, pp III100–III109.
21. Desaintes C, Demeret C: Control of papillomavirus DNA replication and transcription. Semin Cancer Biol 1996;7:339.
22. Barksdale S, Baker CC: Differentiation-specific alternative splicing of bovine papillomavirus late mRNAs. J Virol 1995;69:6553.
23. Terhune SS, Milcarek C, Laimins LA: Regulation of human papillomavirus type 31 polyadenylation during the differentiation-dependent life cycle. J Virol 1999;73:7185.
24. Zhao C, et al: Identification of nuclear and cytoplasmic proteins that interact specifically with an AU-rich, cis-acting inhibitory sequence in the 3′ untranslated region of human papillomavirus type 1 late mRNAs. J Virol 1996;70:3659.
25. zur Hausen H: Roots and perspectives of contemporary papillomavirus research. J Cancer Res Clin Oncol 1996;122:3.
26. Sibbet G, et al: Alpha6 integrin is not the obligatory cell receptor for bovine papillomavirus type 4. J Gen Virol 2000;81:327.
27. Roden RB, et al: Interaction of papillomaviruses with the cell surface. J Virol 1994;68:7260.
28. Volpers C, et al: Binding and internalization of human papillomavirus type 33 virus-like particles by eukaryotic cells. J Virol 1995;69:3258.
29. Booy FP, et al: Two antibodies that neutralize papillomavirus by different mechanisms show distinct binding patterns at 13 A resolution. J Mol Biol 1998;281:95.
30. Stubenrauch F, Laimins LA: Human papillomavirus life cycle: Active and latent phases. Semin Cancer Biol 1999;9:379.
31. Grassmann K, et al: Identification of a differentiation-inducible promoter in the E7 open reading frame of human papillomavirus type 16 (HVP-16) in raft cultures of a new cell line containing high copy numbers of episomal HPV-16 DNA. J Virol 1996;70:2339.
32. Leng X, Wilson VG: Genetically defined nuclear localization signal sequence of bovine papillomavirus E1 protein is necessary and sufficient for the nuclear localization of E1-beta-galactosidase fusion proteins. J Gen Virol 1994;75:2463.
33. Zanardi TA, et al: Modulation of bovine papillomavirus DNA replication by phosphorylation of the viral E1 protein. Virology 1997;228:1.
34. Liu JS, et al: The functions of human papillomavirus type 11 E1, E2, and E2C proteins in cell-free DNA replication. J Biol Chem 1995;270:27283.
35. Gillette TG, Lusky M, Borowiec JA: Induction of structural changes in the bovine papillomavirus type 1 origin of replication by the viral E1 and E2 proteins. Proc Natl Acad Sci USA 1994;91:8846.
36. Kuo SR, et al: Cell-free replication of the human papillomavirus DNA with homologous viral E1 and E2 proteins and human cells extracts. J Biol Chem 1994;269:24058.
37. Russell J, Botchan MR: cis-Acting components of human papillomavirus (HPV) DNA replication: Linker substitution analysis of the HPV type 11 origin. J Virol 1995;69:651.
38. Demeret C, et al: The human papillomavirus type 18 (HPV18) replication protein E1 is a transcriptional activator when interacting with HPV18 E2. Virology 1998;242:378.
39. Hubbert NL, et al: Bovine papilloma virus-transformed cells contain multiple E2 proteins. Proc Natl Acad Sci USA 1988;85:5864.
40. Yang L, et al: Transcription factor E2 regulates BPV-1 DNA replication in vitro by direct protein-protein interaction. Cold Spring Harb Symp Quant Biol 1991;56:335.
41. Gauthier JM, Dillner J, Yaniv M: Structural analysis of the human papillomavirus type 16-E2 transactivator with antipeptide antibodies reveals a high mobility region linking the transactivation and the DNA-binding domains. Nucleic Acids Res 1991;19:7073.
42. Hegde RS, et al: Crystal structure at 1.7 A of the bovine papillomavirus-1 E2 DNA-binding domain bound to its DNA target. Nature 1992;359:505.
43. Moskaluk CA, Bastia D: The bovine papillomavirus type 1 transcriptional activator E2 protein binds to its DNA recognition sequence as a dimer. Virology 1989;169:236.
44. Steger G, Corbach S: Dose-dependent regulation of the early promoter of human papillomavirus type 18 by the viral E2 protein. J Virol 1997;71:50.
45. McBride AA, Romanczuk H, Howley PM: The papillomavirus E2 regulatory proteins. J Biol Chem 1991;266:18411.
46. Ustav E, et al: The bovine papillomavirus origin of replication requires a binding site for the E2 transcriptional activator. Proc Natl Acad Sci USA 1993;90:898.
47. Blitz IL, Laimins LA: The 68-kilodalton E1 protein of bovine papillomavirus is a DNA binding phosphoprotein which associates with the E2 transcriptional activator in vitro. J Virol 1991;65:649.
48. Hibma MH, et al: The interaction between human papillomavirus type 16 E1 and E2 proteins is blocked by an antibody to the N-terminal region of E2. Eur J Biochem 1995;229:517.
49. Bouvard V, et al: Characterization of the human papillomavirus E2 protein: Evidence of trans-activation and trans-repression in cervical keratinocytes. EMBO J 1994;13:5451.
50. Dong G, Broker TR, Chow LT: Human papillomavirus type 11 E2 proteins repress the homologous E6 promoter by interfering with the binding of host transcription factors to adjacent elements. J Virol 1994;68:1115.
51. Kovelman R, et al: Enhanced transcriptional activation by E2 proteins from the oncogenic human papillomaviruses. J Virol 1996;70:7549.
52. Dowhanick JJ, McBride AA, Howley PM: Suppression of cellular proliferation by the papillomavirus E2 protein. J Virol 1995;69:7791.
53. Desaintes C, et al: Expression of the papillomavirus E2 protein in HeLa cells leads to apoptosis. EMBO J 1997;16:504.
54. Hwang ES, et al: Inhibition of cervical carcinoma cell line proliferation by the introduction of a bovine papillomavirus regulatory gene. J Virol 1993;67:3720.
55. Frattini MG, et al: Abrogation of a mitotic checkpoint by E2 proteins from oncogenic human papillomaviruses correlates with increased turnover of the p53 tumor suppressor protein. EMBO J 1997;16:318.
56. Law MF, et al: Mouse cells transformed by bovine papillomavirus contain only extrachromosomal viral DNA sequences. Proc Natl Acad Sci USA 1981;78:2727.
57. Gilbert DM, Cohen SN: Bovine papillomavirus plasmids replicate randomly in mouse fibroblasts throughout S phase of the cell cycle. Cell 1987;50:59.
58. Ustav M, Stenlund A: Transient replication of BPV-1 requires two viral polypeptides encoded by the E1 and E2 open reading frames. EMBO J 1991;10:449.
59. Melendy T, Sedman J, Stenlund A: Cellular factors required for papillomavirus DNA replication. J Virol 1995;69:7857.
60. Hummel M, Lim HB, Laimins LA: Human papillomavirus type 31b late gene expression is regulated through protein kinase C-mediated changes in RNA processing. J Virol 1995;69:3381.
61. Brown DR, et al: Virus-like particles and E1^E4 protein expressed from the human papillomavirus type 11 bicistronic E1^E4^L1 transcript. Virology 1996;222:43.
62. Ozbun MA, Meyers C: Characterization of late gene transcripts expressed during vegetative replication of human papillomavirus type 31b. J Virol 1997;71:5161.
63. Schwartz S: Cis-acting negative RNA elements on papillomavirus late mRNAs. Semin Vir 1998;8:291.
64. Pray TR, Laimins LA: Differentiation-dependent expression of E1^E4 proteins in cell lines maintaining episomes of human papillomavirus type 31b. Virology 1995;206:679.
65. Palermo-Dilts DA, Broker TR, Chow LT: Human papillomavirus type 1 produces redundant as well as polycistronic mRNAs in plantar warts. J Virol 1990;64:3144.
66. Doorbar J, Gallimore PH: Identification of proteins encoded by the L1 and L2 open reading frames of human papillomavirus 1a. J Virol 1987;61:2793.
67. Icenogle J: Analysis of the sequences of the L1 and L2 capsid proteins of papillomaviruses. In Meyers G, et al (eds): Human Papillomaviruses: A Compilation and Analysis of Nucleic Acid and Amino Acid Sequences. Los Alamos, NM, Los Alamos National Laboratory, 1995, pp III73–III89.
68. Doorbar J, Coneron I, Gallimore PH: Sequence divergence yet conserved physical characteristics among the E4 proteins of cutaneous human papillomaviruses. Virology 1989;172:51.
69. Doorbar J, et al: Identification of the human papillomavirus-1a E4 gene products. EMBO J 1986;5:355.

70. Stoler MH, Broker TR: In situ hybridization detection of human papillomavirus DNAs and messenger RNAs in genital condylomas and a cervical carcinoma. Hum Pathol 1986;17:1250.

71. Brown DR, et al: Expression of the human papillomavirus type 11 E5A protein from the E1^E4, E5 transcript. Intervirology 1998;41:47.

72. Brown DR, Chin MT, Strike DG: Identification of human papillomavirus type 11 E4 gene products in human tissue implants from athymic mice. Virology 1988;165:262.

73. Tomita Y, et al: Human papillomavirus type 6 and 11 E4 gene products in condyloma acuminata. J Gen Virol 1991;72:731.

74. Brown DR, et al: Human papillomavirus type 11 E1^E4 and L1 proteins colocalize in the mouse xenograft system at multiple time points. Virology 1995;214:259.

75. Doorbar J, et al: Specific interaction between HPV-16 E1–E4 and cytokeratins results in collapse of the epithelial cell intermediate filament network. Nature 1991;352:824.

76. Doorbar J, Medcalf E, Napthine S: Analysis of HPV1 E4 complexes and their associations with keratins in vivo. Virology 1996;218:114.

77. McCarthy MP, et al: Quantitative disassembly and reassembly of human papillomavirus type 11 viruslike particles in vitro. J Virol 1998;72:32.

78. de Villiers EM: Human pathogenic papillomavirus types: An update. Curr Top Microbiol Immunol 1994;186:1.

79. Flanagan SP: 'Nude,' a new hairless gene with pleiotropic effects in the mouse. Genet Res 1966;8:295.

80. Bosma GC, Custer RP, Bosma MJ: A severe combined immunodeficiency mutation in the mouse. Nature 1983;301:527.

81. Bedell MA, et al: Amplification of human papillomavirus genomes in vitro is dependent on epithelial differentiation. J Virol 1991;65:2254.

82. Ozbun MA, Meyers C: Temporal usage of multiple promoters during the life cycle of human papillomavirus type 31b. J Virol 1998;72:2715.

83. Meyers C, Mayer TJ, Ozbun MA: Synthesis of infectious human papillomavirus type 18 in differentiating epithelium transfected with viral DNA. J Virol 1997;71:7381.

84. Lorincz AT, et al: Human papillomavirus infection of the cervix: Relative risk associations of 15 common anogenital types. Obstet Gynecol 1992;79:328.

85. Gissmann L, et al: Human papillomavirus types 6 and 11 DNA sequences in genital and laryngeal papillomas and in some cervical cancers. Proc Natl Acad Sci USA 1983;80:560.

86. Bosch FX, et al: Prevalence of human papillomavirus in cervical cancer: A worldwide perspective. International biological study on cervical cancer (IBSCC) Study Group. J Natl Cancer Inst 1995;87:796.

87. zur Hausen H: Papillomavirus infections - a major cause of human cancers. Biochim Biophys Acta 1996;1288:F55.

88. Crum CP, et al: Human papillomavirus type 16 and early cervical neoplasia. N Engl J Med 1984;310:880.

89. Cullen AP, et al: Analysis of the physical state of different human papillomavirus DNAs in intraepithelial and in invasive cervical neoplasm. J Virol 1991;65:606.

90. Smotkin D, Wettstein FO: Transcription of human papillomavirus type 16 early genes in a cervical cancer and a cancer-derived cell line and identification of the E7 protein. Proc Natl Acad Sci USA 1986;83:4680.

91. Banks L, et al: Identification of human papillomavirus type 18 E6 polypeptide in cells derived from human cervical carcinomas. J Gen Virol 1987;68:1351.

92. Alvarez-Salas LM, et al: Inhibition of HPV-16 E6/E7 immortalization of normal keratinocytes by hairpin ribozymes. Proc Natl Acad Sci USA 1998;95:1189.

93. Arbeit JM, et al: Progressive squamous epithelial neoplasia in K14-human papillomavirus type 16 transgenic mice. J Virol 1994;68:4358.

94. Barbosa MS, Lowy DR, Schiller JT: Papillomavirus polypeptides E6 and E7 are zinc-binding proteins. J Virol 1989;63:1404.

95. Grossman SR, Laimins LA: E6 protein of human papillomavirus type 18 binds zinc. Oncogene 1989;4:1089.

96. Kanda T, et al: Human papillomavirus type 16 E6 proteins with glycine substitution for cysteine in the metal-binding motif. Virology 1991;185:536.

97. Lee SS, Weiss RS, Javier RT: Binding of human virus oncoproteins to hD1g/SAP97, a mammalian homolog of the Drosophila discs large tumor suppressor protein. Proc Natl Acad Sci USA 1997;94:6670.

98. Werness BA, Levine AJ, Howley PM: Association of human papillomavirus type 16 and 18 E6 proteins with p53. Science 1990;248:76.

99. Li X, Coffino P: High-risk human papillomavirus E6 protein has two distinct binding sites within p53, of which only one determines degradation. J Virol 1996;70:4509.

100. Dulic V, et al: p53-dependent inhibition of cyclin-dependent kinase activities in human fibroblasts during radiation-induced G1 arrest. Cell 1994;76:1013.

101. Thomas JT, Laimins LA: Human papillomavirus oncoproteins E6 and E7 independently abrogate the mitotic spindle checkpoint. J Virol 1998;72:1131.

102. Liu Y, et al: Multiple functions of human papillomavirus type 16 E6 contribute to the immortalization of mammary epithelial cells. J Virol 1999;73:7297.

103. Inoue T, et al: Dispensability of p53 degradation for tumorigenicity and decreased serum requirement of human papillomavirus type 16 E6. Mol Carcinog 1998;21:215.

104. Nakagawa S, et al: Mutational analysis of human papillomavirus type 16 E6 protein: Transforming function for human cells and degradation of p53 in vitro. Virology 1995;212:535.

105. Thomas M, et al: HPV-18 E6 mediated inhibition of DNA binding activity is independent of E6 induced degradation. Oncogene 1995;10:261.

106. Stoppler MC, et al: Natural variants of the human papillomavirus type 16 E6 protein differ in their abilities to alter keratinocyte differentiation and to induce p53 degradation. J Virol 1996;70:6987.

107. Zehbe I, et al: Human papillomavirus16 E6 variants are more prevalent in invasive cervical carcinoma than the prototype. Cancer Res 1998;58:829.

108. Matlashewski GJ, et al: Primary structure polymorphism at amino acid residue 72 of human p53. Mol Cell Biol 1987;7:961.

109. Thomas M, et al: Two polymorphic variants of wild-type p53 differ biochemically and biologically. Mol Cell Biol 1999;19:1092.

110. Storey A, et al: Role of a p53 polymorphism in the development of human papillomavirus-associated cancer. Nature 1998;393:229.

111. Giannoudis A, et al: p53 codon 72 ARG/PRO polymorphism is not related to HPV type or lesion grade in low- and high-grade squamous intra-epithelial lesions and invasive squamous carcinoma of the cervix. Int J Cancer 1999;83:66.

112. Zehbe I, et al: Codon 72 polymorphism of p53 and its association with cervical cancer. Lancet 1999;354:218.

113. Hsu EM, et al: Quantification of HPV-16 E6–E7 transcription in cervical intraepithelial neoplasia by reverse transcriptase polymerase chain reaction. Int J Cancer 1993;55:397.

114. Sedman SA, et al: The full-length E6 protein of human papillomavirus type 16 has transforming and trans-activating activities and cooperates with E7 to immortalize keratinocytes in culture. J Virol 1991;65:4860.

115. Pim D, Massimi P, Banks L: Alternatively spliced HPV-18 E6* protein inhibits E6 mediated degradation of p53 and suppresses transformed cell growth. Oncogene 1997;15:257.

116. Dyson N, et al: The human papillomavirus-16 E7 oncoprotein is able to bind to the retinoblastoma gene product. Science 1989;243:934.

117. Dyson N, et al: Homologous sequences in adenovirus E1A and human papillomavirus E7 proteins mediate interaction with the same set of cellular proteins. J Virol 1992;66:6893.

118. Heck DV, et al: Efficiency of binding the retinoblastoma protein correlates with the transforming capacity of the E7 oncoproteins of the human papillomaviruses. Proc Natl Acad Sci USA 1992;89:4442.

119. Huang PS, et al: Protein domains governing interactions between E2F, the retinoblastoma gene product, and human papillomavirus type 16 E7 protein. Mol Cell Biol 1993;13:953.

120. DeGregori J, Kowalik T, Nevins JR: Cellular targets for activation by the E2F1 transcription factor include DNA synthesis- and G_1/S-regulatory genes. Mol Cell Biol 1995;15:4215.

121. Halbert CL, Demers GW, Galloway DA: The E7 gene of human papillomavirus type 16 is sufficient for immortalization of human epithelial cells. J Virol 1991;65:473.

122. Martin LG, Demers GW, Galloway DA, Disruption of the G1/S transition in human papillomavirus type 16 E7-expressing human cells is associated with altered regulation of cyclin E. J Virol 1998;72:975.

123. Straight SW, et al: The E5 oncoprotein of human papillomavirus type 16 transforms fibroblasts and effects the downregulation of the epidermal growth factor receptor in keratinocytes. J Virol 1993;67:4521.

124. Jarrett WF, et al: Studies on vaccination against papillomaviruses: the immunity after infection and vaccination with bovine papillomaviruses of different types. Vet Rec 1990;126:473.

125. Shope RE: Immunization of rabbits to infectious papillomatosis. J Exp Med 1937;65:219.

126. Kidd JG: The course of virus-induced rabbit papillomas as determined by virus, cells, and host. J Exp Med 1938;67:551.

127. Balmelli C, et al: Nasal immunization of mice with human papillomavirus type 16 virus-like particles elicits neutralizing antibodies in mucosal secretions. J Virol 1998;72:8220.

128. Harro CD, et al: Safety and immunogenicity trial in adult volunteers of a human papillomavirus 16 L1 virus-like particle vaccine. J Natl Cancer Inst 2001;93:284.

129. Feltkamp MC, et al: Vaccination with cytotoxic T lymphocyte epitope-containing peptide protects against a tumor induced by human papillomavirus type 16-transformed cells. Eur J Immunol 1993;23:2242.

130. Alexander M, et al: Generation of tumor-specific cytolytic T lymphocytes from peripheral blood of cervical cancer patients by in vitro stimulation with a synthetic human papillomavirus type 16 E7 epitope. Am J Obstet Gynecol 1996;175:1586.

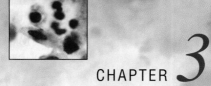

CHAPTER 3

The Papanicolaou Smear

A

• Mark Spitzer
• Cynda Johnson

Terminology in Cervical Cytology: The Bethesda System

The introduction of evaluation of cellular material from the cervix and vagina for the diagnosis of cervical carcinoma is generally attributed to George N. Papanicolaou, an anatomist. In 1928, he published a report titled "New Cancer Diagnosis." Collaborating with Herbert Traut, a gynecologist, he refined the technique of collecting cellular material from the vaginal pool. Another gynecologist, J. Ernest Ayre, introduced the use of a wooden spatula to scrape the cervix and harvest cells directly from the transformation zone.

George Papanicolaou devised the first system of reporting cervical cytology results and based the classification on the degree of certainty that malignant cells were present.

George Papanicolaou himself devised the first system of reporting results of cervical cytology testing in 1954. The system included five classifications, based on the degree of certainty that malignant cells were present. In 1968, a new system was created that was based on morphologic criteria. This system, known as "descriptive," was embraced by the World Health Organization (WHO).

Class 2 cytology was described by various forms of atypia; class 3 was divided into mild, moderate, and severe dysplasia; and class 4 encompassed carcinoma in situ. Ten years later, Richart introduced the concept of cervical intraepithelial neoplasia (CIN), which encompassed all the precancerous epithelial lesions of the uterine cervix.[1-3] Although this system described histologic, not cytologic, changes, many used the terms interchangeably to describe both.

The Bethesda System replaced three levels of CIN with two levels, low-grade and high-grade intraepithelial lesions, which could be used to describe any squamous abnormality of the lower genital tract.

The current cytologic terminology, the Bethesda System (TBS), was the result of the work of an expert panel, which convened in 1988 under the auspices of the National Cancer Institute.[4] The panel affirmed that the cytology report should be considered a medical consultation. TBS replaced the three levels of dysplasia and carcinoma in situ with two levels, low-grade squamous intraepithelial lesion (LSIL) and high-grade squamous intraepithelial lesion (HSIL). The designation of squamous intraepithe-

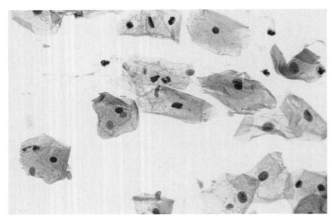

Figure 3–1. Superficial, intermediate squamous epithelial cells as identified in the Papanicolaou smear. Note that the superficial cells have a somewhat pink cytoplasm and a relatively small nucleus, approximately the size of a red blood cell. The intermediate squamous cells have a larger nucleus and, in this stain, a slightly blue cytoplasm.

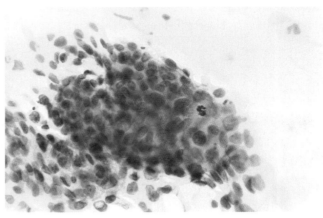

Figure 3–3. Papanicolaou smear: epithelial cell abnormality, high-grade squamous intraepithelial lesion. These cells are consistent with cervical intraepithelial neoplasia grade 3. This group of dysplastic epithelial cells demonstrates marked crowding and overlapping with moderate nuclear pleomorphism. There is nuclear chromatin hyperchromasia, and an apparently abnormal mitotic figure is seen in one cell.

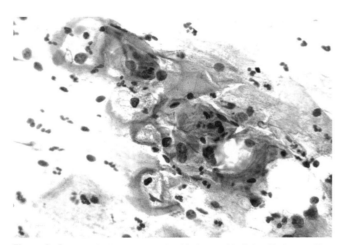

Figure 3–2. Papanicolaou smear classified as epithelial cell abnormality, low-grade squamous intraepithelial lesion. Some koilocytes are evident in this smear, characterized by slightly enlarged nuclei with somewhat irregular nuclear outlines and distinctive perinuclear haloes. Two binucleated squamous cells are also present.

lial lesion (SIL) did not specifically refer to the cervix but could be used to describe any squamous abnormality of the lower genital tract. See Figures 3–1 to 3–3 for examples of normal cytology, LSIL, and HSIL.

> The justification for the term *squamous intraepithelial lesion* was the high spontaneous regression rate of some dysplastic lesions and the lack of predictable progression of these lesions to invasive carcinoma.

The justification for the term *squamous intraepithelial lesion* was the high spontaneous regression rate of some dysplastic lesions and the lack of predictable progression of these lesions to invasive carcinoma. Furthermore, the justification for two categories rather than three or four, as in the CIN and WHO systems, respectively, was the apparent lack of reproducibility for the identification of these categories among different laboratories (interobserver variability) and even by the same cytologist (intraobserver variability). Placing CIN 2/moderate dysplasia, CIN 3/severe dysplasia, and carcinoma in situ into

▼ Table 3–1

Papanicolaou Smear Nomenclature

Papanicolaou Class System (1954)	Descriptive (1968)	CIN (1978)	Bethesda System (1988)
Class 1	Negative for malignant cells	Negative	Within normal limits
Class 2	Inflammatory atypia		Reactive and reparative changes
	Squamous atypia		Atypical squamous cells of undetermined significance
	Koilocytotic atypia		Low-grade SIL; includes condyloma
Class 3	Mild dysplasia	CIN 1	Low-grade SIL; includes condyloma
	Moderate dysplasia	CIN 2	High-grade SIL
	Severe dysplasia	CIN 3	High-grade SIL
Class 4	Carcinoma in situ	CIN 3	High-grade SIL
Class 5	Invasive carcinoma	Invasive carcinoma	Invasive carcinoma

CIN, cervical intraepithelial neoplasia; SIL, squamous intraepithelial lesion.

▼ Table 3–2

1991 Bethesda System for Reporting Cervical/Vaginal Cytologic Diagnoses and Bethesda (2001) Revision

Statement on Specimen Adequacy	Specimen Adequacy
Satisfactory for evaluation	Satisfactory for evaluation (describe presence or absence of endocervical T zone component and any other quality indicators)
Satisfactory for evaluation but limited [reason specified]	[category eliminated*]
Unsatisfactory for evaluation [reason specified]	Unsatisfactory for evaluation (specify reason)
	Specimen may be processed and unsatisfactory or unprocessed
General Categorization (Optional)	
Within normal limits	Negative for intraepithelial lesion or malignancy (NIL)
Benign cellular changes; see descriptive diagnosis	[category eliminated†]
Epithelial cell abnormality; see descriptive diagnoses	Epithelial cell abnormality; see interpretation/result (specify squamous or glandular)
	Other (see interpretation/result)
Descriptive Diagnoses	**Interpretation/Result**
Benign Cellular Changes	*Negative for Intraepithelial Lesion or Malignancy*
Infection	Organisms
Trichomonas vaginalis	*Trichomonas vaginalis*
Fungal organisms morphologically consistent with *Candida* species	Fungal organisms morphologically consistent with *Candida* species
Predominance of coccobacilli consistent with shift in vaginal flora	Shift in vaginal flora suggestive of bacterial vaginosis
Bacteria morphologically consistent with *Actinomyces* species	Bacteria morphologically consistent with *Actinomyces* species
Cellular changes consistent with Herpes simplex virus	Cellular changes associated with Herpes simplex virus
Other	Other non-neoplastic findings (optional to report; list not inclusive)
Reactive and reparative changes	Reactive cellular changes associated with inflammation (includes typical repair), radiation, intrauterine contraceptive device
Reactive cellular changes associated with inflammation (includes typical repair), atrophy with inflammation (atrophic vaginitis), radiation, intrauterine contraceptive device, or other	Atrophy, benign-appearing glandular cells post hysterectomy
Epithelial Cell Abnormalities	*Epithelial Cell Abnormalities*
Squamous cells	Squamous cells
Atypical squamous cells of undetermined significance	Atypical squamous cells
	Of undetermined significance
	Cannot exclude HSIL‡
Low-grade squamous intraepithelial lesion encompassing human papillomavirus/mild dysplasia/CIN 1	Low-grade squamous intraepithelial lesion encompassing human papillomavirus/mild dysplasia/CIN 1
High-grade squamous intraepithelial lesion encompassing moderate and severe dysplasia, CIN 2, and CIN 3/CIS	High-grade squamous intraepithelial lesion encompassing moderate and severe dysplasia, CIS/CIN 2, and CIN 3
	With features suspicious for invasion (if invasion is suspected)
Squamous cell carcinoma	Squamous cell carcinoma
Glandular cells	Glandular cells
Endometrial cells, cytologically benign in postmenopausal women	Category reported as NIL (above)
Atypical glandular cells of undetermined significance	Atypical endocervical cells, endometrial cells, glandular cells
	Atypical glandular/endocervical cells, favor neoplastic
	Endocervical adenocarcinoma in situ
	Adenocarcinoma
Endocervical adenocarcinoma	Endocervical
Endometrial adenocarcinoma	Endometrial
Extrauterine adenocarcinoma	Extrauterine
Adenocarcinoma not otherwise specified	Not otherwise specified
Other Malignant Neoplasms	*Other Malignant Neoplasms (specify)*
Hormonal evaluation (applies to vaginal smears only)	*Educational Notes*
Hormonal pattern compatible with age and history	
Hormonal pattern incompatible with age and history [reason specified]	
Hormonal evaluation not possible owing to [reason specified]	

*These smears are categorized as satisfactory and the limiting factors are described.
†These smears are categorized as either NIL if they are clearly negative or as ASC-US if an epithelial abnormality is suspected.
‡New category.
CIN, cervical intraepithelial neoplasia; CIS, carcinoma in situ.

one category reduces the discordance between interpretations of cytologic and histologic specimens.[5] A statement of the adequacy of the Papanicolaou (Pap) smear for providing an accurate interpretation is also included.[6] Table 3–1 compares the four cytologic classification systems. Further refinements were added to TBS in 1991 and in 2001. Table 3–2 outlines the components of the currently used TBS and the changes implemented in 2001.

ADEQUACY OF THE SPECIMEN

According to TBS, the specimen adequacy must be determined before the cytopathologist proceeds with interpretation of the smear.

According to TBS, the specimen adequacy must be determined before the cytopathologist proceeds with interpretation of the smear.

A smear may be called satisfactory for evaluation if it meets the following four criteria: (1) The patient and the specimen are prominently identified; (2) pertinent clinical history is available, (3) the sample is technically interpretable and of proper cellular composition (no more than 50% of the cells can be obscured by inflammation, debris, or blood), and (4) there is evidence that the cervical transformation zone has been sampled.

The factors that result in a smear being labeled unsatisfactory for evaluation include the following: (1) lack of patient identification on the slide; (2) a broken, unrepairable slide; (3) scant cellularity resulting in less than 10% of the slide being covered by unobscured epithelial cells; and (4) obscuration of 75% or more of the epithelial cells by blood, inflammation, thick areas, air-drying artifact, poor preservation, foreign material, or poor technical detail.

Typical rates of unsatisfactory smears from interlaboratory comparison programs are reported as 0.5% (mean, 0.95%).

Ransdell reviewed the results of smears collected for an 18-month period in 1994 and 1995 at the Universities of Kentucky and Iowa; 208 of 71,872 (0.3%) were found to be unsatisfactory.[7] The significance of unsatisfactory smears was highlighted in this longitudinal study[7] that found that unsatisfactory smears were more likely among high-risk patients and that significantly more had SIL-cancer on follow-up when compared with those with satisfactory smears.

The most common reason for an unsatisfactory smear is scant cellularity, followed by obscuring inflammation and obscuring blood.

TBS 2001 proposed to separate unsatisfactory Paps rejected (not processed) for technical reasons (i.e., unlabeled specimens and broken slides) from those processed but unsatisfactory (i.e., obscuring blood or inflammation). Typical rates of unsatisfactory smears from other interlaboratory comparison programs are reported as 0.5% (mean, 0.95%).[8] The most common reason for an unsatisfactory specimen was scant cellularity, followed by obscuring inflammation and obscuring blood. Two thirds of the patients underwent follow-up sampling, and, of these, a significant number eventually had a diagnosis of SIL or neoplasia.[8]

In TBS 1991, the indications for labeling a smear satisfactory for evaluation but limited by . . . (SBLB) included (1) obscuration of 50% to 75% of the epithelial cells by blood, inflammatory cells, thick areas, drying artifact, poor preservation, foreign material, or poor technical detail; (2) lack of evidence that the transformation zone has been sampled; and (3) lack of pertinent clinical information. The overall rate of SBLB Paps ranges widely among laboratories and averages 24% in one large survey[9] but only 9.3% in another.[10] However, clinicians found this term confusing and viewed the category as an oxymoron—is the specimen satisfactory or is it limited? TBS 2001 workshop eliminated this category. Any limitations on the quality of the smear would be noted in a separate section of the report. Elimination of the category was further supported by retrospective studies that failed to show that partially obscuring factors increase the risk of a false-negative report.[11, 12]

To be considered satisfactory under TBS 1991, a smear needed to contain, at a minimum, two clusters of well-preserved endocervical glandular cells and/ or metaplastic cells. This was supported by studies showing that SIL cells are more likely to be present on smears containing endocervical cells.[13-16] However, retrospective cohort studies have shown that women with smears lacking endocervical cells are not more likely to have squamous lesions on follow-up than women with endocervical cells.[17, 18] Finally, retrospective case-control studies have failed to show an association between false-negative interpretations of smears and lack of endocervical cells.[11, 12] Because TBS 2001 eliminated the category of SBLB, the absence of endocervical cells does not affect specimen adequacy. The lack of endocervical cells is noted in a separate section. If the specimen shows a high-grade lesion or cancer, the presence or absence of endocervical cells is not relevant and not reported.

The American Society of Colposcopy and Cervical Pathology (ASCCP) reviewed these criteria in 1997 and offered algorithms for follow-up of smears that were unsatisfactory (Fig. 3–4).[19]

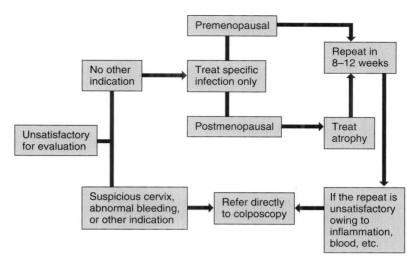

Figure 3–4. Algorithm for smears reported as unsatisfactory for evaluation.

BENIGN CELLULAR CHANGES

Reactive or reparative changes and infection are included under the category of BCC.

The following diagnoses are included under the category of benign cellular changes (BCC): reactive or reparative changes (approximately 90% of cases) and infection (approximately 10% of cases).[20] Placing these diagnoses in the benign category was an intentional effort to remove them from HPV-associated disease. Each of the diagnoses in this group is associated with some predictable cellular changes, but not with neoplasia.

The extent to which inflammation is predictive of an epithelial cell abnormality or a gynecologic infection is debatable.

The most controversial finding in the BCC category is that of inflammation. The extent to which inflammation described on the Pap smear is predictive of epithelial cell abnormality or gynecologic infection remains a question, but management of this condition need not be as intense as that for epithelial cell abnormalities. Several studies found a correlation between sexually transmitted diseases and the presence of inflammation on the Pap smear,[21–26] whereas others did not.[27–29] In those studies that found a correlation, the inflammatory changes appeared to be more predictive of infection in populations at high risk for sexually transmitted diseases. Several investigators noted that the presence of genital infection did not increase the rates of inadequate smears, and they recommended that the Pap smear not be delayed until after treatment of the infection.[24, 30] It is important that the opportunity for obtaining a smear not be missed in this group of infected women.

If inflammation is associated with atrophy, the inflammatory response usually resolves with adequate estrogen therapy.

Although some authors have cited an association between inflammation on the Pap smear and epithelial cell abnormalities, most of these abnormalities were of low grade, and the smear had not been evaluated according to TBS.[31, 32] In smears with persistence of significant inflammation, the association may be greater.[33, 34] However, if atrophy is present, the inflammatory response usually resolves with adequate estrogen therapy.

Reparative changes are often encountered with estrogen deficiency, surgery, radiotherapy, sexual intercourse, or tampon use.

Reactive or reparative changes are listed in Bethesda 2001 in the category of negative for intraepithelial lesion or malignancy (NIL) under the subheading of other non-neoplastic findings and include cellular alterations associated with reparative processes. Reparative processes are often encountered with estrogen deficiency, surgery, radiotherapy, intercourse, IUD use, or tampon use. Chronic radiation effects reflected in the cytologic smear include nuclear and cellular enlargement, cytoplasmic vacuolation, and multinucleation. These differ from postirradiation dysplasia.[35–37] Typical changes associated with the presence of an intrauterine device include inflammation, hyperplasia and papillary proliferation of endocervical epithelium, multinucleation, and increased squamous metaplasia.[38, 39]

The significance of the category BCC in TBS 1991 was unclear. The sensitivity and specificity of cytologic evidence of these conditions are not well known in most cases. Furthermore, the term BCC was felt to be ambiguous by most clinicians. TBS 2001 eliminated the term BCC and reduced the number of general categories from three to two (negative for intraepithelial lesion or malignancy [NIL] and epithelial cell abnormality). Those cases that are clearly reactive should be downgraded to a negative diagnosis, and those that are questionably neoplastic should be upgraded to the epithelial cell abnormality category. Reactive cellular changes may be reported in a separate section.

Infections listed under the BCC category in TBS 1991 would be listed under a subcategory of NIL called organisms. Table 3–3 summarizes an approach to the cytologic diagnosis of BCC in TBS 1991 or the organisms listed in TBS 2001.

ATYPICAL SQUAMOUS CELLS

TBS 1988 separated epithelial cell abnormalities into atypical squamous cells of undetermined significance (ASCUS) and SIL. In the 1991 revision of TBS,[60] pathologists were asked to predict the etiology of the atypical cells in the ASCUS category. The subcategories included ASCUS favoring a reactive process (ASCUS-FR), ASCUS favoring a dysplastic/neoplastic process (ASCUS-FN), and ASCUS not otherwise specified (ASCUS-NOS).

> **The diagnosis of ASCUS is too subjective, poorly reproducible, and overutilized as part of the practice of defensive medicine. Furthermore, it creates management problems for the clinician, anxiety for the patient, and increased cost for the health care system.**

▼ Table 3–3

The Bethesda System: Comments and Recommended Responses to "Infections"

Organism	Comments	Recommended Response
Trichomonas vaginalis	False positives result from the observation of suspicious but nonmotile organisms. Sensitivity is in the 60% range; specificity is 70–80%, with a positive predictive value of 40% in an average-risk population.[40–42]	Offer treatment to the patient after alerting her to the possibility of a false-positive result. Confirm by wet mount or culture if she prefers not to be treated without confirmatory results.
Fungal organisms morphologically consistent with *Candida* species	Sensitivity of Pap smear compared with culture is about 50%. The presence of *Candida* cell forms on the Pap smear has improved correlation with culture results when normal lactobacillary flora is present, when *Trichomonas vaginalis* is absent, and when the infecting *Candida* colonization is *C. albicans*.[43, 44]	Inform the patient of the finding. Recommend treatment if she is symptomatic. Offer her treatment or definitive testing if she is asymptomatic and desires further intervention.
Predominance of coccobacilli consistent with shift in vaginal flora	The "organism" described is equivalent to a diagnosis of bacterial vaginosis. The Bethesda criteria for this diagnosis include (1) filmy background of small coccobacilli; (2) individual squamous cells covered by a layer of coccobacilli, particularly along the margin of the cell membrane, forming the so-called clue cells; and (3) conspicuous absence of lactobacilli. Compared with Gram stain of vaginal discharge, cervical cytologic test results have a sensitivity of 55% to nearly 90% in most studies. Specificity is in the 98% range when read by a single examiner. The respective positive predictive and negative predictive values are 90–96% and 78–99%.[45–49]	Inform the patient of the finding. Treat high-risk patients. Offer treatment to others. Further testing may be offered but is usually not necessary owing to a high degree of specificity of the Pap smear result compared with wet mount testing.
Bacteria morphologically consistent with *Actinomyces* species	These are best recognized on cytologic smear by branching gram-positive filaments. Their presence is strongly associated with the presence of an intrauterine contraceptive device.[50–52]	Patient management is controversial. If she is asymptomatic, responses range from no intervention to removal of the IUD and treatment with antibiotics. Most recommend doing nothing. For the symptomatic woman, treatment options include removal of the IUD, treatment with antibiotics, or both.
Cellular changes consistent with herpes simplex virus	It can be difficult to distinguish viral alterations from the multinucleation and atypia noted in reactive or neoplastic conditions. Sensitivity of cytologic diagnosis of HSV compared with culture has been reported from 30–80% with specificity in the 85% range.[53–55]	It is essential to report this finding to the patient. Further testing may not be needed if the result is consistent with clinical findings. Further testing may be offered if she is asymptomatic, but even that may not be definitive if viral shedding has ceased. The health care provider must be sensitive to the social implications of acquired HSV infection.

▼ Table 3–3

The Bethesda System: Comments and Recommended Responses to "Infections" *(Continued)*

Organism	Comments	Recommended Response
Other	Evidence of a variety of other organisms may be found on the Pap smear. Amoebae have been found in association with the presence of an IUD, as has *Eubacterium nodatum,* which mimics *Actinomyces.*[56, 57] Rarely, viral inclusion bodies suggestive of cytomegalovirus are found.[58] The presence of *Chlamydia trachomatis* is indicated by characteristic inclusion bodies; the sensitivity and specificity of this finding are unclear.[59]	Although each of these findings should be dealt with on a case-by-case basis, the patient must be informed of the result in all cases. Because of the nature of chlamydia as a sexually transmitted disease, the patient should be treated or re-evaluated if treatment on the basis of the Pap smear is declined.

HSV, herpes simplex virus; IUD, intrauterine device; Pap, Papanicolaou.

Since its creation, this category has been the focus of tremendous controversy. (For a more thorough discussion of the significance of an ASCUS smear, see Chapter 25.) Many pathologists and clinicians have argued for the elimination of the ASCUS category. They argue that the diagnosis is too subjective, poorly reproducible, and over-utilized as part of the practice of defensive medicine. Furthermore, it creates management problems for the clinician, anxiety for the patient, and increased cost for the health care system. Those in favor of the category have argued that a "gray zone" is required to indicate uncertainty and the need for vigilance, especially because almost half of all high-grade lesions are found in this category.[61] A preliminary study suggested that eliminating ASCUS would result in increased reporting of LSIL.[62] Others have suggested that the sensitivity for detecting underlying LSIL and HSIL would also decrease.[63, 64]

> **TBS 2001 recommended the elimination of the ASCUS-FR category. Pap smears that were not negative but did not meet the criteria for SIL would be called atypical squamous cells (ASC) and would be subclassified either as of undetermined significance (ASC-US) or as suggestive of a high-grade SIL (ASC-H).**

TBS 1991 recommended that ASCUS smears be categorized as ASCUS-FR, ASCUS-FN, and ASCUS-NOS. ASCUS-FN is associated with a higher percentage of biopsy-confirmed disease, including high-grade disease, than ASCUS-FR. About 2% of ASCUS-FR are associated with high-grade SIL, compared with 9.5% of ASCUS-NOS and 11.2% of ASCUS-FN.[65] However, because there are so many more smears with ASCUS-FR and ASCUS-NOS, they contain a numerically significant number of high-grade lesions. A new category called ASCUS suggestive of a high-grade SIL lesion accounts for only a small percentage of the total number of ASCUS smears but has a high positive predictive value for underlying high-grade SIL.[66–69] However, in one study, the detection of HPV in women with ASCUS-FR was similar to that in benign cellular changes, and the interobserver reproducibility in classifying ASCUS was relatively poor.[70] Based on this evidence, the participants of TBS 2001 recommended the elimination of the ASCUS-FR category. Pap smears that were not negative but did not meet the criteria for SIL would be called atypical squamous cells (ASC) and would be subclassified either as of undetermined significance (ASC-US) or as suggestive of a high-grade SIL (ASC-H). Smears previously classified as ASCUS-FR would be redistributed into either the negative category or the ASC-US category based on the pathologist's impression.

SQUAMOUS INTRAEPITHELIAL LESIONS

> **Most participants at TBS 2001 felt that regrouping CIN 2 into the LSIL category would lead to widespread confusion among clinicians and might result in overtreatment of LSIL lesions. Therefore, the two-tiered system was retained and CIN 2 was left as part of HSIL.**

TBS 1988 separated SIL into low-grade and high-grade categories. Low-grade lesions encompass the cellular changes associated with HPV cytopathic effect (so-called koilocytotic atypia) and mild dysplasia/CIN 1. High-grade lesions encompass moderate dysplasia, severe dysplasia, and carcinoma in situ/CIN 2–3. Since its adoption in 1988, the two-tiered terminology used by TBS has received widespread criticism. It was argued that the two-tiered terminology is not reproducible[71] and provided less information to clinicians than did the three-tiered CIN terminology (CIN 1, CIN 2, and CIN 3).[72] Many clinicians felt that the natural history of CIN 2 was closer to that of CIN 1 than to that of CIN 3, with which it was paired.[73] Furthermore, many European countries pair CIN 2 with CIN 1 for treatment purposes rather than with CIN

3. However, in the final analysis, most participants at TBS 2001 felt that regrouping CIN 2 into the LSIL category would lead to widespread confusion among clinicians and might result in overtreatment of LSIL lesions. Therefore, the two-tiered system was retained. At the other extreme, some cytologists proposed that koilocytotic atypia be separated from the LSIL category. Several studies have demonstrated lower rates of biopsy-confirmed HSIL in women referred to colposcopy on the basis of Pap smears showing only koilocytotic changes as compared with those showing CIN 1.[74] However, other studies have found that the criteria used to distinguish these two findings are not reproducible. Therefore, no modification was made in TBS 2001 in this regard. Finally, the participants at TBS 2001 supported the concept of adding the phrase "invasion cannot be ruled out" to cases of HSIL in which there is nondiagnostic cytologic evidence of invasion. This was added as a subcategory of squamous epithelial cell abnormalities.

GLANDULAR CELLS

The reporting of glandular abnormalities in TBS 1991[60] has been problematic. Glandular abnormalities were divided into three general categories: cytologically benign endometrial cells in a postmenopausal woman, atypical glandular cells of undetermined significance (AGUS), and adenocarcinoma. AGUS was divided into AGUS favoring a reactive process (AGUS-FR), AGUS favoring a neoplastic process (AGUS-FN), and AGUS not otherwise specified (AGUS-NOS). Whenever possible, adenocarcinoma was classified based on its cell of origin.

TBS 1991 defined AGUS as cells that demonstrate changes that exceed obvious reactive and reparative changes but lack unequivocal features for invasive carcinoma.[60] The problem with this definition is that, unlike squamous disease, which was divided into ASCUS, LSIL, HSIL, and cancer, in TBS 1991 there were no intermediary categories between AGUS and adenocarcinoma. This meant that benign causes of AGUS such as polyps, intrauterine devices, cervical endometriosis, previous cervical conization, tubal metaplasia, inflammatory changes, microglandular hyperplasia, and pregnancy-associated changes were intermixed with low- and high-grade SIL involving glands, adenocarcinoma in situ of the cervix, endometrial hyperplasia, and various cancers whose cytologic appearance did not hint to their malignant histologic origins.[75] Unlike ASCUS, which is found in 3% to 5% of all Pap smears, the incidence of AGUS cytology ranges from 0.1% to 0.4% of all smears.[76–80] Furthermore, unlike ASCUS cytology, there is a very high rate of preinvasive and invasive cancer found among women with AGUS Pap smears.[75–90] Therefore, it is extremely important to evaluate all these patients thoroughly.

A further difficulty is that AGUS cytology is only marginally sensitive in identifying glandular disease. A third to a half of all adenocarcinoma in situ and cervical adenocarcinoma are detected only after evaluation of a squamous cytologic abnormality.[91] These lesions are discovered accidentally at the edge of a squamous intraepithelial lesion.[87, 92] Furthermore, invasive cervical adenocarcinoma may show less marked cytologic abnormalities than glandular dysplasias owing to irregular shedding of abnormal glandular cells, smaller sizes of these lesions, endocervical location of the lesions, and location of lesions at the base of gland crypts that may be blocked by benign metaplasia. In addition to difficulties in identifying and classifying glandular cytological abnormalities, because these lesions are rare, a practicing cytopathologist may not encounter them frequently enough to be familiar with their features.[93] This, coupled with the lack of distinction among glandular abnormalities in TBS 1991, led to a tremendous amount of overcall in cytologic glandular interpretation.

> **TBS 2001 concluded that the criteria for adenocarcinoma in situ have been shown to be predictive and reproducible and recommended that a separate category be established for these findings. Also, because AGUS-FR did not reflect the potential seriousness of the underlying condition in some of these cases and might mislead the clinician into thinking that the changes were inflammatory in origin and required no further evaluation, they recommended that the term AGUS-FR be eliminated.**

A review of the literature shows that 9% to 40% of AGUS Pap smears are associated with SIL, up to 8% of AGUS smears are associated with adenocarcinoma in situ of the cervix, up to 12% are associated with endometrial hyperplasia, and up to 10% are associated with endometrial cancer.[76, 77, 81, 85, 86, 94, 95] When AGUS is subdivided, AGUS-FR and AGUS-NOS are associated with CIN in 22% and 26% of cases, respectively. About half these cases are high-grade lesions. They are associated with adenocarcinoma in situ of the cervix in 1.4% and 2%, respectively, with adenocarcinoma of the cervix in 0% and 2%, respectively, and with endometrial adenocarcinoma in 1.6% and 5%, respectively.[75–90] In contrast, AGUS-FN is associated with CIN in 18% of cases, of which two thirds are high grade, but is associated with adenocarcinoma in situ of the cervix in 48%, endocervical adenocarcinoma in 12%, and endometrial carcinoma in 2%.[75–90] In reviewing this data, TBS 2001 concluded that AGUS-FN was clearly a different and distinguishable cytologic entity that probably represents adenocarcinoma in situ of the endocervix. They felt that the criteria for adenocarcinoma in situ have been shown to be predictive and reproducible and recommended that a separate category be established for these findings.[96] The participants at TBS 2001 further felt that the terminology AGUS-FR did not reflect the potential seriousness of the underlying condition in some of these cases. They thought that the term conveyed to the clinician the impression that the changes were inflammatory in origin and required no further evaluation. Consequently, the term AGUS-FR was eliminated. This left only those smears in which the atypical glandular cells were truly of undetermined significance to be called atypical glandular cells (AGC). Qualifying statements are added to AGC to indicate cellular origin of the atypical cells (endocervical, endometrial, or glandular-NOS).

> **Because data from the literature show that women with benign glandular cells in specimens after hysterectomy rarely developed neoplastic lesions regardless of the history of prior malignancy, TBS 2001 stated that these smears do not warrant an interpretation of AGUS and should be called negative.**

One of the most perplexing cytologic problems in TBS 1991 was the categorization of benign glandular cells in specimens from women after hysterectomy. Questions have been raised about the origin of these cells and their significance in relationship to preneoplastic and neoplastic lesions. These cells were often categorized as AGUS cytology. However, data from the literature show that these patients rarely developed neoplastic lesions regardless of the history of prior malignancy.[97–99] The likely origins of these benign cells include prolapse of the fallopian tube, vaginal endometriosis, fistula, vaginal adenosis not associated with diethylstilbestrol exposure, or glandular metaplasia associated with prior radiation or chemotherapy.[98, 99] TBS 2001 stated that these smears do not warrant an interpretation of AGUS and should be called negative.

> **In recognizing that cervical cytology is an inaccurate test for the detection of endometrial lesions, TBS 2001 removed this finding from the category of epithelial cell abnormalities.**

Finally, TBS 1991 classified cytologically benign endometrial cells in postmenopausal women as a glandular epithelial abnormality. Although endometrial cells in premenopausal women are rarely associated with significant endometrial pathology and as such need not be reported,[100–102] historically, benign-appearing endometrial cells were considered a harbinger of endometrial pathology in postmenopausal women, warranting endometrial sampling. This was thought to be a way of identifying the small proportion of women with endometrial carcinoma who are asymptomatic. In recognizing that cervical cytology is an inaccurate test for the detection of endometrial lesions, TBS 2001 removed this finding from the category of epithelial cell abnormalities. Cytologically benign endometrial cells in a woman older than 40 years are reported in their own category (neither epithelial cell abnormality nor negative). The decision on follow-up of these smears is left to the clinician.

SUMMARY OF KEY POINTS

- The current cervical cytologic terminology, TBS, was the result of the work of an expert panel that convened in 1988 under the auspices of the National Cancer Institute. It was revised in 1991 and again in 2001.

- TBS replaced three levels of CIN with two levels: low- and high-grade intraepithelial lesions that were not specific for the cervix.

- The designation of satisfactory for evaluation implies that the cytologic sample is technically interpretable and of proper cellular composition.

- The category of satisfactory for evaluation but limited was eliminated by TBS 2001. Instead, these smears are called satisfactory and a comment is added about obscuring factors.

- The category unsatisfactory for evaluation implies that the smear is unreadable for one of the following reasons: the slide is broken, patient identification is lacking, there is obscuration of 75% or more of the epithelial cells, or there is scant cellularity. The most common reason for unsatisfactory smears is scant cellularity, followed by obscuring inflammation or blood.

- The category of benign cellular changes was eliminated by TBS 2001. Instead, these smears were shifted to either the negative category (no evidence of intraepithelial lesion) or the atypical squamous cells category.

- The diagnosis of ASCUS in TBS 1991 was too subjective, poorly reproducible, and overutilized as part of the practice of defensive medicine. Furthermore, it created management problems for the clinician, anxiety for the patient, and increased cost for the health care system.

- TBS 2001 eliminated the ASCUS-FR category. Pap smears that were not negative but did not meet the criteria for SIL would be called atypical squamous cells (ASC) and would be subclassified either as of undetermined significance (ASC-US) or as suggestive of a high-grade SIL (ASC-H).

- Most participants at TBS 2001 felt that regrouping CIN 2 into the LSIL category would lead to widespread confusion among clinicians and may result in overtreatment of LSIL lesions. Therefore, the two-tiered system was retained and CIN 2 was left as part of HSIL.

Continued on following page

- TBS 2001 added the phrase "invasion cannot be ruled out" to cases of HSIL in which there is nondiagnostic cytologic evidence of invasion.

- The problem with the TBS 1991 definition of AGUS is that, unlike squamous disease, which was divided into ASCUS, LSIL, HSIL, and cancer, there were no intermediary categories between AGUS and adenocarcinoma. This meant that benign causes of AGUS were intermixed with premalignant and malignant causes.

- The criteria for adenocarcinoma in situ have been shown to be predictive and reproducible, so TBS 2001 established a separate category for these findings.

- Because AGUS-FR did not reflect the potential seriousness of the underlying condition and might mislead clinicians, TBS 2001 eliminated that term.

- Because data from the literature show that women with benign glandular cells in specimens after hysterectomy rarely developed neoplastic lesions regardless of the history of prior malignancy, TBS 2001 stated that these smears do not warrant an interpretation of AGUS and should be called negative.

References

1. Davey DD, Nielson ML, Rosenstock W, et al: Terminology and specimen adequacy in cervicovaginal cytology: The College of American Pathologists Interlaboratory Comparison Program Experience. Arch Pathol Lab Med 1992;116:903.
2. Koss LG: The New Bethesda System for reporting results of smears of the uterine cervix. J Natl Cancer Inst 1990;82:988.
3. Wilkinson EJ: Pap smears and screening for cervical neoplasia. Clin Obstet Gynecol 1990;33:817.
4. National Cancer Institute Workshop: The 1988 Bethesda System for reporting cervical/vaginal cytological diagnoses. JAMA 1989; 262:931.
5. Kurman RJ, Malkasian GD Jr, Sedlis A, et al: Clinical commentary. From Papanicolaou to Bethesda: The rationale for a new cervical cytologic classification. Obstet Gynecol 1991;77:779.
6. Herbst AL: Editorial: The Bethesda System for cervical/vaginal cytologic diagnoses: A note of caution. Obstet Gynecol 1990;76:449.
7. Ransdell JS, Davey DD, Zaleski S: Clinicopathologic correlation of the unsatisfactory Papanicolaou smear. Cancer 1997;81:139.
8. Davey DD, Woodhouse S, Styer P, et al: Atypical epithelial cells and specimen adequacy: Current laboratory practices of participants in the college of American pathologists interlaboratory comparison program in cervicovaginal cytology. Arch Path Lab Med 2000;124:203.
9. Papillo JL: Unpublished survey of ASC members reported at TBS 2001.
10. Davey DD, Woodhouse S, Styer P, et al: Atypical epithelial cells and specimen adequacy: Current laboratory practice: The College of American Pathologists interlaboratory comparison program in cytology. Arch Pathol Lab Med 2000;124:203.
11. Mitchell H, Medley G: Differences between Papanicolaou smears with correct and incorrect diagnoses. Cytopathology 1995;6:368.
12. O'Sullivan JP, A'Hern RP, Chapman PA, et al: A case-control study of true-positive versus false-negative cervical smears in women with cervical intraepithelial neoplasia (CIN) III. Cytopathology 1998;9:155.
13. Mintzer MP, Curtis P, Resnick JC, Morrell D: The effect of the quality of Papanicolaou smears on the detection of cytologic abnormalities. Cancer Cytopathol 1999;87:113.
14. Kristensen GB, Skyggebjerg KD, Hølund B, et al: Analysis of cervical smears obtained within three years of the diagnosis of invasive cervical cancer. Acta Cytologica 1991;35:47.
15. Elias A, Linthorst G, Bekker B, et al: The significance of endocervical cells in the diagnosis of cervical epithelial changes. Acta Cytologica 1983;27:225.
16. Vooijs PG, Elias A, van der Graaf Y, et al: Relationship between the diagnosis of epithelial abnormalities and the composition of cervical smears. Acta Cytologica 1985;29:323.
17. Kivlahan C, Ingram E: Papanicolaou smears without endocervical cells. Are they inadequate? Acta Cytologica 1986;30:258.
18. Mitchell H, Medley G: Longitudinal study of women with negative cervical smears according to endocervical status. Lancet 1991; 337:265.
19. Cox JT. ASCCP practice guidelines: Management issues related to quality of the smear. J Lower Genital Tract Dis 1997;1:100.
20. Wilkinson EJ: ASCCP practice guidelines: Management guidelines for follow-up of cytology interpreted as benign cellular changes on Papanicolaou smear of the cervix or vagina. J Lower Genital Tract Dis 2000;4:93.
21. Eckert LO, Koutsky LA, Kiviat NB, et al: The inflammatory Papanicolaou smear: What does it mean? Obstet Gynecol 1995;86: 360.
22. Mali B, Joshi J: Interpreting inflammatory changes in cervical smears. BMJ. 1993;307:383.
23. Wilson JD, Robinson AJ, Kinghorn SA, et al: Implications of inflammatory changes on cervical cytology. BMJ 1990;300:638.
24. Edwards SK, Sonnex C: Influence of genital infection on cervical cytology. Sex Transm Infect 1998;74:271.
25. Singh V, Gupta MM, Latyanarayana L, et al: Association between reproductive tract infections and cervical inflammatory epithelial changes. Sex Transm Dis 1994;25.
26. Kelly BA, Black AS: The inflammatory cervical smear: A study in general practice. Br J Gen Pract 1990;238:240.
27. Bertolino JG, Rangel JE, Blake RL, et al: Inflammation on the cervical Papanicolaou smear: The predictive value for infection in asymptomatic women. Clin Res Method 1992;24:447.
28. Dimian C, Nayagam M, Bradbeer C: The association between sexually transmitted diseases and inflammatory cervical cytology. Genitourin Med 1992;68:305.
29. Parsons WL, Godwin M, Robbins C, et al: Prevalence of cervical pathogens in women with and without inflammatory changes on smear testing. BMJ 1993;306:1173.
30. Schwebke JR, Zajackowski ME: Effect of concurrent lower genital tract infections on cervical cancer screening. Genitourin Med 1997;73:383.
31. Lawley TB, Lee RB, Kapela R: The significance of moderate and severe inflammation on class I Papanicolaou smear. Obstet Gynecol 1990;76:997.
32. Parashari A, Singh V, Gupta MM, et al: Significance of inflammatory cervical smears. APMIS 1995;103:273.
33. McLachlan N, Patwardhan JR, Ayer B, et al: Management of suboptimal cytologic smears: Persistent inflammatory smears. Acta Cytologica 1994;38:531.
34. Seçkin NC, Turhan NÖ, Özmen Ş, et al: Routine colposcopic evaluation of patients with persistent inflammatory cellular changes on Pap smear. Int J Gynecol Obstet 1997;59:25.
35. Davey DD, Gallion H, Jennings CD: DNA cytometry in postirradiation cervical-vaginal smears. Hum Pathol 1992;23:1027.
36. Frierson HF. Jr, Covell JL, Andersen WA: Radiation changes in endocervical cells in brush specimens. Diagn Cytopathol 1990;6: 243.
37. Shield PW: Chronic radiation effects: A correlative study of smears and biopsies from the cervix and vagina. Diagn Cytopathol 1995;13:107.
38. Kaplan B, Orvieto R, Hirsch M, et al: The impact of intrauterine

contraceptive devices on cytological findings from routine Pap smear testing. Eur J Contracept Reprod Health Care 1998;3:75.

39. Pillay B, Gregory ARA, Subbiah M: Cytopathologic changes associated with intrauterine contraceptive devices: A review of cervicovaginal smears in 350 women. Med J Malaysia 1994;49:74.

40. Kreiger JN, Tam MR, Stevens CE, et al: Diagnosis of trichomoniasis: Comparison of conventional wet-mount examination with cytologic studies, cultures, and monoclonal antibody staining of direct specimens. JAMA 1988;259:1223.

41. Paterson BA, Tabrizi SN, Garland SM, et al: The tampon test for trichomoniasis: A comparison between conventional methods and a polymerase chain reaction for *Trichomonas vaginalis* in women. Sex Transm Infect 1998;74:136.

42. Weinberger MW, Harger JH: Accuracy of the Papanicolaou smear in the diagnosis of asymptomatic infection with *Trichomonas vaginalis*. Obstet Gynecol 1993;82:425.

43. Shurbaji MS, Burja IT, Sawyer WL: Clinical significance of identifying Candida on cervicovaginal (Pap) smears. Diagn Cytopathol 1999;21:14.

44. Donders GGG, van Straeten D, Hooft P, et al: Detection of *Candida* cell forms in Pap smears during pregnancy. Eur J Obstet Gynecol Reprod Biol 1992;43:13.

45. Davis JD, Connor EE, Clark P, et al: Correlation between cervical results and Gram stain as diagnostic tests for bacterial vaginosis. Am J Obstet Gynecol 1997;177:532.

46. Giacomini G, Calcinai A, Moreti D, et al: Accuracy of cervical/vaginal cytology in the diagnosis of bacterial vaginosis. Sex Transm Dis 1998;25:24.

47. Lamont RF, Hudson EA, Hay PE, et al: A comparison of the use of Papanicolaou-stained cervical cytological smears with Gram-stained vaginal smears for the diagnosis of bacterial vaginosis in early pregnancy. Int J STD AIDS 1999;10:93.

48. Platz-Christensen JJ, Larsson PG, Sundstrom E, et al: Detection of bacterial vaginosis in wet mount, Papanicolaou stained vaginal smears and in gram stained smears. Acta Obstet Gynecol Scand 1995;74:67.

49. Prey M: Routine Pap smears for the diagnosis of bacterial vaginosis. Diagn Cytopathol 1998;21:10.

50. Fiorino AS: Reviews—intrauterine contraceptive device-associated actinomycotic abscess and actinomyces detection on cervical smear. Obstet Gynecol 1996;87:142.

51. Lippes J: Pelvic actinomycosis: A review and preliminary look at prevalence. Am J Obstet Gynecol 1999;180:265.

52. Perlow JH, Wigton T, Yordan EL, et al: Disseminated pelvic actinomycosis presenting as metastatic carcinoma: Association with the Progestasert intrauterine device. Rev Infect Dis 1991;13:1115.

53. Ashley RL: Laboratory techniques in the diagnosis of herpes simplex infection. Geritourin Med 1993;69:174.

54. Masood S, Hosein I, Pitcher M, et al: Potential value of immunoperoxidase technique in assessment of genital herpes. J Fla Med Assoc 1990;77:516.

55. Maccato ML, Kaufman RH: Herpes genitalis. Dermatol Clin 1992;10:415.

56. Arroyo G, Quinn JA: Association of amoebae and *Actinomyces* in an intrauterine contraceptive device user. Acta Cytologica 1989;33:298.

57. Hill GB: *Eubacterium nodatum* mimics *Actinomyces* in intrauterine device: Associated infections and other settings within the female genital tract. Obstet Gynecol 1992;79:534.

58. Gideon K, Zaharopoulou P: Cytomegalovirus endocervicitis diagnosed by cervical smear. Diagn Cytopathol 1991;7:625.

59. Reyes-Maldonado E, Diáz-Fuente LA, González-Bonilla CV, et al: Detection of *Chlamydia trachomatis* by immunofluorescence, Papanicolaou and immunoperoxidase in women with leucorrhea. Rev Latinam Microbiol 1996;38:65.

60. National Cancer Institute Workshop: The Bethesda System for reporting cervical/vaginal cytologic diagnoses. Acta Cytol 1993;37:115.

61. Kinney WK, Manos MM, Hurley LB, Ransley JE: Where's the high-grade cervical neoplasia? The importance of minimally abnormal Papanicolaou diagnoses. Obstet Gynecol 1998;91:973.

62. Cahill LA, Brainard JA, Frable WJ: Life without ASCUS: The cytotechnologist's and cytopathologist's perspective. Acta Cytol 2000;44:853.

63. Setzer C, Flynn K, Clark I, Rimm DL: Atypical squamous cells of

undetermined significance (ASCUS): Who needs it? Acta Cytol 2000;44:853.

64. Pitman MB, Cibas ES, Powers CN, Frable WJ: Consequences of eliminating ASCUS. Mod Pathol 2001;14:143A.

65. Manos MM, Kinney WK, Hurley LB, et al: Identifying women with cervical neoplasia: Using human papillomavirus DNA testing for equivocal Papanicolaou results. JAMA 1999;281:1605.

66. Quddus MR, Sung CJ, Steinhoff MM, et al: Atypical squamous metaplastic cells. Cancer Cytopathol 2001;93:16.

67. Schoolland M, Sterrett GF, Knowles SAS, et al: The "inconclusive–possible high grade epithelial abnormality" category in Papanicolaou smear reporting. Cancer Cytopathol 1998;84:208.

68. Sherman ME, Kelly D: High-grade squamous intraepithelial lesions and invasive carcinoma following the report of three negative Papanicolaou smears: Screening failures or rapid progression? Mod Pathol 1992;5:337.

69. Hatem F, Wilbur DC: High-grade squamous intraepithelial lesions following negative Papanicolaou smears: False negative cervical cytology rapid progression. Diagn Cytopathol 1995;12:135.

70. Woodhouse SL, Stastny JF, Styer PE, et al: Interobserver variability in subclassification of squamous intraepithelial lesions: Results of the American Pathologists Interlaboratory Comparison Program in Cervicovaginal Cytology. Arch Pathol Lab Med 1999;123:1079.

71. Crum CP, Genest DR, Krane J, et al: Subclassifying atypical squamous cells in ThinPrep cervical cytology correlates with detection of high-risk human papillomavirus DNA. Am J Clin Pathol 1999;112:384.

72. Pinto AP, Crum CP: Natural history of cervical neoplasia: Defining progression and its consequences. Clin Obstet Gynecol 2000;43:352.

73. Selvaggi SM: Is it time to revisit the classification system for cervicovaginal pathology? Arch Pathol Lab Med 1999;123:993.

74. Lonky NM, Sadeghi M, Tzadik GW, Pettiti D: The clinical significance of the poor correlation of cervical dysplasia and cervical malignancy with referral cytologic results. Am J Obstet Gynecol 1999;181:560.

75. Lee KR, Manna EA, St. John T: Atypical endocervical glandular cells: Accuracy of cytology diagnosis. Diagn Cytopathol 1995;13:202.

76. Eddy GL, Stumpf KB, Wojtowycz MA, et al: Biopsy findings in five hundred thirty one patients with atypical glandular cells of uncertain significance as defined by the Bethesda System. Am J Obstet Gynecol 1997;177:1188.

77. Goff BA, Atanasoff P, Brown E, et al: Endocervical glandular atypia in Papanicolaou smears. Obstet Gynecol 1992;79:101.

78. Kim TJ, Kim HS, Park CT, et al: Clinical evaluation of follow-up methods and results of atypical glandular cells of undetermined significance (AGUS) detected on cervicovaginal pap smears. Gynecol Oncol 1999;73:292.

79. Manetta A, Keefe K, Lin F, et al: Atypical glandular cells of undetermined significance in cervical cytologic findings. Am J Obstet Gynecol 1999;180:883.

80. Raab SS, Isacson C, Layfield LJ, et al: Atypical glandular cells of undetermined significance: Cytologic criteria to separate clinically significant from benign lesions. Am J Clin Pathol 1995;104:574.

81. Nasu I, Meurer W, Fu YS: Endocervical glandular atypia and adenocarcinoma: A correlation of cytology and histology. Int J Gynecol Pathol 1993;12:208.

82. Raab SS, Snider TE, Potts SA, et al: Atypical glandular cells of undetermined significance: Diagnostic accuracy and interobserver variability using select cytologic criteria. Am J Clin Pathol 1997;107:299.

83. Ronnette B, Manos MM, Ransley JE, et al: Atypical glandular cells of undetermined significance (AGUS): Cytopathologic features, histopathologic results, and human papillomavirus DNA detection. Hum Pathol 1999;30:816.

84. Schindler S, Pooley RJ, De Frias DVS, et al: Follow-up of atypical glandular cells in cervical-endocervical smears. Ann Diagn Pathol 1998;312.

85. Taylor RR, Guerrieri JP, Nash JD, et al: Atypical cervical cytology: Colposcopic follow-up using the Bethesda System. J Reprod Med 1993;38:443.

86. Veljovich DS, Stoler MH, Andersen WA, et al: Atypical glandular cells of undetermined significance: A five-year retrospective histopathologic study. Am J Obstet Gynecol 1998;179:382.

87. Korn AP, Judson PL, Zaloudek CJ: The importance of atypical glandular cells of uncertain significance in cervical cytology smear. J Reprod Med 1998;43:774.

88. Burja IT, Thompson SK, Sawyer WL, Shurbaji MS: Atypical glandular cells of undetermined significance in cervical smear. Acta Cytol 1999;43:351.

89. Gornall RJ, Singh N, Noble W, et al: Glandular abnormalities on cervical smear: A study to compare the accuracy of cytologic diagnosis with underlying pathology. Eur J Gynaecol Oncol 2000; 21:49.

90. Roberts JM, Thurloe JK, Bowditch RC, et al: Comparison of ThinPrep and Pap smear in relation to prediction of adenocarcinoma in situ. Acta Cytol 1999;43:74.

91. Wilbur DC: Endocervical glandular atypia: A new problem for the cytologist. Diagn Cytopathol 1995;13:463.

92. Maini M, Lavie O, Comeerci G, et al: The management and followup of patients with high-grade cervical glandular intraepithelial neoplasia. Int J Gynecol Cancer 1988;8:287.

93. Mody DR: Agonizing over AGUS. Cancer 1999;87:243.

94. Kennedy AW, Salmieri SS, Wierth SL, et al: Results of the clinical evaluation of atypical glandular cells of undetermined signifi-

95. Zweizig S, Noller K, Real EF, et al: Neoplasia associated with atypical glandular cells of undetermined significance on cervical cytology. Gynecol Oncol 1997;65:314.

96. Solomon DS, Frable WJ, Vooijs GP, et al: ASCUS and AGUS criteria: IAC Task Force Summary. Acta Cytol 1998;42:16.

97. Ponder TB, Easley KO, Davila RM: Glandular cells in vaginal smears from posthysterectomy women. Acta Cytol 1997;41:1701.

98. Tambouret R, Pitman MB, Bell DA: Benign glandular cells in posthysterectomy vaginal smears. Acta Cytol 1998;42:1403.

99. Ramirez MC, Sastry LK, Pisharodi, LR: Benign glandular and squamous metaplastic-like cells seen in vaginal Pap smears of posthysterectomy patients: Incidence and patient profile. Eur J Gynaecol Oncol 2000;21:43.

100. Gray J, Nguyen GK: Cytologic detection of endometrial pathology by Pap smears. Diagn Cytopathol 1999;20:181.

101. Gondos B, King EB: Significance of endometrial cells in cervico-vaginal smears. Ann Clin Lab Sci 1977;7:486.

102. Ng ABP, Reagan JW, Hawliczek S, et al: Significance of endometrial cells in the detection of endometrial carcinoma and its precursors. Acta Cytol 1974;18:356.

cance (AGCUS) detected on cervical cytology screening. Gynecol Oncol 1996;63:14.

 B

• Cynda Johnson

Conventional Cytology

FREQUENCY OF PAP SMEAR TESTING

There is no overriding consensus about the most optimal frequency of cytologic screening.

As demonstrated in Table 3–4, an increased frequency of cytologic sampling can result in a greater reduction in the cumulative rate of invasive cervical cancer. Many factors, especially cost-effectiveness, are considered for any group's statement on the optimal frequency of sampling within a target population. Controversy over the optimal interval for cervical cytology led to a 1987 joint statement from the American Cancer Society and the American College of Obstetricians and Gynecologists: "All women who are, or have been, sexually active, or have reached age 18, should have an annual Pap test and pelvic examination. After a woman has had three or more consecutive satisfactory examinations, the Pap test may be performed less frequently at the discretion of her physician." Table 3–5[1] describes factors that might place a woman at high risk for an abnormal Pap smear and thus in a group where annual Pap testing should probably be continued. Although many health care professionals would like more guidance, no other overriding consensus exists at this time.

▼ Table 3–4

Percentage Reduction in Cumulative Rate of Invasive Cervical Cancer with Different Frequencies of Screening (Age Range 35–65 Years)*

Screening Frequency (yr)	Reduction in Cumulative Rate (%)	No. of Tests
1	93.3	30
2	92.5	15
3	91.4	10
5	83.9	6
10	64.2	3

* Assuming the screen occurs at age 35 years and that a previous screen was performed.

Data from IARC Working Group: Screening for Cancer of the Uterine Cervix. Lyon, France, Internation Agency for Research on Cancer, 1986, p 141.

Several groups have rendered an opinion about further cytologic sampling in the group of women who have undergone a total hysterectomy. Before 1995, only the Canadian Task Force had a position statement on Pap testing after hysterectomy. They concluded that "women who have had a hysterectomy for benign conditions with adequate pathology documentation that the cervical epithelium has been totally removed, and with known previously normal smears, do not need to be screened."[2] In

▼ Table 3–5

Risk Factors for Abnormal Papanicolaou Smear

Exposure to diethylstilbestrol in utero	History of human papillomavirus
History of abnormal Papanicolaou smear	Partner with history of human papillomavirus
Initiation of early sexual activity	Promiscuous male partner
More than one sexual partner (ever)	Illicit drug use
	Smoking habit
History of sexually transmitted disease	Infection with human immunodeficiency virus

1995, Piscitelli et al studied a 10-year retrospective cohort of 697 patients after hysterectomy for benign conditions. Over 9074 woman-years, only 33 abnormal smears were found, of which only 2 were clinically significant. The authors concluded that the low incidence of vaginal dysplasia and carcinoma, combined with the high false-positive rate, supported decreasing the number of smears performed in low-risk women.[3] Pearce et al came to a similar conclusion the following year.[4]

> **There is insufficient evidence to recommend routine vaginal smear screening in women after total hysterectomy for benign disease.**

In the same year, Fetters et al reviewed the literature from English language studies published between 1966 and 1995. They concluded that there were conflicting guidelines on screening after hysterectomy and conflicting data on the risk of vaginal carcinoma after total hysterectomy for benign disease. They concluded that the best-designed research showed no association. In summary, there was insufficient evidence to recommend routine vaginal smear screening in women after total hysterectomy for benign disease.[5]

Finally, in 1999, Fox et al reported that in 5330 smears from a group of hysterectomized women 50 years of age and older, only 9 smears were abnormal. Eight of the nine showed atypical squamous cells of undetermined significance (ASCUS), and one was read as LSIL.[6]

The preponderance of evidence would suggest that woman who have had a total hysterectomy for benign disease do not need further Pap smear testing. Of course, women who have had a supracervical hysterectomy should be tested according to guidelines for nonhysterectomized women.

SAMPLE COLLECTION

> **The cytologic sample should not be collected during the menstrual period.**

Timing

The cytologic sample should not be collected during menses. The patient should avoid vaginal medications, vaginal contraceptives, or douches during the 48 hours before the appointment, and intercourse is not recommended on the night before or the day of the examination.

From the standpoint of obtaining ideal cytology, postpartum Pap smears should not be performed until at least 6 or even 8 weeks after delivery, by which time the cervix has undergone reparative changes, less inflammation is present, and fewer smears will be reported as less than satisfactory.[7] Because of practical constraints relating to a woman's need to see her health care provider to obtain contraception, postpartum visits are often scheduled earlier and the Pap smear is sometimes suboptimal.

If the woman is postmenopausal and previous smears have lacked endocervical cells or have demonstrated atrophy with inflammation, the cervix may be primed with 3 weeks of treatment with intravaginal estrogen cream followed by repeat cytologic sampling.

Technique

Use of a combination of the Ayre spatula for sampling the ectocervix and a brush for sampling the endocervix has been shown to be superior to other techniques for obtaining a conventional Pap smear.[8–13] This combination results in samples that are more likely to be satisfactory for interpretation, with adequate cellularity and an endocervical component, than those prepared using other sampling devices. Different techniques vary in their ability to collect squamous and endocervical cells and to transfer a representative sample onto the glass slide. These differences may make one collection technique (Ayre spatula and cytobrush) more appropriate for conventional cytology, whereas another (broom device) is more appropriate for liquid-based cytology. (See Chapter 3C for a more detailed discussion of this subject.)

> **The quality of the smear can be improved by using the spatula first, followed by the endocervical brush, because fewer smears will be obscured by blood.**

The quality of the smear can be improved by using the spatula first, followed by the endocervical brush, because fewer smears will be obscured by blood.[14] The spatula is first placed at the cervical os, using the end that best conforms to the cervical anatomy. It is rotated 360 degrees about the circumference of the os, maintaining contact with the ectocervix. Optimally, the sample is held and smeared on the slide after the endocervical sample is collected because the slide must be fixed immediately; only a single slide is then needed for both samples. Both sides of the spatula should be smeared on the slide.

The brush is then inserted into the os and rotated 180 degrees, maintaining contact with the cervical canal. If the canal is quite narrow, simply inserting and removing the brush or rotating it only a quarter of a turn may collect sufficient cells. Rotating the brush more than 180 degrees increases the likelihood of bleeding. Similarly, the brush should be inserted along the axis of the cervix. Inserting the brush at an angle to the endocervical canal will drive it into the delicate endocervical stroma, traumatizing it and causing bleeding. The sample is unrolled onto the slide in the opposite direction from which it was collected by twirling the handle of the brush

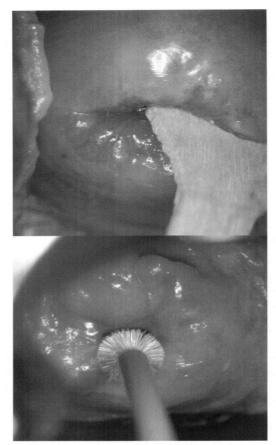

Figure 3–5. Cervical sampling with spatula and brush.

(Figs. 3–5 and 3–6). Although blood is often seen macroscopically on the brush, it rarely interferes with the interpretation of the specimen. The manufacturer of the endocervical brush originally cautioned against its use in

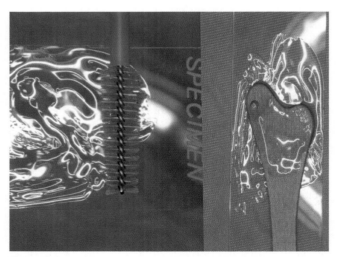

Figure 3–6. To transfer cervical material to the slide for a spatula, smear the sample with a single stroke using moderate pressure to thin out clumps of cells and mucus. Excessive force or manipulation will damage cells. To transfer material from a brush, roll the bristles across the slide by twirling the brush handle.

pregnancy, but its safety and improved Pap smear adequacy over other techniques have been confirmed during pregnancy.[15]

EVALUATION OF THE CONVENTIONAL PAP SMEAR AS A SCREENING TECHNIQUE

The U.S. Preventive Services Task Force has given cytologic screening an "A" recommendation even though there are no randomized trials demonstrating its effectiveness.

The incidence of cervical cancer in the United States has declined from 44 cases per 100,000 women in 1947 to fewer than 8 cases per 100,000. Much of the credit for this decline goes to detection of premalignant disease by organized Pap smear screening programs. The incidence of cervical cancer and mortality decreased 40% after 1973, when mass screening was initiated. It is significant that the U.S. Preventive Services Task Force has given Pap screening an "A" recommendation even though there are no randomized trials demonstrating its effectiveness. However, problems remain. The sensitivity of conventional cytology is low for a screening test, but it was not known how low it was until more recently.

Based on a meta-analysis of 84 appropriately designed and conducted studies, the Agency for Health Care Policy and Research reported that conventional cytology has a specificity of 98% and a sensitivity of 51%.

The Agency for Health Care Policy and Research (AHCPR), through its evidence-based centers, sponsored the development of an evidence-based report on the evaluation of cervical cytology.[16] The report compared new technologies for cervical cytological screening with conventional cytology screening with respect to diagnostic accuracy, costs, and effectiveness in adult women of average cervical cancer risk. The study was based on published literature. On the basis of 84 studies that met quality criteria, conventional cytology screening has a specificity of 98% (95% confidence interval [CI]; 97% to 99%) and a sensitivity of 51% (95% CI; 37% to 66%). The report stressed that the accuracy is increased when the goal is detection of higher-grade lesions (HSIL) as opposed to LSIL or ASCUS. Higher disease prevalence is also associated with greater sensitivity but reduced specificity.

Although the federal government under CLIA has required that 10% of cytologic smears be rescreened, there has been only limited reduction in the false-negative rate of the Pap smear.

It has become clear that the sensitivity of conventional cytology is even lower than traditionally recognized. Suggestions have been offered that practitioners and cytologists alike strive to achieve ideal conditions when taking and processing a Pap smear to reduce the rate of false negativity. Overt lesions should be biopsied without regard for the cytology results.[17] The Federal government under the Clinical Laboratory Improvement Act (CLIA) has required that 10% of smears be rescreened, but this has resulted in only limited reduction in the rate of false-negative smears.[18]

In 1997, an international Task Force on Cell Preparation Methods and Criteria for Sample Adequacy reported that inadequate sampling and inappropriate sample transfer through traditional methods are the major causes of false-negative results, accounting for approximately 50% of missed significant lesions.[19] The finding that, with conventional cytology, much of the cell sample remains on the collection instrument has been a major impetus to study the liquid-based preparation techniques described later in this chapter.

DeMay reviewed studies of false-negative smears in patients who were later found to have cervical cancer. Errors were often related to the presence of few, bland-appearing, or small abnormal cells. Others were related to the cytologist offering an interpretation of a smear that on rescreening should have been read as unsatisfactory or limited in its acceptability for interpretation. Cells with tissue fragments rather than single cells also resulted in false-negative interpretation.[20]

The greatest success of TBS may be the elimination of the unsatisfactory smear from interpretation by those who adhere to careful criteria.

The greatest success of TBS may be the elimination of the unsatisfactory smear from interpretation by those who adhere to careful criteria. In a study by Spires, the interobserver agreement for an unsatisfactory smear was very good. On the other hand, interobserver agreement was only fair for smears read as satisfactory, but limited. The greatest variability was in the definition of adequate minimum cellularity and in the estimation of the number of cells obscured.[21]

Despite this success, the rate of false negativity cannot be reduced beyond a certain level. Quality assurance studies indicate that skilled screening cytologists have an irreducible false-negative fraction of at least 5%.[22] The Pap stain renders certain tumor types, such as lymphomas and sarcomas, harder to diagnose. Cells from necrotic tumors may not be recognizable, and certain small or bland-appearing cells may be overlooked. Sampling might still miss lesions if they are small or eccentric on the cervix or high in endocervical canal. Given these sources of error, the greatest sensitivity that can be expected is in the range of 90%.[23]

In addition to evaluating diagnostic accuracy of conventional cytology, the AHCPR addressed the cost of Pap testing to determine the cost-effectiveness of the procedure.[16] For women 20 to 64 years of age, the total cost (including office visit cost and processing cost) in 1997 dollars was $38.68. The estimate was higher for women 65 years and older at $47.73, unless Medicare reimbursement was considered, which reduced the amount to $35.01.

According to the AHCPR, improved sensitivity on initial screening or rescreening can result in an acceptable cost per life saved at 3-year Pap screening intervals.

Estimate of cost-effectiveness of conventional cytology screening every 3 years compared with no Pap screening was $4097 per life-year saved. If the false-negative rate were reduced by 60% at a technology cost of $10 per slide, the cost per life-year saved would increase to $22,010 but would rise to more than $50,000 with more frequent screening intervals. If the false-negative rate were reduced by 85%, with technology applied to rescreening of all Pap smears initially read as negative, with an incremental cost per slide of $10 and Pap screening every 3 years, the cost per life-year saved would be $45,375. According to the AHCPR, either approach—improved sensitivity on initial screening or rescreening as described—can result in an acceptable cost per life saved at 3-year Pap screening intervals.[16] The current challenge is to assess the new technologies to determine which, if any, will become part of the new standard of care in screening for cervical cancer.

SUMMARY OF KEY POINTS

- An increased frequency of cytologic sampling can result in a greater reduction in the cumulative rate of invasive cervical cancer. There is, however, no overriding consensus about how often sampling should be performed.

- There is insufficient evidence in the literature to recommend routine vaginal sampling in women who have undergone hysterectomy for benign disease. Women who have had a supracervical hysterectomy should be tested according to the recommendations for nonhysterectomized women.

- Women should avoid use of intravaginal medication and douches during the 48 hours before cytologic sampling and should not engage in sexual intercourse the night before or the day of the examination.

- For conventional cytology, use of both the Ayre spatula and the endocervical brush results in samples that are more likely than those prepared using other sampling devices to be satisfactory for interpretation, with adequate cellularity including an endocervical component.

- It has been shown that the sensitivity of the Pap test is lower than traditionally thought. The AHCPR report demonstrated that the conventional smear has a sensitivity of 51% (95% CI; 37% to 66%) and a specificity of 98% (95% CI; 97% to 99%). The accuracy of conventional cytology is increased when the goal is detection of higher-

Continued on following page

grade lesions. Higher disease prevalence is also associated with greater sensitivity but reduced specificity.

• Inadequate sampling and sample transfer by traditional methods are the major causes of false-negative results, accounting for approximately 50% of missed significant lesions.

References

1. Fink DJ: Changes in ACS checkup guidelines for the detection of cervical cancer. CA Cancer J Clin 1988;38:127.
2. Mandelblatt J: Papanicolaou testing following hysterectomy. Questions and answers. JAMA 1991;266:1289.
3. Piscitelli JT, Bastian LA, Wilkes A, et al: Cytologic screening after hysterectomy for benign disease. Am J Obstet Gynecol 1995;173:424.
4. Pearce KF, Haefner HK, Sarwar SF, et al: Cytopathological findings on vaginal Papanicolaou smears after hysterectomy for benign gynecologic disease. N Engl J Med 1996;335:1559.
5. Fetters MD, Fischer G, Reed BD: Effectiveness of vaginal Papanicolaou smear screening after total hysterectomy for benign disease. JAMA 1996;275:940.
6. Fox J, Remington P, Layde P, et al: The effect of hysterectomy on the risk of an abnormal screening Papanicolaou test result. Am J Obstet Gynecol 1999;180:1104.
7. Rarick TL, Tchabo JG: Timing of the postpartum Papanicolaou smear. Obstet Gynecol 1994;83:761.
8. Boon ME, de Graaff JC, Rietveld WJ: Analysis of five sampling methods for the preparation of cervical smears. Acta Cytologica 1989;33:843.
9. Koonings PP, Dickinson K, d'Ablaing G III, et al: A randomized clinical trial comparing the cytobrush and cotton swab for Papanicolaou smears. Obstet Gynecol 1992;80:241.
10. Murata PJ, Johnson RA, McNicoll KE: Controlled evaluation of implementing the cytobrush technique to improve Papanicolaou smear quality. Obstet Gynecol 1990;75:690.
11. Reissman SE: Comparison of two Papanicolaou smear techniques in a family practice setting. J Fam Pract 1988;26:525.
12. Ruffin MT IV, Van Noord GR: Improving the yield of endocervical elements in a Pap smear with the use of the cytology brush. Fam Med 1991;23:365.
13. Toffler WL, Pluedeman CK, Sinclair AE, et al: Comparative cytologic yield and quality of three Pap smear instruments. Clin Res Method 1993;25:403.
14. Eisenberger D, Hernandez E, Tener T, et al: Order of endocervical and ectocervical cytologic sampling and the quality of the Papanicolaou smear. Obstet Gynecol 1997;90:755.
15. Paraiso MFR, Brady K, Helmchen R, et al: Evaluation of the endocervical cytobrush and cervex-brush in pregnant women. Obstet Gynecol 1994;84:539.
16. Agency for Healthcare Policy and Research: Evidence Report/Technology Assessment, Number 5. Evaulation of Cervical Cytology. Maryland, AHCPR Publication No. 99-E010, February 1999.
17. Featherston WC: False-negative cytology in invasive cancer of the cervix. Clin Obstet Gynecol 1983;26:929.
18. Koss LG: The Papanicolaou test for cervical cancer detection. A triumph and a tragedy. JAMA 1989;261:737.
19. McGoogan E, Colgan TJ, Ramzy I, et al: Cell preparation methods and criteria for sample adequacy. IAC Task Force summary. Acta Cytologica 1996;42:25.
20. DeMay RM: Cytopathology of false negatives preceding cervical carcinoma. Am J Obstet Gynecol 1996;175:1110.
21. Spires SE, Banks ER, Weeks JA, et al: Assessment of cervicovaginal smear adequacy: The Bethesda System guidelines and reproducibility. Am J Clin Pathol 1994;102:54.
22. Austin RM: Results of blinded rescreening of Pananicolaou smears versus biased retrospective review. Arch Pathol Lab Med 1997;121:311.
23. DeMay RM: Common problems in Papanicolaou smear interpretation. Arch Pathol Lab Med 1997;121:229.

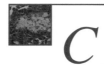

• Juan Felix

Liquid-Based, Thin-Layer Cytology

George Papanicolaou introduced cervical cytology into clinical practice in 1940.[1] In 1945, the Papanicolaou (Pap) smear received the endorsement of the American Cancer Society as an effective method for the prevention of cervical cancer. The widespread use of this test has been largely credited for the drastic reduction in the incidence and mortality of cervical cancer in the United States, Canada, and much of Western Europe in the last 50 years.[2–5] The ingenious technique of collecting exfoliated cells from the cervix, placing them on a glass slide, and examining them under the microscope remained largely unchanged for more than 50 years. It was only in the 1980s that a combination of events spurred a re-evaluation of the efficacy of the Pap smear and an explosion of technology in the field that has culminated in liquid-based thin-layer cytology.

The first documented incident of deficiencies in gynecologic cytology laboratories was reported by the United States Air Force. Allegations claiming inaccuracies in Pap smear diagnosis performed by a contract laboratory between 1972 and 1977 resulted in an investigation into the matter by government agencies. These investigations led to the discovery of large numbers of underdiagnoses of test results of Air Force personnel and their dependents that were largely attributed to poor regulation of laboratory personnel and large workloads.[6] In 1987, a highly publicized investigative report published in *The Wall Street Journal* denounced the egregious practices of a few cytology laboratories in the eastern United States.[7] The report exposed the policies of several high-volume, low-cost laboratories that encouraged excessive productivity of their screening cytotechnologists at the cost of accuracy. Similar problems had been documented in other laboratories yet had not received such widespread attention.[8]

Greatly spurred on by public outcry, further government investigations into these and other allegations brought forth by the report led to the recommendation of guidelines for the practice of cytology that culminated in an amendment to the Clinical Laboratories Improvement Act (CLIA) in 1988[9]. (See Chapter 3D). CLIA 88 established workload limits on cytotechnologists screening slides and instituted performance standards for both laboratories and laboratory professionals. The regulations passed as part of this act limited the number of cytology slides that a cytotechnologist could screen in a 24-hour period to 100, established a minimum of 10% rescreen of slides initially deemed normal by a cytotechnologist, and mandated remediation of cytotechnologists for clinically significant underdiagnoses.

> **The sensitivity of the conventional Pap smear for the detection of cervical cancer precursors is less than 50%. Screening errors are a less common cause of false-negative cytology than are errors of sampling.**

In subsequent years, results of numerous studies evaluating the sensitivity of the Pap smear were published in peer-reviewed medical literature. Published figures on the sensitivity of the Pap smear ranged widely from 31% to 89%, largely depending on the design, population, and end point of the study.[10–18] Interestingly, in the three series in which the cause of the false-negative result was investigated, screening errors were less common than were errors of sampling, in which the slides were carefully rescreened and no abnormal cells were found.[11, 12, 19] These data strongly indicated that the limitations of the conventional Pap smear were caused by more than just poor laboratory practice or human error on the part of cytotechnologists. The systematic evaluation of the conventional Pap smear culminated with the publication of two meta-analyses of the world literature.[20, 21] Both these studies established that the sensitivity of the conventional Pap smear for the detection of cervical cancer precursors was less than 50%.

Advances in image analysis and increased speed of computer processors allowed for efforts to develop computerized instruments that could assist or even replace human cytotechnologists in the tedious chore of screening Pap smears. Although several efforts were undertaken to design devices that would evaluate the conventional Pap smear, other groups believed that there were limitations inherent to a conventionally prepared slide that posed insurmountable impediments to computer analysis. The limitations identified could be divided into sampling limitations and preparation limitations.

LIMITATIONS OF THE CONVENTIONAL PAP SMEAR

> **Commonly used devices for performance of the Pap smear collect between 600,000 and 1.2 million cervical epithelial cells, but fewer than 20% of these collected cells are transferred onto the glass slide.**

> **The transfer of cells to a glass slide is a random event and is statistically prone to error if the population of abnormal cells is not homogeneously distributed throughout the specimen.**

The efficacy of the conventional Pap smear is predicated on the presumption that if an abnormality exists on the cervix, a Pap smear device will collect abnormal cells and transfer them onto the glass slide. This presupposes either that all the cells collected are deposited to the glass slide or that the population transferred onto the slide contains an adequate representation of the abnormal cells. The first of these premises was proven incorrect by Hutchinson and coworkers, who showed that commonly used devices for the performance of the Pap smear collected between 600,000 and 1.2 million cervical epithelial cells but that fewer than 20% of these collected cells were transferred onto the glass slide[22] (Fig. 3–7). The knowledge that most of the epithelial cell sample was never transferred to the slide that was screened by cytotechnologists provided

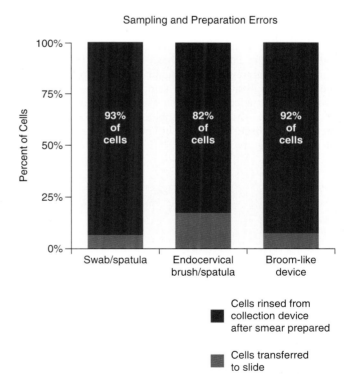

Figure 3–7. Each bar in this graph shows the total number of cells collected by the three most common cervical sampling devices: the Ayre spatula and cotton swab, the Ayre spatula and endocervical brush, and the broom device. The portion of the sample that adheres to the glass slide is represented in green, whereas the portion in blue remains on the device and is destined to be discarded.

a viable explanation for the high prevalence of true false-negative rate reported in the previously mentioned studies. Particularly disturbing was the realization that the transfer of cells to the glass slide is a random event and therefore statistically prone to error if the population of abnormal cells is not homogeneously distributed throughout the specimen.

> **Preparation of the conventional Pap smear by the clinician is a highly variable and poorly controlled technique. Optimal application of cells onto a glass slide should be done rapidly and in a systematic fashion to promptly fix the specimen and avoid air drying and degeneration and evenly spread the epithelial cells across the entire surface of the slide.**

Preparation of the conventional Pap smear by the clinician is a highly variable and poorly controlled technique. Optimal application of cells onto a glass slide should be done in a systematic fashion to evenly spread the epithelial cells across the entire surface of the slide and maximize the transfer of cells while minimizing clumping. Importantly, the transfer of cells onto the slide must be done rapidly to promptly fix the specimen and avoid air-drying or degeneration. In addition to these technical challenges, uncontrollable variables exist that affect the optimization of the conventional Pap smear. The presence of inflammatory cells and blood will compete for available area on the glass slide. In severe cases, the inflammatory cells or blood could replace or obscure the epithelial cells, creating an impediment to visual analysis (Fig. 3–8). Finally, inflamed epithelial cells and normal epithelial cells in the late luteal phase will form thick, three-dimensional aggregates that again pose an obstruction to the clear visualization of the sample (Fig. 3–9). Studies evaluating the adequacy of the Pap smear report that an excess of 15% of all Pap smears are limited owing to the presence of obscuring blood, inflammation, or thick areas of overlapping epithelial cells.[23, 24]

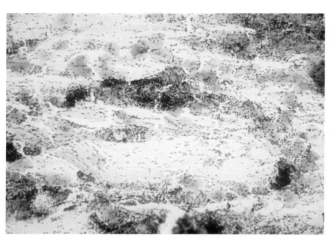

Figure 3–9. Photomicrograph of a conventional Papanicolaou smear showing aggregation of epithelial cells. Some aggregates are associated with inflammatory cells, whereas other areas are composed only of aggregates of epithelial cells (magnification ×100).

The stated limitations of the conventional Pap smear were believed by many to pose insurmountable obstacles to the successful development of a computer-assisted screening device. Inherent limitations of the conventional Pap smear needed to be addressed and overcome to create a computer-assisted technology that was superior to the conventional Pap smear. Liquid-based, thin-layer technology was conceived out of the necessity to improve the physical state of the Pap smear to allow for accurate evaluation by a computerized device.

PRINCIPLES OF EFFICACY OF LIQUID-BASED CYTOLOGY

> **Liquid-based, thin-layer technology was developed to address the five major limitations posed by the conventional Pap smear: failure to capture the entire specimen, inadequate fixation, random distribution of abnormal cells, obscuring elements, and technical variability in the quality of the smear.**

Liquid-based, thin-layer technology was developed to overcome the technical limitations of the conventional Pap smear. The technology was developed to specifically address the five major limitations posed by the conventional Pap smear: failure to capture the entire specimen obtained, inadequate fixation, random distribution of abnormal cells, obscuring elements, and technical variability in the quality of the smear. Collecting cells directly into a liquid fixative addresses the first two limitations. By immersing the cervical collection device into the liquid fixative, the cells are fixed instantly, avoiding the damaging contact with the dry slide and minimizing postcollection degeneration and air-drying. In addition, if proper technique is observed, the vast majority of the cells retrieved

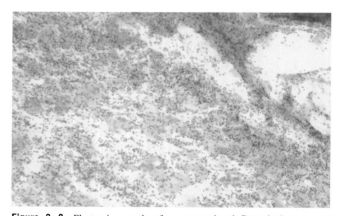

Figure 3–8. Photomicrograph of a conventional Papanicolaou smear showing numerous red blood cells and inflammatory cells overlying the cervical epithelial cells, obstructing clear vision of cellular detail (magnification ×100).

by the sampling devices are rinsed into the liquid media, capturing virtually the entire sample obtained from the patient into the vial.[25]

> **Mechanical mixing of the cells creates a homogenous sample in which abnormal cells are evenly distributed throughout the sample.**

Mechanical mixing of the cells follows collection of cells into liquid fixative. Although the different products that use this technology have different methods of mixing, the principle is the same; mixing the cells creates a homogenous sample in which abnormal cells, if present, are evenly distributed throughout the sample. Specimen homogeneity directly addresses the false-negative conventional Pap smears potentially caused by a failure to include nonrandomly distributed abnormal cells on the glass slide. Sample homogeneity is critical, because no slide will capture the entire sample collected from the patient but rather will contain only a relatively small amount of the collection. The efficacy of this process was demonstrated by Hutchinson et al, who produced multiple slides from abnormal samples and identified abnormal cells in virtually all the slides.[25] Liquid collection and sample mixing seem to facilitate the consistent identification of lesions, regardless of the method used. Khalbuss et al used a modified electric toothbrush to mix liquid-fixed residual cells obtained after a conventional Pap smear. Usable samples were produced by simple cytocentrifugation onto glass slides. Despite the simplicity of the procedure, diagnostic equivalency to the conventionally prepared Pap smear was demonstrated.[26]

The final two limitations of the conventional Pap smear, obscuring elements and thick sample, are addressed in very different fashions by the products currently available. The ThinPrep (Cytyc Corp., Boxborough, Massachusetts) uses a polycarbonate cylinder that holds a membrane with an 8-μm pore size at the end to mix and subsequently suction the media. As the collection fluid of the sample passes through this semipermeable barrier, the membrane detains epithelial cells and infectious organisms, but much of the debris as well as some inflammatory cells are allowed to pass. When sufficient epithelial cells accumulate on the membrane, as determined by a pressure sensor, the suction is discontinued, and the membrane is placed against the glass slide to transfer the cells.

The Autocyte Prep (TriPath Imaging, Inc., Burlington, North Carolina) uses a liquid gradient onto which the sample is layered following vigorous vortexing. The sample and gradient are then centrifuged. The gradient preferentially concentrates epithelial cells, partially depleting the final sample of extraneous material, blood, and inflammatory cells. Some of this filtrate is then pipetted onto a chamber by a robotic pipetter, and the sample is allowed to settle by gravity onto the slide. Both techniques result in consistent, thin-layer preparations of epithelial cells that are depleted of extraneous elements. Both products produce slides containing 50,000 to 75,000 cells per slide in circular areas.

EFFICACY OF LIQUID-BASED, THIN-LAYER TECHNOLOGY

> **Despite the limitations of the current data, more than 500,000 subjects have been studied, with a preponderance of data indicating a significant benefit of liquid-based, thin-layer technology in the detection of cervical cancer precursor lesions and in the improvement of specimen adequacy.**

The efficacy of liquid-based thin-layer cytology has been assessed by numerous clinical trials. Two types of study designs account for most of the published studies—the split-sample design and the intended use, direct-to-vial design. The split-sample studies accrue patients in whom a single sample collection is performed. The sample is used to prepare a conventional Pap smear. The residual material remaining on the collection device is then rinsed in the collection media and sent for thin-layer preparation. This study design suffers from a beneficial bias in favor of the conventional Pap smear, because it is prepared first and may deplete the remaining sample of abnormal cells for thin-layer preparation. The second type of study is the intended use, direct-to-vial design in which women enrolled have their cervical sample directly deposited to the liquid collection media. Comparison of the technology with its conventional counterpart is performed by obtaining matched populations of historical controls. This type of study also suffers from numerous biases, including differences in the populations studied, selection bias on the basis of ability to afford a more expensive technology, and high-risk patient selection to a test perceived to have superior sensitivity. To date, no published data evaluating prospective, randomized trials comparing these technologies with the conventional Pap smear exist. Despite the limitations of the current data, the number of patients studied is now more than 500,000, with a preponderance of data indicating a significant benefit of liquid-based, thin-layer technology over the conventional Pap smear in the detection of cervical cancer precursor lesions and in the improvement of specimen adequacy.

Early clinical studies comparing the ThinPrep and the Autocyte Prep (formerly known as the CytoRich) were performed on early versions of the devices that later underwent significant modifications. These studies will not be reviewed in detail here because the devices tested were replaced with newer versions that are the only ones clinically available. The importance of these early trials was in the demonstration of diagnostic equivalence to the conventional Pap smear despite the adverse bias introduced by the split-sample study design.[19, 27–37]

> **Only one published study to date failed to find more squamous intraepithelial lesion in the liquid-based slides than in the conventional smear, showing a nonsignificant 3% decrease in the detection of squamous intraepithelial lesions.**

Most of the more recent studies use versions of the automated devices approved by the U.S. Food and Drug Ad-

▼ Table 3–6

Performance of the ThinPrep in Split-Sample Studies

Reference	No. of Cases	SIL		% Increase	ASCUS		Unsatisfactory		SBLB	
		Conv.	*TP*		*Conv.*	*TP*	*Conv.*	*TP*	*Conv.*	*TP*
Lee, 1996	6747	8%	9.4%	18.4	7.7%	7.4%	1.6%	1.9%	27.8%	19.8%
Roberts, 1997	35,560	2%	2.3%	11.7	N/A	N/A	3.5%	0.7%	8.3%	20%
Corkill, 1998	1583	2.7%	5.6%	109.5	3.7%	5.1%	N/A	N/A	2.2%	0.3%
Shield, 1999	300	7%	8.3%	19.1	N/A	N/A	17.3	6.3%	N/A	15.3%
Wang, 1999	972	4.4%	6%	34.9	N/A	N/A	N/A	N/A	N/A	N/A
Hutchinson, 1999	8636	4.9%	5.2%	6	1.8%	7.5%	N/A	N/A	N/A	N/A

ASCUS, atypical squamous cells of undetermined significance; Conv., conventional; SBLB, satisfactory but limited by; SIL, squamous intraepithelial lesion; TP, ThinPrep.

ministration (FDA) and are reviewed and summarized in Tables 3–6 through 3–9. The studies are listed by design and divided into those studies done in a split-sample fashion and those done in the intended-use, direct-to-vial design. Examination of the data summarized reveals that liquid-based cytology outperformed the conventional Pap smear in the detection of cervical cancer precursors. In fact, only one study published failed to find more squamous intraepithelial lesions (SIL) in the liquid-based slides than in the conventional smear, showing a nonsignificant 3% decrease in the detection of SIL.[37] The equivalent or superior performance of liquid-based thin-layer slides is particularly impressive in the split-sample studies, where cases in which the conventional smear showed no lesions

were found to represent SIL on the leftover cells. The range of improvement afforded by liquid-based cytology in these split-sample studies ranged from a low of 6% to a high of 110% improvement with the ThinPrep technology and from a low of −3% to a high of 137% with the Autocyte Prep technology (Tables 3–6 and 3–7). On average, the improvement seen with the ThinPrep device, summarized from these studies, was 15%,[38–43] with a similar 18% improvement in the series of samples summarized from the Autocyte Prep studies.[23, 37, 44–47]

Summary of the direct-to-vial studies for the ThinPrep shows a 140% improvement in the detection of SIL over the historical, conventional Pap smear controls[24, 48–54] (Table 3–8). These clinical data strongly support the

▼ Table 3–7

Performance of Autocyte Prep in Split-Sample Studies

Reference	No. of Cases	SIL		Increase	ASCUS		Unsatisfactory		SBLB	
		Conv.	*Prep*		*Conv.*	*Prep*	*Conv.*	*Prep*	*Conv.*	*Prep*
Vassilakos, 1996	560	3.8%	4.6%	24%	12.9%	7.7%	5.4%	3.8%	28.3%	8.4%
Takahashi, 1997	2000	3.5%	3.4%	−3%	1.1%	4.6%	N/A	N/A	N/A	N/A
Wilbur, 1997	286	4.2%	9.1%	117%	13.6%	13.3%	3.5%	1.1%	30%	16%
Bishop, 1998	8983	5.2%	5.9%	13%	6.2%	6%	1%	0.6%	28.1%	15.8%
Kunz, 1998	554	1.4%	3.4%	137%	9.6%	3.3%	19%	12%	N/A	N/A
Minge, 2000	14,539	4.4%	5.8%	32%	6.9%	5.9%	0.9%	0.6%	N/A	N/A

ASCUS, atypical squamous cells of undetermined significance; Conv., conventional; SBLB, satisfactory but limited by; SIL, squamous intraepithelial lesion.

▼ Table 3–8

Performance of the ThinPrep in Direct-to-Vial Studies

Reference	No. of Cases	SIL		Increase	ASCUS		Unsatisfactory		SBLB	
	Conv./TP	*Conv.*	*TP*		*Conv.*	*TP*	*Conv.*	*TP*	*Conv.*	*TP*
Weintraub, 1997	13,067/18,247	1%	2.9%	190%	1.6%	2.7%	0.7%	0.3%	30.9%	10.9%
Papillo, 1998	18,569/8541	1.6%	2.5%	56%	9%	6.6%	0.2%	0.4%	4.8%	4.4%
Bolick, 1998	39,408/10,694	1.1%	2.9%	164%	2.3%	2.9%	1%	0.3%	17.8%	11.6%
Dupree, 1998	22,323/19,351	1.2%	1.7%	40%	4.9%	4.6%	2%	3.8%	N/A	N/A
Guidos, 1999	5423/9583	1.3%	4.7%	262%	2%	3.4%	1.2%	0.5%	21.4%	0.7%
Carpenter, 1999	5000/2727	7.7%	10.5%	36%	12.5%	6.9%	0.6%	0.3%	19.4%	10.5%
Diaz-Rosario, 2000	74,756/56,339	1.8%	3.2%	79%	4.8%	4.5%	0.2%	0.7%	22%	18.7%
Weintraub, 2000	129,619/39,455	0.6%	2.3%	141%	1.5%	2.4%	0.3%	0.2%	27.8%	8.1%

ASCUS, atypical squamous cells of undetermined significance; Conv., conventional; SBLB, satisfactory but limited by; SIL, squamous intraepithelial lesion; TP, ThinPrep.

▼ Table 3–9

Performance of the Autocyte Prep in Direct-to-Vial Studies

Reference	No. of Cases Conv./Prep	SIL Conv.	SIL Prep	Increase	ASCUS Conv.	ASCUS Prep	Unsatisfactory Conv.	Unsatisfactory Prep	SBLB Conv.	SBLB Prep
Vassilakos, 1998	15,402/32,655	1.1%	3.6%	224%	3.7%	1.6%	1.9%	0.4%	13.4%	2.7%
Vassilakos, 1999	88,569/111,358	2%	3.2%	63%	3%	1.2%	1.5%	0.2%	4.6%	1.2%
Vassilakos, 2000	19,923/81,120	1.2%	3.4%	283%	3.5%	1.9%	N/A	N/A	N/A	N/A
Tench, 2000	10,367/2231	1%	1.7%	67%	3.8%	5.5%	2.9%	0.4%	31%	16%

ASCUS, atypical squamous cells of undetermined significance; Conv., conventional; SBLB, satisfactory but limited by; SIL, squamous intraepithelial lesion.

FDA labeling stating that the ThinPrep is superior to the conventional Pap smear for the detection of cervical cancer precursor lesions.

Summary of the direct-to-vial studies for the Autocyte Prep is similarly impressive, with more than a 200% increase in the detection of SIL over historical, conventional controls[55–58] (Table 3–9). It is necessary to mention that three of the four direct-to-vial Autocyte Prep studies did not use the FDA-approved instrument to produce the slides, but rather used manual pipetting.[56, 57] However, the one direct-to-vial study for the Autocyte Prep that did use the FDA-approved instrument and procedure showed an increase in the detection of SIL of 67%.[55]

Direct-to-vial studies using the ThinPrep revealed such marked improvements in the detection of SIL that much of the medical community began to suspect that the increased diagnoses of SIL may have been the result of "overcalls" on the part of overzealous cytopathologists in these studies rather than true detection of abnormalities. Confirmation that this increase in SIL is true detection of dysplasia rather than overcalls by cytopathologists can be found in several studies in which subsets of patients with biopsy follow-up are available. Papillo et al found a statistically significant increase in specificity of a diagnosis of SIL with the ThinPrep (81%) over the conventional Pap smear (72%).[52] Diaz-Rosario et al found equivalent specificity, as determined by biopsy-proven dysplasia, between the ThinPrep (74%) and the conventional Pap (79%).[49] Finally, Hutchinson et al also reported biopsy correlation data from a population-based study in Costa Rica.[39] In this study, the specificity of the ThinPrep diagnosis was 85.4% when compared with biopsy results. By comparison, conventional cytology had a slightly better correlation to biopsy of 88.8%. In all three studies, the superior sensitivity, combined with the specificity reported, led to a significant increase in the detection of biopsy-proven dysplasia. Although fewer data exist for the Autocyte Prep, two reports comment on biopsy correlation. Vassilakos et al reported a statistically significant improvement in correlation between the Autocyte Prep diagnosis and the biopsy result when compared with the conventional Pap smear.[58] The improvement in correlation was particularly notable among cases diagnosed by the Autocyte Prep slide as high-grade SIL, where 90% of biopsies confirmed the diagnosis.

The final concern voiced regarding liquid-based, thin-layer technology was directed at the rise in the diagnosis of atypical squamous cells of undetermined significance (ASCUS) in a few of the series. Although many series report an absolute decrease in the frequency of a diagnosis of ASCUS, all the series report a decrease in the ASCUS-to-SIL ratio. This parameter is considered a more representative measure of performance because the detection of more disease will be accompanied by the detection of all abnormalities, including nondiagnostic abnormalities such as ASCUS. The improvement in nondiagnostic abnormalities seen in the ASCUS category is also seen for the diagnosis of atypical glandular cells of undetermined significance (AGUS). Ashfaq et al reported a significant improvement in the detection of adenocarcinoma of the cervix, with a 65% decrease in the false-negative rate for the diagnosis of adenocarcinoma by ThinPrep over the conventional Pap smear, as well as a 64% increase in the specificity of a diagnosis of AGUS or adenocarcinoma.[59]

THIN-LAYER–BASED COMPUTER-ASSISTED SCREENING

When used in conjunction with thin-layer slides, computer-assisted screening devices offer tremendous promise.

Computer-assisted screening devices have been shown to reduce the incidence of false-negative Pap tests when used in a quality control mode to rescreen cases with a diagnosis of "within normal limits."[60, 61] In addition, one instrument (the Autopap 300) is approved by the FDA for primary screening, with the capability of rendering machine-only diagnoses of within normal limits for 25% of the lowest-risk tests in a non–high-risk screening population. Usage issues regarding the definition of the "high-risk patient" and the unacceptability of many slides to be read by the device, combined with the increase in cost and low reimbursement rates by insurance carriers, have delayed the widespread acceptance of this technology. Computer-assisted screening devices designed to screen liquid-based, thin-layer slides circumvent many of the technical problems faced in screening the conventional Pap smear. Clinical trials evaluating these devices are few and are in early phases. In a series of 583 patients, Takahashi et al found that an interactive computer analysis system, the Autocyte Screen, yielded a false-negative rate of only 1.8% (detecting 55 of 56 cases of SIL) while triaging only 21% of cases for pathologist review.[62] In a series of 1676 thin-layer preparations, Bishop et al reported that the Autocyte Screen had an improved sensitivity in the detection of SIL, with the computer-assisted screening yielding a 98% sensitivity compared with an 89% sensitivity by manual screening alone.[63] Although larger clinical trials are needed, these early results offer great promise for an improvement in screening sensitivity while reducing human effort and time spent. Thin-layer technology has largely reduced obstacles to the use of computer imaging, allowing optical analysis of single cells rather than of clusters. When used in conjunction with thin-layer slides, computer-assisted screening devices offer tremendous promise, particularly as human cytotechnologists are decreasing in number while demand for screeners is increasing.

MOLECULAR TESTING OUT OF RESIDUAL MATERIAL LEFT IN THE VIAL

> To date, successful out-of-vial testing has been shown for human papillomavirus, *Chlamydia trachomatis*, and herpes simplex virus.

An unexpected benefit of liquid-based thin-layer technology was discovered on the realization that abundant cellular material remained in the vial after production of the slide. It is estimated that, on average, one tenth or less of the cellular material is used to make the test slide. The remainder of the cellular material was originally destined to be discarded. However, with the advancement of molecular testing, biologists began using the residual material to test for the presence of infectious organisms. To date, successful out-of-vial testing has been shown for human papillomavirus (HPV), *Chlamydia trachomatis* (CT), and herpes simplex virus (HSV). The ability to detect infections in the residual volume of the collection fluid offers numerous opportunities for simplification of collection devices and minimization of routing errors, found commonly with multiple samples from one patient. The most exemplary benefit of this adjunct technology is seen in the case of HPV testing for women with a cytologic diagnosis of ASCUS. Results of two large clinical trials have shown that detection of high–oncogenic risk HPV DNA types using the Hybrid Capture II (HC II) assay effectively separates patients with a cytologic diagnosis of ASCUS into one group with a higher likelihood of having cervical intraepithelial neoplasia (CIN) grade 2 or 3 and another group at no increased risk of harboring high-grade CIN. Women with a diagnosis of ASCUS who test positive for high oncogenic risk HPV are at increased risk of harboring high-grade CIN. In contrast, women with a diagnosis of ASCUS who test negative for high oncogenic risk HPV have a risk of high-grade SIL comparable with that of women who have a normal Pap smear result.[64, 65] The HPV DNA test using the HC II assay can be performed by separately collecting a sample of cells into transport media or by using the residual cell sample from the liquid-based cytology sample. The latter option

offers the clinically desirable benefit of automatically testing the sample of patients with a cytologic diagnosis of ASCUS without the necessity of an additional patient visit or patient-clinician interaction. If a patient is found to be HPV DNA positive, she is referred for colposcopy. If the patient is HPV DNA negative, the risk of a high-grade SIL is low enough to recommend screening at the routine interval. This triage strategy has been shown to reduce unnecessary colposcopic examinations in 45% to 60% of women with ASCUS cytology, reducing the morbidity, anxiety, and cost associated with that procedure.[64, 65] Cost analyses of triage strategies have shown a cost savings in the management of patients using HPV testing over previous cytology-based or colposcopy-based strategies.[64] Results from the National Cancer Institute's ASCUS–Low Grade SIL Triage Study (ALTS) show a statistically significant improvement in the detection CIN 2 and CIN 3 for patients triaged to either immediate colposcopy or HC II HPV DNA detection when compared with patients followed up with Pap smears.[65] These data have encouraged us to advocate the use of high–oncogenic risk HPV DNA testing in patients with a cytologic diagnosis of ASCUS to define the likelihood of dysplasia in the patient and the need for a colposcopic workup.

CYTOLOGIC CRITERIA

> Microscopic evaluation of liquid-based thin-layer slides differs somewhat from examination of conventionally prepared Pap smears. There is a reduction in obscuring inflammation and blood, the slides lack a smearing pattern, and the nuclei appear crisp and lack degenerative changes.

Microscopic evaluation of liquid-based thin-layer slides differs somewhat from examination of conventionally prepared Pap smears. The process of producing slides consistently having a thin layer of epithelial cells with a reduction in obscuring inflammation and blood results in significant changes in the appearance of the slide. Because the slides are machine made, they lack a smearing pattern (Fig. 3–10). The obliteration of this pattern initially worried cytotechnologists, who relied on these features to aid them in the identification of abnormalities. Similarly, the excellent fixation of the cells produces clear, crisp-appearing nuclei that lack degenerative changes. Again, some cytotechnologists relied on these degenerative changes that produced extremely dark nuclei to aid them in identifying abnormalities. Although these phenomena do still occur, the benefits of a better-fixed sample without obstructing debris greatly outweigh any detriment that these side effects produce. As evidenced by the large body of clinical data showing increased detection of abnormalities using liquid-based technology, minimal retraining of cytotechnologists is effective in ensuring excellent diagnostic accuracy.

Optimal fixation minimizes degenerative nuclear changes. For this reason, abnormal cells often lack degenerative

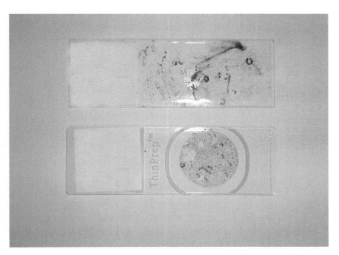

Figure 3–10. Comparison of the appearance of conventional Papanicolaou (Pap) smear versus a machine-made, thin-layer preparation. Note the uniformity in the distribution of cells throughout the machine-made slide *(bottom)* compared with the streaking and aggregating of cellular material seen in the conventional Pap smear *(top).*

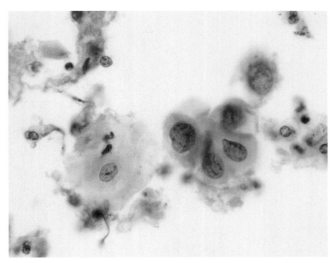

Figure 3–12. A ThinPrep Papanicolaou test showing a high-grade squamous intraepithelial lesion. Note that although hyperchromasia is slight to absent, the chromatin is irregularly distributed and the nuclear outlines are markedly irregular, ensuring the abnormal diagnosis (magnification ×600).

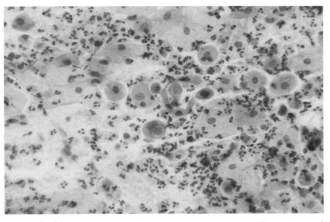

Figure 3–11. Conventional Papanicolaou smear revealing abnormal squamous cells. The nuclei show dark chromatin with little internal detail. This "smudged" appearance to the chromatin is characteristic of degenerative change (magnification ×200).

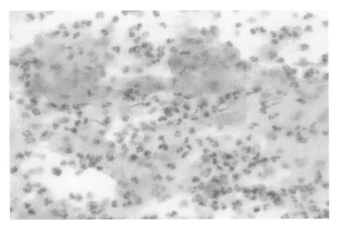

Figure 3–13. A conventional Papanicolaou smear showing several abnormal squamous cells among normal epithelial cells, inflammatory cells, and blood. Scrutiny of the abnormal cells, once identified, reveals them to be diagnostic of a high-grade squamous intraepithelial lesion (magnification ×400).

hyperchromasia (Fig. 3–11). Instead, the nuclei appear euchromatic but demonstrate the marked nuclear irregularities that characterize dysplasia (Fig. 3–12). Although machine-made slides eradicate the smear pattern, the even dispersal of cells allows abnormal cells to be seen clearly against a clear background. No longer are abnormal cells obscured by inflammation or sheets of normal epithelial cells (Fig. 3–13). Unlike many cases of conventional cytology where obscuring elements made thorough screening virtually impossible, systematic screening of thin-layer slides virtually always results in the identification of abnormal cells by the cytotechnologist.

LOW-GRADE SQUAMOUS INTRAEPITHELIAL LESIONS

Liquid-based cytology enhances both the nuclear irregularities and the chromatin pattern seen in low-grade SIL; more importantly, it highlights the cytoplasmic cavity, enhancing the true internal border of the koilocytic clearing.

Low-grade SIL is most prevalent in women in their early reproductive years (ages 16 to 26 years) or at the

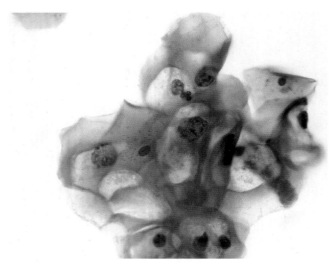

Figure 3–14. A ThinPrep Papanicolaou test showing a low-grade squamous intraepithelial lesion. Note the clarity of both cytoplasmic and nuclear detail afforded by the liquid fixation as well as the absence of extraneaous material (magnification ×600).

onset of sexual activity.[66–69] They are uncommon in women in the remainder of their reproductive lives but become somewhat more common in mid- to late menopause (age older than 58). The cytologic diagnosis of low-grade SIL is made on the identification of abnormal squamous cells that are equivalent in size to a normal superficial or intermediate cell. Diagnostic abnormalities include enlargement of the nucleus, irregularity of the nuclear membrane, and irregular chromatin distribution. Additional features that aid in the diagnosis and are frequently seen include hyperchromasia, as well as cavitation of the cytoplasm immediately surrounding the nucleus to form a well-demarcated internal cytoplasmic border. The latter cytoplasmic changes, commonly referred to as koilocytosis, should not be equated with a low-grade SIL in the absence of the diagnostic nuclear features. Liquid-based cytology enhances both the nuclear

irregularities and the chromatin pattern seen in low-grade SIL; more importantly, it highlights the cytoplasmic cavity, enhancing the true internal border of the koilocytic clearing (Figs. 3–14 and 3–15). When findings are inconclusive, the diagnosis of ASCUS should be entertained (see later discussion).

HIGH-GRADE SQUAMOUS INTRAEPITHELIAL LESIONS

Although liquid-based cytology reduces degenerative hyperchromasia, it does not affect hyperchromasia caused by aneuploidy. The enhancement induced by the optimal fixation of liquid-based slides also ensures that high-grade abnormalities will exhibit identifiable nuclear irregularities not seen in benign mimics.

High-grade SIL is most prevalent in women in their mid- to late reproductive years (ages 26 to 48 years), although they may be seen at any age after the onset of sexual activity.[66, 70, 72] The cytologic diagnosis of high-grade SIL relies on the presence of abnormal squamous cells that are smaller than those seen in low-grade lesions. The average size of a high-grade SIL is equivalent to that of a normal parabasal cell. Diagnostic abnormalities include nuclear enlargement, marked increase in nuclear-to-cytoplasmic ratio, irregularity of the nuclear membrane, and irregular chromatin distribution. Commonly encountered features that aid the diagnosis also include marked hyperchromasia and abnormal nuclear shapes. Although liquid-based cytology reduces degenerative hyperchromasia, it does not affect hyperchromasia caused by aneuploidy (Figs. 3–16 to 3–17). The enhancement brought about by the optimal fixation of liquid-based slides practically guarantees that abnormal high-grade cells will ex-

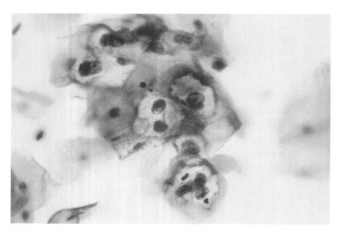

Figure 3–15. An Autocyte Prep Papanicolaou test showing a low-grade lesion. Note the sharpness of the cytoplasmic borders forming the koilocytic cavity and the excellent nuclear detail (magnification ×600).

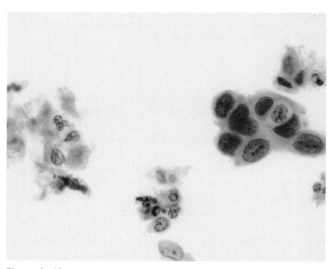

Figure 3–16. A ThinPrep Papanicolaou test showing a high-grade lesion. Note that although marked hyperchromasia is present, nuclear detail is preserved, indicating the true rather than the degenerative nature of the increase in chromatin (magnification ×600).

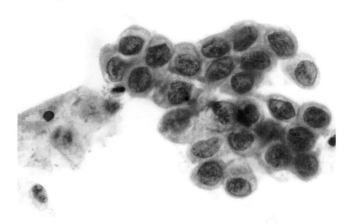

Figure 3–17. A ThinPrep Papanicolaou test showing a high-grade lesion. This cluster represents a true syncytium of abnormal cells. The individual nuclei are easily distinguishable, as are the nuclear irregularities and the irregular chromatin distribution (magnification ×600).

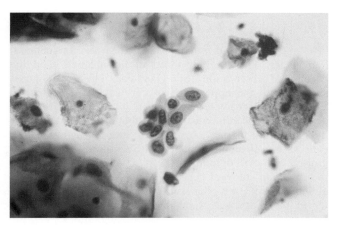

Figure 3–18. An Autocyte Prep Papanicolaou test showing a high-grade lesion. The abnormal cells are easily identified among normal epithelial cells. The absence of debris, inflammatory cells, and blood greatly facilitates their identification (magnification ×200).

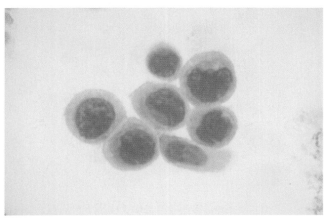

Figure 3–19. An Autocyte Prep Papanicolaou test showing a high-grade lesion. Note the readily identifiable nuclear convolutions seen in these abnormal nuclei. Nuclear convolutions and irregularities are expected with liquid-based fixation (magnification ×600).

hibit identifiable nuclear irregularities not seen in benign mimics.

ATYPICAL SQUAMOUS CELLS OF UNDETERMINED SIGNIFICANCE

Liquid-based cytology has been shown to aid in reducing the proportion of ASCUS diagnoses, probably based on improvements in both the fixation and the quality of the slide.

The diagnosis of ASCUS is an undesirable but inevitable diagnosis that results from the morphologic variability of squamous cells in different physiologic and pathologic states. Although inevitable, the frequency with which the diagnosis of ASCUS is made should be minimized because its clinical management is fraught with controversy.[72] The percentage of women with a cytologic diagnosis of ASCUS who harbor biopsy-proven dysplasia is generally accepted to be around 20%.[71, 73] Importantly, some series show that more cases of high-grade SIL are identified in patients with a cytologic diagnosis of ASCUS than are identified in patients with a cytologic diagnosis of high-grade SIL.[74, 75] Although criteria exist to separate most cervical cancer precursor lesions from lesions that are reactive in nature, no single criterion or combination of criteria will effectively do so in all cases. The category of ASCUS is therefore reserved for lesions in which a clear distinction between reactive and neoplastic cells cannot be made. Liquid-based cytology has been shown to aid in reducing the proportion of ASCUS diagnoses, probably on the basis of improvements in both the fixation and the quality of the slide. Improved slide quality allows for more cases to be correctly classified as either normal or SIL (Figs. 3–20 and 3–21).

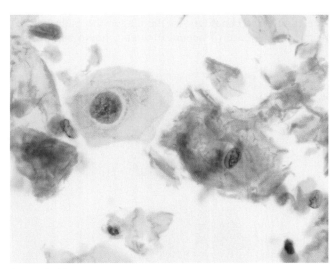

Figure 3–20. An Autocyte Prep Papanicolaou test showing atypical squamous cells of undetermined significance. The nuclear enlargement and increase in chromatin content mark this cell as abnormal. The absence of nuclear convolutions or irregularities and the presence of a small nucleolus puts into question the diagnosis of squamous intraepithelial lesion (magnification ×600).

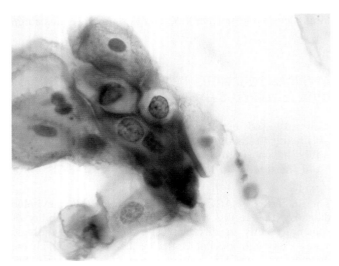

Figure 3–21. A ThinPrep Papanicolaou test showing atypical squamous cells of undetermined significance (ASCUS). The nuclear enlargement and cytoplasmic cavitation suggest squamous intraepithelial lesion; however, the finely distributed, delicate chromatin and the absence of nuclear irregularities place it in the ASCUS category (magnification ×600).

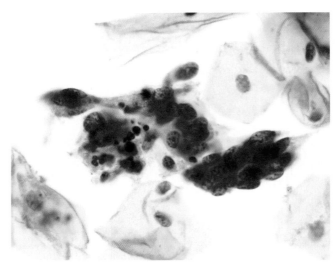

Figure 3–23. A ThinPrep Papanicolaou test showing abnormal endocervical glandular cells with marked nuclear enlargement, hyperchromasia, and nuclear crowding. The cells have lost their orderly relationship to each other, characteristic of adenocarcinoma in situ (magnification ×600).

CYTOLOGY OF CERVICAL ADENOCARCINOMA

With liquid-based, thin-layer technology, the even dispersal of normal cells and the excellent preservation of glandular clusters contrast sharply with the appearance of adenocarcinoma.

Glandular lesions of the cervix are not as easily detected on cytologic examination as are squamous lesions.[76] Speculation as to the reason for the decreased sensitivity of the Pap smear for adenocarcinoma of the cervix and its precursor lesions vary widely. It is possible that the cytologic features of early adenocarcinoma are so subtle that they are prone to not being recognized by the screening cytotechnologist or the diagnosing pathologist.[77] Again, in the case of adenocarcinoma, liquid-based, thin-

layer technology has proven superior to the conventional Pap smear. The even dispersal of normal cells and the excellent preservation of glandular clusters contrast sharply with the appearance of cervical adenocarcinoma. The cytologic characteristics that allow for a diagnosis of cervical adenocarcinoma include abundant glandular cellular material, marked crowding of endocervical glandular cells within clusters, architectural aberrations of glandular groups, and cytologic atypia (Figs. 3–22 to 3–24).[77] In a retrospective study of cervical adenocarcinoma, Ashfaq et al showed both a higher sensitivity and a higher specificity in the diagnosis of adenocarcinoma using the ThinPrep method over conventionally prepared slides.[78]

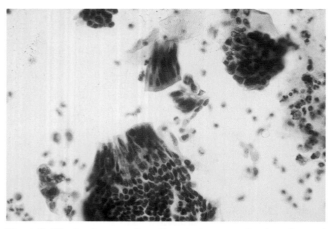

Figure 3–22. An Autocyte Prep Papanicolaou test showing abnormal endocervical glandular aggregates. The cells show marked crowding, stratification, and nuclear enlargement. Findings are indicative of cervical adenocarcinoma in situ (magnification ×200).

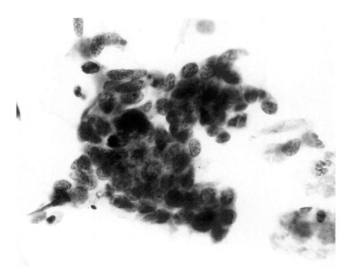

Figure 3–24. A ThinPrep Papanicolaou test showing abnormal endocervical glandular cells. The aggregate shows crowding and peripheral loss of polarity of the nuclei (feathering), characteristic of adenocarcinoma in situ (magnification ×600).

SUMMARY OF KEY POINTS

- Screening errors are a less common cause of false-negative cytology than are errors of sampling.

- Commonly used devices for the performance of the Pap smear collect between 600,000 and 1.2 million cervical epithelial cells, but fewer than 20% of these collected cells are transferred onto the glass slide.

- In conventional cytology, the transfer of cells to a glass slide is a random event and is statistically prone to error if the population of abnormal cells is not homogeneously distributed throughout the specimen.

- Preparation of the conventional Pap smear by the clinician is a highly variable and poorly controlled technique.

- The transfer of cells onto a slide must be done rapidly to promptly fix the specimen and avoid air-drying or degeneration.

- More than 15% of all Pap smears are limited owing to the presence of obscuring blood, inflammation, or thick areas of overlapping epithelial cells.

- Liquid-based, thin-layer technology was developed to address the five major limitations posed by the conventional Pap smear: failure to capture the entire specimen, inadequate fixation, random distribution of abnormal cells, obscuring elements, and technical variability in the quality of the smear.

- Mechanical mixing of the cells creates a homogenous sample in which abnormal cells are evenly distributed throughout the sample.

- Successful out-of-vial testing has been shown for HPV, CT, and HSV.

- Microscopic evaluation of liquid-based, thin-layer slides differs somewhat from examination of conventionally prepared Pap smears.

- Liquid-based cytology enhances both the nuclear irregularities and the chromatin pattern and highlights the cytoplasmic cavity, enhancing the true internal border of koilocytic clearing.

- Liquid-based cytology has been shown to aid in reducing the proportion of ASCUS diagnoses, probably based on improvements in both the fixation and the quality of the slide.

References

1. Widra, EA, Dookhan D, Jordan A, et al: Evaluation of the atypical cytologic smear. Validity of the 1991 Bethesda System. J Reprod Med 1994;39:682.
2. Benedet JL, Anderson GH: Cervical intraepithelial neoplasia in British Columbia: A comprehensive program for detection, diagnosis, and treatment. Gynecol Oncol 1981;12:S280.
3. Cramer DW: The role of cervical cytology in the declining morbidity and mortality of cervical cancer. Cancer 1974;34:2018.
4. Laara E, Day NE, Hakama M: Trends in mortality from cervical cancer in the Nordic countries: Association with organised screening programmes. Lancet 1987;1:1247.
5. Macgregor JE, Moss S, Parkin DM, Day NE: Cervical cancer screening in north-east Scotland. IARC Sci Publ 1986;76:25.
6. New Papanicolaou test suggested for Air Force dependents. U.S. Med 1978:1.
7. Bogdanich W: Lax laboratories: The Pap test misses much cervical cancer through labs' errors. The Wall Street Journal, November 11, 1987:1.
8. Chapman B: Crisis in Newport. CAP Today 1994;8:26.
9. Meisels A: Cytologic diagnosis of human papillomavirus. Influence of age and pregnancy stage. Acta Cytol 1992;36:480.
10. Giles JA, Hudson E, Crow J, et al: Colposcopic assessment of the accuracy of cervical cytology screening. BMJ 1988;296:1099.
11. Joseph MG, Cragg F, Wright VC, et al: Cyto-histological correlates in a colposcopic clinic: A 1-year prospective study. Diagn Cytopathol 1991;7:477.
12. Kristensen GB, Skyggebjerg KD, Holund B, et al: Analysis of cervical smears obtained within three years of the diagnosis of invasive cervical cancer. Acta Cytol 1991;35:47.
13. MacCormac L, Lew W, King G, Allen PW: Gynaecological cytology screening in South Australia: A 23-year experience. Med J Aust 1988;149:530.
14. Mitchell H, Medley G, Giles G: Cervical cancers diagnosed after negative results on cervical cytology: Perspective in the 1980s. BMJ 1990;300:1622.
15. Plott AE, Martin FJ, Cheek SW, et al: Measuring screening skills in gynecologic cytology. Results of voluntary self-assessment. Acta Cytol 1987;31:911.
16. Soost HJ, Lange HJ, Lehmacher W, Ruffing-Kullmann B: The validation of cervical cytology. Sensitivity, specificity and predictive values. Acta Cytol 1991;35:8.
17. van der Graaf Y, Vooijs GP, Gaillard HL, Go DM: Screening errors in cervical cytologic screening. Acta Cytol 1987;31:434.
18. Yobs AR, Plott AE, Hicklin MD, et al: Retrospective evaluation of gynecologic cytodiagnosis. II. Interlaboratory reproducibility as shown in rescreening large consecutive samples of reported cases. Acta Cytol 1987;31:900.
19. Hutchinson ML, Cassin CM, Ball HG III: The efficacy of an automated preparation device for cervical cytology. Am J Clin Pathol 1991;96:300.
20. Agency for Health Care Policy and Research: Evidence Report/Technology Assessment No. 5, Evaluation of Cervical Cytology. 1999, Report No. 99-E010.
21. Fahey MT, Irwig L, Macaskill P: Meta-analysis of Pap test accuracy. Am J Epidemiol 1995;141:680.
22. Hutchinson ML, Isenstein LM, Goodman A, et al: Homogeneous sampling accounts for the increased diagnostic accuracy using the ThinPrep processor. Am J Clin Pathol 1994;101:215.
23. Bishop JW, Bigner SH, Colgan TJ, et al: Multicenter masked evaluation of AutoCyte Prep thin layers with matched conventional smears. Including initial biopsy results. Acta Cytol 1998;42:189.
24. Bolick DR, Hellman DJ: Laboratory implementation and efficacy assessment of the ThinPrep cervical cancer screening system. Acta Cytol 1998;42:209.
25. Hutchinson ML, Zahniser DJ, Sherman ME, et al: Utility of liquid-based cytology for cervical carcinoma screening: Results of a population-based study conducted in a region of Costa Rica with a high incidence of cervical carcinoma. Cancer 1999;87:48.
26. Khalbuss WE, Rudomina D, Kauff ND, et al: SpinThin, a simple, inexpensive technique for preparation of thin-layer cervical cytology from liquid-based specimens: Data on 791 cases. Cancer 2000;90:135.
27. Aponte-Cipriani SL, Teplitz C, Rorat E, et al: Cervical smears prepared by an automated device versus the conventional method. A comparative analysis. Acta Cytol 1995;39:623.
28. Awen C, Hathway S, Eddy W, et al: Efficacy of ThinPrep preparation of cervical smears: a 1,000-case, investigator-sponsored study. Diagn Cytopathol. 1994;11:33.
29. Bur M, Knowles K, Pekow P, et al: Comparison of ThinPrep preparations with conventional cervicovaginal smears. Practical considerations. Acta Cytol 1995;39:631.
30. Ferenczy A, Robitaille J, Franco E, et al: Conventional cervical cytologic smears vs. ThinPrep smears. A paired comparison study on cervical cytology. Acta Cytol 1996;40:1136.

31. Geyer JW, Hancock F, Carrico C, Kirkpatrick M: Preliminary evaluation of Cyto-Rich: An improved automated cytology preparation. Diagn Cytopathol 1993;9:417.

32. Laverty CR, Thurloe JK, Redman NL, Farnsworth A: An Australian trial of ThinPrep: A new cytopreparatory technique. Cytopathology 1995;6:140.

33. McGoogan E, Reith A: Would monolayers provide more representative samples and improved preparations for cervical screening? Overview and evaluation of systems available. Acta Cytol 1996;40:107.

34. Sprenger E, Schwarzmann P, Kirkpatrick M, et al: The false negative rate in cervical cytology. Comparison of monolayers to conventional smears. Acta Cytol 1996;40:81.

35. Wilbur DC, Cibas ES, Merritt S, et al: ThinPrep processor. Clinical trials demonstrate an increased detection rate of abnormal cervical cytologic specimens. Am J Clin Pathol 1994;101:209.

36. Wilbur DC, Dubeshter B, Angel C, Atkison KM: Use of thin-layer preparations for gynecologic smears with emphasis on the cytomorphology of high-grade intraepithelial lesions and carcinomas. Diagn Cytopathol 1996;14:201.

37. Takahashi M, Naito M: Application of the CytoRich monolayer preparation system for cervical cytology. A prelude to automated primary screening. Acta Cytol 1997;41:1785.

38. Corkill ME, Knapp D, Hutchinson ML: Improved accuracy for cervical cytology with the ThinPrep method and the endocervical brush-spatula collection procedure. J Lower Fem Gen Tract 1988;167:466.

39. Hutchinson ML, Zahniser DJ, Sherman ME, et al: Utility of liquid-based cytology for cervical carcinoma screening: Results of a population-based study conducted in a region of Costa Rica with a high incidence of cervical carcinoma. Cancer 1999;87:48.

40. Lee KR, Ashfaq R, Birdsong GG, et al: Comparison of conventional Papanicolaou smears and a fluid-based, thin-layer system for cervical cancer screening. Obstet Gynecol 1997;90:278.

41. Roberts JM, Gurley AM, Thurloe JK, et al: Evaluation of the ThinPrep Pap test as an adjunct to the conventional Pap smear. Med J Aust. 1997;167:466.

42. Shield PW, Nolan GR, Phillips GE, Cummings MC: Improving cervical cytology screening in a remote, high risk population. Med J Aust. 1999;170:255.

43. Wang TY, Chen HS, Yang YC, Tsou MC: Comparison of fluid-based, thin-layer processing and conventional Papanicolaou methods for uterine cervical cytology. J Formos Med Assoc 1999;98:500.

44. Kunz J, Rondez R, Yoshizaki C, et al: [Comparison of conventional Pap smears with thin layer specimen (liquid-based Pap test) and correlation with cytopathological findings with HPV status using the Hybrid Capture system]. Schweiz Rundsch Med Prax 1998;87:1434.

45. Minge L, Fleming M, VanGeem T, Bishop JW: AutoCyte Prep system vs. conventional cervical cytology. Comparison based on 2,156 cases. J Reprod Med 2000;45:179.

46. Vassilakos P, Cossali D, Albe X, et al: Efficacy of monolayer preparations for cervical cytology: Emphasis on suboptimal specimens. Acta Cytol 1996;40:496.

47. Wilbur DC, Facik MS, Rutkowski MA, et al: Clinical trials of the CytoRich specimen-preparation device for cervical cytology. Preliminary results. Acta Cytol 1997;41:24.

48. Carpenter AB, Davey DD: ThinPrep Pap test: Performance and biopsy follow-up in a university hospital. Cancer 1999;87:105.

49. Diaz-Rosario LA, Kabawat SE: Performance of a fluid-based, thin-layer Papanicolaou smear method in the clinical setting of an independent laboratory and an outpatient screening population in New England. Arch Pathol Lab Med 1999;123:817.

50. Dupree WB, Suprun HZ, Beckwith DG, et al: The promise and risk of a new technology: The Lehigh Valley Hospital's experience with liquid-based cervical cytology. Cancer 1998;84:202.

51. Guidos BJ, Selvaggi SM: Use of the ThinPrep Pap test in clinical practice. Diagn Cytopathol 1999;20:70.

52. Papillo JL, Zarka MA, St John TL: Evaluation of the ThinPrep Pap test in clinical practice. A seven-month, 16,314-case experience in northern Vermont. Acta Cytol 1998;42:203.

53. Weintraub J: The coming revolution in cervical cytology: A pathologist's guide for the clinician. Ref Gynecol Obstet 1997;5:2.

54. Weintraub J, Morabia A: Efficacy of a liquid-based thin layer method for cervical cancer screening in a population with a low incidence of cervical cancer. Diagn Cytopathol 2000;22:52.

55. Tench W: Preliminary assessment of the AutoCyte Prep. Direct-to-vial performance. J Reprod Med 2000;45:912.

56. Vassilakos P, Griffin S, Megevand E, Campana A: CytoRich liquid-based cervical cytologic test. Screening results in a routine cytopathology service. Acta Cytol 1998;42:198.

57. Vassilakos P, Saurel J, Rondez R: Direct-to-vial use of the AutoCyte Prep liquid-based preparation for cervical-vaginal specimens in three European laboratories. Acta Cytol 1999;43:65.

58. Vassilakos P, Schwartz D, de Marval F, et al: Biopsy-based comparison of liquid-based, thin-layer preparations to conventional Pap smears. J Reprod Med 2000;45:11.

59. Ashfaq R, Gibbons D, Vela C, et al: ThinPrep Pap test. Accuracy for glandular disease. Acta Cytol 1999;43:81.

60. Duggan MA: Papnet-assisted, primary screening of cervico-vaginal smears. Eur J Gynaecol Oncol 2000;21:35.

61. Wilbur DC, Prey MU, Miller WM, et al: Detection of high grade squamous intraepithelial lesions and tumors using the AutoPap system: Results of a primary screening clinical trial. Cancer 1999;87:354.

62. Takahashi M, Kimura M, Akagi A, Naitoh M: AutoCyte screen interactive automated primary cytology screening system. A preliminary evaluation. Acta Cytol 1998;42:185.

63. Bishop JW, Kaufman RH, Taylor DA: Multicenter comparison of manual and automated screening of AutoCyte gynecologic preparations. Acta Cytol 1999;43:34.

64. Vassilakos P, Cossali D, Albe X, et al: Efficacy of monolayer preparations for cervical cytology: Emphasis on suboptimal specimens. Acta Cytol 1996;40:496.

65. Solomon D, Schiffman M, Tarone R: Comparison of three management strategies for patients with atypical squamous cells of undetermined significance: Baseline results from a randomized trial. J Natl Cancer Inst 2001;93:293.

66. Carson HJ, DeMay RM: The mode ages of women with cervical dysplasia. Obstet Gynecol 1993;82:430.

67. Luthra UK, Prabhakar AK, Seth P, et al: Natural history of precancerous and early cancerous lesions of the uterine cervix. Acta Cytol 1987;31:226.

68. Meisels A: Cytologic diagnosis of human papillomavirus. Influence of age and pregnancy stage. Acta Cytol 1992;36:480.

69. Burghardt E: Early histological diagnosis of cervical cancer. Major Probl Obstet Gynecol 1973;6:1.

70. Fabiani G, Pittino M, D'Aietti V, et al: [Cervical dysplasias. Comparative study of the cytological picture, anatomo-pathologic and age stage]. Minerva Ginecol 1987;39:629.

71. Cramer DW: The role of cervical cytology in the declining morbidity and mortality of cervical cancer. Cancer 1974;34:2018.

72. Widra EA, Dookhan D, Jordan A, et al: Evaluation of the atypical cytologic smear. Validity of the 1991 Bethesda System. J Reprod Med 1994;39:682.

73. Wilbur DC, Facik MS, Rutkowski MA, et al: Clinical trials of the CytoRich specimen-preparation device for cervical cytology. Preliminary results. Acta Cytol 1997;41:24.

74. Benedet JL, Anderson GH: Cervical intraepithelial neoplasia in British Columbia: A comprehensive program for detection, diagnosis, and treatment. Gynecol Oncol 1981;12(2 pt 2):S280.

75. Awen C, Hathway S, Eddy W, et al: Efficacy of ThinPrep preparation of cervical smears: A 1,000-case, investigator-sponsored study. Diagn Cytopathol 1994;11:33.

76. Raab SS: Can glandular lesions be diagnosed in Pap smear cytology? Diagn Cytopathol 2000;23:127.

77. Biscotti CV, Gero MA, Toddy SM, et al: Endocervical adenocarcinoma in situ: An analysis of cellular features. Diagn Cytopathol 1997;17:326.

78. Ashfaq R, Gibbons D, Vela C, et al: ThinPrep Pap test. Accuracy for glandular disease. Acta Cytol 1999;43:81.

• Edward J. Wilkinson

Clinical Laboratories Improvement Act

In the United States, pathologists as well as cytotechnologists are directly involved in the delivery of cytopathology services. This chapter will cover issues in training, accreditation, laboratory inspection, and laboratory quality assurance.

> **To receive a certificate of special competency in cytopathology, physicians who have completed a 5-year residency in anatomic and clinical pathology must take an extra year of training in a cytopathology fellowship approved by the Accreditation Council for Graduate Medical Education and pass the American Board of Pathology examination in cytopathology.**

Cytopathology is a subspecialty of anatomic pathology. Physicians completing a pathology residency today typically have 5 years of training in anatomic and clinical pathology and are eligible for board certification in anatomic and clinical pathology from the American Board of Pathology (ABP). Certification is achieved by passing the ABP examinations. Those whose primary interest is in cytopathology can receive a certificate of special competency in cytopathology by taking an extra year of training in a cytopathology fellowship approved by the Accreditation Council for Graduate Medical Education (ACGME) and passing the ABP examination in cytopathology.

Cytotechnologists must complete a 1-year cytotechnology training program accredited by the Committee on Allied Health Education and Accreditation or another credentialing organization as established in the Clinical Laboratories Improvement Act (CLIA) Section 493.1483. Requirements for entry include either a bachelor of science or a bachelor of arts degree, with sufficient science background as established by the credentialing organization. Successful completion of 1 year of training in an accredited program, beyond college graduation, is required for a person to be eligible for examination for certification as a cytotechnologist by the American Society of Clinical Pathologists (ASCP). To work as a cytotechnologist, a current cytotechnologist license must be held in the state in which the laboratory is located. In addition to the ASCP and the College of American Pathologists (CAP) there are three other major organizations in the United States that support cytopathology and cytotechnology. These are the American Society of Cytopathology (ASC),

the Papanicolaou Society, and the International Academy of Cytology (IAC). The IAC represents approximately 51 international cytology organizations throughout the world, and the United States is represented primarily by the ASC.

One of the major hurdles for the delivery of cervical cytopathology services is the labor-intensive nature of the screening process. Today, the interpretation of a cervical cytology sample is not an automated process. Rather, for each smear, a vast number and variety of cells must be individually and painstakingly screened for a variety of benign as well as neoplastic changes. Cells from other areas, including the vagina, rectum, endometrium, fallopian tube, peritoneum, and ovary may also be seen in cervical smears. In addition, a number of neoplastic, metaplastic, reactive, and inflammatory changes may be encountered. Many infectious organisms are also identified on the cervical cytology sample. As a result, proper interpretation of a cervical cytology smear requires a substantial degree of knowledge and experience to provide meaningful information.

Cytopathologists and cytotechnologists providing cervical cytology services typically do so within a certified cytopathology laboratory, in accordance with CLIA: "All cytology slide preparations are evaluated on the premises of a laboratory certified to conduct testing in the subspecialty of cytology."[1]

> **With the emergence in the United States of health maintenance organizations and large commercial laboratories, cytopathology services may be subcontracted to secondary laboratories that provide cytopathology services.**

Cytopathology laboratories are of several types. They may be part of a larger hospital-based laboratory system; a hospital may own an affiliated laboratory that is not necessarily inside the hospital, but rather immediately adjacent or in proximity to it; the cytopathology laboratory may be privately owned; or the laboratory may be a commercial venture where pathologists and cytotechnologists are employed. With the emergence in the United States of health maintenance organizations (HMOs) and large commercial laboratories, cytopathology services may be subcontracted to secondary laboratories that provide cytopathology services. A comprehensive discussion of the impact of these practices is beyond the scope of this chapter; however, it is an important issue, and some aspects of it will be discussed along with laboratory quality assurance issues.

> **A laboratory director oversees issues such as budget, personnel, space, and operational aspects of the laboratory. A medical director is responsible for all the medical aspects of the laboratory. A cytotechnology supervisor supports the laboratory's cytotechnologists and technicians and assists the medical director with quality assurance and continued quality improvement issues.**

Most cytopathology laboratories are structured in the same manner. There is usually a general laboratory director who oversees issues such as budget, personnel, space, and operational aspects of the laboratory. In large laboratories, there may be a separate laboratory manager who deals specifically with operational issues. There is a medical director who is responsible for all the medical aspects of the laboratory. In some settings, the medical director and the laboratory director are the same individual. The cytotechnology supervisor reports to the laboratory director and may also serve as laboratory manager. In most states, cytotechnology supervisors hold a supervisor's license, which requires them to have some years of experience and to pass a laboratory supervisor examination. The roles of the supervisor include support of the laboratory's cytotechnologists and technicians and responsibility for quality assurance and continued quality improvement issues, in concert with the work of the medical director and the delivery of cytopathology services. In smaller laboratories, the cytotechnology supervisor may also be the manager. Within larger laboratories, there is usually a technician who assists the cytotechnologists in the preparation of cytologic materials, including staining the smears, placing coverslips on the slides, and preparing the slides from liquid-based material. Most hospital-based and hospital-affiliated laboratories provide cervical cytopathology services as well as medical cytology services. As a result, preparation techniques can be quite variable, depending on the nature of the specimen.

> **Papanicolaou smears deemed "within normal limits" by a licensed cytotechnologist may be reported as such without further review.**

In most laboratories, cytology samples are first reviewed by cytotechnologists. Papanicolaou (Pap) smears deemed "within normal limits" (WNL) by a licensed cytotechnologist may be reported as such without further review. Under CLIA 88 guidelines, all other smears (other than those WNL) must be reviewed by the cytopathologist. In small laboratories, the pathologist may perform the screening and report the diagnosis.

> **Each individual engaged in the evaluation of cytology preparations by nonautomated microscopic technique may not examine more than 100 conventional slides in a 24-hour period, irrespective of the site or laboratory.**

Specific workload limits are designated by CLIA 88 under Section 493.1257, as follows:

- "Each individual engaged in the evaluation of cytology preparations by non-automated microscopic technique examines no more than 100 slides (one patient per slide, gynecologic or non-gynecologic, or both) in a 24 hour period, irrespective of the site or laboratory. This limit represents an absolute maximum number of slides and is not to be employed as a performance target for each individual."[1]
- "Liquid-based slide preparatory techniques which result in cell dispersion over one-half or less of the total available slide area and which is examined by non-automated microscopic technique count as one-half slide."[1]

Laboratories are required to retain cytology slides for 5 years and reports for 10 years.[1]

QUALITY ASSURANCE, COMPETENCY ASSESSMENT, AND PROFICIENCY TESTING IN THE CYTOPATHOLOGY LABORATORY

> **As mandated by CLIA 88, no fewer than 10% of the cervical cytology cases reported as WNL must be rescreened and re-reviewed.**

Cervical cytology specimens undergo quality assurance review as mandated by CLIA 88 (Section 493.1257). No fewer than 10% of the cervical cytology cases reported as WNL must be rescreened and re-reviewed. This review must include slides from patients considered high risk. "The laboratory must establish a program that includes a review of slides from at least 10 percent of the gynecologic cases interpreted to be negative for reactive, reparative, atypical, premalignant or malignant conditions as defined."[1]

The supervisor of the cytology laboratory generally performs rescreening, with support from the medical director.[2] A meta-analysis of 14 studies dealing with rescreening of Pap smears originally reported as WNL reported 0.18% as abnormal. Of the smears originally reported as WNL, 0.7% were reclassified as squamous intraepithelial lesions of all types, and 0.2% were reclassified as high-grade squamous intraepithelial lesions.[3] A new technique is being studied as an alternative to rescreening 10% or more of the slides classified as WNL. This technique is called rapid review. Unlike the conventional rescreening that intensely examines 10% of the cases reported as WNL, chosen randomly (including slides from high-risk patients), rapid review scans all the slides originally reviewed by the cytotechnologists and classified as WNL. The review excludes those cases that have recognized cellular abnormalities but may include cases with extensive inflammation, somewhat limited sample, or other issues. Rapid review is a 30- to 120-second review of the entire slide, as compared with a full rescreen that takes approximately 5 minutes.[2] Re-examination of the slide is usually done by the supervisory cytotechnologist or a designated experienced cytotechnologist. There is debate among cytopathologists as to which of these rescreening processes is more effective. In meta-analysis, rapid review reported a false-negative rate of 2%, as compared with 0.8% for the conventional 10% rescreening.[2]

> For each patient with a current high-grade intraepithelial lesion or a more severe lesion, the laboratory must review all gynecologic specimens received within the previous 5 years if they are available in the laboratory. If significant discrepancies are found that may affect patient care, the laboratory must notify the patient's physician and issue an amended report.

When a patient is identified with a cervical cytologic sample classified as a high-grade squamous intraepithelial lesion or a more severe lesion, CLIA 88 mandates the following: "For each patient with a current high grade intraepithelial lesion or above (moderate dysplasia or CIN-2 or above), the laboratory must review all normal or negative gynecologic specimens received within the previous five years, if available in the laboratory (either on-site or in storage). If significant discrepancies are found that would affect patient care, the laboratory must notify the patient's physician and issue an amended report."[1]

Cytopathology laboratories throughout the United States that provide cytopathology services billable to Medicare and third-party payers must be accredited. Accreditation for cytopathology laboratories requires inspection by the licensing body or licensing body's designee. In many states, the inspection process is assigned to the CAP's Clinical Laboratory Inspection Program, a highly structured and carefully maintained program operated by the CAP and staffed by pathologists who volunteer their time to add to these important programs.[4] In addition, hospital-based laboratories undergo inspection by the Joint Commission on Accreditation of Health Care Organizations (JCAHO), the Occupational Safety and Health Administration (OSHA), and other inspection agencies relevant to the operations of hospitals and hospital laboratories. The standards of commitment to quality assurance, accuracy, and review promote the highest level of patient care services.[5-7]

The CAP operates an intralaboratory comparison program in cervical-vaginal pathology.[8, 9] The ASCP also operates a laboratory assessment program.[10] Both these programs operate in the United States, and most cytopathology laboratories participate in one or both. These programs measure interlaboratory reproducibility and also provide an opportunity for evaluating competency within an individual laboratory. Within a given laboratory, the cytotechnologists, cytotechnology supervisor, medical director, and other pathologists involved in the cervical cytopathology laboratory participate in these programs.[11, 12] However, these programs do not measure a given laboratory's performance, because they do not permit intralaboratory consultation on difficult cases or permit responses to questions when there are specific issues. Although these programs do not measure individual skills within the laboratory, this measurement may be done internally using the programs' quality assurance materials.

Significant efforts are under way by pathologists and pathology-related professional organizations to maintain and improve the Pap smear. These efforts include the proficiency testing program developed and managed by the CAP interlaboratory comparison program in cervico-vaginal cytology.

> Under the present paradigm of HMOs, cytopathology and cervical biopsy services are often "carved out" from local laboratories, and specimens are sent to a commercial laboratory that holds the HMO's laboratory contract. This significantly impedes the communication between the clinician and the pathologist who rendered the diagnosis.

A particularly valuable quality assurance and quality improvement resource for cytopathology laboratories is their ability to correlate subsequent cervical biopsy findings with the Pap smear that prompted that biopsy.[13] However, under the present paradigm of HMOs, cytopathology and cervical biopsy services are often "carved out" from the local laboratories and the pathologists with whom physicians ordinarily interact. Instead, the specimens are sent to a commercial laboratory that holds the HMO's laboratory contract. This disrupts the internal review process as well as the interaction between the pathologist and the clinician. This problem is further compounded by the fact that the clinician does not have immediate access to the pathologist responsible for the report or to the relevant cervical cytology and biopsy materials. This significantly impedes the practice of evidence-based medicine because it disrupts the correlation of the colposcopy findings with the biopsy and cytology findings and hinders the development of a treatment plan with the support of the pathologist who rendered the diagnosis.

SUMMARY

Clinical cytopathology services in the United States today are highly regulated. Individuals are extensively trained, and the quality of their work and that of the laboratories is extensively tested and inspected. Nevertheless, the pressures from HMOs for cost containment have led to large commercial laboratories centralizing and subcontracting cytology services, which, in turn, has interfered with the critical communication between the cytopathologist and the clinician.

SUMMARY OF KEY POINTS

- To receive a certificate of special competency in cytopathology, physicians who have completed a 5-year residency in anatomic and clinical pathology must take an extra year of training in an ACGME-approved cytopathology fellowship and pass the ABP examination in cytopathology.

- A laboratory director oversees issues such as budget, personnel, space, and operational aspects of the laboratory. A medical director is responsible for all the medical aspects of the laboratory. A cytotechology supervisor supports the laboratory's cytotechnologists and technicians and assists the medical director with quality assurance and continued quality improvement issues.

- Pap smears deemed WNL by a licensed cytotechnologist may be reported as such without further review.

- Each individual engaged in the evaluation of cytology preparations by nonautomated microscopic technique may not examine more than 100 conventional slides in a 24-hour period, irrespective of the site or laboratory.

- As mandated by CLIA 88, no fewer than 10% of the cervical cytology cases reported as WNL must be rescreened and re-reviewed.

- For each patient with a current high-grade intraepithelial lesion or a more severe lesion, the laboratory must review all gynecologic specimens received within the previous 5 years, if they are available in the laboratory. If significant discrepancies are found that may affect patient care, the laboratory must notify the patient's physician and issue an amended report.

- Under the present paradigm of HMOs, cytopathology and cervical biopsy services are often carved out from the local laboratories, and specimens are sent to a commercial laboratory that holds the HMO's laboratory contract. This significantly impedes the communication between the clinician and the pathologist who rendered the diagnosis.

- In large commercial laboratories, cytopathology services may be subcontracted to secondary laboratories that provide cytopathology services.

References

1. Clinical Laboratory Improvement Amendments of 1988 (CLIA 88) (Public Law 100-578). Fed Register 1990;55:9538.
2. Arbyn M, Schenck U: Detection of false negative Pap smears by rapid reviewing: A meta analysis. Acta Cytol 2000;44:949.
3. Coleman DV, Baker R: Sensitivity of partial re-screening in cervical cytology. Acta Cytol 1997;41:1631.
4. College of American Pathologists on line: Available at http://www.cap.org
5. Joint Commission on Accreditation of Health Care Organizations on line: Available at http://www.jcaho.org
6. Occupational Safety and Health Administration: Occupational exposure to blood borne pathogens. Fed Register 1996;60(30).
7. Occupational Safety and Health Administration: Occupational exposures to chemicals in laboratories. Laboratory standard. Fed Register 1990.
8. Jones BA, Davey DD: Quality management in gynecologic cytology using interlaboratory comparison. Arch Pathol Lab Med 2000;124:672.
9. College of American Pathologists: Commission on Laboratory Accreditation Inspection Checklist. Northfield, IL, Cytopathology, 2000.
10. Triol JH (ed): ASCT Cytopathology Quality Assurance Guide, vols. I and II. Raleigh, NC, American Society for Cytotechnology, 1992.
11. Davey DD, McGoogan E, Somarak TM, et al: Competency assessment and proficiency testing. Acta Cytol 2000;44:939.
12. Davey DD, Nielsen ML, Frable WJ, et al: Improving accuracy in gynecologic cytology: Results of the College of American Pathologists interlaboratory comparison program in cervicovaginal cytology (PAP). Arch Pathol Lab Med 1993;117:1193.
13. Jones BA, Novis DA: Cervical biopsy-cytology correlation: A College of American Pathologists Q-Probes study of 22,439 correlations in 348 laboratories. Arch Pathol Lab Med 1996;120:523.

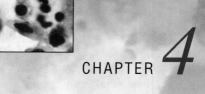

CHAPTER *4*

Adjunctive Testing

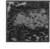

A

- Gregory L. Brotzman
- Mark Spitzer

Cervicography

For more than 50 years, the Papanicolaou (Pap) smear has been the primary screening test for the detection of invasive cervical cancer and precancerous lesions. This test represents one of the greatest successes in gynecology and one of the most important achievements in cancer prevention. In 1989, the success of the Pap smear in reducing cervical cancer led Leopold G. Koss to write that the cervical smear is an effective tool of cancer detection, "perhaps the only effective cancer screening test known today."[1] Yet in a more recent study by the Agency for Health Care Policy and Research (AHCPR), it was determined that, in unbiased studies, the actual sensitivity of the Pap smear is approximately 51%.[2] Early reports hinted at the low sensitivity of cervical cytology and prompted a search for alternatives.

> Cervicography has been proposed as an adjunctive test that would increase the sensitivity and specificity of the Pap smear for detection of precancerous and invasive cervical lesions.

One means of improving the detection of cervical cancer and its precursor lesions is the use of an adjunctive test that increases the sensitivity and specificity of cervical screening when it is combined with the Pap smear. Such a test, if used appropriately, could possibly reduce the overall cost of cervical cancer prevention. One of the first technologies proposed as an adjunctive test to the Pap smear was cervicography. This chapter discusses cervicography, the Cervicography Cervical Cancer Screening System, and their impact on cervical cancer screening. (Please note that the terms Cerviscope Camera, Cervigram Slide, Cervigram Picture, and Cervicography Cervical Cancer Screening System are either registered trademarks or service marks of NTL Processing, Inc.)

INTRODUCTION OF CERVICOGRAPHY

In 1980, Adolf Stafl, a colposcopist and photographer at the Medical College of Wisconsin, invented a diagnostic method he called cervicography using an apparatus he called the cervicograph. Cervicography is a method of detecting cancer and other cervical abnormalities by projecting a photographic image of the cervix onto a screen, where it is evaluated by an expert reviewer.

Stafl emphasized that successful colposcopy depended on the expertise of the examiner and that colposcopy in the hands of the inexperienced practitioner may result in misdiagnosis of a cervical lesion, thus endangering the life of the patient with invasive cancer. Stafl developed the cervicograph, an inexpensive optical instrument that he believed allowed permanent objective documentation of the cervical findings. He proposed that the instrument be used for evaluation of patients with an abnormal cytologic diagnosis and for cervical cancer screening along with the Pap smear. He believed that the cervicograph offered a unique opportunity for critical assessment of colposcopic expertise and provided permanent documentation of cervical findings.

The cervicograph is an optical instrument that takes a picture of the cervix for permanent documentation of the cervical findings.

In order to achieve these goals, cervicography would need magnification comparable to normal colposcopic magnification ($\times$16), maximal depth of focus, the highest possible resolution, the ability to visualize the entire cervix in one view, easy portability, and a sufficiently intense light source to permit a short exposure time.

The Cerviscope Camera is a 35-mm camera with a fixed focal-distance telephoto macrolens, an illumination source, and a strobe flash mounted on a handheld platform. Following placement of an intravaginal speculum, the cervix is visualized, cleaned with dry gauze, and moistened with 4% acetic acid. The cervicograph is focused on the cervix by moving the instrument back and forth. When the cervix is in focus, a picture is taken.

Cervigrams are the cervicograph slides projected on a screen and observed by the evaluator from a distance of 3 feet.

The Cervigram Slide is projected on a screen 10 feet or greater in width and is observed from a distance of 3 feet. The cervicographic findings were originally divided into four groups: negative—the entire squamocolumnar junction is fully visible, no abnormal lesion is present; suspicious—an abnormal lesion (white epithelium, punctation, mosaic, atypical vessels) is present; unsatisfactory—the squamocolumnar junction is not visible; and technically defective—picture is out of focus, underexposed, or overexposed or the entire cervix is not visible.

Stafl originally reported the results of a study of 700 women who underwent cervicography.[3] The women were from two study groups. The first group consisted of 296 women referred to a colposcopy clinic for evaluation of abnormal cervical cytology. The second group consisted of 404 patients presenting for routine screening who had no previous or current history of abnormal cervical cytology. Colposcopically directed biopsies were performed to ascertain histologic evidence of disease. The study demonstrated that the histologic differences between colposcopy and cervicography were not significant and that both methods had comparable diagnostic accuracy. Cervicography missed some "out of sight" lesions when the evaluation was unsatisfactory (i.e., the squamocolumnar junction was not visible) but identified patients with low- and high-grade disease who were missed by cytology. The study also demonstrated that individuals not experienced in colposcopy could easily obtain a satisfactory cervigram.

In December 1983, cervicography was licensed to a commercial firm that eventually became National Testing Laboratories (NTL) Worldwide. NTL developed the system that was used in all cervicography studies from that point forward.

INITIAL STUDIES

In the initial study by Tawa et al, the cervigram was determined to be significantly more sensitive than the Pap smear, whereas the Pap smear was significantly more specific than the cervigram in detecting cervical intraepithelial neoplasia.

The first large study of cervicography was performed by Tawa et al.[4] In this study, a total of 3271 gynecology patients between the ages of 18 and 50 years were simultaneously screened for cervical intraepithelial neoplasia (CIN) and invasive cervical cancer with cytology and with cervicography. The accuracy of each screening test result, when positive or suspicious, was evaluated independently, and the results were compared with colposcopically directed biopsy results. The cervigram was determined to be significantly more sensitive than the Pap smear, whereas the Pap smear was determined to be significantly more specific than the cervigram in detecting CIN.

Results indicated that 5.1 times more CIN lesions were detected by the cervigrams than by the Pap smears.

Results of the study demonstrated that 5.1 times more CIN lesions were detected by the cervigrams than by the Pap smears. Seventy-two CIN lesions were detected by the cervigram, and 14 were detected by the Pap smear. The 4:1 ratio for the detection of CIN 2 and CIN 3 by the cervigram and the Pap smear was similar to the cervigram's overall increased rate of CIN detection. The authors concluded that the cervigram was just as effective in detecting CIN 2 and CIN 3 as it was in detecting CIN 1.

The results of the Tawa et al study also pointed out that cervicography and cytology were complementary. Some CIN lesions were detected with both tests, a few CIN lesions were detected on the Pap smear alone, but a significant number of CIN lesions were detected only by the cervigram. These findings were similar to the results of studies where colposcopy and Pap smears were combined for screening.[5-7] The outcomes are not surprising, because cervical cytology evaluates cellular abnormalities, whereas the cervigram and colposcopy evaluate the appearance of the cervical epithelium.

Cervical cytology evaluates cellular abnormalities, whereas cervicography and colposcopy evaluate the appearance of the cervical epithelium.

Jones et al[8] conducted a prospective study of 236 patients with "atypical" but not dysplastic Pap smears who were evaluated by colposcopy and directed biopsies to assess the significance of the atypical smear. Cervicography was compared with repeat cytology and with the results of the colposcopic assessment. Fifty-eight patients (25%) had biopsy-proved CIN. Repeat cytology identified only 17% of these patients. Colposcopy noted "atypical transformation zones" in 97% of the patients with CIN.

Cervigrams identified 81% of the CIN lesions but had a 15% method failure (unsatisfactory—transformation zone not seen in 6%, and technically defective—uninterpretable in 9%).

Results of the Jones study demonstrated that five patients with biopsy-proved CIN had cervigrams that were judged to be negative, but the transformation zone was not entirely seen. In this study, all CIN 2 and CIN 3 lesions were identified by both colposcopy and cervicography, provided the cervicography was satisfactory. Additionally, results demonstrated that colposcopy and cervicography were sufficiently sensitive to be considered as potential intermediate screening procedures, although cervicography had greater specificity and a higher positive predictive value than did colposcopy.

If cervicography is used as an intermediate screening test, all patients with unsatisfactory cervicography results must be evaluated further, and technically defective studies must be repeated.

Jones and colleagues suggested that simply repeating the Pap smear as the sole method of evaluating patients with atypical cytologic diagnoses should be abandoned. They further concluded that if cervicography is used as an intermediate screening test, all patients with unsatisfactory cervicography results must be evaluated further and that technically defective studies must be repeated. Patients with normal cervigrams should not be considered disease free on the basis of cervicography alone.

At the same time, Spitzer et al[9] performed a similar study comparing cervicography, colposcopy, and cytology. They also concluded that repeat cytology alone was an inadequate method of evaluating patients with atypical cytologic diagnoses and that intermediate triage with cervicography was superior. However, in their high-risk population, direct referral for colposcopy was a more cost-effective strategy. In settings where colposcopy resources are limited, intermediate triage with cervicography is an appropriate alternative.

ADDITIONAL STUDIES

Subsequent to these studies, many other studies of cervicography have been done in various parts of the world. The results have consistently demonstrated that cervicography is more sensitive and less specific than cytology. The later studies evaluated modifications to the system used to report cervicography results that were intended to increase the specificity of cervicography.

In several studies, cervicography has detected cervical cancer when the cervical cytology was normal.

An early study by Blythe[10] evaluated 578 patients using cervicography and cytology. The study confirmed the lack of sensitivity of the Pap smear and corroborated data on cervicography presented earlier by Stafl. But, more importantly and for the first time, one patient with cervi-

cal cancer was diagnosed by cervicography although the Pap smear was normal. This was the first of several studies in which cervicography detected cervical cancer when the cervical cytology was normal.[11, 12]

The technically defective rate of the Cervicography Cervical Cancer Screening System is less than 2%.

One finding highlighted in the Blythe study[10] was the high rate of unsatisfactory and technically defective cervigrams. In this study, 27.5% of the Cervigram Slides were technically defective, and 26.4% were unsatisfactory. The problem of technically defective cervigrams was resolved when NTL improved the training of practitioners to whom it sold cervicography equipment (the Cerviscope Camera). Most studies completed subsequently reflected a technically defective rate of less than 2%. In a study by Schneider et al, a large population-based study of 8460 women in Costa Rica, the technically defective rate was 1.3%.[11] The problem of unsatisfactory Cervigram Slides was also resolved with changes in the system by which cervicography results are reported. This issue will be discussed later in the chapter.

After the changes in the cervigram report form, the specificity of cervicography increased significantly. The first of the studies to reflect the increased specificity was by Kesic et al.[13] The authors found that cervicography correctly identified 24 of 27 women with CIN or invasive cancer, whereas cytology detected only 14, a sensitivity of 89% for cervicography versus 52% for cytology. They also found that cervicography was only slightly less specific than cytology, 92% versus 94%, respectively. In the study by Schneider et al,[11] the specificity of cervicography in detecting high-grade CIN and cancer was 95% versus 94.2% for cytology. But as the changes in the reporting system improved the specificity of cervicography, its sensitivity relative to cytology diminished. In the latter study, the overall sensitivity of cervicography in detecting high-grade lesions and cancer was only 49.3% compared with 77.2% overall for cytology.[11] Although cervicography was the only test evaluated in this study to detect all 11 of the cervical cancers, its sensitivity was lower than previously reported, whereas that of cytology was higher than previously reported. In their discussion, the authors speculated that the unusually high sensitivity for high-grade squamous intraepithelial lesion (HSIL) and cancer exhibited by conventional cytology in this study (much higher than that previously experienced in the same population) may have been because the cytologic evaluation in this study was optimized by careful clinician training, a strict fixation and staining protocol, and site visits by experts in cytotechnology and cytopathology from the United States. Reasons for the reported lower sensitivity of cervicography may include the definition of disease used in the paper, the indications for a colposcopic examination, and the classification of a positive cervigram when histology was not available.

Eskridge et al[14] performed a study to determine the efficacy of combining repeat cytology with cervicography for the identification of HSIL among patients who previously had atypical squamous cells of undetermined significance (ASCUS) or low-grade squamous intraepithelial lesion (LSIL) on cytology. In this study, the sensitivity for the detection of CIN 2 and CIN 3 in patients with an initial ASCUS smear was 46% (specificity 64%) and 92% (specificity 30%) for the repeat cytology and for cervicography, respectively. The sensitivity for CIN 2 and CIN 3 in those patients with an initial LSIL smear was 78% (specificity 48%) and 89% (specificity 59%) for the repeat Pap smear and the cervicography system, respectively. Repeat cytology led to detection of only 46% of CIN 2 and CIN 3 lesions, whereas cervicography detected 92% of them. One of the conclusions from this study was that the cervicography system was a helpful adjunctive technique for detection of CIN 2 and CIN 3 lesions in patients with previous ASCUS or LSIL Pap smears. Their finding led the authors to question the recommendation of the 1992 National Cancer Institute workshop on the Bethesda System that repeat Pap testing alone is an acceptable follow-up strategy for ASCUS Pap tests. In this study and others, it was suggested that if the cervigram is negative, most of these patients can reasonably be followed up with serial Pap smears, whereas if the cervigram is atypical or positive, closer follow-up or colposcopy should be considered.[15–17]

> **If the cervigram is negative, most of the patients can be followed up with serial Pap smear, whereas if the cervigram is atypical or positive, closer follow-up or colposcopy is recommended.**

Ferris et al,[18] in a study of 1449 women, evaluated the use of cervicography by primary care specialists in community clinical sites to determine whether its use would enhance and complement the Pap smear. They concluded that cervicography detected twice as many patients with premalignant disease as cytology alone detected and that cervicography correctly identified the only invasive cancer in the study, whereas cytology failed to identify the cancer. Additionally, the authors concluded that cervicography as performed by primary care physicians effectively enhanced cervical cytologic screening.

COST-EFFECTIVENESS OF CERVICOGRAPHY

> **Per dollar spent in a screening setting, the Cervicography Cervical Cancer Screening System detected 3.7 times more CIN lesions than did the Pap smear.**

In a health care environment with limited resources, it is imperative that cost be considered in the implementation of any new or different protocol or technology. Several studies have evaluated the cost-effectiveness of cervicography. A study by Tawa et al concluded that per dollar spent in their organization (Kaiser Permanente–Los Angeles), cervicography detected 3.7 times more CIN lesions than did cytology.[4]

August et al[17] compared the cost per CIN detected for patients with atypical Pap smears using three approaches: treat and repeat the Pap smear; perform colposcopy for all women with atypical Pap smears; and use cervicography as an intermediate triage tool for women with atypical Pap smears. They concluded that the cost per case of CIN detected was $3728 for the "treat and repeat" protocol, $3713 when all women underwent colposcopy, and $2005 when intermediate triage with cervicography was used. They concluded that cervicography appears to be the best case-finding technique currently available for the evaluation of the atypical Pap smear.[17]

> **It has been demonstrated that cervicographic findings are significantly reproducible when reviewed by experienced evaluators.**

In the only study of interobserver variability of cervigram evaluations, August et al compared the evaluations of eight evaluators certified by NTL. The Cervigram Slides of 500 patients selected randomly from one of the evaluator's series were independently evaluated by each of eight evaluators who were blinded to the patients' history and physical findings. They concluded that cervigram evaluators had a high degree of interobserver agreement and that this agreement was superior to that previously reported in studies of colpophotography and cervical cytology. It was demonstrated that cervicographic findings are significantly reproducible when reviewed by experienced evaluators.[17]

> **The cervicography system is a standardization of the procedure incorporated into a unified, organized, and quality-controlled method.**

Only expert colposcopists who have been tested and licensed by NTL evaluate the Cervigram Slides. They follow an established evaluation algorithm to maintain standardization in the evaluation process. This ensures the highest possible interobserver and intraobserver correlation results while allowing for professional differences of opinion.

EQUIPMENT AND SUPPLIES

The supplies needed to take a Cervigram Picture include a speculum (any kind, metal or plastic, can be used, but a medium-sized or larger speculum is preferable because it allows for better visualization of the entire cervix); cotton swabs (large rectal swabs about 8 in long and small, cotton-tipped applicators); 5% acetic acid solution; a condom placed over the speculum blades or some other sidewall retractor if necessary to retract the vaginal sidewalls; the Cerviscope Camera and power supply; cervigram film (ASA 200 professional-grade Kodak Ektachrome color slide film); and a patient log sheet.

> **The Cerviscope Camera produces consistent, high-resolution, panoramic photographic images of the cervix.**

The Cerviscope Camera is a specially designed, handheld camera with an attached light source and a fixed-focus macro lens (Fig. 4–1). All settings are preset by NTL, and the focus is obtained by moving the unit closer

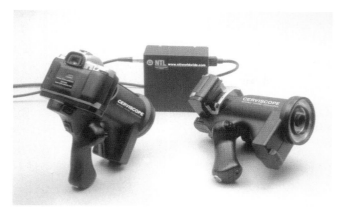

Figure 4–1. Example of a cerviscope, power supply, and power cable.

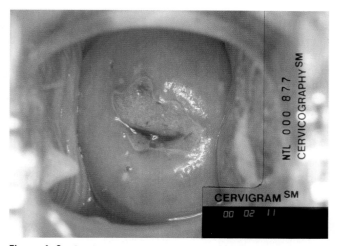

Figure 4–2. Cervigram demonstrating a normal cervix. Patient and clinic identifier information is located on the right side of the slide, resulting from camera databack impression on the film when the image is obtained.

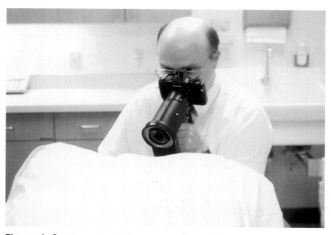

Figure 4–3. Example of how a cervigram is taken. Note that the clinician holds the cerviscope in the left hand. The trigger release is located on the handle so the right hand does not need to be used to snap the picture.

to get a clear and unobstructed view, the cervix is generously soaked with 5% acetic acid for about 15 seconds. Sufficient acetic acid should be used until a pool forms in the posterior vaginal fornix. The cerviscope is refocused and, after 15 seconds, acetic acid is reapplied to the cervix for another 15 seconds from the pool in the posterior fornix. The cerviscope is refocused, and two Cervigram Pictures are taken. The procedure normally adds less than 2 minutes to the examination.

EVALUATING THE CERVIGRAM SLIDE

Cervigrams are evaluated by NTL licensed evaluators (Fig. 4–4) who follow an evaluation algorithm during the evaluation process (Fig. 4–5) and complete the pre-printed, computer-generated cervigram evaluation report form, which is then returned to NTL for processing (Fig. 4–6).

to or farther away from the cervix. The focal distance allows adequate working room. The Cerviscope Camera produces consistent, high-resolution, panoramic photographic images of the cervix and upper vagina (Fig. 4–2).

TAKING A CERVIGRAM PICTURE

The cervigram is normally taken in the office setting at the time of routine cytologic screening after the Pap smear has been obtained (Fig. 4–3). A checklist is used for taking a cervigram (Appendix 1). Two images per patient are usually taken. It is important for the clinician to make certain that he or she has a clear and unobstructed view of the entire cervix and that the cervix is centered in the image. If the entire cervix cannot be included in one image, one side of the cervix should be taken with the first image and the other side with the second image. After ensuring that the cervix is positioned

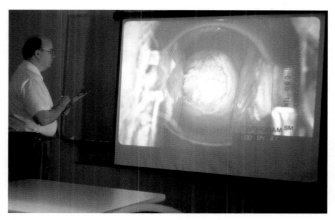

Figure 4–4. The evaluation process. The evaluator stands 3 feet from the screen, giving a magnified, panoramic view of the cervix.

Text continued on page 80

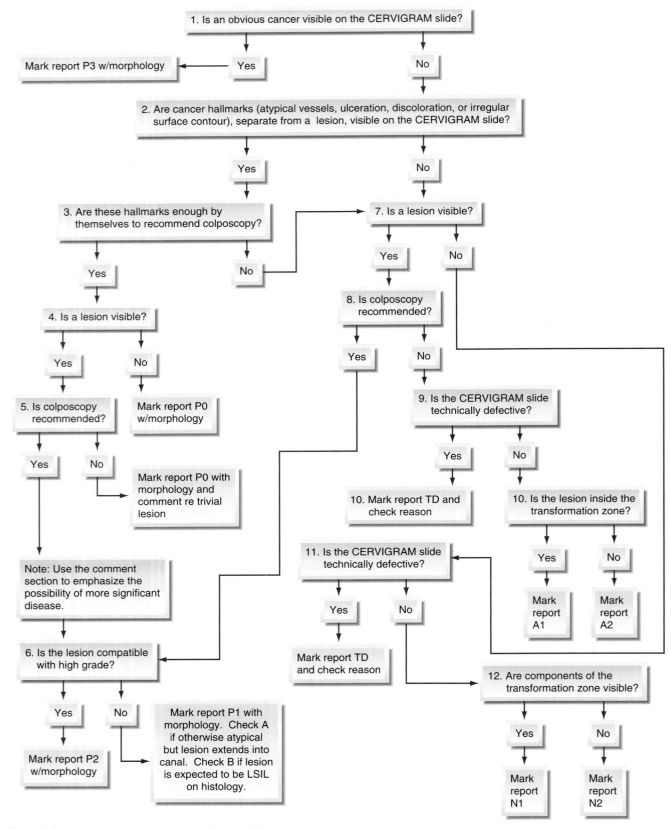

Figure 4–5. Example of the cervigram evaluation algorithm.

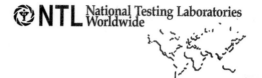

NTL National Testing Laboratories Worldwide

CERVICOGRAPHY℠ System

CERVIGRAM™ Slide

EVALUATION REPORT

NTL PROCESSING, INC.

400 Biltmore Drive, Suite 407
Fenton, MO 63026
(314) 343-4533
(800) 325-9737 or (800) 842-7135

*(SEE REVERSE SIDE OF REPORT FOR IMPORTANT NOTES AND EXPLANATION)

☐ NEGATIVE—Repeat * the CERVIGRAM™ picture and Pap smear on a routine basis.

1. _____ Components of the transformation zone are visible.

2. _____ Components of the transformation zone are not visible.

☐ ATYPICAL—A CERVIGRAM™ picture and Pap smear are recommended* in _____ 6 or _____ 12 months.

1. _____ A lesion of doubtful significance is visible inside the transformation zone.

2. _____ A lesion of doubtful significance is visible outside the transformation zone.

☐ POSITIVE—Colposcopy is recommended.*

0. _____ Probable normal variant; appearance warrants colposcopy to exclude significant disease.

1. _____ Compatible with low grade lesion: _____ A _____ B

2. _____ Compatible with high grade lesion.

3. _____ Compatible with cancer.

_____ Morphology _____

_____ Acetowhite epithelium

_____ Punctation

_____ Mosaic

_____ Atypical vessels

_____ Erosion or ulceration

_____ Discoloration

_____ Irregular surface contour

☐ TECHNICALLY DEFECTIVE—See attached notice and please retake* CERVIGRAM™ picture.

1. _____ View of cervix obscured by: _____ mucus _____ blood _____ position of cervix _____ other: _____

2. _____ Insufficient acetic acid reaction when reaction is anticipated

3. _____ Other problems: _____ Out of focus _____ Overexposed _____ Underexposed

☐ OTHER—(Vagina, vulva, penis, anus - see Comments Section)

COMMENTS—

☐ CERVIGRAM™ slide(s) is satisfactory for evaluation. The quality could have been improved. Please note the item(s) marked in the technically defective category above.

Other: _____

_____

_____

Evaluated By: _____ Date _____

WE ARE UNABLE TO DETECT ABNORMALITIES NOT VISIBLE ON THE CERVIGRAM™ SLIDE

WHITE—FACILITY COPY   YELLOW—NTL COPY
FACILITY   BLUE—EVALUATOR COPY   © 1994 NTL Processing, Inc.

Figure 4–6. Example of a cervigram evaluation form.

Cervigram Evaluation Report Form

Cervigrams are currently reported in the following categories: negative, atypical, positive, and technically defective.

The evaluation report form has undergone several changes over the years since 1982, the latest change being in 1995. Cervigrams are currently reported in 1 of 4 categories: negative (N1 and N2); atypical (A1 and A2); positive (P0—probable normal variant, appearance warrants colposcopy to exclude significant disease; P1—compatible with low-grade lesion; P2—compatible with high-grade lesion; P3—compatible with cancer); or technically defective.

A negative evaluation means no definite lesion is visible to the evaluator. It does not mean that a lesion is not present in the endocervical canal.

A negative evaluation means no definite lesion is visible to the evaluator. It does not indicate the absence of disease. If a lesion is present, it is likely in the endocervical canal. For this reason, it is important to perform endocervical brush cytology at the time a cervigram is taken. The negative category is subcategorized into one of two possibilities depending on whether components of the transformation zone are visible (N1) or not visible (N2) (Figs. 4–7 and 4–8). Except in very high-risk young women, it is recommended that following a negative cervigram, screening with cervicography should be continued every fourth year until about age 50 years. Testing could end sooner if the components of the transformation zone are no longer visible.

An atypical evaluation means that if a lesion is present, it is considered of doubtful significance, and colposcopy is not recommended.

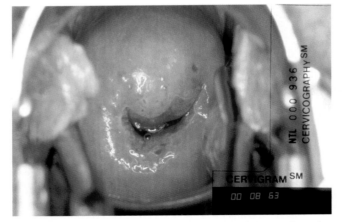

Figure 4–7. N1 (negative) cervigram. Components of the transformation zone are present.

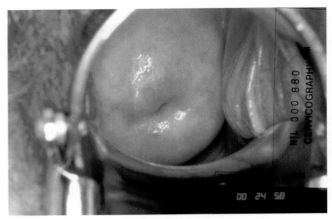

Figure 4–8. N2 (negative) cervigram. Components of the transformation zone are not visible.

The atypical category improves the specificity of cervicography but decreases the sensitivity to some degree.

An atypical evaluation means a lesion is visible, but, based on the site of the lesion, the morphology, and the age of the patient, the lesion is considered to be of doubtful significance. Colposcopy is not normally recommended for an atypical cervigram. The colposcopic evaluation of women with atypical cervigrams would increase the sensitivity of the examination at the expense of decreasing specificity. The atypical category was introduced because many of the previously low-grade positive reports exhibited negative histology even though a colposcopic lesion was definitely visible. It is hypothesized that the lesion in the atypical category may be in a very early stage or is regressing and therefore not detectable by histology. The addition of the atypical category improves the specificity of cervicography but decreases its sensitivity to some degree. The atypical category is subcategorized into one of two possibilities depending on whether the lesion is inside (A1) or outside (A2) the transformation zone (Figs. 4–9 and 4–10). Atypical cervigrams should be repeated in a year unless the smear is ASCUS; then, colposcopy might be considered if the objective is to ensure the highest sensitivity in screening.

The positive evaluation means that a lesion is visible and colposcopy is recommended or that no lesion is visible but the appearance of the cervix warrants colposcopy to exclude significant disease.

A positive evaluation means that a lesion is visible and colposcopy is recommended based on the site and morphology of the lesion and the patient's age or that no definite lesion is visible but the appearance of the cervix warrants colposcopy to exclude significant disease. This latter situation, a P0, is a very infrequent report (Fig. 4–11). The positive category is further subcategorized as P1, P2, or P3. The P1 subcategory has two classifications:

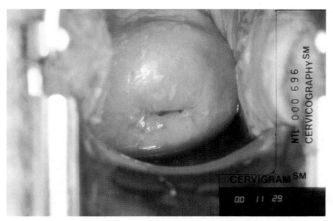

Figure 4–9. Atypical cervigram with faint, white epithelium noted at 12 o'clock.

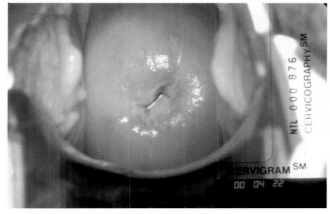

Figure 4–12. P1A cervigram. A geographic area of faint, acetowhite epithelium is noted.

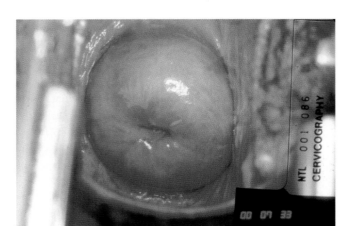

Figure 4–10. Atypical cervigram.

P1A—a lesion extending into the canal, the visible portion of which is considered to be of doubtful significance; and P1B—a lesion compatible with low-grade disease (Figs. 4–12 and 4–13). The P1A classification is included in the positive category instead of the atypical category because the visible portion of the lesion may be a sentinel for more significant disease in the endocervical canal. The P2 classification is compatible with high-grade disease (Figs. 4–14 and 4–15), and the P3 classification is compatible with invasive cancer (Fig. 4–16). After a positive cervigram, colposcopy is recommended.

A technically defective evaluation means that the slide is not adequate for evaluation because the cervix is obscured by mucus, vaginal sidewalls, hair, the speculum, a polyp, or excessive acetic acid pooling in the posterior fornix.

A technically defective evaluation should be repeated.

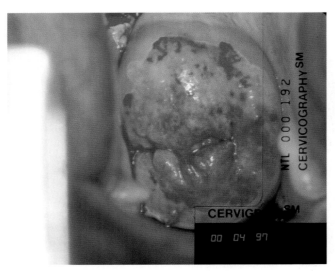

Figure 4–11. P0 cervigram. Biopsies revealed invasive squamous cell cancer.

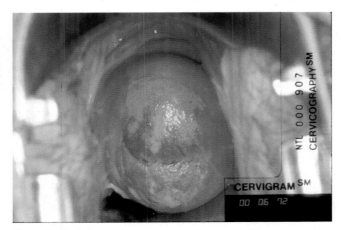

Figure 4–13. P1B cervigram. A geographic area of faint, acetowhite, fine mosaic pattern, suggestive of a low-grade lesion, is noted.

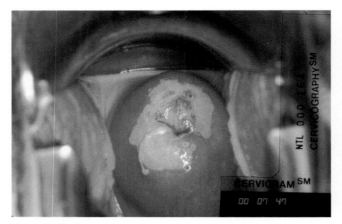

Figure 4–14. P2 cervigram. Large four-quadrant area of dense, aceto-white epithelium consistent with a high-grade lesion.

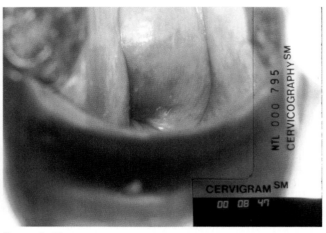

Figure 4–17. Technically defective cervigram owing to obscuring blood.

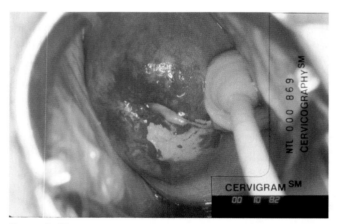

Figure 4–15. P2 cervigram. Lesion noted at 6 o'clock with sharp margins and dense, acetowhite epithelium.

A technically defective evaluation means the slide is not adequate for evaluation, usually when the cervix is obscured by mucus, vaginal sidewalls, hair, the vaginal speculum, a polyp, or excessive acetic acid pooling in the posterior fornix. The technically defective cervigram is an infrequent (less than 2%) occurrence. The evaluator will suggest repeating the cervigram (Fig. 4–17). A technically defective cervigram should be repeated.

OTHER APPLICATIONS FOR THE PROCEDURE/SYSTEM

Cervicography was developed primarily for use as a screening adjunct to the Pap smear, but cervicography can also be used to document the colposcopic appearance of the ectocervix (Fig. 4–18). Cervicography has been a valuable research tool to document the appearance of the cervix before and after treatment with various topical

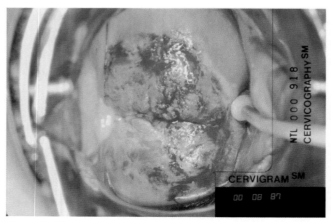

Figure 4–16. P3 cervigram. Dense, acetowhite epithelium, irregular contour, and atypical vessels are appreciated.

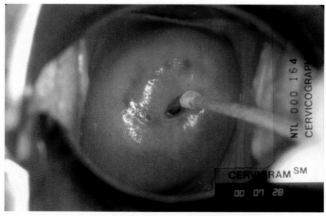

Figure 4–18. Example of postcryotherapy cervix with venous lakes present and a trivial area of acetowhite epithelium noted on the posterior lip of the cervix.

creams and intravaginal devices. Cervigram Slides have also been used for chart documentation, for teaching colposcopy recognition skills, and in the testing and monitoring of colposcopic skills.

CONCLUSION

Cervicography has played an important, although limited, role in the screening of women for cervical cancer and precancerous conditions. Studies have shown that cervicography is useful for routine screening and for the triage of ASCUS Pap smears. Cervicography has a future as a valuable research tool, for chart documentation, for teaching colposcopy recognition skills, and in the testing and monitoring of colposcopic skills.

SUMMARY OF KEY POINTS

- Cervicography has been proposed as an adjunctive test that would increase the sensitivity and specificity of the Pap test in detecting precancerous and invasive cervical disease. Cervicography is not promoted as an independent or stand-alone test.

- Cervicography was invented as a method of detecting cervical cancer and other abnormalities.

- The procedure uses the Cerviscope Camera to take a color picture of the cervix after 5% acetic acid has been applied to it. The film is developed into 35-mm slides, and the resulting slide image is projected onto a screen and evaluated by an expert colposcopist.

- Cervigrams are reported in one of four categories: negative, atypical, positive, and technically defective.

- A negative evaluation means that no lesion is visible to the evaluator. It does not mean that a lesion does not exist in the endocervical canal. The negative category is subdivided based on whether components of the transformation zone are visible (N1) or not visible (N2).

- An atypical evaluation means that a lesion is visible but that, in the opinion of the evaluator, the lesion is of doubtful significance. Colposcopy is not normally recommended for the atypical evaluation.

- A positive evaluation means that a lesion is visible, and colposcopy is recommended. It can also mean that no definite lesion is visible but that the appearance of the cervix warrants colposcopy to exclude significant disease.

- A technically defective evaluation means that the slide is not adequate for evaluation and should be repeated.

- In some studies, cervicography detected invasive cancer not detected by cytology alone.

- Early studies of cervicography reported a sensitivity that ranged from 89% to 92% for the detection of high-grade precursor lesions or invasive disease, but the specificity was low. Changes on the cervigram report form have resulted in increased specificity, but at the expense of a decreased sensitivity—as low as 49.2% in one study.

- Studies show that, per dollar spent, cervicography detects more CIN lesions than conventional cytology.

- In addition to being used as an adjunctive test, cervicography has been used as a valuable research tool, for chart documentation, for teaching colposcopy recognition skills, and in the testing and monitoring of colposcopic skills.

References

1. Koss L: The Papanicolaou test for cervical cancer detection. A triumph and a tragedy. JAMA 1989;261:737.
2. Agency for Health Care Policy and Research: Evidence Report/Technology Assessment No. 5, Evaluation of Cervical Cytology [AHCPR Publication No. 99-E010]. Rockville, MD, U.S. Department of Health and Human Services, 1999.
3. Stafl A: Cervicography: A new method for cervical cancer detection. Am J Obstet Gynecol 1981;139:815.
4. Tawa K, Forsythe A, Cove K, et al: A comparison of the Papanicolaou smear and the cervigram: Sensitivity, specificity, and cost analysis. Obstet Gynecol 1988;71:229.
5. Navratil D, Burghardt E, Bajardi F, et al: Simultaneous colposcopy and cytology used in screening for carcinoma of the cervix. Am J Obstet Gynecol 1958;75:1292.
6. Limburg H: Comparison between cytology and colposcopy in the diagnosis of early cervical carcinoma. Am J Obstet Gynecol 1958;75:1298.
7. Coppelson M, Pixley D, Reid B: Colposcopy: A Scientific and Practical Approach to the Cervix in Health and Disease. Springfield, IL, Charles C Thomas, 1971.
8. Jones D, Creasman W, Dombroski R, et al: Evaluation of the atypical Pap smear. Am J Obstet Gynecol 1987;157:544.
9. Spitzer M, Krumholz BA, Chernys AE, et al: The comparative utility of repeat Pap smears, cervicography and colposcopy in the management of patients with atypical Pap smears. Obstet Gynecol 1987;69:731.
10. Blythe J: Cervicography: A preliminary report. Am J Obstet Gynecol 1985;152:192.
11. Schneider D, Herrero R, Bratti C, et al: Cervicography screening for cervical cancer among 8460 women in a high-risk population. Am J Obstet Gynecol 1999;180:290.
12. Spitzer M, Krumholz B, Seltzer V, Molho L: Cervical cancer detected by cervicography in a patient with negative cervical cytology. Obstet Gynecol 1986;68:68S.
13. Kesic V, Soutter P, Sulovic V, et al: A comparison of cytology and cervicography in cervical screening. Int J Gynecol Cancer 1993;2:395.
14. Eskridge C, Begneaud W, Landwehr C: Cervicography combined with repeat Papanicolaou test as triage for low-grade cytologic abnormalities. Obstet Gynecol 1998;92:351.
15. Allen D, Ashton P, Wintle M, et al: The use of cervicography in the follow-up of cervical intraepithelial neoplasia treated by CO_2 laser. Austral NZ J Obstet Gynaecol 1995;35:349.
16. ASCCP Practice Guideline: Management guidelines for follow-up of atypical squamous cells of undetermined significance ASCUS. Colposcopist 1996;27:1.
17. August N: Cervicography for evaluating the "atypical" Papanicolaou smear. J Reprod Med 1991;36:89.
18. Ferris D, Payne P, Frisch L, et al: Cervicography: Adjunctive cervical cancer screening by primary care clinicians. J Fam Pract 1993;37:158.

▼ *Appendix 1*

Taking Cervigram Pictures: A Checklist

[ ] Obtain supplies needed—appropriate speculum, large and small cotton swabs, 5% acetic acid, condom, Cerviscope Camera, power supply and cords, patient log sheet, and clipboard.

[ ] Insert the speculum.

[ ] The cervix must be in view and positioned appropriately.

[ ] Visualize the cervix, especially the transformation zone, if applicable.

[ ] Move any hair that crosses the speculum opening.

[ ] Perform a Pap smear.

[ ] Using a soaked large cotton swab, cleanse the cervix of any discharge or mucus.

[ ] Using a soaked cotton swab, stop any bleeding.

[ ] Remove any mucus, discharge, and blood from the posterior fornix.

[ ] Thoroughly soak a large cotton swab with 5% acetic acid and form a pool of acetic acid in the posterior fornix by dabbing the cervix.

[ ] Apply the first applications of 5% acetic acid with a thoroughly soaked large cotton swab for at least 15 seconds. After dabbing the cervix four or five times, the cotton becomes dry. Use the pool of acetic acid in the posterior fornix to resoak the cotton. Continue this routine for at least 15 seconds.

[ ] Observe the acetic acid effect, if applicable.

[ ] Pick up the Cerviscope Camera and ascertain that film is in the camera and properly loaded and that the cervigram number agrees with the patient log sheet. The cervigram number you see in the cervigram number display is the number that will be imprinted when you press the shutter release.

[ ] Properly grip the Cerviscope Camera with your left hand.

[ ] Sit close to the patient so you do not have to lean too far forward.

[ ] Hold the speculum handle with your right hand.

[ ] Align the Cerviscope Camera in the same axis as the speculum.

[ ] Position your nose perpendicular to the Cerviscope Camera databack, look through the viewfinder, center the cervix in the viewfinder, focus on the cervical os, and rest your left elbow against your chest for better stability.

[ ] View the cervix with the Cerviscope Camera, *but do not take a Cervigram Picture.* You are only allowing time for the first applications of 5% acetic acid to begin taking effect and looking for possible obstructions in the form of blood and mucus.

[ ] Again, thoroughly soak a large cotton swab with 5% acetic acid.

[ ] Apply the second applications of 5% acetic acid with a thoroughly soaked large cotton swab for at least 15 seconds. Remember that after dabbing the cervix four or five times, the cotton becomes dry. Use the pool of acetic acid in the posterior fornix to resoak the cotton. Continue this routine for at least 15 seconds.

[ ] You must see an acetic acid effect, if applicable.

[ ] Stop any bleeding that may have occurred.

[ ] Remove any mucus.

[ ] Adjust the position of the cervix, if necessary.

[ ] Hold the speculum handle with your right hand.

[ ] Align the Cerviscope Camera in the same axis as the speculum.

[ ] Position your nose perpendicular to the Cerviscope Camera databack, look through the viewfinder, center the cervix in the viewfinder, focus on the cervical os, and rest your left elbow against your chest.

[ ] Take the first Cervigram Picture. *Remember, what you see is what you get!*

[ ] Stop any bleeding that may have occurred.

[ ] Remove any mucus.

[ ] Adjust the position of the cervix, if necessary.

[ ] Reapply the 5% acetic acid, if necessary.

[ ] Hold the speculum handle with your right hand.

[ ] Align the Cerviscope Camera in the same axis as the speculum.

[ ] Position your nose perpendicular to the Cerviscope Camera databack, look through the viewfinder, center the cervix in the viewfinder, focus on the cervical os, and rest your left elbow against your chest.

[ ] Take the second Cervigram Picture. *Remember, what you see is what you get!*

[ ] Turn off the Cerviscope examination lights.

[ ] Complete the patient log sheet.

[ ] Record the cervigram numbers in the patient chart.

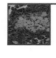

B

• Attila T. Lorincz

Human Papillomavirus Testing

Papillomaviruses are small DNA tumor viruses (Fig. 4–19) that infect the skin of many different animal species and typically produce warty lesions. The human papillomaviruses (HPV) are the largest known subgroup, with more than 100 types. Some are carcinogenic, whereas the majority cause benign epithelial lesions (warts, condylomas, papules, macules, etc.) that are rarely, if ever, malignant. HPV types are classified on the basis of genome homology, originally requiring liquid hybridization analysis to define a new type. However, it has been accepted that HPV types can be classified by sequence comparisons of the L1 region, with a novel HPV type defined as any complete genomic clone that shares less than 90% nucleotide sequence identity with any other known type.[1] Because HPV is difficult to culture, most investigations and all routine diagnostics have relied on one or more of three nucleic acid–based tests for detecting and typing HPV in specimens. These tests are polymerase chain reaction (PCR), the Hybrid Capture 2 system (HC2, Digene Corp., Gaithersburg, Maryland), and in situ hybridization (ISH).

> **Because HPV is difficult to culture, one or more of three nucleic acid–based tests have been used for detecting and typing HPV in specimens: the polymerase chain reaction, the Hybrid Capture 2 system, and in situ hybridization.**

It is now widely recognized that HPV causes essentially all cervical cancers worldwide[2-7] and that HPV infection precedes the appearance of neoplastic disease by many years.[8-13] Studies have shown the merit of HPV DNA testing for routine clinical use, including the management of women with Papanicolaou (Pap) smears showing atypical squamous cells of undetermined significance (ASCUS) and the population screening of women older than 30 years.[9, 14-22]

A number of arguments that include the following points can be made for the case of routine HPV DNA testing of clinical specimens from the female lower genital tract:

1. HPV is a necessary cause of cervical cancer.
2. HPV is an excellent marker of women at risk for neoplasia.
3. The best medical practice requires identification of etiologic agents.
4. HPV testing is an objective and reproducible means of assessing risk.
5. HPV testing improves cost-effectiveness.
6. The Pap smear is not a test for HPV.

> **HPV testing has been shown to be 15% to 20% more sensitive than the conventional Pap smear and at least 10% more sensitive than liquid-based Pap smears while exhibiting an equivalent specificity in the relevant defined subgroups of women.**

A strong impetus driving the clinical adoption of HPV testing is the recognition that the conventional Pap smear is prone to irreducible errors. The Pap smear is an old test and is difficult to execute with high quality in routine practice.[23-29] HPV DNA testing is 15% to 20% more sensitive than the conventional Pap smear[9, 14, 17, 19-21, 30] and at least 10% more sensitive than liquid-based cytology Pap smears (Atypical Squamous Cells of Undetermined Significance/Low-Grade Squamous Intraepithelial Lesions Triage Study [ALTS][31]) while exhibiting an equivalent specificity *in the relevant defined subgroups of women.* Colposcopic placement of biopsies is often considered to be 100% accurate, leading to the opinion that the true "gold standard" for disease definition is colposcopy. This misconception is more related to the arbitrary definition of the gold standard than to the actual accuracy

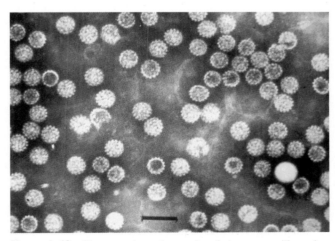

Figure 4–19. Electron photomicrograph of human papillomavirus (HPV) virions. HPVs are small icosahedral viruses of 55 nm in diameter that have a double-stranded DNA genome of approximately 8000 base pairs. (Photo courtesy of A Bennett Jenson, Georgetown University, Washington, DC.)

of colposcopy. In an ideal scenario with highly expert colposcopists, the technique is very accurate, but even in experienced hands, colposcopy may not find the most significant disease in up to 15% of cases (Belinson et al, unpublished data from the Shanxi Province Cervical Cancer Screening Study [SPOCCS]). Thus, HPV testing can help colposcopists to more accurately define a cervix lacking neoplastic changes: a colposcopically normal-appearing cervix that is negative by a highly sensitive HPV DNA test like HC2 or by PCR is very unlikely to harbor occult disease. Finally, cost-modeling studies by various groups have led to the conclusion that HPV testing is a more effective means of managing women with ASCUS Pap smears.

> **A colposcopically normal-appearing cervix that is negative by a highly sensitive HPV DNA test is very unlikely to harbor occult disease.**

BASICS OF PROBE TECHNOLOGY

> **Fundamental to all nucleic acid probe tests is an exquisitely specific recognition of target nucleic acid sequences by complementary probe nucleic acid sequences.**

DNA and RNA are the raw materials of nucleic acid–based probe tests. As they exist in cells or cell lysates, these molecules can be conceptualized as long, thin strings resembling microscopic strands of hair. The molecules exist most commonly as single strands or in closely attached pairs, the so-called hybrids. The process of hybridization can be manipulated by the probe scientists and is the key step in HPV detection. Fundamental to all probe tests is an exquisitely specific recognition of target nucleic acid sequences by complementary probe nucleic acid sequences. The ways in which molecules of DNA and RNA behave in aqueous solution, as they pertain to the essentials of probe tests, have been described in detail in earlier reviews.[32-36] Under normal physiologic conditions that can be further fine-tuned in the test tube, nucleic acid molecules exhibit a strong attraction for their partners and preferentially exist as stable, double-stranded pairs. These double-stranded molecules can be separated into single-stranded forms by well-known physical or chemical means. Then, as desired, the partners can be induced again to form pairs. If one of the partners is outcompeted by an excess of labeled complementary sequence produced in the laboratory, the pairing reaction can be used to reveal the presence of the target sequence (Fig. 4–20).

This reaction represents one of the most sophisticated lock-and-key mechanisms available in nature. The integrity of this system has been dictated by the need for organisms to transmit vast quantities of useful genetic information to their offspring. In probe test parlance, the key is the probe, the lock is the target, and the locking step is analogous to the hybridization of probe and target, which liberates stored kinetic energy. Once paired, the duplex persists in a favored, thermodynamic, lower energy state until it is disturbed by conditions that induce separation of the partner strands. In practical use, it rarely matters which genetic information is in the probe as long as its complementary sequence is in the target. The choice of which nucleic acid strand constitutes the probe is mainly at the discretion of the probe test development scientists.

TYPES OF PROBE TESTS

> **The early, nonamplified probe tests, which have since been abandoned, were difficult to perform, and good sensitivity and specificity were only obtained in a few expert laboratories, leading to an overabundance of poor data and a massive amount of misinformation about HPV.**

Probe tests can be divided into in vitro and in situ tests (e.g., ISH) and can be further subdivided into three broad groups: (1) nonamplified tests, (2) target amplification-based tests, and (3) signal amplification-based tests. In the 1970s and early 1980s, nonamplified tests were the sole route to HPV DNA detection. Unfortunately, these tests were difficult to perform and delivered good sensitivity and specificity in only a few expert laboratories. This led to an overabundance of poor data in the literature and a massive amount of misinformation about HPV that is only now being dispelled. The nonamplified tests have been all but abandoned in favor of target amplification-based (PCR) and signal amplification-based (HC2) tests; thus only the PCR and HC2 in vitro tests and ISH will be discussed.

> **The general rule for obtaining an adequate sample for HPV DNA testing is that a good sample for the Pap smear is also a good sample for HPV testing.**

An important consideration for every test is the collection of a good clinical specimen. Although it is quite easy to collect exfoliated cells for use in HC2 or PCR, there is still the need for some training and care. The general rule is that a good sample for the Pap smear is also a good sample for HPV DNA testing. In the case of a Pap specimen collected for a liquid-based cytology test, a 2-mL aliquot can be processed for HPV DNA testing by a simple procedure that involves pelleting the cells by centrifugation.[37] In the case of a conventional Pap smear, an accompanying HC2 HPV DNA test requires collection of a second specimen with a specially designed conical brush (Fig. 4–21).

Hybrid Capture 2

> **HC2 is an in vitro, solution hybridization, signal amplification–based test for detecting DNA and RNA targets.**

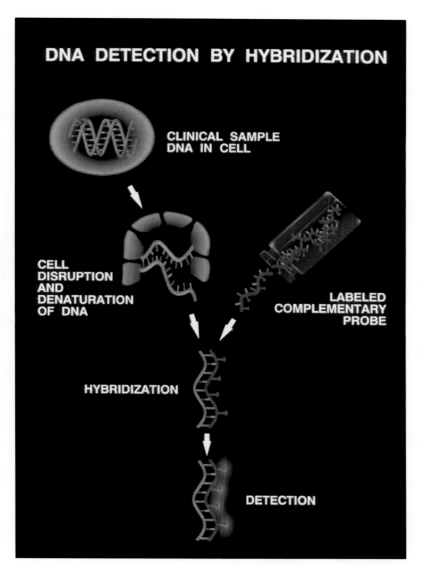

DNA DETECTION BY HYBRIDIZATION

CLINICAL SAMPLE
DNA IN CELL

CELL
DISRUPTION
AND
DENATURATION
OF DNA

LABELED
COMPLEMENTARY
PROBE

HYBRIDIZATION

DETECTION

Figure 4–20. Basic principles of DNA hybridization tests. The diagram shows a cell in the upper left corner that contains a highlighted DNA target of a virus. The cell is disrupted to release its contents (typically accomplished by heating in alkali of 0.25 M or above or by digestion with detergents and proteases). The DNA strands become separated in the first step by action of either the alkali (pH > 13) or heating (~100°C) or both. The separated DNA strands are then contacted by a labeled complementary single-stranded probe prepared in the laboratory. The probe hybridizes to the DNA, forming a probe-target hybrid, which must then be separated from the unreacted probes by physical (washing) or chemical (degradation of unprotected probe) means. There are many ways of labeling the probe, and the label dictates the method for detecting the hybrids. In the figure, the probe is labeled with a fluorophore that, when irradiated with light of a specific wavelength, will emit light of a longer wavelength that can be detected by a photomultiplier tube.

HC2 is an in vitro, solution hybridization, signal amplification-based test for detecting DNA or RNA targets (Fig. 4–22). For HPV detection, it is formatted as a solution hybridization of RNA probes with HPV DNA genomic targets that is followed by an immunologically based back end similar to an enzyme-linked immunosorbent assay (ELISA).[38] Table 4–1 shows the temporal sequence of steps in the HC2 test. The test derives its high sensitivity from several independent sources. In HC2, the entire genome of the virus is the usual target of choice.

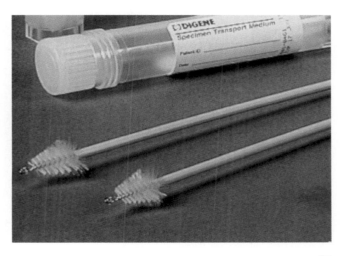

Figure 4–21. Hybrid Capture human papillomavirus (HPV) test cervical sampler, a conical brush for collecting a specimen of exfoliated cells from the uterine cervix. After clearing the cervical transformation zone of mucus, the brush is inserted into the os until the large outer bristles are barely visible. The brush is turned slowly counterclockwise for three full turns and slowly removed. It is placed into the liquid in the accompanying transport tube. The shaft is broken at the marked score line, and the tube is capped for shipping to the HPV testing laboratory.

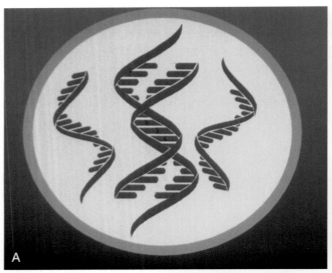
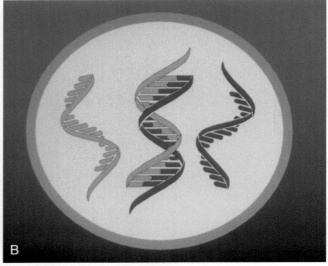
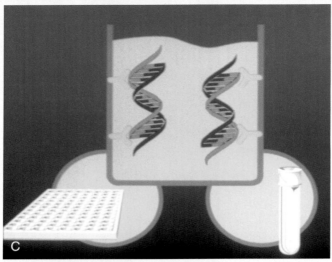
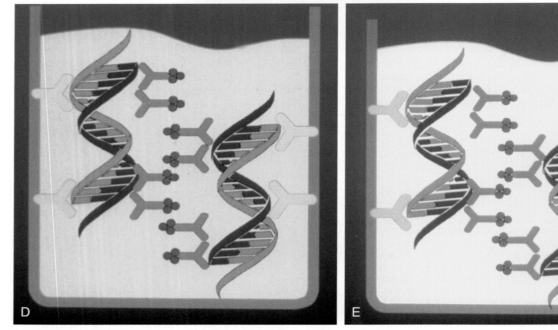

Figure 4-22. The key steps of the Hybrid Capture procedure. *A*, Release and denature nucleic acids. *B*, Hybridize single-stranded RNA (e.g., for human papillomavirus targets) or DNA (e.g., for human immunodeficiency virus targets) probe with target nucleic acid. *C*, Capture RNA:DNA hybrids onto a solid phase (in tube or microplate format). *D*, Allow reaction of captured hybrids with multiple antibody conjugates. *E*, Detect enhanced chemiluminescent signal.

▼ Table 4–1

Hybrid Capture 2 Procedure

Assay Step	Time	Temperature
Sample denaturation	45 min	65°C
Hybridization with full genomic RNA probes	1 hr	65°C
Capture on the surface of plate coated with RNA:DNA antibody	1 hr	Ambient
Detection react with reagent 1 alkaline phosphatase RNA:DNA antibody conjugate	30 min	Ambient
Wash (six times)	3–5 min	Ambient
Detection react with reagent 2 chemiluminescent substrate	15 min	Ambient
Read in plate luminometer	3 min	Ambient
Total time	~4.5 hr	

Long, unlabeled, single-stranded RNA probes are prepared by in vitro transcription and used to hybridize efficiently with all 8000 nucleotides of the HPV DNA genome. RNA-DNA hybrids are more stable than are DNA-DNA hybrids, and the use of single-stranded RNA probes avoids unwanted side reactions such as re-pairing of the two complementary strands of a typical DNA probe. A source of added sensitivity for HC2 is the use of RNA-DNA antibodies that are conjugated to multiple molecules of alkaline phosphatase. These antibody conjugates recognize short stretches of RNA-DNA hybrid in a specific but non–sequence-dependent manner such that hundreds of antibodies can coat a single genomic hybrid of HPV DNA. Each immobilized alkaline phosphatase enzyme reacts with thousands of molecules of the chemiluminescent dioxetane substrate to produce a steady stream of photons that are counted by the photomultiplier tube of a luminometer (Fig. 4–23). The HC2 test readily accepts large amounts (5% to 10% or more) of clinical material into the reaction without inhibition of the reaction.

The HC2 test derives its high sensitivity from the reaction produced by using single-stranded RNA probes to hybridize with all 8000 nucleotides of the HPV-RNA genome, thus producing RNA-DNA hybrids that are more stable than DNA-DNA hybrids and avoiding undesired side reactions. HC2 can detect 13 different carcinogenic HPV types that represent virtually all important cancer-causing HPV types known worldwide.

The first generation Hybrid Capture test (HCT) was replaced in 1996 by an improved HC2 version with greater sensitivity and ease of use. HC2 employs a removable strip microtiter plate and four additional probes for high-risk HPV types. HC2 can detect 13 different carcinogenic HPV types (types 16, 18, 31, 33, 35, 39, 45, 51, 52, 56, 58, 59, and 68) that represent virtually all important cancer-causing HPV types worldwide. Other formulation changes and an improved luminometer have increased the analytic sensitivity of HC2 by about 50-fold over that of HCT, such that HC2 can detect as few as 1000 HPV genomes per assay. However, for clinical use, the actual sensitivity increase is about 10-fold, with the lower limit for HC2 being 5000 genomes per assay. A valuable attribute of HC2 is its dynamic range of quantitation of over four logs.[9, 38, 39] The test is highly robust and reproducible and is used in more than 500 laboratories across the world.[9, 17, 19–22, 37, 39–46] HC2 was the HPV test of choice for the ALTS study[37] and demonstrated excellent reproducibility across all five university centers (four test sites and one quality-control laboratory). HC2 is approved by the U.S. Food and Drug Administration (FDA) for routine clinical use. Indications for use of HC2 can be summarized as follows:

1. To aid in the diagnosis of sexually transmitted HPV infections

2. To screen patients with ASCUS Pap smear results to determine the need for referral to colposcopy

3. To aid the physician in risk assessment of women

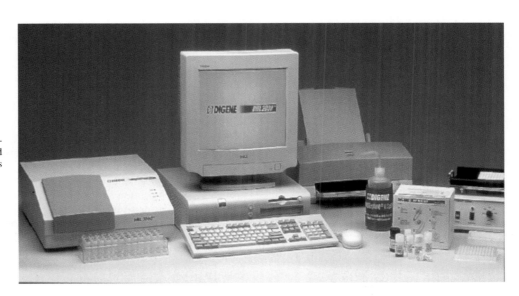

Figure 4–23. Equipment for detecting reaction results of the Hybrid Capture 2 test. The luminometer is the low instrument on the left.

with low-grade squamous intraepithelial lesion (LSIL) or high-grade squamous intraepithelial lesion (HSIL) cytology results before colposcopy

Polymerase Chain Reaction

> **In the PCR test, the target DNA is selectively amplified by enzymatic means through repeated cycles of denaturation, primer hybridization, and primer extension.**

The approach taken by target-amplified tests is to create extra copies of the desired target sequence before detection of these amplicons by more traditional methods (Fig. 4–24). In PCR[47–49] the target DNA is selectively amplified by enzymatic means through repeated cycles of denaturation, primer hybridization, and primer extension. Target DNA concentration rises exponentially, and after 30 cycles more than 1 million copies of the target DNA are produced. Hence, as few as 10 to 100 HPV DNA molecules can be amplified and detected within a portion of a biopsy or smear containing 5×10^4 cells. PCR has been used to detect HPV DNA in a diversity of specimen types including fresh or fixed exfoliated cell preparations and biopsies, such as Pap smears and sections of paraffin-embedded tissue biopsies from cervical intraepithelial neoplasia (CIN) and cervical cancer.[50] There are many ways to detect the amplified products (amplicons). For example, amplicons may be spotted on membranes or electrophoresed in gels to resolve bands of various sizes.

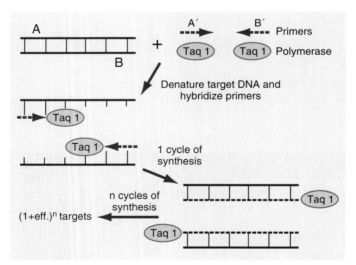

Figure 4–24. Performance of one cycle of polymerase chain reaction (PCR) synthesis. Double-stranded target DNA is denatured by heating to approximately 100°C and then cooled to 50°C to 70°C, to allow the two primers (A′ and B′) to hybridize specifically to their complementary DNA target sequences (A and B), usually a few hundred nucleotides apart. The primers direct synthesis of new DNA toward each other by means of a polymerase enzyme such as Taq 1, converting the initial two DNA target strands into four target strands, upon which another full PCR cycle can be performed. After *n* cycles, one target will become $(1 + eff)^n$ amplicons (or targets), where eff is the efficiency of the amplification and *n* is a number between 0 and 1. In an ideal PCR with 100% efficiency, eff = 1. Usually, the value of eff is 0.7 to 0.8. (From Lorincz AT: Molecular methods for the detection of human papillomavirus infection. Obstet Gynecol Clin North Am 1996;23:707.)

In gel-based procedures, detection may be accomplished by fluorescent dye (e.g., ethidium bromide, cyber green) staining followed by photography or direct digitization of the gels or photographs. For added sensitivity and specificity, the amplicons may be treated like targets and hybridized with large probes in conventional nonamplified formats (dot blot or Southern blot) or with oligonucleotide probes in an ELISA format.

> **During the PCR amplification process, target DNA concentration rises exponentially, and after 30 cycles more than 1 million copies of the target DNA are produced.**

There are also real-time detection versions of PCR; one popular method is dubbed the TaqMan test.[51] In this method, the signal is generated during the reaction by use of a signal oligonucleotide probe that contains a fluorescent nucleotide molecule juxtaposed with a quenching nucleotide molecule. As a PCR reaction proceeds in the presence of target, the quenching nucleotide is digested by the Taq polymerase exonuclease activity and is separated from the fluorophore, which can then be read by a modified fluorescent reader.[8, 11]

Several alternative sets of primers are used for detecting HPV by PCR. Two commonly used sets are the consensus primer pair MY09/MY11 (the MY set)[52] and the general primers GP5/GP6[53]; both primer sets amplify regions in the conserved L1 open reading frame. Several other sets of primers have been reported in the literature, such as the MY variants PGMY,[54] the consensus E1 primers[55] and the type-specific E6 primers.[56] Most of these alternative primers have been insufficiently validated to recommend their use; for example, the PGMY primers do not seem to offer a major advantage over the improved MY set (R. Burk et al, personal communication). The MY primers produce a PCR amplicon of about 450 nucleotides, whereas the GP primer pair produces an amplicon of about 140 nucleotides from an area of L1 that overlaps with the MY region. Debate continues as to which HPV PCR method is better. Both methods are fairly equivalent for in vitro use, but the GP primers are better for amplification of targets from paraffin-embedded sections, because the longer MY amplicons are not synthesized as efficiently owing to formalin cross-linking in the tissue.

The MY primers are designed with many positions of nucleotide code degeneracy so that alternative sequences present in different HPV types can be accommodated. Thus, in reality, the MY primers represent a family of related molecules, some of which will hybridize efficiently with HPV 16 and others with HPV 18. The original primer pairs have undergone successive improvements to broaden the spectrum of HPV types recognized. A more recent improvement[57] permits a more efficient recognition of HPV 51. There is some variability in the sensitivity with which the various HPV types are detected,[58] and some types are detected only poorly if at all, such as HPV 43 and HPV 44. However, all important carcinogenic types are detected with reasonably constant efficiency. Differences in efficiency may become important in quantitative PCR applications when studies are performed to compare relative amounts of different specific types. For qualitative use, the differences are less important and mainly affect the accuracy with which low levels of HPV DNA are detected in clinical specimens.

The literature describes several ways in which HPV amplicons can be detected and the HPVs typed. Originally, the amplicons were electrophoresed in sizing gels so that the specific products could be detected. Different HPV types give amplicons with either MY or GP primers that are difficult to distinguish in size by gel electrophoresis; thus, this simplistic method is difficult and inaccurate for typing. An improvement on the method employs amplicon digestion with specific restriction endonucleases to give band patterns that can distinguish among HPV types; however, even this improvement does not give ideal results. Additional PCR test development has led to fairly robust oligonucleotide probe-based ELISA procedures that can give accurate typing information.[52, 59] The use of oligonucleotide probes, in effect, results in a loss of some of the sensitivity normally available to tests that use larger probes in solution, but because the target region is amplified up to 1 million times, the loss in sensitivity is usually not a problem. Versions of PCR that amplify long regions of up to 10 kb are now available,[60] but this process is less efficient than amplifying short regions, and there is little or no gain in overall sensitivity. PCR methods that amplify regions of target DNA that are only 100 to 400 nucleotides long remain the most popular tests for diagnostic purposes.

PCR methods that amplify regions of target DNA that are only 100 to 400 nucleotides long remain the most popular tests for diagnostic purposes.

PCR amplicon detection in a reverse blot format (e.g., the "line blot" test) is gaining popularity, as it allows the identification and simultaneous typing of more than 25 different HPV types. In the line blot test, the probes are immobilized in a grid pattern on a solid surface (e.g., a nylon filter membrane, a glass or silicon chip) and the targets (amplicons) are added in solution to the supports to allow hybridization, which may then be detected by chemiluminescence or color deposition. In positive specimens, there is a variable pattern of hybrids seen on the solid support, with different patterns corresponding to various HPV types or sets of types. Two such line blot systems have been described in the literature, one using the MY primers or variants of these primers and another using the SPF set of primers.[61, 62]

Some research groups are sequencing amplicons from various regions of the HPV genome as a means of differentiating between minor type variants and mutants.[63] These sequence-based methods have provided excellent epidemiologic information on the spread of variants through human populations and for studies of viral persistence in various groups of women.

Sequencing amplicons from various regions of the HPV genome as a means of differentiating between minor type variants and mutants has provided data on the spread of HPV variants through human populations and for studies of viral persistence in certain groups of women.

Theoretically, it is possible to make PCR even more sensitive by combining target amplification with highly sensitive signal amplification. In a research setting, this may be desirable. Generally, ultra-high sensitivity is not needed in the clinical context, because excessive sensitivity quickly becomes a liability that markedly reduces the utility of the results owing to concerns over contamination (analytic false positives)[64, 65] or detection of true but inconsequential amounts of HPV DNA (clinical false positives).[47, 66]

In Situ Hybridization

ISH is usually applied to histology sections or cell smears and can provide excellent morphologic detail of tissue or cellular contents.

ISH is usually applied to histology sections or cell smears and, if performed carefully, can provide not only the exact localization of target sequences but also excellent morphologic detail of tissue or cellular contents (Fig. 4–25). Basically, thin tissue sections or cells are perme-

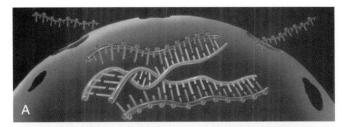
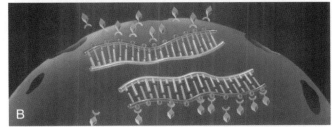
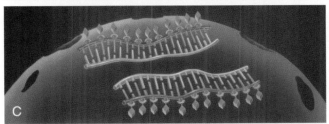

Figure 4–25. Key steps in the in situ hybridization procedure. A, Probes are drifting into the cell nucleus through pores created by detergent and/or protease treatment. The probe molecules are starting to hybridize with a partially unraveled HPV DNA target in the cell nucleus. B, Two probe molecules have fully formed hybrids with each strand of an original target duplex. Enzyme molecules (diamonds with curved attachments) are starting to attach to the hybrids via the label on the probes (one example might be biotin on the probes binding streptavidin-conjugated alkaline phosphatase). C, Fully decorated hybrids containing numerous enzymes per hybrid. These enzymes will then catalyze deposition of colored precipitates that will stain the nuclei of HPV-infected cells, as shown in Figure 4–26. HPV, human papillomavirus.

abilized by a gentle process involving enzymes, detergents, or both, so that small pores permit access of probes to the nucleus. Hybridization of probe to target occurs within the permeabilized nuclei or other organelles. Although morphology is retained generally intact, some distortions do occur, and these depend for the most part on the method of tissue fixation and the nature of the permeabilization process. Neutral-buffered 10% formalin is a particularly good tissue fixative that is compatible with ISH. Many variations of ISH are in use.[32, 67–71]

> **ISH is less sensitive than PCR or HC2 and is better used as a confirmatory test on equivocal biopsies of suspected LSIL, for which the test shows its highest sensitivity and best clinical benefit.**

Because ISH is so different from in vitro tests, it is difficult to draw direct comparisons. A disadvantage of ISH is that it is relatively labor-intensive and does not lend itself readily to high throughput manual testing or automation. It is usually limited to research laboratories and expert pathology laboratories but is becoming more widespread with a growing appreciation of its benefits. As performed in most laboratories, ISH is less sensitive than PCR or HC2 and is better used as a confirmatory test on equivocal biopsies of suspected LSIL, for which the test shows its highest sensitivity and best clinical benefit. The presence of a nuclear HPV signal confirms the nature of the lesion, and a negative result indicates the converse (Fig. 4–26). High-grade CINs and cancers typically have low levels of HPV per cell and are often negative by ISH, which usually requires 5 or 10 genomes or more per cell to show a positive result. Typically, 10% to 30% of cancers and CIN 2 and CIN 3 positive by HC2 or PCR are negative by ISH.[68, 70, 71] Fortunately, ISH can be enhanced by sophisticated fluorescence-based confocal microscopy with digitized image detection and computer enhancement.

> **Typically, 10% to 30% of cancers and CIN 2 and CIN 3 positive by HC2 or PCR are negative by ISH.**

There is also a relatively new signal-amplified version of ISH that employs tyramide deposition to enhance the signal (Fig. 4–27). With these modifications, ISH can achieve the ultimate sensitivity of one copy of HPV per cell, but the methods are still expensive and difficult for routine use.

Another limitation of ISH is that it tends to show greater cross-reactivity between HPV types. In particular, some versions that employ biotin-labeled DNA probes can be misleading for type determination in the hands of inexperienced users. However, careful attention to reagent preparation, to hybridization and washing conditions, and to slide interpretation can overcome most problems and provide accurate typing.

CAUTIONS IN TEST INTERPRETATION

> **There are many reasons for the reported variability of the performance of the HPV probe tests, including interference with amplication of the DNA sequences, false-positive results, and cross-reactivity of the tests.**

A review of the literature shows a substantial variation in the reported performance of HPV probe tests relative to each other and to histology. In many studies, the HC2 and PCR tests show excellent sensitivity and specificity for detecting disease.[2, 9, 17, 20, 45, 72] In other studies, the correlations are not as good.[16, 65, 66, 73] There are many possible reasons for these variations. PCR, in particular, is prone to inhibitory substances that can interfere with amplification and lower sensitivity. With HC2, inhibition is not of concern; in fact, in many studies HC2 is more sensitive than PCR. Historically, PCR was associated with excessive false positives, but this has lessened. With HC2, analytic false positives are not common, representing less than 1% of positive results. Cross-reactivity in HC2 can present some problems in epidemiologic studies.

> **Sample adequacy is critical to avoid false-negative results in both HC2 and PCR.**

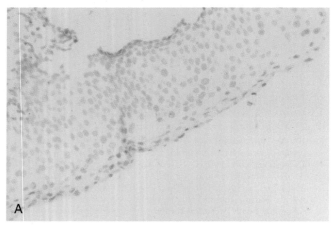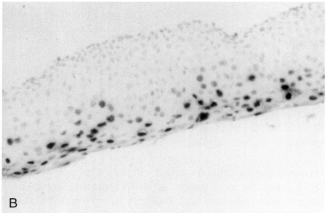

Figure 4–26. An in situ hybridization showing sections from the same tissue biopsy of CIN hybridized with (*A*) negative control probe (pBR322 plasmid) and (*B*) HPV probe. The positive reaction can be seen by the darkly staining nuclei of the superficial epithelial cells. HPV, human papillomavirus.

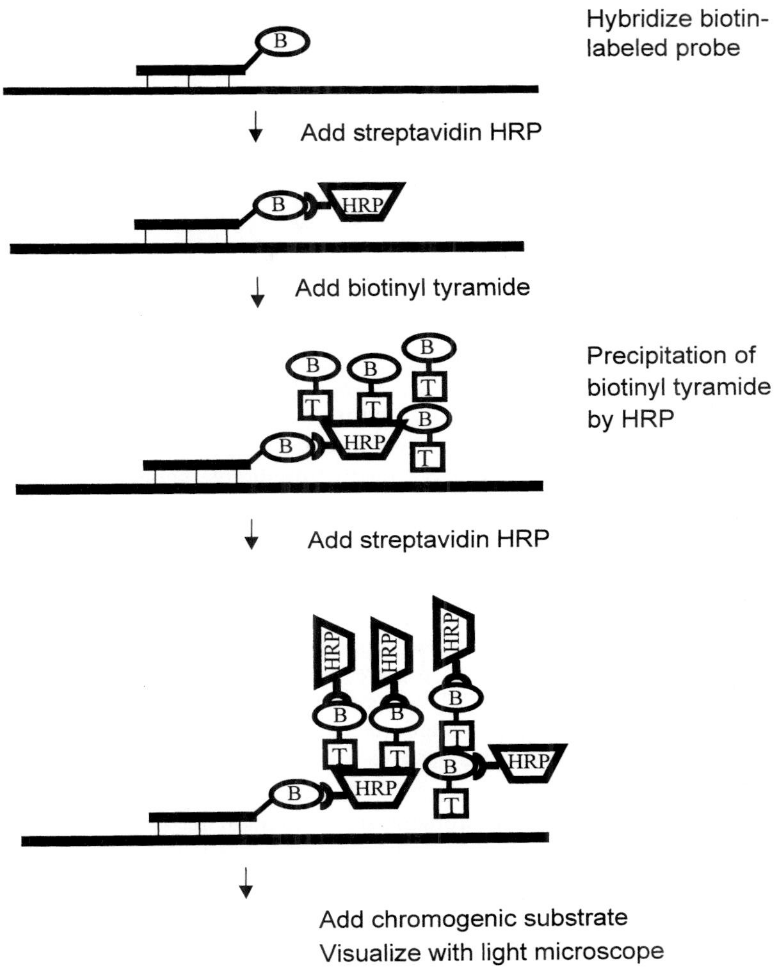

Figure 4–27. In situ hybridization procedure employing an indirect tyramide signal amplification (TSA) method.[81] TSA can be used to enhance sensitivity in either direct (not shown) or indirect formats. Typically, both formats use biotinylated nucleic acid probes. After wash steps, the slides are reacted with streptavidin-labeled horseradish peroxidase (HRP). In the direct TSA assay, fluorescent-labeled tyramide molecules (e.g., tyramide-fluorescein, tyramide-cyanine-3) are added, and the HRP catalyzes the accumulation of the fluorescent-labeled tyramide molecules onto the surface where they can be viewed by fluorescent microscopy. In the indirect method, biotin-labeled tyramide molecules are added and immobilized to the probe site by HRP catalysis. The slide is washed and incubated with streptavidin HRP molecules. After removal of the unbound streptavidin-HRP, a chromogenic HRP substrate is added and viewed by light microscopy. Both methods result in a substantial improvement in sensitivity, and because the signal amplification is localized to the probe region, there is little to no loss in signal resolution. (From Anthony JG, Linske-O'Connell L, Lorincz AT: Nucleic acid hybridization. In Specter S, Hodinka RL, Young SA [eds]: Clinical Virology Manual, 3rd ed. Washington, DC, ASM Press, 2000, pp 169–181.)

Specimen adequacy is critical to avoid false negatives in both HC2 and PCR. In the author's experience, sampling is an important area that requires careful attention. Some essential elements to consider are proper access to CIN 2 and CIN 3 lesions deep in the endocervical canal, especially in older women. Brush devices are better at cutting through mucus or other material to access HPV-infected cells (see Figure 4–21). Careful and standardized sampling should be learned by every clinician attempting to use HPV tests in screening and patient management. Dacron swabs are not optimal but may be acceptable for self-sampling or for use in pregnant women. The use of cotton swabs for taking specimens should be avoided.

One reason for poor agreement between accurate HPV DNA tests may be the subjectivity of histopathology that can result in underdiagnosis or overdiagnosis of the biopsy.

Another reason for poor agreement between accurate HPV DNA tests and histology may be related to the subjectivity of the histopathology.[26] CIN 2 is usually lumped with CIN 3, and it is possible that overcall on histology may place some CIN 1 into the CIN 2–CIN 3 group. Because CIN 1 is sometimes caused by only low-risk or novel HPV types, the result will be interpreted as false negative for a probe test that detects only carcinogenic HPV types. In some instances, variants of immature squamous metaplasia or other artifacts may be misread as CIN 2 or CIN 3.

CLINICAL UTILITY OF HPV TESTING

The frequent occurrence of HPV infection in young women who are at lowest risk for neoplastic disease requires that HPV testing be applied differently according to the age of the patient.

Carcinogenic HPV types are strong determinants of cervical cancer, with infection producing estimated relative risks approaching 100.[7, 10, 74–76] The emerging picture indicates that HPV is highly prevalent in young, sexually active populations, with an incidence of up to 20%.[77, 78] Infection is mostly transient with a mean duration of about 8 months for low-risk HPV types and 13 months for carcinogenic HPV types. In a minority of infected individuals, carcinogenic HPV types become persistent and predispose the women to cancer 10 to 40 years later.

In light of these facts and, in particular, of the frequent occurrence of HPV infection in young women who are at lowest risk for neoplastic disease, it is apparent that HPV

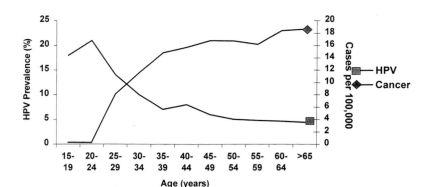

Figure 4–28. HPV prevalence[82] and cervical cancer incidence by age.[83] Although the HPV data are from the Netherlands and the cancer data are from the United States, these populations are quite similar, and thus this representation is also generally true for the U.S. population. The same trends have been observed in many other geographic locations, such as Costa Rica[9] and Canada.[84] HPV, human papillomavirus.

testing will be applied differentially with respect to age. In general, clinical management decisions in women with abnormal Pap smears can integrate HPV testing regardless of age. This is because, in women with ASCUS Pap smears, HPV testing has a good positive predictive value at all ages, and the very high (>99%) negative predictive value of the HPV test is tremendously useful in quickly reassuring clinicians and women who test HPV negative that there is a very low probability of missed disease[14, 17, 22, 31] (Pretorius et al, unpublished data). In contrast, for screening of normal populations, it is best to avoid testing younger women for predominantly transient HPV infection. Thus, most HPV screening strategies call for HPV DNA testing in women older than 30 years (Fig. 4–28)[9, 19–21] (Belinson et al, unpublished SPOCCS data).

> **HPV testing does not appear to be beneficial in young women, who are known to have predominantly transient HPV infection.**

The most compelling data for clinical utility of HPV DNA testing in patient management relates to women with ASCUS Pap smears. The test has been employed in three major ASCUS Pap triage studies involving more than 4000 women and more than 300 cases of high-grade cervical disease[17, 31] (Pretorius et al, unpublished data), as well as numerous smaller studies.[14, 22, 44] The results showed that immediate HPV-based triage had a sensitivity of 90% to 96%, compared with 75% to 85% for the repeat Pap smear. The specificities of the HC2 HPV test and the Pap test were equivalent. In hypothetical management programs relying on immediate reflex HPV testing or 6-month repeat Pap testing, similar numbers of women (about 40%) would be referred to colposcopy on the basis of a triage HC2 test or a liquid-based cytology Pap test (ThinPrep, Cytyc Corp., Roxborough, Massachusetts). Cost calculations performed by one of the participating institutions (Kaiser Permanente, California) demonstrated that HPV testing was more effective than either repeat Pap testing or immediate colposcopy.

> **Based on data, the immediate HPV-based triage of ACSUS would result in a sensitivity of 90% to 96%, compared with 75% to 85% for the repeat Pap smear.**

In addition to using HPV testing for managing women with ASCUS Pap smears, the test can also be used in a number of worrisome situations to provide more information to the clinician and the patient in a timely manner. These other uses include follow-up after treatment as a "test of cure,"[79, 80] to help resolve discordant cytology, colposcopy, and histology findings,[43] and as a reassurance tool in combination with colposcopy to more effectively rule out the possibility of missed disease (Belinson et al, unpublished SPOCCS data; Pretorius et al, unpublished data).

> **The median sensitivity of HPV testing for women with CIN 2 or CIN 3 and invasive disease was 93%, compared with 75% for the conventional Pap smear.**

> **The Pap smear was slightly more specific than HPV DNA testing for the presence of high-grade cervical disease.**

HC2 testing has been employed in more than 10 large population screening trials from various countries, with a combined total of more than 50,000 women. A few of these studies have been published, whereas others are still under way or with manuscripts in preparation.[9, 19–21] The median sensitivity of HPV testing for women with high-grade (CIN 2 or CIN 3) disease and cancer was 93%; for the Pap smear it was 75%. In contrast, the Pap smear was slightly more specific than HPV DNA testing when considering the presence of cervical high-grade disease. However, future disease developing from HPV infections was not counted in the calculations. The important tasks now relate mainly to exploring algorithms that will allow an optimal combination of Pap and HPV testing to further lower cancer incidence in developed countries and to cost-effectively stem the massive incidence of cervical cancer in the developing world.

FUTURE DIRECTIONS

The incorporation of HPV testing into routine clinical practice is accelerating, and the potential for its use in both developed and developing nations is being investigated. Automation will make routine HPV testing for triage and mass screening less expensive and more accurate than repeat Pap smears, because it will virtually eliminate human error and the subjectivity of interpretation. HPV testing may be done in conjunction with the Pap test, or in some situations HPV testing may be a superior alternative to Pap testing, especially in countries that lack sufficient numbers of qualified cytotechnicians, who can take years to train. In countries where there is no routine Pap screening and also, to some extent, in countries with established screening programs, there is likely to be better compliance if women can submit specimens to testing laboratories from the privacy of their homes and avoid regular invasive sampling procedures. Self-sampling for HPV shows great promise.[19, 41, 46] (Belinson et al, unpublished SPOCCS data). The frequency of Pap smears might be reduced to intervals of 3 years or less if supplemented by a home HPV test in the intervening years.

CONCLUSIONS

Tests for HPV have become accurate, objective, and highly reproducible. Currently, three tests are available: HC2, PCR, and ISH. With these methods, it is possible to detect more than 100 different HPV types. However, from a clinical perspective, only tests for the core group of 13 carcinogenic HPV types are likely to be used frequently. Test procedures and equipment are evolving quickly. The ultimate goal is superior sensitivity and specificity in a simple, automated format with fully comprehensive software for test runs, data analysis, and report generation. The overall outlook is that automated, molecular-based tests are likely to play a key role in predicting, detecting, and confirming most human diseases and are becoming indispensable in all major medical disciplines.

SUMMARY OF KEY POINTS

- HPV types are classified by DNA sequence comparison of the L1 region. A novel HPV type is defined as any complete genomic clone that shares less than 90% nucleotide sequence identity with any other known type.
- Because HPV is considered essential to the etiology of cervical cancer, it may be argued that HPV is an excellent marker of women at risk for neoplasia.
- In a woman with a colposcopically normal cervix, the absence of HPV by a highly sensitive HPV DNA test implies that it is unlikely that occult disease is present.
- The fundamental basis of DNA probe technology is the exquisitely specific recognition of target nucleic acid sequences by complementary probe nucleic acid sequences.
- The low-sensitivity, nonamplified HPV tests initially developed have been abandoned in favor of the target amplification-based (PCR) and signal amplification-based (HC2) tests now in current use.
- The HC2 test is a signal amplification test. It relies on RNA-DNA "hybrids" that are recognized by RNA-DNA antibodies conjugated to alkaline phosphatase. The antibody conjugates recognize the RNA-DNA hybrids, and hundreds of antibodies can coat a single genomic hybrid. Each alkaline phosphatase enzyme reacts with chemiluminescent substrate to produce a steady stream of photons that are counted by a luminometer. The test has demonstrated highly reproducible results across study sites.
- Cross-reactivity can be a problem in HC2.
- PCR is a target-amplified test. It uses technology that creates extra copies of the desired target sequence before detection of the amplified products, or amplicons, by more traditional methods. Sequencing amplicons from various regions of the HPV genome has produced the ability to differentiate between minor type variants present in different populations and to better understand the persistence of HPV in various groups of women.
- PCR is prone to inhibitory substances that can interfere with amplification and decrease sensitivity.
- ISH is usually applied to histology sections or cell smears and can provide the exact localization of target sequences and excellent morphologic detail of tissue or cellular contents. It is a labor-intensive test and cannot easily be automated.
- ISH is less sensitive than PCR or HC2 and is better used as a confirmatory test on equivocal biopsies of LSIL for which the test shows its highest sensitivity and best clinical benefit.
- Typically, 10% to 30% of CIN 2 and CIN 3 and cancer are negative by ISH but positive by PCR and HC2.
- Specimen adequacy is critical to avoid false negatives in both HC2 and PCR. Careful, standardized sampling is important, and brush devices produce better samples than swabs. Dacron swabs are not optimal but can be used for self-sampling or if the patient is pregnant. Cotton swabs should be avoided.
- HPV testing is not an effective test in young women with transient HPV infections.
- Most HPV screening strategies include testing in women older than 30 years and in women with ASCUS for whom the test has a high negative predictive value.
- Data have demonstrated that immediate HPV-based triage of ASCUS Pap smears has a sensitivity of 90% to 96%, compared with 75% to 85% for the repeat Pap smear performed, on average, 6 months later with comparable specificity.
- The median sensitivity of HPV testing for routine screening of women with CIN 2 or CIN 3 and cancer is 93%, compared with 75% for the Pap smear. The Pap smear is slightly more specific than HPV DNA testing when considering the presence of high-grade cervical disease.

References

1. Delius H, Saegling B, Bergmann K, et al: The genomes of three of four novel HPV types, defined by differences of their L1 genes, show high conservation of the E7 gene and the URR. Virology 1998;240:359.

2. Bosch F, Xavier M, Michele M, et al: Prevalence of human papillomavirus in cervical cancer: A worldwide perspective. J Natl Cancer Inst 1995;87:796.

3. Boshart M, Gissmann L, Ikenberg H, et al: A new type of papillomavirus DNA, its presence in genital cancer biopsies and in cell lines derived from cervical cancer. EMBO 1984;3:1151.

4. Durst M, Gissmann L, Ikenberg H, zur Hausen H: A papillomavirus DNA from a cervical carcinoma and its prevalence in cancer biopsy samples from different geographic regions. Proc Natl Acad Sci U S A 1983;80:3812.

5. Fuchs PG, Girardi F, Pfister H: Human papillomavirus DNA in normal, metaplastic, preneoplastic and neoplastic epithelia of the cervix uteri. Int J Cancer 1988;41:41.

6. Lorincz AT, Temple GF, Kurman RJ, et al: Oncogenic association of specific human papillomavirus types with cervical neoplasia. J Natl Cancer Inst 1987;79:671.

7. Lorincz AT, Reid R, Jenson AB, et al: Human papillomavirus infection of the cervix: Relative risk associations of 15 common anogenital types. Obstet Gynecol 1992;79:328.

8. Josefsson AM, Magnusson PKE, Ylitalo N, et al: Viral load of human papilloma virus 16 as a determinant for development of cervical carcinoma in situ: A nested case-control study. Lancet 2000;355:2189.

9. Schiffman M, Herrero R, Hildesheim A, et al: HPV DNA testing in cervical cancer screening: Results from women in a high-risk province of Costa Rica. JAMA 2000;283:87.

10. Wallin KL, Wiklund F, Angstrom T, et al: Type-specific persistence of human papillomavirus DNA before the development of invasive cervical cancer. N Engl J Med 1999;341:1633.

11. Ylitalo N, Sorensen P, Josefsson AM, et al: Consistent high viral load of human papillomavirus 16 and risk of cervical carcinoma in situ: A nested case-control study. Lancet 2000;355:2194.

12. Koutsky LA, Holmes KK, Critchlow CW, et al: A cohort study of the risk of cervical intraepithelial neoplasia grade 2 or 3 in relation to papillomavirus infection. N Engl J Med 1992;327:1272.

13. Lorincz AT, Schiffman MH, Jaffurs WJ, et al: Temporal associations of human papillomavirus infection with cervical cytologic abnormalities. Am J Obstet Gynecol 1990;162:645.

14. Cox JT, Lorincz AT, Schiffman MH, et al: Human papillomavirus testing by hybrid capture appears to be useful in triaging women with a cytologic diagnosis of atypical squamous cells of undetermined significance. Am J Obstet Gynecol 1995;172:946.

15. Cuzick J, Szarewski A, Terry G, et al: Human papillomavirus testing in primary cervical screening. Lancet 1995;345:1533.

16. Wright TC, Sun XW, Koulos J: Comparison of management algorithms for the evaluation of women with low-grade cytologic abnormalities. Obstet Gynecol 1995;85:202.

17. Manos MM, Kinney WK, Hurley LB, et al: Identifying women with cervical neoplasia: Using human papillomavirus DNA testing for equivocal Papanicolaou results. JAMA 1999;281:1605.

18. Krumholz BA: Value of human papillomavirus testing. Am J Obstet Gynecol 2000;182:479.

19. Wright TC Jr, Denny L, Kuhn L, et al: HPV DNA testing of self-collected vaginal samples compared with cytologic screening to detect cervical cancer. JAMA 2000;283:81.

20. Cuzick J, Beverley E, Ho L, et al: HPV testing in primary screening of older women. Br J Cancer 1999;81:554.

21. Clavel C, Masure M, Bory JP, et al: Hybrid capture II-based human papillomavirus detection, a sensitive test to detect in routine high-grade cervical lesions: A preliminary study on 1518 women. Br J Cancer 1999;80:1306.

22. Kuperman L, Krumholz BA: The triage of women with ASCUS cytology using human papillomavirus DNA testing. J Lower Genital Tract Dis 2000;4:1.

23. Davey DD, Nielsen ML, Frable WJ, et al: Improving accuracy in gynecologic cytology: Results of the College of American Pathologists interlaboratory comparison program in cervicovaginal cytology. Arch Pathol Lab Med 1993;117:1193.

24. Duca P, Braga M, Chiappa L, et al: Intralaboratory reproducibility of interpretation of Pap smears: Results of an experiment. Tumori 1988;74:737.

25. Klinkhamer PJJM, Vooijs GP, de Haan AFJ: Intraobserver and interobserver variability in the diagnosis of epithelial abnormalities in cervical smears. Acta Cytologica 1988;32:794.

26. Robertson AJ, Anderson JM, Beck JS, et al: Observer variability in histopathological reporting of cervical biopsy specimens. J Clin Pathol 1989;42:231.

27. Sherman ME, Schiffman MH, Lorincz AT, et al: Toward objective quality assurance in cervical cytopathology: Correlation of cytopathologic diagnoses with detection of high-risk human papillomavirus types. Am J Clin Pathol 1994;102:182.

28. McCrory DC, Matchar DB, Bastian L, et al: Evaluation of Cervical Cytology. Rockville, MD, Agency for Health Care Policy and Research, 1999.

29. Fahey MT, Irwig L, Macaskill P: Meta-analysis of Pap test accuracy. Am J Epidemiol 1995;141:680.

30. Clavel C, Bory JP, Rihet S, et al: Comparative analysis of human papillomavirus detection by hybrid capture assay and routine cytologic screening to detect high-grade cervical lesions. Int J Cancer 1998;75:525.

31. Solomon D, Schiffman M, Tarone B, for the ALTS Group. Comparison of three management strategies for patients with atypical squamous cells of undetermined significance (ASCUS): Baseline results from a randomized trial. J Natl Cancer Inst 2001;93:293.

32. Hames BD, Higgins SJ (eds): Nucleic Acid Hybridisation: A Practical Approach. Oxford, IRL Press, 1985.

33. Lorincz AT: Human papillomavirus detection tests. In Holmes KK, Mardh PA, Sparling P, et al (eds): Sexually Transmitted Diseases, 2nd ed. New York, McGraw-Hill, 1990, pp 953–959.

34. Meinkoth J, Wahl G: Hybridization of nucleic acids immobilized on solid supports. Anal Biochem 1984;138:267.

35. Lorincz AT: Molecular methods for the detection of human papillomavirus infection. Obstet Gynecol Clin North Am 1996;23:707.

36. Anthony JG, Linske-O'Connell L, Lorincz AT: Nucleic acid hybridization. In Specter S, Hodinka RL, Young SA (eds): Clinical Virology Manual, 3rd ed. Washington, DC, ASM Press, 2000, pp 169–181.

37. The Atypical Squamous Cells of Undetermined Significance/Low-Grade Squamous Intraepithelial Lesions Triage Study (ALTS) Group: Human papillomavirus testing for triage of women with cytologic evidence of low-grade squamous intraepithelial lesions: Baseline data from a randomized trial. J Nat Cancer Inst 2000;92:397.

38. Lorincz A: Hybrid capture™ method for detection of human papillomavirus DNA in clinical specimens. Papillomavirus Rep 1996;7:1.

39. Nindl I, Lorincz A, Mielzynska I, et al: Human papillomavirus detection in cervical intraepithelial neoplasia by the second generation hybrid capture microplate test, comparing two different cervical specimen collection methods. Clin Diagn Virol 1998;10:49.

40. Lin C-T, Tseng C-J, Lai C-H, et al: High-risk HPV DNA detection by hybrid capture II: An adjunctive test for mildly abnormal cytologic smears in women ≥50 years of age. J Reprod Med 2000;45:345.

41. Hillemanns P, Kimmig R, Huttermann U, et al: Screening for cervical neoplasia by self-assessment for human papillomavirus DNA. Lancet 1999;354:1970.

42. Ronnett BM, Manos MM, Ransley JE, et al: Atypical glandular cells of undetermined significance (AGUS): Cytopathologic features, histopathologic results, and human papillomavirus DNA detection. Human Pathol 1999;30:816.

43. Fait G, Daniel Y, Kupferminc MJ, et al: Does typing of human papillomavirus assist in the triage of women with repeated low-grade, cervical cytologic abnormalities? Gynecol Oncol 1998;70:319.

44. Ferris DG, Wright TC Jr, Litaker MS, et al: Comparison of two tests for detecting carcinogenic HPV in women with Papanicolaou smear reports of ASCUS and LSIL. J Fam Pract 1998;46:136.

45. Peyton CL, Schiffman M, Lorincz AT, et al: Comparison of PCR- and hybrid capture-based HPV detection systems using multiple cervical specimen collection strategies. J Clin Microbiol 1998;36:3248.

46. Sellors JW, Lorincz AT, Mahony JB, et al: Comparison of self-collected vaginal, vulvar and urine samples with physician-collected cervical samples for human papillomavirus testing to detect high-

grade squamous intraepithelial lesions. Can Med Assoc J 2000;163: 513.

47. Bauer HM, Ting Y, Greer CE, et al: Genital human papillomavirus infection in female university students as determined by a PCR-based method. JAMA 1991;265:472.

48. Mullis K, Faloona F, Scharf S, et al: Specific enzymatic amplification of DNA in vitro: The polymerase chain reaction. Cold Spring Harb Symp Quant Biol 1986;51:263.

49. Mullis KB, Faloona FA: Specific synthesis of DNA in vitro via a polymerase-catalyzed chain reaction. Methods Enzymol 1987;155: 335.

50. Griffin NR, Dockey D, Lewis FA, Wells M: Demonstration of low frequency of human papillomavirus DNA in cervical adenocarcinoma and adenocarcinoma in situ by the polymerase chain reaction and in situ hybridization. Intl J Gynecol Pathol 1991;10:36.

51. Josefsson A, Livak K, Gyllensten U: Detection and quantitation of human papillomavirus by using the fluorescent 5' exonuclease assay. J Clin Microbiol 1999;37:490.

52. Ting Y, Manos MM: Detection and typing of genital human papillomaviruses. In Innis MA, Gelfand DH, Sninsky JJ, White TJ (eds): PCR Protocols: A Guide to Methods and Applications. San Diego, Academic Press, 1990, pp 356–367.

53. van den Brule AJC, Meijer CJLM, Bakels V, et al: Rapid detection of human papillomavirus in cervical scrapes by combined general primer-mediated and type-specific polymerase chain reaction. J Clin Microbiol 1990;28:2739.

54. Gravitt PE, Peyton CL, Alessi TQ, et al: Improved amplification of genital human papillomaviruses. J Clin Microbiol 2000;38:357.

55. Gregoire L, Arella M, Campione-Piccardo J, Lancaster WD: Amplification of human papillomavirus DNA sequences by using conserved primers. J Clin Microbiol 1989;27:2660.

56. Shibata DK, Arnheim N, Martin WJ: Detection of human papilloma virus in paraffin-embedded tissue using the polymerase chain reaction. J Exp Med 1988;167:225.

57. Hildesheim A, Schiffman MH, Gravitt PE, et al: Persistence of type-specific human papillomavirus infection among cytologically normal women. J Infect Dis 1994;169:235.

58. Goldsborough MD, McAllister P, Reid R, et al: A comparison study of human papillomavirus prevalence by the polymerase chain reaction in low risk women and in a gynaecology referral group at elevated risk for cervical cancer. Mol Cell Probes 1992;6:451.

59. Lungu O, Sun XW, Wright TC Jr, et al: A polymerase chain reaction-enzyme-linked immunosorbent assay method for detecting human papillomavirus in cervical carcinomas and high-grade cervical cancer precursors. Obstet Gynecol 1995;85:337.

60. Cohen J: "Long PCR" leaps into larger DNA sequences. Science 1994;263:1564.

61. Gravitt PE, Peyton CL, Apple RJ, Wheeler CM: Genotyping of 27 human papillomavirus types by using L1 consensus PCR products by a single-hybridization, reverse line blot detection method. J Clin Microbiol 1998;36:3020.

62. Kleter B, van Doorn LJ, Schrauwen L, et al: Development and clinical evaluation of a highly sensitive PCR-reverse hybridization line probe assay for detection and identification of anogenital human papillomavirus. J Clin Microbiol 1999;37:2508.

63. Xi LF, Demers W, Koutsky LA, et al: Analysis of human papillomavirus type 16 variants indicates establishment of persistent infection. J Infect Dis 1995;172:747.

64. Kwok S, Higuchi R: Avoiding false positives with PCR. Nature 1989;339:237.

65. Tidy J, Farrell PJ: Retraction: Human papillomavirus subtype 16b. Lancet 1989 Dec;2(8678–8679):1535.

66. Hinchliffe SA, van Velzen D, Korporaal H, et al: Transcience of cervical HPV infection in sexually active, young women with normal cervicovaginal cytology. Br J Cancer 1995;72:943.

67. Beckmann AM, Myerson D, Daling JR, et al: Detection and localization of human papillomavirus DNA in human genital condylomas by in situ hybridization with biotinylated probes. J Med Virol 1985;16:265.

68. Chapman WB, Lorincz AT, Willett GD, et al: Evaluation of two commercially available in situ hybridization kits for detection of human papillomavirus DNA in cervical biopsies: Comparison to Southern blot hybridization. Mod Pathol 1993;6:73.

69. Moench TR: In situ hybridization. Mol Cell Probes 1987;1:195.

70. Nagai N, Nuovo G, Friedman D, Crum CP: Detection of papillomavirus nucleic acids in genital precancers with the in situ hybridization technique. Int J Gynecol Pathol 1987;6:366.

71. Schneider A, Oltersdorf T, Schneider V, Gissmann L: Distribution pattern of human papilloma virus 16 genome in cervical neoplasia by molecular in situ hybridization of tissue sections. Int J Cancer 1987;39:717.

72. Morrison EAB, Ho GYF, Vermund SH, et al: Human papillomavirus infection and other risk factors for cervical neoplasia: A case-control study. Int J Cancer 1991;49:6.

73. Hatch KD, Schneider A, Abdel-Nour MW: An evaluation of human papillomavirus testing for intermediate- and high-risk types as triage before colposcopy. Am J Obstet Gynecol 1995;172:1150.

74. Lorincz AT: Human papillomaviruses. In Lennette EH, Smith TF (eds): Laboratory Diagnosis of Viral Infections, 3rd ed. New York, Marcel Dekker, 1999, pp 635–663.

75. Kjaer SK, van den Brule AJC, Bock JE, et al: Determinants for genital human papillomavirus (HPV) infection in 1000 randomly chosen young Danish women with normal Pap smear: Are there different risk profiles for oncogenic and nononcogenic HPV types? Cancer Epidemiol Biomarkers Prev 1997;6:799.

76. Nobbenhuis MAE, Walboomers JMM, Helmerhorst TJ, et al: Relation of human papillomavirus status to cervical lesions and consequences for cervical-cancer screening: A prospective study. Lancet 1999;354:20.

77. Ho GYF, Bierman R, Beardsley L, et al: Natural history of cervicovaginal papillomavirus infection in young women. N Engl J Med 1998;338:423.

78. Franco EL, Villa LL, Sobrinho JP, et al: Epidemiology of acquisition and clearance of cervical human papillomavirus infection in women from a high-risk area for cervical cancer. J Infect Dis 1999;180:1415.

79. Bollen LJM, Tjong-A-Hung SP, van der Velden J, et al: Clearance of cervical human papillomavirus infection by treatment for cervical dysplasia. Sex Transm Dis 1997;24:456.

80. Elfgren K, Bistoletti P, Dillner L, et al: Conization for cervical intraepithelial neoplasia is followed by disappearance of human papillomavirus deoxyribonucleic acid and a decline in serum and cervical mucus antibodies against human papillomavirus antigens. Am J Obstet Gynecol 1996;174:937.

81. Wiedorn KH, Kuh H, Galle J, et al: Comparison of in-situ hybridization, direct and indirect in-situ PCR as well as tyramide signal amplification for the detection of HPV. Histochem Cell Biol 1999;111:89.

82. Melkert PWJ, Hopman E, van den Brule AJC, et al: Prevalence of HPV in cytomorphologically normal cervical smears, as determined by the polymerase chain reaction, is age-dependent. Int J Cancer 1993;53:919.

83. National Cancer Institute: SEER Program Self Instructional Manual for Cancer Registrars. Book 7: Statistics and Epidemiology for Cancer Registries. Bethesda, MD, National Institutes of Health, 1994.

84. Sellors JW, Mahony JB, Kaczorowski J, et al, for the Survey of HPV in Ontario women (SHOW) Group: Prevalence and predictors of human papillomavirus infection in women in Ontario, Canada. Can Med Assoc J 2000;163:503.

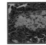

• Neal M. Lonky

Cervical Screening with in Vivo and in Vitro Modalities: Speculoscopy Combined with Cytology

EVOLUTION OF VISUALIZATION OF THE CERVIX AND LOWER GENITAL TRACT FROM A DIAGNOSTIC TO A SCREENING ROLE

All visual inspection techniques, including colposcopy, are limited to examination of the areas that are overtly visible. Cervical cytology remains useful for the discovery of endocervical and small lesions not visible to the unaided eye of the examiner.

The performance of colposcopy involves significant clinician time and financial expenditures. Colposcopy requires special training, is expensive, and is not available in the majority of clinical settings. Therefore, it has not been used during routine screening. If colposcopy was widely available and cost-effective, it would likely be used as a routine screening examination, either in place of or, more likely, in tandem with the Papanicolaou (Pap) smear. However, all visual inspection techniques, including colposcopy, are limited to the examination of the areas that are overtly visible, making adequate evaluation of the endocervical canal problematic. Cervical cytology remains useful in the discovery of endocervical and small lesions not visible to the unaided eye of the examiner, especially when the endocervical sampling brush is used.

In this traditional role, colposcopy is a *diagnostic* test. However, visual tests may also be used as *screening* tools.

As it is currently used, colposcopy is reserved for women who are already deemed at risk by virtue of the first abnormal screening test. In this traditional role, colposcopy is a *diagnostic* test. However, visual tests may also be used as *screening* tools. When visual tests are used in screening, vascular patterns and tissue characteristics are not considered, making the test simpler and leading to a dichotomous "positive" or "negative" result.

To appreciate the value of tissue visualization in the screening process, one must understand that screening tests are not fully diagnostic of the underlying histologic grade. They merely identify women at risk for having cervical dysplasia or cancer and require a further diagnostic test to make the final diagnosis. Furthermore, to properly evaluate the value of a screening test, we must decide whether there is value in identifying all women with precursor lesions or just those with high-grade disease or early invasive carcinoma.

ENHANCED SCREENING WITH CERVICAL VISUALIZATION: EVIDENCE-BASED ANALYSIS

Acetic acid denatures nuclear proteins and dehydrates cellular cytoplasm, causing tissues with increased nuclear-to-cytoplasmic ratios to reflect projected white light and appear white. This effect can also be appreciated during magnified or unaided (naked eye) examinations following the application of 4% to 6% acetic acid. This has been the basis for use in screening women for cervical disease (predominantly in underdeveloped countries where Pap smear programs are not feasible) and has been called "downstaging" by some.[1-3] The appearance of well-demarcated acetowhite cervical lesions in women undergoing screening for cervical cancer correlates with underlying cervical neoplasia, but this correlation is not perfect. In the study by Van Le et al,[1] nurse practitioners, physicians, and physician assistants screened clinic attendees with downstaging and Pap smears. Eighty-five additional patients (with negative Pap smears) were referred for colposcopy owing to the presence of acetowhite cervical lesions seen during screening. Thirty-five of 85 (41%) patients had dysplasia on directed biopsies. The number of women screened, which generated those 85 additional referrals, was not reported; therefore, the number of women referred for colposcopy who were subsequently found to have normal findings could not be calculated.

Adding visualization identified more patients with dysplastic cervical lesions (that cytology had missed), but with an increase in the number of patients referred for colposcopy who were subsequently found to have a normal colposcopy or biopsy.

A study from the University of Zimbabwe/JHPIEGO Cervical Cancer Project[4] studied 2203 screening patients referred for colposcopy with either abnormal cytology or visual inspection and downstaging. Downstaging (called VIA in this study) detected 76.7% (95% confidence interval, 70.3% to 82.3%) of the cervical cancer precursor lesions. Adding visualization identified more patients with dysplastic cervical lesions (that cytology had missed), but with an increase in the number of patients referred for colposcopy who were subsequently found to have a normal colposcopy or biopsy. Because "screen negative" women were not evaluated with colposcopy and biopsy, true sensitivity and specificity were not determined.

Slawson et al[3] evaluated 2872 women eligible for screening without a previous history of cervical disease. Each patient received a conventional Pap smear and downstaging as previously defined. There were 140 cases of biopsy-proven cervical intraepithelial neoplasia (CIN) discovered (prevalence, 4.9%), 33 (24%) of which were discovered solely because of abnormal downstaging (Pap smear was negative).

> **The false-positive rate of a visual screening tool may appear higher if the "gold standard" (colposcopically directed biopsy) misses some disease.**

False-positive visual screening cases may occur for two major reasons. Benign conditions such as inflammatory atypia or immature metaplasia may turn white after the application of acetic acid, or the biopsy may be misdirected. In both instances, the clinician may conclude that the visual screen was false positive, but in the second scenario this false-positive result is due to examiner error. This conclusion is supported by three studies[5–7] in which patients had directed biopsies for presumed high-grade visually suspicious lesions, followed immediately by electrosurgical loop excision of the entire transformation zone. In at least one third of the cases, the loop excision specimen documented a more severe change than did the directed biopsy. The false-positive rate of a visual screening tool may appear higher if the "gold standard" (colposcopically directed biopsy) misses some disease.

OVERCOMING THE LIMITATIONS OF THE CONVENTIONAL PAP SMEAR

> **The failure of some cervical lesions to be represented in the cellular analysis performed in the laboratory may be due to examiner error, laboratory error, or failure of these neoplastic lesions to exfoliate. However, some lesions inside the endocervical canal cannot be visualized and may be reached and sampled only by cytologic brush techniques.**

Although the performance of exfoliative cytology has improved our ability to indirectly identify cervical neoplasia, it has limitations. One study documents a high false-negative rate (50%) of a single conventional Pap smear examination.[8] Enhancements to the conventional Pap smear, such as thin-layer preparations and computerized Pap smear reading, resulted in improved collection, fixation, and inspection steps of this in vitro process. However, there is evidence that some cervical lesions are not represented in the cellular analysis performed in the laboratory. This may be due to failure of these neoplastic lesions to exfoliate, to examiner error, or to laboratory error. Some lesions that cannot be detected with cytology-based screening may be visualized. However, some lesions inside the cervical canal cannot be visualized and may be reached and sampled only through cytologic brushing for microscopic analysis. The most sensitive screening procedure to detect both types of lesions would combine visual (in vivo) and laboratory cytology-based (in vivo) methodologies. The objective is to increase the sensitivity of a single examination without reducing test accuracy through loss of specificity or referring an excessive number of patients for colposcopy, which might make the test too impractical or too expensive. This approach combines enhanced lesion visualization (speculoscopy) with the conventional Pap smear.

Magnified Visualization with Chemiluminescence: Speculoscopy and the Evidence-Based Literature

> **Speculoscopy visualizes the cervix with blue-white chemiluminescent illumination and low-power, portable magnification following the application of dilute acetic acid.**

Speculoscopy visualizes the cervix with blue-white chemiluminescent illumination and low-power, portable magnification ($\times4-6$ magnification loupe or monocular) following the application of dilute (4% to 6%) acetic acid. Speculoscopy is different in that it uses the unique spectral frequency, placement, and energy emitted from the chemiluminescent light source. In two studies where the chemiluminescent light source was compared with magnified inspection using projected white- and blue-filtered, incandescent illumination of the cervix (PIL), speculoscopy disclosed more biopsy-proven dysplastic lesions of the cervix than did PIL.[9, 10] In more than 10,000 published cases from a wide array of clinical settings and examiners (colposcopists, noncolposcopists, physicians, and nurse clinicians), the addition of speculoscopy to the conventional Pap smear resulted in a greater than twofold rise in sensitivity (from 40.7% for the Pap smear alone to 92.2% using the combined approach). This involved the detection of all grades of cervical dysplasia or malignancy.[11]

> **Speculoscopy disclosed more biopsy-proven dysplastic lesions of the cervix than did projected white- and blue-filtered, incandescent illumination of the cervix.**

The addition of speculoscopy to the conventional Pap smear in routine screening was studied prospectively. The first multicenter study was specifically designed to include colposcopy for all study participants. Mann et al reported on 243 screening patients (no history of cervical or vaginal pathology or treatment) from 12 clinical sites.[12] All patients had both a screening Pap smear and speculoscopy. The Pap smear detected 9 of 29 (31%) women with cervical dysplasia or condyloma, whereas the combination of the Pap smear and speculoscopy (called magnified chemiluminescent illumination in that study) detected 24 of 29 cases (83%) (p < 0.001). The negative predictive value of the combined visual-cytologic test was 99%. Polatti et al replicated this study design in Italy, where 600 patients were screened.[13] Colposcopy was performed in all participants, and colposcopically directed biopsy was used to establish the tissue diagnosis. The Pap smear alone detected 23.7% of cervical dysplasia or carcinoma, whereas the combination of Pap smear and speculoscopy increased the detection rate to 78.8%. Cytology failed to detect about one third of biopsy-proven high-grade CIN that was discovered by speculoscopy alone (10 of 33 cases). Although the majority of the false-negative Pap smears represented low-grade disease, one third of the cases were high grade.

When evaluating visual screening adjuncts, one must balance the enhancement of sensitivity with the propensity toward referring healthy women for colposcopy.

In a larger study by Wertlake et al, the question of examiner expertise was addressed.[14] More than 180 practitioners, including physicians and nonphysicians (most were not colposcopy trained) evaluated 5692 screening patients (as previously defined). Only women with a positive screening test were referred for colposcopic evaluation, so the true sensitivity and specificity could not be determined. Of the women screened who completed the protocol, speculoscopy alone (patients with negative Pap smear results) detected 11 of 32 cases of high-grade dysplasia and 154 of 191 low-grade dysplasias. Once again, one third of the high-grade dysplasias would have been missed if speculoscopy were omitted during screening. The authors concluded that combined visual-cytologic screening is appropriate for all clinicians currently performing the conventional Pap smear procedure, not just colposcopists.

According to published data, screening with chemiluminescence, as opposed to other light sources, imparts the lowest overcall rate.

Colposcopy is a more sensitive test than speculoscopy for very small lesions.

When evaluating visual screening adjuncts, one must balance the enhancement of sensitivity with the propensity toward referring healthy women for colposcopy (overcall) because of an abnormal screening test. According to published data, screening with chemiluminescence (as opposed to other light sources) imparts the lowest overcall rate. Overcall rates ranged from 6% to 8% in most series, as compared with studies using projected nonchemiluminescent light sources with overcall rates of 10% to 20%.[12-14] Photographic documentation and in-

spection of the cervix (cervicography), which employs magnification and projected illumination, exhibited lower sensitivity and higher overcall.[15] When speculoscopy is added to conventional cytology, one can expect the specificity of screening to decrease from 95% to 80% to 85%. If speculoscopy was removed from the screening setting and compared directly with colposcopy for higher-risk women already referred for colposcopy, examiners were twice as likely to overcall suspicious lesions with colposcopy as compared with speculoscopy.[16] Colposcopy is a more sensitive test than speculoscopy for very small lesions. When examiners are trained to distinguish sharp acetowhite lesions from "look-alike" faint lesions with indistinct borders, they are less apt to identify benign lesions as suspicious under chemiluminescent illumination, making speculoscopy more suitable for screening than colposcopy.

When examiners are trained to distinguish sharp acetowhite lesions from "look-alike" faint lesions with indistinct borders, they are less apt to identify benign lesions as suspicious under chemiluminescent illumination, making speculoscopy more suitable for screening than colposcopy.

SPECULOSCOPY AS PART OF THE PAPSURE PROCEDURE: INDICATIONS FOR USE AND METHOD OF PROCEDURE

The appearance of intravaginal structures is improved using chemiluminescent light energy, compared with using bright room light.

Visualization of the cervix and lower genital tract with speculoscopy is indicated whenever a patient is having a Pap smear for cervical cancer screening. The chemiluminescent Speculite light source and other tools needed to perform speculoscopy are shown in Figure 4–29. The examiner may choose a monocular or binocular, low-power magnification loupe to visualize the cervix and vagina during the inspection phase of the procedure. The Speculite device (capsule of chemiluminescent chemicals) is activated by bending the outer capsule, which fractures a more brittle inner capsule, allowing chemicals to intermix (Fig. 4–30). The Speculite capsule should be shaken vigorously for 10 to 15 seconds, allowing the chemicals to mix and activating the blue-white chemiluminescent illumination (Fig. 4–31). The Speculite is then attached to the inner, middle aspect of the upper blade of the vaginal speculum using double-sided tape (Fig. 4–32). Following insertion of the vaginal speculum and gross inspection, an endocervical and exocervical Pap smear specimen is obtained, and the tissues are then rinsed with a dilute (4% to 6%) acetic acid solution. The ambient room light is dimmed or extinguished. To avoid a completely dark room environment, the examiner may leave a light source illuminated in the corner of the room or a window shade drawn to allow only a small amount of ambient room light. The unique blue-white illumination can be noted in Figure 4–33.

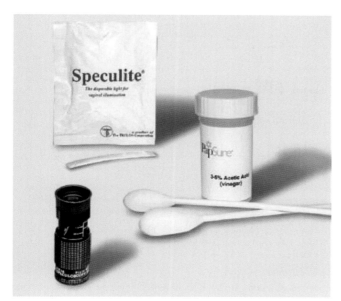

Figure 4–29. Speculoscopy requires the foil packet containing the Speculite, acetic acid solution, and ×4–6 magnification.

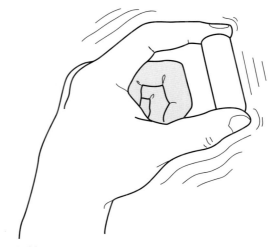

Figure 4–31. Vigorously shake the capsule to intermix the chemicals to accelerate the chemical reaction and create bright light.

Vascular abnormalities may be distinguished, but owing to the low-power magnification and low-energy light source, they are not specifically used to grade lesions already seen under Speculite illumination.

The appearance of intravaginal structures is improved using chemiluminescent light energy, compared with using projected conventional light. The tissues appear brighter, and visualization of the landmarks needed to evaluate the condition of the cervix and vagina is facilitated when the room light is dimmed or extinguished. The cervix and vagina are inspected for the presence of

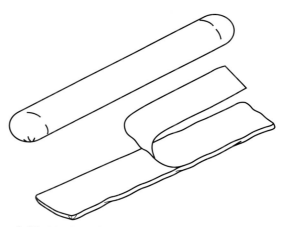

Figure 4–32. The Speculite is attached to the double-sided tape. The other side is attached to the inner aspect of the upper speculum blade.

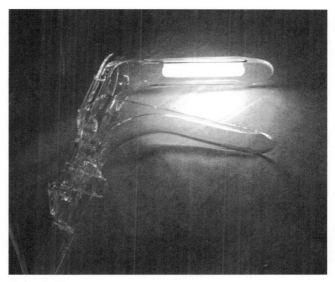

Figure 4–33. Speculoscopy is ideally performed in a low, ambient, room light setting. This permits the lesions to become faintly luminescent and be more easily visualized.

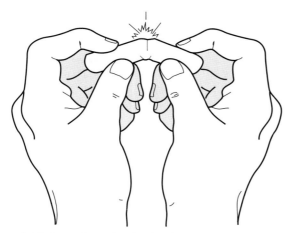

Figure 4–30. To activate the chemiluminescent light, bend the outer flexible capsule to fracture the brittle inner capsule, thereby mixing the chemicals and creating blue-white light.

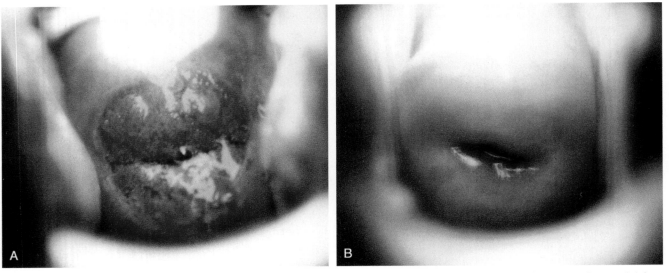

Figure 4-34. *A,* Cervix under speculoscopy with a normal transformation zone devoid of lesions. Bright areas of reflection appear glossy and deform or disappear when depressed with a cotton-tipped applicator. *B,* Normal cervix without lesions appears uniform and is pink-blue in color under speculoscopy. No well-demarcated lesions are seen.

exophytic or endophytic lesions, acetowhite epithelium, ulcers, or masses and changes associated with cervical cancer or its precursors. Vascular abnormalities may be distinguished, but owing to the low-power magnification and low-energy light source, they are not specifically used to grade lesions already seen under Speculite illumination.

> **A positive speculoscopy result is defined as the presence of at least one acetowhite lesion that appears bright and distinct with at least one sharply marginated border on the cervix or vagina.**

The results are interpreted as either positive or negative. A positive speculoscopy result is defined as the presence of at least one acetowhite lesion that appears bright and distinct with at least one sharply marginated border on the cervix or vagina. The lesions may stand out from the surrounding dark-red or blue-tinged normal epithelium that does not reflect the chemiluminescent light. A negative speculoscopy result is one in which the cervix or lower genital tract is devoid of any sharply marginated acetowhite lesion and the cervix coloration is uniformly pink with a bluish hue. Faint lesions with indistinct borders should be considered negative and often represent benign areas of squamous metaplasia or inflammation.

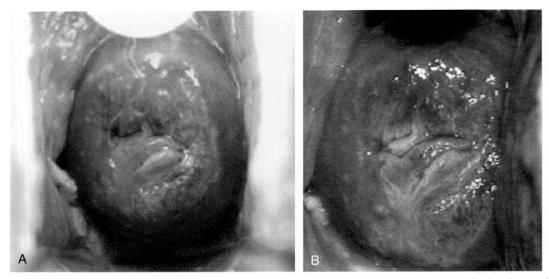

Figure 4-35. *A,* This cervix represents a variant of normal. A small area of metaplasia at 3 o'clock is faintly acetowhite, but the margins are poorly defined or fuzzy bordered. This would be a look-alike, potentially false-positive examination to the untrained examiner. *B,* The same cervix during colposcopy appears normal. There are no suspicious lesions seen.

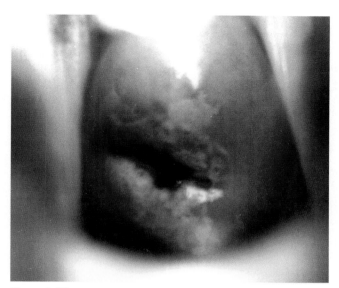

Figure 4–36. A large lesion under speculoscopy with sharp borders defines a positive screening examination.

A negative speculoscopy result is one in which the cervix or lower genital tract is devoid of any sharply marginated acetowhite lesion and the cervix coloration is uniformly pink with a bluish hue. Faint lesions with indistinct borders should be considered negative and often represent benign areas of squamous metaplasia or inflammation.

Figure 4–34A demonstrates a negative speculoscopy result where the cervix shows a normal transformation zone devoid of lesions. Light reflection can be easily distinguished from true lesions because they appear glossy and change shape when depressed with a cotton-tipped applicator. Figure 4–34B shows a negative result as well. Figure 4–35A also shows a negative speculoscopy result, but there is an indistinct lesion with a fuzzy border at 3 o'clock. Metaplastic or inflammatory lesions appear as indistinct, faint, acetowhite changes, distinct from dysplasia that appears sharp and well demarcated. Figure 4–35B shows the corresponding colpophotograph. Figures 4–36 and 4–37A demonstrate positive speculoscopy results with at least one sharply marginated lesion. Figure 4–37A can be compared with the corresponding colpophotograph in 4–37B showing a mosaic pattern. Positive speculoscopy and colposcopy results are compared in Figure 4–38. The lesions are larger and more numerous under speculoscopy. This may be due to the lower energy of the speculoscopy light source permitting a lower reflectivity and a higher tissue penetration. The biopsies from the anterior and posterior cervix showed CIN 2 and CIN 3 in this case. A combined visual-cytologic test (called PapSure) is positive when either the speculoscopy result or the cytology result is abnormal, and it is negative when both results are normal.

A combined visual-cytologic test (called PapSure) is positive when either the speculoscopy result or the cytology result is abnormal, and it is negative when both results are normal.

Chemiluminescence: Properties That Enhance the Detection of True Cervical Neoplasia

The sensitivity and specificity of screening with chemiluminescence were superior when compared with those of projected incandescent or halogen illumination, with a lower overall rate.

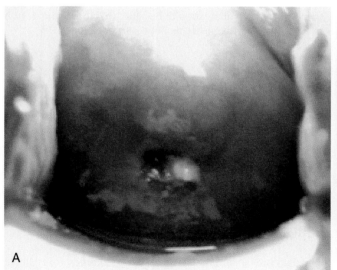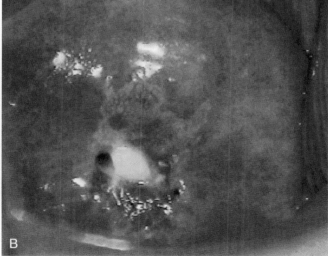

Figure 4–37. *A,* A bright, well-demarcated lesion on the anterior lip can be seen under speculoscopy. This screening test is positive. *B,* The same cervix under colposcopy is also positive with a suspicious lesion near 12 o'clock. Owing to the high-power illumination and magnification, mosaic can be appreciated and serves as the landmark for a directed biopsy. The biopsy showed high-grade dysplasia.

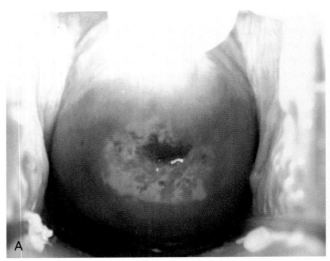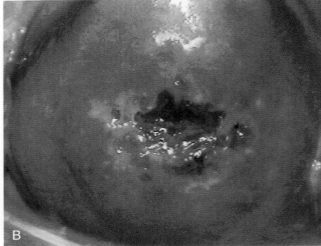

Figure 4–38. Photograph of a neoplastic lesion seen under speculoscopy (*A*) and colposcopy (*B*). The lesions are larger and more numerous under speculoscopy owing to the lower-energy light source and deeper tissue penetration. These were low-grade lesions on biopsy.

Two studies have shown that simply filtering projected incandescent illumination (with a blue or green filter) toward the cervical portio will not duplicate the ability of chemiluminescence to disclose CIN lesions.[12, 13] In these studies, the sensitivity and specificity of screening with chemiluminescence were superior when compared with those of projected incandescent or halogen illumination, with a lower overall rate.

> **The physical properties of chemiluminescent light that are thought to be responsible for disclosing lesions under the epithelial surface are low energy, diffuse light emission, intravaginal placement of the light, proximity to the cervical mucosa, and ideal color spectrum that contrasts tissues with differing reflective indices.**

The physical properties of chemiluminescent light that are thought to be responsible for disclosing lesions under the epithelial surface are low energy, diffuse light emission, intravaginal placement of the light, proximity to the cervical mucosa, and ideal color spectrum that contrasts tissues with differing reflective indices. When using the intravaginal chemiluminescent light capsule, the following pitfalls and remedies exist:

1. Instead of projecting light toward the cervical portio, the light capsule should be attached to the inner upper speculum blade. This is akin to "lighting the room" from the ceiling as opposed to projecting light from the "doorway" to view the object at the distal end. The bar of light may reflect off the moist mucosal surface. The reflection takes on a glossy appearance and may be distinguished from a true cervical lesion by the clinician's gently rotating the speculum or depressing the area with a moist cotton-tipped applicator. True lesions should remain white and uniform, whereas light reflection will change in shape and appearance or may entirely disappear when the speculum and light are moved or the tissue is depressed.

2. Patients with a large cervix or acentric portio may obstruct the light and may require manipulation of the speculum or the cervix to achieve adequate visualization. Replacement of the light onto the lower speculum blade may be necessary if the cervix is displaced anteriorly.

3. Neoplastic lesions appear to have an opaque or matte surface texture, whereas light reflection appears quite shiny or glossy in appearance.

4. The borders of neoplastic lesions are sharp, whereas lesions with indistinct or fuzzy borders more likely represent metaplastic or inflammatory changes. Nabothian cysts are more rounded and also exhibit indistinct borders.

5. When one discovers ulcerations, erosions, or vascularized areas that are suspicious for cancer, the presence or absence of acetowhite change is of secondary importance. The examiner should be sure to biopsy the lesion to establish the diagnosis as soon as possible.

> **When one discovers ulcerations, erosions, or vascularized areas that are suspicious for cancer, the presence or absence of acetowhite change is of secondary importance. The examiner should be sure to biopsy the lesion to establish the diagnosis as soon as possible.**

INTERPRETATION AND TRIAGE OF PAPSURE SCREENING RESULTS

The PapSure examination uses two modalities to evaluate a patient's risk for cervical or lower genital tract neoplasia. The clinician must use the results of in vitro cytologic data as well as the result of in vivo visual inspection. Table 4–2 shows the potential findings based on the data obtained with two tests. A positive Pap smear is defined as evidence of a low-grade squamous intraepithelial lesion (LSIL) or a higher-grade abnormality. The presence of atypical glandular cells of undetermined significance (AGUS) should also be defined as abnormal in this management algorithm.

In Table 4–2, patients in group A should be referred for colposcopy by virtue of the Pap smear abnormality alone, and speculoscopy does not add new information regarding their risk status. Patients in group B also require colposcopy, but experience shows that they compose the smallest referral group. If dysplasia is found, these patients usually have small lesions on the portio, or endocervical disease. Patients in group C are newly discovered to be at risk because they have positive speculoscopy despite negative Pap smear results. If colposcopy is performed within a few weeks, biopsies show CIN 1 or worse in over 60% of cases. Research has shown that colposcopy may be safely deferred for 6 months in women deemed reliable for follow-up and otherwise low risk. In women with persistent speculoscopic lesions 6 months later, the yield of colposcopic biopsy increased to more than 90%.[17] All the cases of high-grade dysplasia missed by the Pap smear should be discovered in group C, except for the remote case of isolated endocervical disease. Patients in group D receive negative evaluations on both cytology and speculoscopy. This provides reassurance to patients because the negative predictive value is more than 99%. It may be possible to widen screening intervals for women who are screen negative for the PapSure procedure. Groups E and F demonstrate the value of speculoscopy in the triage of patients with atypical squamous cells of undetermined significance (ASCUS) Pap smears.

In a study where all women received speculoscopy, conventional cytology, and colposcopy, Massad et al found that in those with ASCUS results, 53% had lesions seen under speculoscopy, and 96% of women with positive speculoscopy had positive colposcopy. In addition, 97% of all patients with biopsy-proven intraepithelial neoplasia were discovered.[18] The remaining 3% of cases with ASCUS results, negative speculoscopy, and positive colposcopy showed biopsies no worse than CIN 1. This study suggests that performing primary PapSure examinations could assist in effective triage when ASCUS Pap smear results are encountered (without requiring an additional clinic visit or laboratory [human papillomavirus] test).

Impact on Cost-Effectiveness of Screening

Speculoscopy can be effectively performed by all clinicians currently performing Pap smears, including nurse practitioners, with an improvement in screening sensitivity of 200% to 300%.[14, 19] The added cost of the equipment and added service (approximately $20 to $25 per examination) is offset by the improvement in sensitivity (cost per case of CIN or cancer detected). In populations where ASCUS Pap smears lead to unnecessary colposcopic referral, the prior knowledge of speculoscopy results can lead to more effective triage, delaying or eliminating colposcopy in those with a negative speculoscopy examination.[18] The negative predictive value of the combined speculoscopy and Pap smear (PapSure) is more than 99% and provides the option of widened screening intervals in women who test negative. By reassuring low-risk patients, health care providers in all settings can more appropriately focus resources on women who are at high risk for cervical cancer. The savings reaped from not having to repeatedly screen those women who are at low risk for cervical disease can be reinvested in outreach to the underserved and underscreened and in screening with the combined in vitro and in vivo modalities. A study comparing the conventional Pap test performed annually with PapSure performed biannually showed PapSure to be cost-effective while reducing the cervical cancer prevalence and death rate using a Markov prediction model.[20]

▼ Table 4–2

Combined Visual/Cytologic Examination Using Speculoscopy and Cytology (PapSure)*

Group	Pap Smear Result	Speculoscopy Result	PapSure Result
A	(+)	(+)	(+)
B	(+)	(−)	(+)
C	(−)	(+)	(+)
D	(−)	(−)	(−)
E	ASCUS	(+)	Consider high risk
F	ASCUS	(−)	Consider low risk

* It may be possible to widen screening intervals for women who are "screen negative" for the PapSure procedure. Colposcopy may be advised for patients with positive or high-risk PapSure results.

ASCUS, atypical squamous cells of undetermined significance; Pap, Papanicolaou.

SUMMARY OF KEY POINTS

- Adding an adjunctive visualization technique to routine Pap smear screening identifies more patients with dysplastic cervical lesions (that cytology had missed), but with an increase in the number of patients referred for colposcopy who are subsequently found to have a normal colposcopy or biopsy.

- The false-positive rate of a visual screening tool may appear higher if the gold standard (colposcopically directed biopsy) misses some disease.

- False-negative Pap smears may be due to failure of the neoplastic lesions to exfoliate, to examiner error, or to laboratory error.

- Some lesions inside the cervical canal cannot be visualized and may be reached and sampled only through cytologic brushing for an endocervical smear.

- Speculoscopy visualizes the cervix with blue-white chemiluminescent illumination and low-power, portable magnification following the application of dilute acetic acid.

continued on following page

- The sensitivity and specificity of screening with chemiluminescence were superior when compared with those of projected incandescent or halogen illumination, with a lower overcall rate.

- Colposcopy is a more sensitive test than speculoscopy for very small lesions.

- When examiners are trained to distinguish sharp acetowhite lesions from look-alike faint lesions with indistinct borders, they are less apt to identify benign lesions as suspicious under chemiluminescent illumination.

- A positive speculoscopy result is defined as the presence of at least one acetowhite lesion that appears bright and distinct with at least one sharply marginated border on the cervix or vagina.

- A negative speculoscopy is one in which the cervix or lower genital tract is devoid of any sharply marginated acetowhite lesion and the cervix coloration is uniformly pink with a bluish hue. Faint lesions with indistinct borders should be considered negative and often represent benign areas of squamous metaplasia or inflammation.

- A combined visual-cytologic test (called PapSure) is positive when either the speculoscopy result or the cytology result is abnormal, and it is negative when both are normal.

- The physical properties of chemiluminescent light that are thought to be responsible for disclosing lesions under the epithelial surface are low energy, diffuse light emission, intravaginal placement of the light, proximity to the cervical mucosa, and ideal color spectrum that contrasts tissues with differing reflective indices.

- When one discovers ulcerations, erosions, or vascularized areas that are suspicious for cancer, the presence or absence of acetowhite change is of secondary importance. The examiner should be sure to biopsy the lesion to establish the diagnosis as soon as possible.

- Speculoscopy aids in identifying women with neoplastic lesions, including high grade, whose Pap smears are negative (normal) or atypical (ASCUS), because it does not rely on exfoliation or in vitro laboratory analysis.

- It may be possible to widen screening intervals for women who are screen negative for the PapSure procedure.

References

1. Van Le L, Broekhuizen F, Janzer-Steele R, et al: Acetic acid visualization of the cervix to detect cervical dysplasia. Obstet Gynecol 1993;81:293.
2. Nene B, Deshpande S, Jayant K, et al: Early detection of cervical cancer by visual inspection: A population-based study in rural India. Int J Cancer 1996;68:770.
3. Slawson D, Bennett J, Herman J: Are Papanicolaou smears enough? Acetic acid washes of the cervix as adjunctive therapy: A HARNET study. J Fam Pract 1992;35:271.
4. University of Zimbabwe/JHPIEGO Cervical Cancer Project: Visual inspection with acetic acid for cervical-cancer screening: Test qualities in a primary-care setting. Lancet 1999;353:869.
5. Buxton E, Luesley D, Shafi M, Rollason M: Colposcopically directed punch biopsy: A potentially misleading investigation. Br J Obstet Gynecol 1991;98:1273.
6. Chappatte O, Byrne D, Raju K, et al: Histological differences between colposcopic-directed biopsy and loop excision of the transformation zone (LETZ): A cause for concern. Gynecol Oncol 1991;43:46.
7. Massad L, Halperin C, Bitterman P: Correlation between colposcopically directed biopsy and cervical loop excision. Gynecol Oncol 1996;60:400.
8. Agency for Health Care Policy and Research: Evidence Report/Technology Assessment No. 5, Evaluation of Cervical Cytology, AHCPR Publication No. 99-E010, January 1999.
9. Lonky N, Edwards G: Comparison of chemiluminescent light versus incandescent light in the visualization of acetowhite epithelium. Am J Gynecol Health 1992;6:11.
10. Suneja A, Mahishee, Agarwal N, Misra K: Comparison of magnified chemiluminescent examination with incandescent light examination and colposcopy for detection of cervical neoplasia. Indian J Cancer 1998;35:81.
11. U.S. Food and Drug Administration: Monograph: Papanicolaou Smear Plus Speculoscopy, 1997.
12. Mann W, Lonky N, Massad S, et al: Papanicolaou smear screening augmented by a magnified chemiluminescent exam. Int J Gynecol Obstet 1993;43:289.
13. Polatti F, Giunta P, Migliora P, et al: Speculoscopy combined with Pap smear in the cervical-vaginal screening. Current Obstet Gynecol 1994;3:178.
14. Wertlake P, Francus K, Newkirk G, Parham G: Effectiveness of the Papanicolaou smear and speculoscopy as compared with the Papanicolaou smear alone: A community-based clinical trial. Obstet Gynecol 1997;90:421.
15. Baldauf JJ, Dreyfus M, Ritter J, et al: Cervicography. Does it improve cervical cancer screening? Acta Cytol 1997;41:295.
16. Lonky N, Mann W, Massad L, et al: Ability of visual tests to predict underlying cervical neoplasia. J Reprod Med 1995;40:530.
17. Parham GP, Andrews NR, Lee ML: Comparison of immediate and deferred colposcopy in a cervical screening program. Obstet Gynecol 2000;95:340.
18. Massad L, Lonky N, Mutch D, et al: Use of speculoscopy in the evaluation of women with atypical Papanicolaou smears. J Repro Med 1993;38:163.
19. Edwards G, Rutkowski C, Palmer C: Cervical cancer screening with Papanicolaou smear plus speculoscopy by nurse practitioners in a health maintenance organization. J Low Gen Tract Dis 1997;3:141.
20. Taylor L, Sorensen S, Ray N, et al: Cost-effectiveness of the conventional Pap smear test with a new adjunct to cytological screening for squamous cell carcinoma of the uterine cervix and its precursors. Arch Fam Med 2000;9:713.

D

• Swee Chong Quek
• Albert Singer

TruScan (Polarprobe)

The TruScan (Polarprobe) device employs a real-time approach to the detection of tissue abnormalities.

Despite its success, cytologic screening for cervical cancer has been plagued by several problems. There are concerns about the false-negative rate of cervical cytology. Another disadvantage is the delay between the time the test is taken and when the results are eventually available. Consequently, alternative methods have been developed in an attempt to address these issues. The TruScan (Polarprobe) device employs a real-time approach to the detection of tissue abnormalities. Traditionally, diagnostic and screening tests rely on biochemical information or on the recognition of abnormalities based on cell morphology (e.g., cytology) or tissue structure (e.g., histopathology, radiology, ultrasonography). The TruScan device is an in vivo system that uses the electrical and optical properties of cervical tissue to arrive at its diagnosis.

TECHNOLOGY

The instrument uses a software-implemented tissue classifier, which provides the operator with instantaneous feedback without requiring tissue sampling for cytologic analysis.

The main components of the device include a pen-shaped handpiece that contains the tissue stimulation and sensor elements. The handpiece is connected by a cable to a console that contains a microprocessor control module and a digital signal processor. The instrument uses a software-implemented tissue classifier, which provides the operator with instantaneous feedback without requiring tissue sampling for cytologic analysis.

The handheld device makes contact with the cervix, emitting low-level electrical pulses and optical signals. The measured response, or tissue "signature," is digitized and compared in real time with a data bank of previously determined tissue types using a tissue-matching algorithm. If a match is found, the results are then classified into one of three categories: normal, low-grade abnormality, and high-grade abnormality or cancer.

Cervical tissue is stimulated with low-level electrical pulses and optical signals. Responses to those stimuli are categorized by comparing them with responses to similar stimuli stored in a training database.

The design of the system follows a phenomenologic approach in which cervical tissue is stimulated with low-level electrical pulses and optical signals. Responses to those stimuli are categorized by comparing them with responses to similar stimuli stored in a training database. As the system operates to discriminate among tissue types, a statistical matching operation is performed against the training database. The discriminant parameters that feed the tissue-matching algorithm are chosen from a wide array of possibilities on the basis that they demonstrate maximum variability over the range of tissue types of interest and minimum variability within any particular tissue type of interest.[1]

The concept of using electrical parameters to detect malignant tissue has several precedents. Fricke and Morse, in 1926, conducted a study looking at electrical measurements of breast tumors.[2] Subsequently, Langman and Burr studied electromagnetic measurements of cervical tissue and found "significant differences in cancerous and non-cancerous tissue."[3, 4] However, these early techniques were not amenable to general in vivo use, partly because of the size and amount of equipment required. Significant advances in electronics, optics, and computerization have been made, and these have subsequently enabled the miniaturization and implementation of these technologies to make in vivo testing a reality. In addition, much more is now known about the structural organization within both benign and malignant cells.

Description

The handpiece contains the tissue stimulator and sensor elements.

The handpiece is a 170-mm long, pen-shaped instrument that tapers at its distal end to a tip of approximately 5 mm in diameter; it contains the tissue stimulator and sensor elements (Fig. 4–39). The tip incorporates three

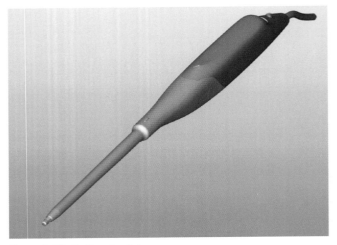

Figure 4–39. TruScan handpiece.

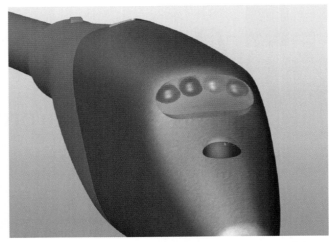

Figure 4–41. Rear of the TruScan handpiece showing indicator lights.

kidney-shaped gold electrodes at its periphery (Fig. 4–40, labeled E), surrounding four light-emitting diodes (Fig. 4–40, labeled R, G, and IR) that are separated by optical fiber spacers. A detector photodiode (Fig. 4–40, labeled SiDet) is at the center. At the proximal end of the handpiece, an array of lights indicates the result to the operator (Fig. 4–41). A cable connects the handpiece to the console.

The console contains a microprocessor module and a digital signal processor.

The console contains a microprocessor module and a digital signal processor. The microprocessor handles the data to and from the digital signal processor that implements the complex floating arithmetic necessary for operation of the tissue classifier. The console allows patient information to be entered and stored and incorporates a

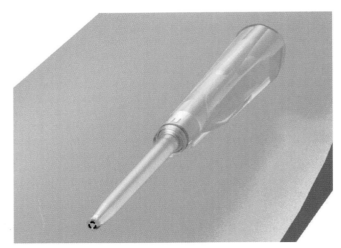

Figure 4–42. Single-use sleeve designed to fit over the handpiece.

printer for the screening results. The unit may be battery powered or AC powered and is designed to operate with 100-V to 260-V supplies.

The initial prototypes of TruScan were subject to a high-level disinfection procedure using 2% glutaraldehyde solution. More recent prototypes use a disposable sleeve that is designed to fit over the probe tip and contains optical windows, to allow the transmission and detection of light, and electrodes for the electrical readings (Fig. 4–42).

Electrical Discriminators

When an electrical voltage is applied to tissue and then turned off abruptly, the tissue behaves like a decaying battery, lasting for a fraction of a second.

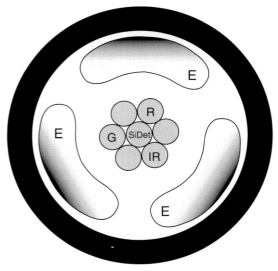

Figure 4–40. TruScan probe tip.

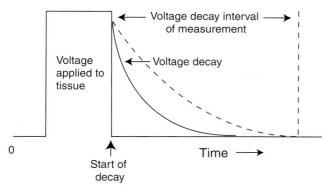

Figure 4-43. Electrical decay curve. Two curves are shown depicting different decay constants.

The cell membranes and varying internal structures of any tissue form a complex of capacitors and resistors. When an electrical voltage is applied to tissue and then turned off abruptly, the tissue behaves like a decaying battery, lasting for a fraction of a second. Because both the decay time and the waveform will differ among different types of tissue, the voltage decay waveform can provide a dynamic signature of the tissue that assists in its classification.[5] TruScan applies low-voltage pulses (0.8 V of 260-μs duration) to the cervix via a combination of its three electrodes, and the resultant electrical decay curve is measured and analyzed (Fig. 4-43).

Optical Discriminators

The initial analyses of cervical tissue types based on electrical decay curves were unable to distinguish unambiguously among the different cervical tissue types, because there was a degree of overlap with their electrical characteristics. Additional parameters were required to provide complementary information, and this led to the implementation of selective wavelength spectroscopy.

Different types of tissue vary predictably with respect to reflectance, transmittance, absorbance, and scattering of electromagnetic radiation.

TruScan uses the transmission and scattering properties of tissue in a process called diffuse reflectance.

Different types of tissue vary predictably with respect to reflectance, transmittance, absorbance, and scattering of electromagnetic radiation. TruScan uses the transmission and scattering properties of tissue in a process called diffuse reflectance. Four light-emitting diodes transmit light at specific wavelengths within the electromagnetic spectrum—two red diodes (600 nm), a green diode (525 nm), and an infrared diode (940 nm). These are activated in sequence, and the tissue response is detected by a detector photodiode at the excitation as well as at the off-excitation frequency, thus producing a relatively broadband spectrum for analysis (Fig. 4-44).

By combining the electrical decay and spectroscopic information, the TruScan is able, by means of a classification algorithm, to categorize the tissue.

By combining the electrical decay and spectroscopic information from a particular area on the cervix, TruScan is able, by means of a classification algorithm, to categorize the tissue.

TISSUE CLASSIFICATION ALGORITHM

The final output is a result of algorithmic operation on three levels: an observation level, a "spot" level, and a whole-patient screening result.

The tissue classification algorithm is a pattern-matching expert system. The final output is a result of algorith-

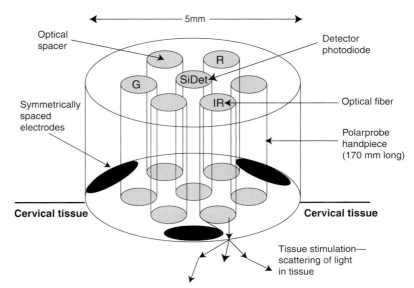

Figure 4-44. Optical fibers convey light of different wavelengths to the probe tip, where cervical tissue is stimulated and the response is detected.

mic operation on three levels—an observation level, a "spot" level, and a whole-patient screening result.

Observation Level Algorithm

Tissue "observations" are conducted 14 times per second, and a preliminary diagnosis is made as the observation is completed.

Tissue observations (that is, optical and electrical stimuli and measurements) are conducted 14 times per second. Approximately 70 optical and electrical parameters are measured for each observation. Conceptually, each of these parameters defines an axis of multidimensional phase space in which the characteristic optoelectronic signatures of each of the various cervical tissue types form groups of clusters. The "width" of these clusters in any one dimension is determined by the interobservation and interpatient variation in the parameter of interest. A preliminary diagnosis is made after each tissue observation, and these are kept in the device memory as the examination proceeds.

Spot-Level Algorithm

A "spot" is defined as a series of measurements made with the tip of the probe at one location on the cervix. The spot measurement time is less than 1 second. The spot is delimited by "poor contact" signals before and after the probe tip is applied to the tissue spot. If the operator lifts the probe tip off the cervix before the spot measurement is complete, the system will signal an error to the operator with the handpiece lights, and the spot measurement will be restarted.

The spot algorithm constructs an array of relative probabilities for each of the possible tissue diagnoses in the spot.

Once data from an entire spot measurement have been gathered, a higher-level algorithm considers all the observation results from a particular spot (approximately 14 observations). This spot-level algorithm then constructs an array of relative probabilities for each of the possible tissue diagnoses for the spot. In this way, repeated observation measurements are used to confirm and build up confidence in the spot results.

Patient-Level Algorithm

The operator moves the tip of the probe around the ectocervix and everted portion of the endocervix. A minimum of 15 spots is required for each patient to ensure coverage of the cervical transformation zone. This generally takes between 2 and 3 minutes.

After visualizing the cervix with a vaginal speculum, the operator moves the tip of the probe, under prompting from the handpiece lights, around the ectocervix and everted portion of the endocervix. A minimum of 15

spots is required for each patient to ensure coverage of the cervical transformation zone; this generally takes between 2 and 3 minutes. When the operator has finished the examination, a button on the handpiece is pressed to signal completion. The patient-level algorithm checks that 15 spot measurements have been performed and, if necessary, prompts the operator that the examination has been inadequate. If the requisite number of spot measurements has been made, the patient-level algorithm proceeds to calculate a final diagnosis. A linear regression analysis is performed, using as input the tissue probability arrays from each spot. This layer of the algorithm assigns 1 of the 17 possible tissue types as the highest grade present on the patient, and then a final patient classification of high grade, low grade, or normal is assigned.

After the requisite number of spot measurements has been made, the patient-level algorithm calculates a final diagnosis.

In summary, the system automatically performs 14 tissue measurements per second, with each measurement involving a complex series of events (Fig. 4–45). Each sequence begins with optical and electrical stimulation of tissue, followed by detection of the tissue response. The specific parameters from the optical and electrical signals are extracted and checked for errors. The extracted parameters are then compared with those in the training data set and classified into various tissue-type categories. The result of the examination of each individual spot is relayed to the operator by a sequence of lights positioned on the probe handle, and the sequence is restarted. At the end of the examination, the overall result is obtained via a printout from the console.

"GOLD STANDARD" REFERENCE DIAGNOSIS

A total of 17 tissue types have been programmed into the system. These tissue types have been further divided into three categories: normal, low-grade abnormality, and cancer or high-grade abnormality.

The recognition algorithm of the TruScan device must be "trained." Therefore, the optical and electrical data must be related to an independent "gold standard" reference diagnosis for a training data set.

The initial data from which subsequent classification systems were developed are part of a series of evaluations that have been ongoing since 1987. These evaluations were of volunteers attending the colposcopy clinics of two hospitals in Sydney, Australia.[6] All these volunteers had a TruScan examination followed by colposcopy and biopsies as appropriate. TruScan is an expert system, and, as for all expert systems, the recognition algorithm must be "trained." Therefore, the optical and electrical data must be related to an independent "gold standard" reference diagnosis for a training data set. The location of the data clusters in multidimensional parameter space for each tissue type is determined by matching each data

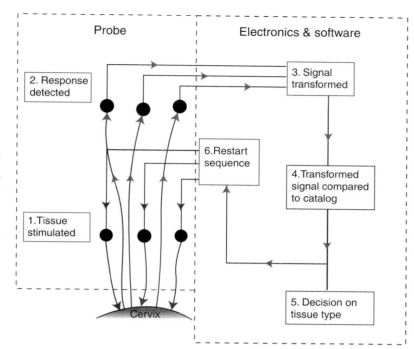

Figure 4–45. TruScan signal processing. (Modified from Coppleson M, Reid BL, Skladnev VN, et al: An electronic approach to the detection of pre-cancer and cancer of the uterine cervix: A preliminary evaluation of the Polarprobe. Int J Gynecol Cancer 1994;4:79.)

cluster to the gold standard diagnosis. For algorithm training, extensive reference data are obtained, including colposcopic and histologic information.

In addition to the original colposcopic diagnosis, a colposcopic video review is performed, with lesion scoring according to Reid's colposcopic index (Chapter 9C). Histology readings are obtained from the local laboratory. In addition, an independent histologist performs digital image capture from the histology slides, and further diagnosis by other histologists may then be performed in a blinded fashion from the digital images.

Obtaining multiple histologic diagnoses for each biopsy allows the final derived gold standard to be more robust against the known interobserver variability associated with histologic readings. The training gold standard is then used in the construction of the expert system tissue classification algorithm.

TISSUE CLASSIFICATION

Because the tip of the probe is 5 mm in diameter, it often spans the junction between two or more cervical tissue types. TruScan detects tissue junctions by means of an imbalance between the electrical measurements as the applied voltage is cycled around the three possible combinations of electrodes. The junctional data are represented as distinct groups of data clusters in the multidimensional optical and electrical parameter phase space.

A total of 17 tissue types have been programmed into the system. For TruScan to be optimized as a screening tool, these tissue types have been further divided into three categories that are of use to the clinician: normal, low-grade abnormality, and cancer or high-grade abnormality.

CLINICAL TRIALS

Of 41 patients with cancer, TruScan correctly identified 40 as having cancer, a sensitivity of 97.6%.

To date, three trials have been conducted using different prototypes of TruScan. The first was a prospective trial to determine the sensitivity and specificity of the device in the detection of cervical neoplasms.[7] The primary objective of the trial was to determine if TruScan could distinguish subjects with overt clinical cervical cancer from those free of cancer. The study was conducted in Recife, Brazil, which has one of the highest rates of cervical cancer in the world.[8] In this study, the TruScan pattern-matching algorithm was specifically set for only the detection of invasive cancer. Forty-one patients with colposcopically and histologically confirmed ectocervical cancer were examined using TruScan, followed by colposcopic evaluation and punch biopsy. A control group of 45 women with negative Papanicolaou (Pap) smears within the preceding 12 months were also recruited. These women, who had no visible significant lesions on the cervix, underwent the same procedure, except that no biopsies were taken. Of the 41 patients with cancer, the TruScan correctly identified 40 as having cancer, a sensitivity of 97.6% (95%; confidence interval [CI] 87.1%, 99.9%). TruScan indicated the possibility of cancer in 4 of the 45 women free of cancer, a specificity of 91.1% (95%; CI 78.7%, 97.5%).

A study comparing a prototype TruScan device with cytology was carried out in 1998 at two centers in the United Kingdom (The Whittington Hospital, London and St. Mary's Hospital, Manchester).[9] The objective of the study was to compare the relative sensitivity and specificity of TruScan with those of the Pap smear for the detection of squamous intraepithelial lesions. Histology from colposcopically directed biopsies was used as the reference standard. A total of 369 consecutive women with abnormal Pap smears who had been referred for colposcopy were recruited. They each underwent a Tru-Scan examination by an operator who was blinded to both the referring Pap smear result and the subsequent colposcopic examination. A second person, blinded to the TruScan result, then performed a Pap smear followed by a colposcopic examination and a biopsy, if indicated. Both the Pap smears and the biopsy specimens were then assessed by local and independent cytopathologists. The independent assessors were blinded to the referral Pap smear results and colposcopic findings. In this study, the TruScan result was considered positive if either a low-grade or a high-grade abnormality was found. Cytology was considered positive if an abnormality greater than or equal to "borderline nuclear changes" (broadly equivalent to atypical squamous cells of undetermined significance [ASCUS]) was reported. Histology from the 369 subjects found 195 to have cervical intraepithelial neoplasia (CIN) grade 1 or greater, with the remaining 174 showing no CIN. The TruScan results were then compared with those of both local and independent cytology.

> **When independent cytology results were used, there was no significant difference between the sensitivity of TruScan and that of repeat cytology for the detection of all grades of CIN.**

When independent cytology results were used, there was no significant difference between the sensitivity of TruScan and that of repeat cytology for the detection of all grades of CIN. In this analysis, the false-positive rate for TruScan was found to be higher than that for repeat cytology.

Using cytology results as reported by the local cytopathologists, there was no significant difference in sensitivity between TruScan and repeat cytology, but in this case the false-positive rate for cytology was significantly higher than that of TruScan.

> **TruScan has a significantly better sensitivity and a lower false-positive rate than does repeat cytology.**

Subsequent to that study, there was a significant design change in the development of TruScan. Both hardware and software modifications were made that essentially digitized all the previously analog processes. The study as described previously was repeated at The Whittington Hospital and was concluded in December 1999 with the recruitment of more than 200 women. The results show that TruScan has a significantly better sensitivity and a lower false-positive rate than does repeat cytology.

ACCEPTABILITY

> **Women experienced less anxiety, less pain, and fewer after-effects like bleeding and discomfort with TruScan than with the Pap smear.**

For screening to work effectively, it is essential for any screening test to consider psychosocial aspects. Cytologic screening in the form of the Pap smear is not uniformly acceptable to all social groups and is influenced by many factors, one of which is the fear or dislike of the idea of a test.[10] A survey was carried out at The Whittington Hospital involving 152 women attending the colposcopy clinic who had experienced both the Pap smear and TruScan examination.[11] They were asked their views on the acceptability, after-effects, and delivery of results associated with the two tests. A questionnaire was devised that included visual analog scales for the assessment of anxiety and pain scores. The findings were that these women experienced less anxiety (mean score 2 of 10 versus 4.5 of 10), less pain (3% versus 33%), and fewer after-effects such as bleeding and discomfort (5% versus 12%) with TruScan than with the Pap smear. Significantly more women—82% (95%; CI 76%, 88%) versus 2% (95%; CI 0%, 4%) preferred TruScan examination to the Pap smear. When asked about the effect of having an immediate result and explanation available to them after the TruScan examination, the majority (98%) felt reassured. In addition, 82% (95%; CI 75%, 88%) of women responded that TruScan would encourage them to attend for screening, versus 18% (95%; CI 12%, 25%) for the Pap smear. The main reasons for this response were the relatively painless application and the immediate result associated with TruScan.

FUTURE DEVELOPMENTS

TruScan studies have been conducted or are being conducted in several centers in Australia, the Philippines, Singapore, South Africa, South America, the United Kingdom, and the United States for data collection to refine the tissue classification algorithm.

A smaller-diameter handpiece is being developed to enable tissue measurements within the endocervical canal. In addition, the technology is potentially applicable to other sites in the body, and it is feasible that sites such as the endometrium, vulva, and vagina may be investigated in a similar way in the future.

SUMMARY OF KEY POINTS

- The TruScan (Polarprobe) device employs a real-time approach to the detection of tissue abnormalities.

- The device includes a pen-shaped handpiece that is connected by a cable to a console containing a microprocessor control module and a digital signal processor.

- The handpiece makes contact with the cervix, emitting low-level electrical pulses and optical signals.

- The probe alerts the operator through the array of lights on the probe handle if proper contact is being made between the probe and the cervix.

- When an electrical voltage is applied to tissue and abruptly turned off, the tissue behaves like a decaying battery, lasting for a fraction of a second.

- Because both the decay time and the waveform will differ among different types of tissue, the voltage decay waveform can provide a dynamic signature of the tissue that can assist in its classification.

- TruScan also uses the transmission and scattering properties of electromagnetic radiation in tissue, in a process called diffuse reflectance.

- By combining the electrical decay and spectroscopic information from a particular area on the cervix, TruScan is able, by means of a classification algorithm, to categorize the tissue.

- Seventeen tissue types have been programmed into the system and divided into three categories: normal, low-grade abnormality, and cancer or high-grade abnormality.

- In a study of 41 patients with cancer, TruScan correctly identified 40 as having cancer, a sensitivity of 97.6%.

- One study indicates that TruScan has a significantly better sensitivity and a lower false-positive rate than does repeat cytology.

- Women experienced less anxiety, less pain, and fewer after-effects such as bleeding and discomfort with TruScan than with the Pap smear.

References

1. Quek SC, Mould T, Canfell K, et al: The Polarprobe—emerging technology for cervical cancer screening. Ann Acad Med Singapore 1998;27:717.
2. Fricke H, Morse S: The electrical capacity of tumors of the breast. J Cancer Res 1926;10:1461.
3. Langman L, Burr HS: A technique to aid in the detection of malignancy of the female genital tract. Am J Obstet Gynecol 1949;57:274.
4. Langman L, Burr HS: Electromagnetic studies in women with malignancy of cervix uteri. Science 1947;105:209.
5. Wundermann I, Coppleson M, Skladnev VN, et al: Polarprobe: A precancer detection instrument. J Gynecol Tech 1995;1:105.
6. Coppleson M, Reid BL, Skladnev VN, et al: An electronic approach to the detection of pre-cancer and cancer of the uterine cervix: A preliminary evaluation of Polarprobe. Int J Gynecol Cancer 1994;4:79.
7. Singer A: Clinical experience with the usage of the Polarprobe. Proceedings of the EUROGIN Third International Congress, 1997 March 24–27, Paris, France. Paris, European Research Organisation on Genital Infection and Neoplasia, 1997.
8. Parkin DM, Muir CS, Whelan SL, et al (eds): Cancer Incidence in Five Continents, vol VI. IARC Scientific Publications No. 120. Lyons, France, International Agency for Research on Cancer, 1992, pp 960–961.
9. Quek SC: A comparative study of the Polarprobe with histopathology and repeat cytology in women with abnormal referral smears. Proceedings of the British Society of Colposcopy and Cervical Pathology Annual Conference, 1999, April 8–10, Sutherland, England. Birmingham, England, British Society of Colposcopy and Cervical Pathology, 1999.
10. Campion MJ, Brown JR, McCance DJ, et al: Psychosexual trauma of an abnormal cervical smear. Br J Obstet Gynaecol 1988;95:175.
11. Mould TAJ, Quek SC, Lovegrove J, et al: The acceptability of cytological screening for cervical cancer compared to a new electronic screening device—the Polarprobe. Proceedings of the EUROGIN Third International Congress, 1997 March 24–27, Paris, France. Paris, European Research Organization on Genital Infection and Neoplasia, 1997.

CHAPTER *5*

Principles and Technique of the Colposcopic Examination

• Barbara S. Apgar
• Mary M. Rubin
• Gregory L. Brotzman

The primary goal of the colposcopist is to ensure that invasive disease is not missed.

The colposcopic examination involves the systematic evaluation of the lower genital tract, with special emphasis on the superficial epithelium and blood vessels of the underlying connective tissue stroma. Although the term *colposcopy* specifically refers to the cervix, it is broadly used to mean the magnified illumination of the entire lower female genital system, including the vulva, vagina, and cervix. Colposcopy allows the examiner to identify specific colposcopic features that distinguish normal from abnormal findings and to form an impression as to whether the features are benign or are the hallmarks of preinvasive or invasive disease. The primary goal of the colposcopist is to ensure that invasive disease is not missed. If the colposcopic examination is performed according to acceptable protocols and is guided by a colposcopic assessment method[1] that allows the grading of epithelial findings, an accurate diagnosis can be obtained.[2]

Today, it is widely accepted that conization should not be performed unless there is some reasonable suspicion that the patient is harboring a high-grade lesion or unless there is any suspicion that she may have an occult invasive cancer.

As a screening test, the role of cervical cytology is to identify patients who have cervical neoplasia so that they may be directed to a diagnostic procedure.[3] An abnormal Papanicolaou (Pap) smear serves as the initial warning sign that neoplasia may be present. Fortunately, colposcopy has largely replaced conization in the initial triage of the abnormal Pap smear.[4] Despite all efforts, however, there remain some instances when conization is the only means of securing an accurate histologic diagnosis. Reasons for performing cervical conization include unsatisfactory colposcopy,[5] normal colposcopy of the lower genital tract with no explanation for the abnormal cytology,[6] existence of a disparity between the cytology and the histology, adenocarcinoma in situ (AIS), or suspicion of microinvasion.[7] However, even these time-tested rules have undergone some refinement. Today, it is widely ac-

cepted that conization should not be performed unless there is some reasonable suspicion that the patient is harboring a high-grade lesion or unless there is any suspicion that she may have an occult invasive cancer.

Although there is less agreement on the subtle differences between the colposcopic features of squamous metaplasia and those of low-grade squamous intraepithelial lesions than there is for the diagnosis of normal epithelium, high-grade squamous intraepithelial lesions, and invasion, similar lack of agreement is found in the histologic diagnosis of these conditions as well.

Colposcopy is subject to interobserver variability roughly equal to that found in other diagnostic procedures, including histopathology. To some, however, colposcopy has been called interpretive, subjective, and fallible.[8] There is no doubt that the prediction of the histologic diagnosis based on specific colposcopic pattern recognition skills requires experience and practice. Nevertheless, the advantages of colposcopy outweigh its disadvantages. There is good interobserver agreement for the colposcopic findings of normal epithelium, high-grade squamous intraepithelial lesions, and invasion.[9] Although there is less agreement on the subtle differences between the colposcopic features of squamous metaplasia and those of low-grade squamous intraepithelial lesions, similar lack of agreement is found in the histologic diagnosis of these conditions as well. Colposcopy also has its limitations among women in whom the transformation zone is not fully visualized.

Because the ability of histology to define the true level of disease on the cervix is dependent on a properly directed biopsy, the histologic interpretation is only as accurate as the skill of the colposcopist in interpreting the colposcopic findings correctly and in properly directing the biopsy.

Each time a colposcopic examination is performed, the principles of practice are the same: excluding the presence of invasive disease and, if indicated, selecting the most appropriate site for biopsy. The interpretation of the colposcopic findings is basic to the decision of whether or not to perform a biopsy.[9] The ability to accurately direct a biopsy to the area of greatest hispathologic abnormality is dependent on the expertise of the colposcopist. Because the ability of histology to define the true level of disease on the cervix is dependent on a properly directed biopsy, the histologic interpretation is only as accurate as the skill of the colposcopist in interpreting the colposcopic findings correctly, in distinguishing between minor and major lesions, and in properly directing the biopsy.[10]

The cornerstone of colposcopic practice is the correlation of cytology, histology, and the colposcopic impression.[11] The use of a systematic approach in colposcopy ensures that each epithelial surface is examined, that the findings are transmitted to the patient, and, if necessary, that follow-up visits are secured. The use of such a systematic approach helps the clinician avoid errors.

The focus of this chapter is the procedural aspects of the colposcopic examination. Pattern recognition skills for normal and abnormal colposcopic findings will be discussed in Chapters 6 and 8 through 13.

PREPARATION FOR INITIATION OF COLPOSCOPY SERVICES

The equipment and supplies needed to perform colposcopy are listed in Tables 5–1, 5–2, and 5–3. Consideration should also be given to the physical space where the colposcopy will be performed. A cramped examination room similar to that used for routine examinations may not have sufficient space for all the additional equipment needed to perform colposcopy and may hinder the ability to comfortably and efficiently examine both routine patients and those undergoing colposcopic examination.

The colposcopist should speak with the pathologist and agree about the transmission of specimens, the interpretation of results, and the consultation guidelines should disagreements or questions arise. This will help avoid misguided therapeutic decisions related to misunderstandings between the pathologist and the clinician.

The choice of a cytology-pathology laboratory is also an important one. Ideally, the laboratory and the patholo-

gist should be accessible to the colposcopist so that they can discuss cases and correlate their findings. The colposcopist should speak with the pathologist and agree about the transmission of specimens, the interpretation of results, and the consultation guidelines should disagreements or questions occur. They should also come to a clear understanding about the classification systems that will be used for cytologic and histologic interpretation, what each diagnosis means, and the clinical implication of that diagnosis. This will help avoid misguided therapeutic decisions related to misunderstandings between the pathologist and the colposcopist.

Competent nursing or medical assistant support is critical in making the colposcopic examination successful. It is ideal if the assistant and the colposcopist share a similar philosophy about colposcopic practice and general care of the patient. The assistant can check the equipment and supplies before each examination, ensuring that supplies are replenished and equipment is available and in good working order.

The colposcopist should develop a new or adapt an existing colposcopic record that contains basic medicolegal documentation (see Appendices 1 to 4 for examples of forms). The demographic and colposcopic findings can be included on the same form or on separate ones. If informed consent is to be obtained, the legal office of the institution will generally approve the forms. In addition to

▼ Table 5–2
Colposcopic Equipment

Colposcope with extra light bulbs
Optional attachments for colposcope (camera, video, teaching head, television monitor, videocassette recorder)
Cervical punch biopsy forceps
Endocervical curette
Endocervical specula of various sizes
Cervical hook
Ring or sponge forceps
Needle holder (long handle)
Surgical scissors (long handle)
Anoscope, clear plastic

▼ Table 5–1
General Equipment for Colposcopy

Examination room
Examination table, preferably with adjustable height and heel cushions
Stand or surgical table for supplies
Examination gloves of various sizes, including latex free gloves
Various-sized specula (Graves', Pedersen's)—metal reusable or plastic disposable
Container for dirty surgical instruments before sterilization
Autoclave for equipment and supplies
Disinfectant solution containing 2% glutaraldehyde

▼ Table 5–3
Specific Supplies for the Colposcopic Examination

Monsel's solution (ferric subsulfate) dehydrated to thick paste
Diluted (quarter or half strength) Lugol's iodine solution
3% to 5% acetic acid (or vinegar) in small container
Small containers for individual patient use
Silver nitrate sticks
Large cotton swabs and small cotton-tipped applicators
Toothpicks
Gauze pads (4 × 4)
Disposable pads for placement under patient's buttocks
Lens paper
Glass slides
Buffered formalin or other laboratory preservative
Fixative for slide preparation
Suture
Local anesthetic (1% lidocaine)

record documentation, a procedure for patient notification should be developed. Patients who are lost to follow-up are often not treated and so fail to benefit from the clinician's screening and diagnostic efforts.

> **Reports indicate that up to 40% of patients are lost to follow-up. Among the barriers that have been identified are transportation, child care, work, fear, and preoccupation with busy life routines.**

It has been shown that there are many barriers to the compliance of patients returning for requested follow-up visits. Reports indicate that up to 40% of patients are lost to follow-up.[12] Among the barriers that have been identified are transportation, child care, work, fear, and preoccupation with busy life routines. Patient lack of understanding about the seriousness of the problem has also been studied.[13] Others have found that compliance with follow-up is more closely correlated with the severity of the disease at the time of colposcopy than with an understanding of the disease process.[14] The authors suggest that greater compliance after colposcopy may be gained by improving the identification of noncompliant patients when they schedule nongynecologic visits.

SPECIFIC EQUIPMENT FOR THE COLPOSCOPIC EXAMINATION

Colposcope

As a procedure, colposcopy has been around since the 1920s, when the colposcope was little more than an inexpensive, optically modified binocular with an illuminator on the upper surface.[15] By the 1930s, colposcopy was widely used in central Europe. After cervical cytologic screening was introduced, the colposcopic examination became a secondary verification technique, even in Europe where the method was first introduced. It was not until the 1970s that colposcopy became an accepted procedure for the verification of cytologic findings in the United States. Colposcopy is now accepted worldwide as the most studied method for detection of early cervical neoplasia.

The modern optical colposcope is a binocular microscope with a built-in light source and a converging objective lens attached to a support appliance. It provides magnification and illumination for colposcopic assessment of the target tissue (Fig. 5–1). Each optical colposcope is equipped with binocular lenses and tubes with individual settings. If desired, the diopters can be set to individually correct the refractive error of each of the colposcopist's eyes so that glasses will not be required during the procedure. If glasses are not worn, the rubber appliances on the eyepieces can produce a seal between the eyes and the binocular tubes that blocks out extraneous light. Other colposcopists prefer to wear their glasses during the procedure and peel back the rubber appliances on the eyepieces. The interpupillary distance can be individually adjusted so that a clear stereoscopic image is displayed.

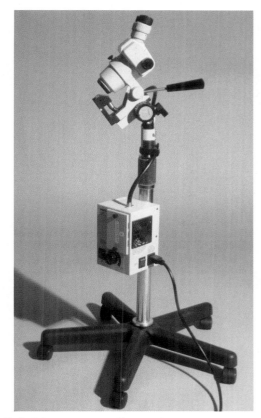

Figure 5–1. Colposcope on a rolling stand.

> **Most colposcopes have a focal length of around 300 mm. If the focal distance is too short, there will be limited room to maneuver instruments in front of the lens. If the focal length is too long, the colposcopist will be placed too far away from the target tissue to comfortably perform the examination.**

The colposcope has a fixed focal distance determined by the objective lens—that is, the working distance between the lens and the target tissue. Most colposcopes have a focal length of around 300 mm. If the focal distance is too short, there will be limited room to maneuver instruments in front of the lens. If the focal length is too long, the colposcopist will be placed too far away from the target tissue to comfortably perform the examination.

Most colposcopes are equipped with the capability for fine and coarse focusing by either moving the colposcope itself or using the fine focus knobs on the instrument. As long as the colposcope is at its fixed focal length, the target tissue should be in relatively good focus. Coarse focus can always be achieved by simply moving the entire colposcope. Finer focus capability can be achieved by turning the fine focus knob (Fig. 5–2). Some colposcopes can achieve par-focal capability so that the focus remains throughout all magnification levels. To obtain par focus, the focus must first be achieved under high magnification.

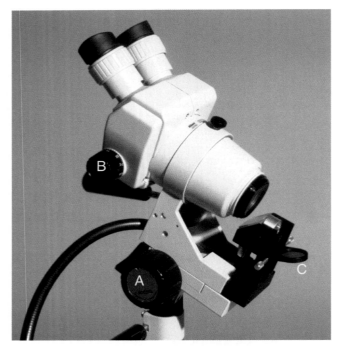

Figure 5-2. Close-up of colposcope head with the fine focus knob noted at the base of the head *(A)* and the zoom focus noted near the oculars *(B)*. The green filter *(C)* flips up to provide green-light examination of the genital skin.

Colposcopes typically provide the capability for variable magnification. Less expensive colposcopes are equipped with a single, fixed magnification. Some colposcopes have a mechanism to change magnifications through separate discrete steps, whereas others are able to zoom through low, medium, and high magnification levels without going through individual steps of magnification. Low-power magnification ($\times 2$ to $\times 6$) is typically used for examination of the vulva and of male genitalia; medium power ($\times 8$ to $\times 15$) is generally used for examination of the vulva, vagina, and cervix, and high power ($\times 15$ to $\times 25$) is especially helpful when assessing the fine detail of vessel patterns, specifically atypical vessels. Changing the magnification will alter the diameter of the field of vision. The higher the magnification, the smaller the field of vision and the less the illumination of the target tissue. Most modern colposcopes provide a totally illuminated field at low magnification.

The green filter absorbs certain wavelengths of light, making the red color of the vessels appear blacker and sharpening the contrast with the surrounding epithelium.

Most colposcopes are equipped with a green filter that serves to enhance the fine detail of the vascular pattern of the target epithelium (see Fig. 5-2). The light may need to be increased while the green filter is being used. The green filter absorbs certain wavelengths of light, making

the red color of the vessels appear blacker and sharpening the contrast with the surrounding epithelium.

The light source on the colposcope may be incandescent, tungsten, xenon, or halogen. The halogen light provides a brighter light that is excellent for photography.

One of the main criticisms of the video colposcope is that the colposcopic image on the video monitor is a two-dimensional rather than a three-dimensional image, making assessment of the contour and density of the lesion more difficult.

Until the introduction of video colposcopy, the basic technique of optical colposcopy had not changed significantly. Video colposcopy is a new method of providing magnification and illumination without use of binocular eyepieces. The system includes a video colposcope and a high-resolution video monitor.[16] The colposcopic image is viewed on a video monitor in a manner similar to laparoscopy. One of the main criticisms of the video colposcope is that the colposcopic image on the video monitor is a two-dimensional rather than a three-dimensional image, making assessment of the contour and density of the lesion more difficult.

It may take some time for a colposcopist to adjust from standard colposcopy to video colposcopy. The adjustment phase is required to allow for the development of new psychomotor skills, especially with regard to the performance of the directed biopsy.[17] In one study, colposcopists were able to assess the grade of colposcopic change equally well with both the optical and the video colposcopes. In this comparison, the nonstereoscopic video monitor did not appear to hinder contour assessment and depth perception. However, there were more unsatisfactory colposcopic examinations of the endocervical canal while the video colposcope was used. The rates of colposcopic impression agreement were not significantly different between the two colposcopes. However, when the colposcopists using the two systems were queried, they preferred visualization, assessment, and sampling through the optical colposcope and judged it to be "easier."

Instruments for Colposcopy

Punch Biopsy Forceps

There are many punch biopsy forceps available and, over time, each colposcopist will select a favorite one to use. Most of the biopsy instruments are named after the designer or manufacturer (Tischler, Burke, Kevorkian, and Eppendorfer), and each obtains a slightly different-shaped specimen. The Tischler forceps has a single anchoring tooth and obtains a rounded specimen. The Eppendorfer forceps has alligator teeth on the anchoring edge and obtains a square specimen. A Baby Tischler forceps retrieves a smaller specimen with potentially less bleeding at the biopsy site (Fig. 5-3). All the punch biopsy forceps are constructed with a handle shank and a biopsy tip or head. The jaws of the head consist of an anchoring device and a cutting edge. Some of the shanks can be

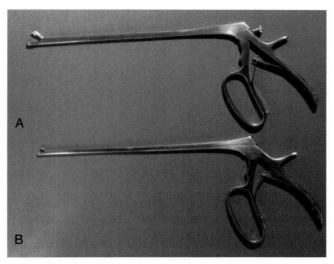

Figure 5–3. Examples of Tischler punch biopsy instruments. Regular size (*A*) and baby Tischlers (*B*).

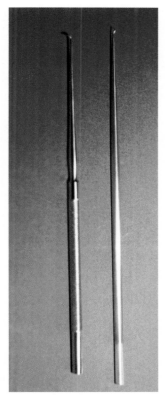

Figure 5–5. Cervical hooks.

rotated 360 degrees so the entire instrument does not have to be rotated during the procedure.

Endocervical Curettes

Endocervical curettes are long, stainless steel sticks consisting of a finger-grip handle and a head or tip with a cutting edge (Fig. 5–4). Only one edge of the tip includes the sharp cutting edge. The other edge is dull and is not used as a cutting surface. The cutting edge of the tip is on the same plane as the finger hold on the handle. The head or tip is made with or without a basket. If a basket is present, the sample may be collected in the basket, but it may prove difficult to remove.

Cervical Hooks

A long surgical hook can be used to "pucker" the tissue so a biopsy sample can be obtained (Fig. 5–5). A hook is especially helpful if the biopsy surface is flat and the punch biopsy forceps cannot be adequately anchored on the tissue. A skin hook can prevent the tissue from slipping away from the biopsy forceps. The bend of the hook

should not be too acute or it will be impossible to grasp the tissue. The tip of the hook should not be too sharp lest the tissue be torn during the process of sampling. It is rare that a hook will be needed on the cervical epithelium. More often, the hook is used to visualize the rugae or lesions in the vagina.

Endocervical Speculum

It is occasionally necessary to visualize the endocervical canal, either because a lesion extends into the canal or because the transformation zone is not fully visualized. In one report, unsatisfactory colposcopy was noted to occur in approximately 1% to 5% of colposcopic examinations.[18] Others have reported that 10% to 15% of premenopausal women younger than 45 years will have an unsatisfactory colposcopic examination.[19] Postmenopausal women may have even higher percentages of unsatisfactory colposcopy because the squamocolumnar junction is located deep in the endocervical canal. Adequate visualization of the entire transformation zone may be facilitated by the use of an endocervical speculum. Additionally, the instrument can be used to examine the endocervical canal for polyps or other lesions. The endocervical speculum is placed into the external os and then opened gently. The blades of the endocervical speculum are available in a variety of sizes and lengths (Fig. 5–6). Different tips are designed specifically for nulliparous, parous, and stenotic cervices.

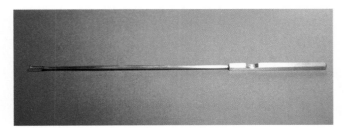

Figure 5–4. Endocervical curette without a basket.

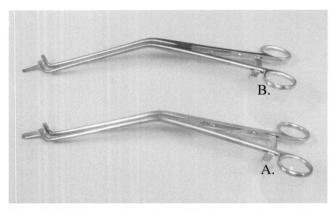

Figure 5–6. Endocervical specula. *A,* Thin line speculum used for a narrowed cervical os. *B,* Regular blade type endocervical speculum.

Vaginal Sidewall Retractors

The vaginal sidewall may obscure visualization of the cervix during the colposcopic examination. Vaginal sidewall retraction is usually unnecessary, but when the vaginal walls are lax and redundant, the ability to retract the sidewall may allow the colposcopist to complete an otherwise impossible examination. Vaginal retractors are specially designed to fit inside the speculum and open with a ratchet mechanism (Fig. 5–7). The problem is that the hinges of the speculum may prevent complete separation of the retractor paddles, so the colposcopist may be unable to achieve the desired visualization of the cervix. Another option is to place a condom or the finger of an examination glove over the speculum blades so that when the speculum is opened, the vaginal walls will be retracted. After the tip is cut off, the condom or latex finger is placed over the closed blades of the speculum (Fig. 5–8). In some situations, especially if the patient is obese, it is difficult to open the speculum with the latex finger or condom in place, and some extra hand strength may be required.

Supplies for Colposcopy

Acetic Acid or Vinegar

> To achieve an acetic acid effect in nonkeratinized epithelium, the 3% to 5% acetic acid must be left in contact with the tissue for at least 1 minute.

Colposcopy is performed after the application of dilute (3% to 5%) acetic acid or vinegar to the cervix. The "acetowhiteness" of the epithelium may indicate a benign or a neoplastic process. The solution is applied copiously with gauze sponges, large cotton-tipped swabs, or a spray bottle. To achieve an acetic acid effect in nonkeratinized epithelium, the 3% to 5% acetic acid must be left in contact with the tissue for at least 1 minute. During the examination, the acetic acid may need to be reapplied to maintain the acetowhite effect. The vessel patterns may be more prominent as the acetowhite reaction begins to fade. The solution may burn, especially if the patient has a vaginal infection. Allergic reactions are rare.

Aqueous Lugol's Solution

> Lugol's solution stains normal squamous epithelium a dark, mahogany color, indicating that glycogen is present in the cells. Absent staining denotes a nonglycogenated state.

Iodine solution is diluted to quarter-strength or half-strength to obtain Lugol's solution. Lugol's solution is unstable on the shelf and should be replaced every 3 to 6 months. Although the dilute solution may produce less drying effect and irritation than full-strength iodine produces, some patients are particularly sensitive. Some will even have an intense allergic reaction. Patients should always be queried about previous allergic reactions to iodine before Lugol's solution is applied. Lugol's solution stains normal squamous epithelium a dark, mahogany color, indicating that glycogen is present in the cells. Absent staining denotes a nonglycogenated state (Fig. 5–

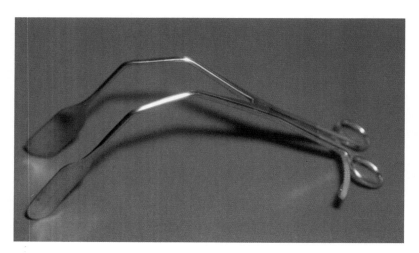

Figure 5–7. Lateral wall retractor.

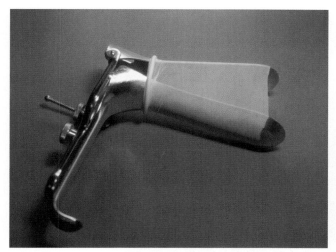

Figure 5–8. Use of a condom over the blades of a speculum can keep the vaginal walls from obscuring the cervix during colposcopy.

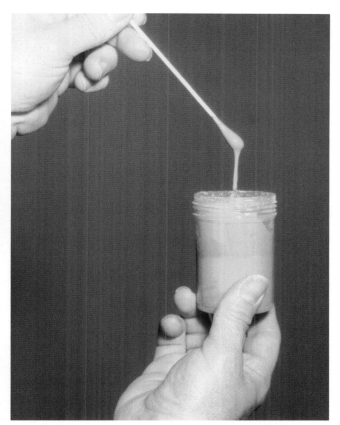

Figure 5–10. Thickened Monsel's solution with a molasses consistency.

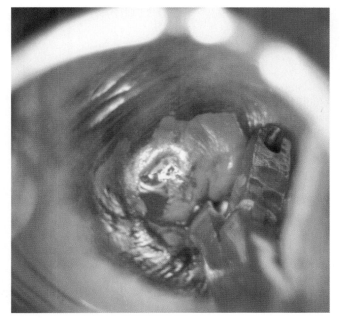

Figure 5–9. Area on the anterior lip of the cervix that rejects iodine. A biopsy forceps is about to sample this area of low-grade cervical intraepithelial neoplasia.

9). Squamous metaplasia may exhibit variegated staining, whereas columnar epithelium stains a mustard-yellow color (see Chapter 9).

Monsel's Solution

> **Monsel's solution and silver nitrate interfere with biopsy interpretation and should not be applied until after all the samples are taken.**

Monsel's (ferric subsulfate) solution (Fig. 5–10) is used to achieve hemostasis after directed biopsy. The solution becomes more effective when it is allowed to dehydrate in the open air until it becomes a thick paste, but if it dehydrates too much, it will solidify and become unusable. After the biopsy is completed, Monsel's solution is applied directly to the biopsy site with a small cotton-tipped applicator. Pressure is applied at the same time with the applicator. When hemostasis is difficult to achieve, the applicator should be held on the biopsy site for a few minutes. Monsel's solution will interfere with biopsy interpretation and should not be applied until after all the samples are taken.[20] Excessive Monsel's solution should be removed from the vagina before the speculum is removed. The patient should be warned that the Monsel's solution may produce a charcoal-like vaginal discharge for several days.

Silver Nitrate

Silver nitrate sticks can be used for hemostasis. They are especially helpful if they are placed directly in the center of the biopsy site. The patient may experience more irritation or burning with silver nitrate than with Monsel's solution. As with Monsel's solution, the silver nitrate will interfere with biopsy interpretation and should be applied only after all biopsies are completed.

See Figure 5–11 for an example of a colposcopy equipment and supply tray.

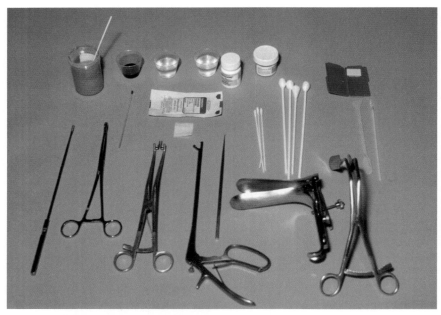

Figure 5–11. Supply and equipment setup for colposcopy. Starting at the left upper corner of the figure, the supplies shown are Monsel's solution, iodine, saline, 5% acetic acid, benzocaine gel, specimen container, silver nitrate sticks, hemostatic gauze, 1 × 1 inch paper towel squares, small and large cotton-tipped applicators, Papanicolaou smear supplies, lateral wall retractor, speculum, cervical hook, biopsy forceps, endocervical speculum, ring forceps, and endocervical curette.

COLPOSCOPICALLY DIRECTED BIOPSY*

There are many important aspects the colposcopist should consider when performing colposcopically directed biopsies. First, the task of colposcopic assessment is accomplished using a grading or assessment system to identify the most severe lesion or lesions requiring biopsy.

> **When there is only one well-visualized and easily accessible lesion, one biopsy is sufficient. Performing additional biopsies causes discomfort to the patient and is unnecessary. Large, complex lesions often require multiple samples to rule out invasive cancer.**

Ensuring that the transformation zone and all the lesions are well visualized will ultimately improve the ability to select which sites to biopsy. The speculum should be opened as wide as the patient can tolerate, using both the bottom pin and the side pin. When there is only one well-visualized and easily accessible lesion, the biopsy can be accomplished relatively easily. Performing additional biopsies causes discomfort to the patient and is unnecessary. However, large, complex lesions often require multiple samples to rule out invasive cancer. When performing multiple biopsies, the clinician should order

the biopsy sites from posterior to anterior to prevent blood from flowing onto other lesions and obscuring subsequent sample sites.[21] Local anesthetic is not usually required for biopsy of the cervix or the upper to middle third of the vagina. It is necessary if the distal third of the vagina or the vulva is biopsied. Some clinicians have found it beneficial to use topical anesthetic, but at least one study offered some evidence that it is not effective.[22]

> **The value of routine endocervical curettage is controversial, and some colposcopists reserve it for selected patients, such as those in whom the transformation zone is not fully visualized, those who have been previously treated, those at high risk for recurrent disease, and those to be treated with ablative therapy. ECC is always contraindicated in the pregnant patient.**

The highest-grade lesions are likely to be found closest to the squamocolumnar junction. When the lesion extends into the endocervical canal, an attempt should be made to manipulate the cervix to sample the proximal aspect of the lesion. The value of a routine endocervical curettage (ECC) is controversial, and some colposcopists reserve it for selected patients such as those in whom the transformation zone is not fully visualized, those who have been previously treated, those at high risk for recurrent disease, and those to be treated with ablative therapy. ECC is always contraindicated in the pregnant patient. Whether to perform ECC before or after the cervical biopsies is a matter of style rather than correct technique. Performing

---

*This section was written by Mary M. Rubin.

the ECC first under colposcopic guidance allows the colposcopist to avoid inadvertently contaminating the ECC with tissue from an ectocervical lesion. This is important when the colposcopy is otherwise satisfactory and the presence of a positive ECC would indicate the need for a deeper excisional procedure rather than an ablative procedure or a shallower excision. However, once done, the ECC may cause bleeding that can obscure the remaining lesions and interfere with properly directing the biopsy.

When the desired biopsy site is found in the vagina, the difficulty of obtaining a biopsy is increased, because the tubular configuration of the vagina does not allow a perpendicular approach to the lesion. The biopsy may be facilitated by slowly withdrawing the speculum and creating a ridge or fold, enabling the clinician to securely grasp the desired site for biopsy.

> **Although a large biopsy cannot be taken with a small-jawed biopsy instrument, a large-jawed biopsy instrument need not take only large biopsies. A small biopsy can be taken using only the tip of the jaw.**

The choice of a punch biopsy instrument is usually one of personal preference. It is important to realize that the size of the jaws should not dictate the size of the biopsy. Although a large biopsy cannot be taken with a small-jawed biopsy instrument, a large-jawed biopsy instrument need not take only large biopsies. A small biopsy can be taken using only the tip of the jaw. In some cases, however, the specific punch biopsy forceps needed to perform colposcopic biopsy is dependent on the size and location of the lesion. If there is concern about microinvasion or frank invasion, a punch biopsy forceps with a wider-opening jaw, such as the Tischler forceps, is necessary to obtain a sample of adequate depth. If the sample is too small and superficial, the pathologist may not be able to rule out invasion. A biopsy forceps with a small basket, such as the baby Tischler forceps, may enable adequate sampling of a lesion extending into the narrow endocervical canal. If the basket of the forceps is larger than the cervical os, it is impossible to enter the endocervical canal.

Small lesions can often be completely excised. In many cases, the exact area to be biopsied in a large, uniformly abnormal lesion may not be critical. However, when there is ulceration present, the colposcopist should attempt to sample an edge of intact epithelium, as well as a portion of the ulcerative bed to more accurately establish the diagnosis.

At times, it is difficult to securely grasp the tissue with the punch biopsy forceps. Depending on the location of the lesion and the configuration of the biopsy forceps, the jaw of the instrument may slide off the tissue, or the cutting edge will not be able to touch the surface of the lesion. Occasionally, the angle required for the cutting edge of the forceps to contact the tissue cannot be achieved within the limited confines of the speculum. It may be easier to turn the biopsy forceps upside down, allowing the longer cutting edge to reach the tissue with less of an angle. Occasionally, a tenaculum or hook is needed to mobilize the cervix or tent the tissue to obtain the sample.[23]

> **A colposcopist who feels the need to locate the biopsy site, push the colposcope aside, and then obtain the sample without the benefit of magnification and illumination has not sufficiently mastered the skills of colposcopy and should not be doing colposcopy without direct supervision.**

A colposcopist who feels the need to locate the biopsy site, push the colposcope aside, and then obtain the sample without the benefit of magnification and illumination has not sufficiently mastered the skills of colposcopy and should not be doing colposcopy without direct supervision. This approach can lead to inadequate sampling of the worst lesion, underdiagnosis, and inappropriate treatment. The biopsy sites should be visualized with the colposcope on completion of the procedure to ensure that the desired area was sampled.[24]

The biopsy forceps should be kept closed until withdrawn from the vagina to avoid dropping the small specimen before it is deposited in the specimen container. Occasionally, especially when a small basket forceps is used, a small specimen will pass right through the basket. It is important to verify that the specimen is present in the basket before applying pressure to the biopsy site to control the bleeding. The specimen will sometimes be found on the blade of the speculum and can be easily retrieved and deposited in the appropriate specimen container, rather than lost in the trash on a cotton swab. The basket may also be empty when a complete cut through the tissue has not been achieved. One small edge of the specimen may still be attached at the biopsy site. This usually occurs when the punch biopsy forceps is dull. The biopsy instruments will need to be sharpened on a regular basis. Care should be taken not to crush or overmanipulate the specimen, and it should be placed immediately in the preservative to avoid air-drying. Both situations can lead to difficulty in interpretation and diagnosis.[25]

Monsel's solution achieves optimal hemostasis when it is used as a thickened paste. The need to biopsy multiple sites warrants a word of caution about the application of hemostatic agents. All samples should be obtained before applying Monsel's solution or silver nitrate. The caustic nature of these chemicals can interfere with the histologic reading of the sample.[20] Immediate pressure after each biopsy with a large cotton swab will also decrease blood loss and may obviate the need for additional hemostatic agents.

Ideally, the colposcopist should place each biopsy in a separate, labeled container. This enables the colposcopist to correlate the colposcopic impression with the histologic results. The grade and location of the lesion can affect the choice of treatment. However, the cost considerations of separate pathology charges for each specimen may obviate the use of this approach. Labeling the specimens is critical, and it is the colposcopist's responsibility to ensure that all samples are correctly labeled before they are removed from the examination room.

TECHNIQUE OF COLPOSCOPIC EXAMINATION

1. The supplies and equipment are checked before the examination is begun.

2. The proper documentation forms are stamped with the patient identification card, and, if applicable, informed consent is obtained.

3. The patient is placed in the dorsal lithotomy position and properly draped.

4. The colposcopist sits comfortably at the colposcope, the interpupillary distance of the binoculars is set, and the colposcope is turned on.

5. The vulva is inspected with the colposcope. Three percent to five percent acetic acid or vinegar may be used to enhance the epithelial findings. If an abnormal area is identified, vulvar biopsy may be performed at this time. Some colposcopists defer colposcopy and biopsy of the vulva to the end of the examination.

6. The largest size of intravaginal speculum that the patient can tolerate is placed in the vagina.

7. If necessary, vaginal sidewall retraction is achieved with a vaginal retractor placed inside the speculum or by a condom or latex glove finger applied over the speculum blades (tip of condom or glove must be cut off!).

8. The cervix must be adequately visualized. Gentle wiping of mucus may be necessary. If the cervix is not in a satisfactory position and it is impossible to view the cervix, moistened, rolled-up gauze pads can be placed in the fornix with ring forceps.

9. If applicable, cytologic sampling is performed. If bleeding follows, a cotton-tipped applicator gently placed in the endocervical canal will usually stop the bleeding. Monsel's solution should not be applied at this time.

10. The cervix is viewed with white light (and saline if it is dry) under low power ($\times 4$ to $\times 8$) magnification. Gross findings and the presence of leukoplakia are noted.

11. The vessel pattern is examined with the green filter. The vessels are examined under low and high magnification. Three percent to five percent acetic acid should not be applied until after the vascular pattern is assessed.

12. A copious amount of 3% to 5% acetic acid (or vinegar) is applied to the cervix with saturated cotton swabs, gauze, cotton balls on a ring forceps, or a spray bottle. Excessive rubbing or patting of the cervix should be avoided. Gently placing the cotton balls, gauze, or swabs on the cervix and allowing the solution to thoroughly soak the tissue avoids unnecessary abrasions or bleeding. A second application of acetic acid should follow the first application to ensure an appropriate aceto-white reaction. Once the cervix is thoroughly soaked, the excess mucus can be easily removed.

13. The cervix is assessed for epithelial findings after the acetic acid application (acetowhite reaction) with low, intermediate, and high magnification. The aceto-white reaction will begin to fade slowly or quickly depending on the severity of the epithelial abnormality. As the acetowhite reaction fades, the vessel patterns (mosaic and punctation) become more distinct because of the contrast with the surrounding tissue. If vessel patterns are present, they should be examined under high-power magnification. Use of the green filter again may confirm vessel patterns.

14. The normal and abnormal epithelial and blood vessel patterns should be mentally mapped, because it will be necessary to recall the findings when it is time to complete the documentation forms.

15. If the patient is not allergic to iodine, the cervix may be stained with dilute Lugol's solution. An assessment of the epithelial patterns is dependent on the interaction between cellular glycogen and iodine. Lugol's can have a drying effect on the vagina, and it will stain the patient's underclothing.

16. If applicable, endocervical sampling is accomplished with an endocervical curette or cytobrush. The curette is held like a pencil and inserted through the external os, and the entire endocervical canal is sampled with definitive strokes. Care should be taken not to contaminate the sample with ectocervical lesions. While it is in the endocervical canal, the sample is spun onto the tip of the curette, and the curette is removed straight from the canal. A cytobrush or ring forceps can be used to remove the remainder of the sample from the canal. The entire sample is placed in fixative, and the specimen bottle is labeled with patient identification.

17. If applicable, colposcopically directed biopsies are performed. The biopsy site is selected, and the sample is obtained with the cervical biopsy punch. The anchoring edge of the biopsy punch firmly grasps the tissue so the lesion will not slip away while the biopsy is performed. The posterior surface of the cervix is biopsied first to avoid blood obscuring the biopsy site. The sample should not be pulled from the biopsy site. Additional samples are obtained if there is remaining tissue at the biopsy site. If the tooth of the biopsy punch cannot anchor the tissue, a skin hook is used to create a fold of tissue so the jaws of the punch can close around it. The cervix is checked to make sure all biopsies have been successfully obtained. The biopsy specimens are removed from the biopsy punch and placed in fixative. The specimen bottles are labeled with the patient identification information.

18. Monsel's solution is applied to achieve hemostasis after all the biopsies are obtained. Occasionally, only pressure will be required. The Monsel's solution should contact the actual tissue rather than only the blood oozing from the biopsy site. Silver nitrate sticks can also be used. The blood and Monsel's solution should be cleaned from the fornices with a cotton swab before the speculum is removed.

19. The vagina is inspected as the speculum is removed. Application of Lugol's solution is helpful to delineate abnormal epithelium. If Lugol's solution is not used, the vagina should be grossly inspected as the speculum is removed. A skin hook can be used to see between the vaginal rugae.

20. If applicable, vulvar biopsy can be accomplished at this time.

21. The patient is informed about the preliminary colposcopic impression. She is also instructed about the mechanism and time frame for reporting her results. Educational material may be given to her before she leaves the office.

22. The specimens are checked to ensure that patient identification has been properly applied. Laboratory forms are completed, and the specimen is prepared for transportation to the laboratory.

23. The documentation forms are completed. The cervical diagram should indicate satisfactory or unsatisfactory colposcopy, presence of normal and abnormal findings, and location of colposcopically directed biopsies.

24. The colposcope is cleaned and the supplies replenished. Surgical instruments are prepared for sterilization.

Table 5–4 lists the steps and the expected findings for site-specific colposcopy of the cervix, vagina, and vulva.

DOCUMENTATION OF COLPOSCOPIC FINDINGS

Demographic information, clinical findings and recommendations for follow-up visits or referral should all be included in the colposcopic record.

Documentation of clinical findings is an important part of the systematic colposcopic procedure. It is recommended that the colposcopic record be an independent part of the patient's chart and that it be readily retrievable. Consideration should be given to preprinting the colposcopic record forms so that all information is completed in a systematic manner at the time of each examination. Demographic information, clinical findings, and recommendations for follow-up visits or referrals should all be included in the colposcopic record (Table 5–5). The demographic information should include name, address, and telephone number of the patient (or contact person); date of the last menstrual period; pertinent sexual history; menstrual history; and current contraceptive methods, if applicable. The clinician should then obtain a history of the current complaint, including a history of previous abnormal Pap tests, a history of previous sexually transmitted diseases, and a history of sexually transmitted diseases in sexual partners (see Appendices 1 to 4 for examples of forms).

In recording the clinical findings, the location of the squamocolumnar junction and the external os should be

▼ Table 5–4A

Site-Specific Colposcopy: Cervix

Steps in Colposcopic Assessment	The Kind of Observations You Can Expect to Make at This Step of the Examination	
	Normal Findings	*Abnormal Findings*
1. Clean the cervix with saline.*	Mature squamous and columnar epithelia	Leukoplakia Polyps Nabothian cysts
2. Assess the cervix with a green filter before the application of 3%–5% acetic acid.*		Abnormal vascular patterns Atypical vessels

3. Assess the cervix after the application of 3%–5% acetic acid.	Gland openings
	Squamous metaplasia
	Squamocolumnar junction
	Nonspecific acetowhite changes
		Condyloma acuminatum
		Acetowhite changes specific for preinvasive and invasive disease
		  CIN 1, 2, 3
		  Cervical carcinoma
		Abnormal vascular patterns
		Atypical vessels

4. Assess the cervix after the application of diluted Lugol's iodine solution.*	Dark, mahogany staining (glycogenated epithelium)	Nonstaining Variegated (nonglycogenated epithelium)
5. Perform endocervical sampling* (ECC, cytobrush).		
6. Perform colposcopic-directed biopsy* (cervical biopsy punch).		
7. Perform hemostasis (pressure, Monsel's solution, silver nitrate).*		

* Not required.
CIN, cervical intraepithelial neoplasia; ECC, endocervical curettage.

Table continued on following page

▼ Table 5–4B

Site-Specific Colposcopy: Vagina

Steps in Colposcopic Assessment	The Kind of Observations You Can Expect to Make at This Step of the Examination	
	Normal Findings	*Abnormal Findings*
1. Clean the vagina with saline* and assess.	Squamous epithelium (no glands)	Adenosis Vaginal polyps Vaginal cysts DES morphology
2. Assess the vagina with a green filter before the application of 3%–5% acetic acid.*		Abnormal vascular patterns (punctation) Atypical vessels Patches of superficial erosions (strawberry spots caused by vaginitis)
3. Assess the vagina after the application of 3%–5% acetic acid.	Nonspecific acetowhite epithelium	Acetowhite epithelium specific for preinvasive or invasive disease VAIN 1, 2, 3 Vaginal carcinoma
4. Assess the vagina after the application of diluted Lugol's iodine solution.	Dark, mahogany staining (glycogenated epithelium)	Nonstaining (nonglycogenated epithelium) Variegated
5. Perform colposcopic-directed biopsy* (vaginal biopsy punch, local anesthesia, excision).		
6. Perform hemostasis (pressure, Monsel's solution, silver nitrate).		

* Not required.
DES, diethylstilbestrol; VAIN, vaginal intraepithelial neoplasia.

identified on the diagram of the cervix. The colposcopic impressions of both normal and abnormal findings on the cervix, vulva, vagina, and rectum should be displayed on the colposcopic record. These include acetowhite epithelium, leukoplakia, mosaic, punctation, and atypical vessels. A label that indicates the position of the finding should designate each abnormal area.

The clinician should also record any cytologic specimens or cultures that were sent or biopsies that were performed at the time of colposcopy. The record of col-

▼ Table 5–4C

Site-Specific Colposcopy: Vulva

Steps in Colposcopic Assessment	The Kind of Observations You Can Expect to Make at This Step of the Examination	
	Normal Findings	*Abnormal Findings*
1. Assess before the application of 3%–5% acetic acid.	Hart's line Hair-bearing and non–hair-bearing squamous epithelium Sebaceous hyperplasia	Benign epithelial abnormalities (lichen sclerosus, lichen planus, squamous cell hyperplasia) Lentigo maligna Bartholin's cyst/abscess Epithelial cysts
2. Assess with 3% acetic acid.	Micropapillomatosis labialis Nonspecific acetowhite epithelium	Condyloma acuminatum Acetowhite epithelium specific for preinvasive disease or invasion VIN 1, 2, 3 Vulvar carcinoma
3. Perform colposcopic-directed biopsy* (local anesthesia, punch, excision).		
4. Perform hemostasis (direct pressure, Monsel's solution [small amount, wipe away excess]).		
5. Apply protective dressing.*		

* Not required.
VIN, vulvar intraepithelial neoplasia.

▼ Table 5-5

Documentation, Laboratory Forms, and Patient Education

Colposcopic record
Demographic form if it is separate from the colposcopic record
Informed consent if it is an institutional requirement
Laboratory forms for cytopathology and surgical pathology
General laboratory forms (cultures, β-hCG, wet smear preparation)
Preoperative and postoperative patient information sheets
3 × 5 card for "tickler" file if there is no computer database
Patient reminder card, addressed at clinic visit
Educational brochures

β-hCG, beta-human chorionic gonadotropin.

poscopic findings should include a statement about whether the transformation zone was fully visualized, whether there was suspicion of invasive cancer, and whether all the abnormal lesions were visualized in their entirety. Finally, the recommendations for follow-up visits or referrals are recorded, including the return visit interval. If the patient fails to return for the appropriate follow-up visit(s), the method of notification should be recorded. If all attempts to reach the patient fail, a registered letter should be sent, with documentation of the mailing placed in the medical record.

SUMMARY OF KEY POINTS

- The primary goal of the colposcopist is to ensure that invasive disease is not missed.

- Conization should not be performed unless there is some reasonable suspicion that the patient is harboring a high-grade lesion or unless there is any suspicion that she may have an occult invasive cancer.

- The subtle differences between the features of squamous metaplasia and those of low-grade intraepithelial lesions make both the colposcopic and the histologic diagnosis of these conditions difficult.

- Because the ability of histology to define the true level of disease on the cervix is dependent on a properly directed biopsy, the histologic interpretation is only as accurate as the skill of the colposcopist in properly directing the biopsy.

- The colposcopist and the pathologist should agree about the transmission of specimens, the interpretation of results, and the consultation guidelines in case disagreements or questions occur. This will help avoid misguided therapeutic decisions related to misunderstandings between the pathologist and the clinician.

- Up to 40% of patients are lost to follow-up. Among the barriers that have been identified are transportation, child care, work, fear, and preoccupation with busy life routines.

- Most colposcopes have a focal length of around 300 mm. If the focal distance is too short, there will be limited room to maneuver instruments in front of the lens. If the focal length is too long, the colposcopist will be too far away from the target tissue to comfortably perform the examination.

- The green filter absorbs certain wavelengths of light, making the red color of the vessels appear blacker and sharpening the contrast with the surrounding epithelium.

- The colposcopic image on video colposcope is two-dimensional rather than three-dimensional, making assessment of the contour and density of the lesion more difficult.

- To achieve an acetic acid effect in nonkeratinized epithelium, the 3% to 5% acetic acid must be left in contact with the tissue for at least 1 minute.

- Lugol's solution stains normal squamous epithelium a dark, mahogany color, indicating that glycogen is present in the cells. Absent staining denotes a nonglycogenated state.

- Monsel's solution and silver nitrate interfere with biopsy interpretation and should not be applied until after all the samples are taken.

- When there is only one well-visualized and easily accessible lesion, one biopsy is sufficient. Performing additional biopsies causes discomfort to the patient and is unnecessary. Large, complex lesions often require multiple samples to rule out invasive cancer.

- The value of a routine ECC is controversial, and some colposcopists reserve it for selected patients, such as those in whom the transformation zone is not fully visualized, those who were previously treated, those at high risk for recurrent disease, and those to be treated with ablative therapy.

- ECC is always contraindicated in the pregnant patient.

- Although a large biopsy cannot be taken with a small-jawed biopsy instrument, a large-jawed biopsy instrument need not take only large biopsies. A small biopsy can be taken using only the tip of the jaw.

- Demographic information, clinical findings, and recommendations for follow-up visits or referrals should all be included in the colposcopic record.

References

1. Reid R: A Rapid method for improving colposcopic accuracy. Colposcopy Gynecol Laser Surg 1987;3:139.
2. Townsend DE, Richart RM: Diagnostic errors in colposcopy. Gynecol Oncol 1981;12:259.
3. Benedet JL, Anderson GH, Boyes DA: Colposcopic accuracy in the

diagnosis of microinvasive and occult invasive carcinoma of the cervix. Obstet Gynecol 1985;65:557.

4. Kohan S, Beckman EM, Bigelow B, et al: Colposcopy and the management of cervical intraepithelial neoplasia. Gynecol Oncol 1977;5:27.

5. Rome RM, Chanen W, Ostor AG: Preclinical cancer of the cervix: Diagnostic pitfalls. Gynecol Oncol 1983;22:302.

6. Noller KL, Stanhope CR: Colposcopic accuracy: Comparison of satisfactory examinations with results of conization. Colposcopy Gynecol Laser Surg 1984;1:181.

7. Roman LD, Felix JC, Muderspach, LI et al: Risk of residual invasive disease in women with microinvasive squamous cancer in a conization specimen. Obstet Gynecol 1997;90:759.

8. Homesley HD: Assessment of colposcopic skills. Colposcopy Gynecol Laser Surg 1987;3:135.

9. Hopman EH, Voorhorst FJ, Kenemans P, et al: Observer agreement on interpreting colposcopic images of CIN. Gynecol Oncol 1995;58:206.

10. Anderson MC: Are we vapourising microinvasive lesions? Colposcopy Gynecol Laser Surg 1987;3:33.

11. Skehan M, Soutter WP, Lim K, et al: Reliability of colposcopy and directed punch biopsy. Br J Obstet Gynecol 1990;97:811.

12. Laedtke TW, Dignan M: Compliance with therapy for cervical dysplasia among women of low socioeconomic status. South Med J 1992;8:5.

13. Lerman C, Hanjani P, Caputo C, et al: Telephone counseling improves adherence to colposcopy among lower-income minority women. J Clin Oncol 1992;80:330.

14. Gold MA, Dunton CJ, Macones GA, et al: Knowledge base as a predictory of follow-up compliance after colposcopy. J Lower Genital Tract Dis 1997;1:132.

15. Ferenczy A, Hilgarth M, Jenny J, et al: The place of colposcopy and related systems in gynecologic practice and research. J Reprod Med 1988;33:737.

16. Ferris DG: Video colposcopy. J Lower Genital Tract Dis 1997;1:15.

17. Ferris DG, Ho TH, Guijon F, et al: A comparison of colposcopy using optical and video colposcopes. J Lower Genital Tract Dis 2000;4:65.

18. Yandell RB, Hannigan EV, Dinh TV, et al: Avoiding conization for inadequate colposcopy: Suggestions for conservative therapy. J Reprod Med 1996;4:135.

19. Rochelson B, Krumholtz B: The unsatisfactory colposcopy examination. J Reprod Med 1983;28:131.

20. Spitzer M, Chernys AE: Monsel's solution-induced artifact in the uterine cervix. Am J Obstet Gynecol 1996;175:1204.

21. Campion M, Ferris D, diPaola F, et al: Systematic Approach to Colposcopy. Augusta, GA, Educational Systems, 1991.

22. Ferris D, Harper D, Callahan B, et al: The efficacy of topical benzocaine gel for providing anesthesia prior to cervical biopsy and endocervical curettage. J Lower Genital Tract Dis 1997;1:221.

23. Burghardt E: The colposcopic examination. In Burghardt E, Pickel H, Girardi F (eds): Colposcopy-Cervical Pathology Textbook and Atlas, 2nd ed. New York, Georg Thieme Verlag, 1991, p 125.

24. Burke L, Antonioli D, Ducatman B: Instrumentation and biopsy technique. In Burke L, Antonioli D, Ducatman B (eds): Colposcopy Text and Atlas. Norwalk, CT, Appleton and Lange, 1991, p 7.

25. Kolstadt P, Stafl A: Diagnostic criteria. In Kolstadt P, Stafl A (eds): Atlas of Colposcopy, 2nd ed. Baltimore, University Park Press, 1977, p 23.

▼ *Appendix 1*

Colposcopy Form

Patient ID#: _____

Examiner Name(s): _____ **Date:** _____ **Primary Care Physician:** _____

Reason(s) for colposcopy: _____

_____

Colposcopic Findings:

LK—leukoplakia, WE—white epithelium, PN—punctation, MO—mosaic, AV—atypical vessel, SCJ—squamocolumnar junction, X—biopsy sites

Pap smear done: _____ Yes _____ No

_____ ECC _____ Biospy of _____ Cervix _____ Vagina _____ Vulva

_____ HPV testing _____ Wet prep _____ Other _____

Colposcopy findings:

*Vulva, vagina, perineum, perianal area normal: _____ Yes _____ No

If no, describe: _____

*Entire SCJ seen: _____ Yes _____ No

*Limits of lesion seen: _____ Yes _____ No _____ NA

*Invasive cancer seen: _____ Yes _____ No

Colposcopic Diagnosis: _____

Cytology Diagnosis: _____

Biopsy Diagnosis: _____

Final Impression:

_____ Low-grade CIN

_____ High-grade CIN

_____ Invasive carcinoma

_____ Condyloma acuminatum

_____ Ectropion

_____ Squamous metaplasia

_____ Endocervical polyp   _____ Endometrial polyp

_____ Other _____

Remarks: _____

_____

● Results and plan discussed with patient: _____ Yes _____ No

　by _____ Phone _____ Letter _____ Other (　　　　　　　) Date: _____

● Treatment options discussed, including:

　_____ LEEP _____ LEEP cone _____ Laser _____ Cryo _____ CKC _____ TCA _____ Observation _____ Other

Management option selected: _____

● Follow-up date: _____

● Note sent to Primary Care Physician: _____ Yes Date: _____   _____

　　　　　　　　　　　　　　　　　　　　　　　　　　　　　　　　　　　　Colposcopist Signature

▼ *Appendix 2*

Colposcopy Information Sheet

What is colposcopy? It is close-up examination of the cervix using a special microscope called a colposcope.

Why do I need it? It will help identify the cause of your abnormal Papanicolaou (Pap) smear. An abnormal Pap smear may indicate cancerous and precancerous conditions, as well as some relatively harmless conditions. The Pap smear alone, however, cannot give a definitive diagnosis. The cervix must be magnified many times by the colposcope to look for the source of the abnormal cells. A small segment of each of these areas is then obtained for study by a pathologist. This is called a biopsy.

Is any preparation necessary? You should not douche, use any vaginal creams, or have intercourse 2 days before the examination. You should not have your period at the time of the examination. It is ideal to perform the colposcopy just after your period has ended. Many women find it helpful to take three ibuprofen tablets 1 to 2 hours before their appointment to reduce any cramping associated with a biopsy (do not use ibuprofen if you are allergic to it or to aspirin or if you are pregnant).

What is the examination like? It is like a regular pelvic examination, except that instead of looking at the cervix with the naked eye, the clinician will be looking through the colposcope. The entire examination takes approximately 20 to 30 minutes. If a biopsy is obtained, a slight pinching sensation may be experienced. The final step is to do a scraping of the inside of the cervix. This is called an endocervical curettage. This part of the examination lasts only about 15 seconds and is usually associated with some cramping.

What happens after the examination? You will be given a sanitary napkin to wear. No time off from work is needed. Intercourse should be avoided until all bleeding stops. No other limitation of activities is needed. The biopsy results will be back within 2 weeks, at which time your clinician will contact you to discuss treatment plans, if necessary, as well as what follow-up is needed. Please contact your clinician if she or he has not contacted you within 2 weeks of your appointment. If your phone number or address changes, please inform _____ at _____ so that we can update your chart.

▼ *Appendix 3*

Patient Intake Form

Referred by: _____ Your name: _____

Your address: _____ City/State: _____ Zip code: _____

Home telephone: _____ Work telephone: _____

Your age now: _____ Date of your last menstrual period: _____

- -

Please answer the following questions. Your answers will remain strictly confidential.

Reason(s) for referral: _____ Abnormal Pap smear

_____ Vaginal discharge

_____ Vaginal bleeding

_____ DES exposure

_____ Warts   For how long? _____

_____ Other _____

Any prior treatment for abnormal Pap smears? _____ Yes _____ No

   If yes, please list date and type of treatment: _____

Marital status: _____ Married _____ Single _____ Divorced

Age at first intercourse: _____   (0 = not applicable)

Total number of sexual partners in your lifetime: _____

Total # of pregnancies: _____   # of Miscarriages or abortions: _____

Type of birth control currently used: _____ Birth control pill

                                     _____ IUD

                                     _____ Tubal ligation

                                     _____ Norplant

                                     _____ Vasectomy in partner

                                     _____ Barrier method

                                     _____ Other   What? _____

Do you smoke cigarettes? _____ Yes _____ No

   If yes, how many packs a day? _____   For how many years? _____

Have you ever been treated for any of the following:

_____ Herpes   _____ Chlamydia _____ Trichomoniasis _____ Other _____

_____ Gonorrhea _____ Syphilis   _____ Warts   _____ No

Has your sexual partner ever been treated for the following:

_____ Herpes   _____ Chlamydia _____ Trichomoniasis _____ Other _____

_____ Gonorrhea _____ Syphilis   _____ Warts   _____ No

Have you ever taken an AIDS test? _____ Yes _____ No

   If yes, was the result _____ positive or _____ negative?

Do you use intravenous drugs presently? _____ Yes _____ No

   In the past? _____ Yes _____ No

Do you have a history of a bleeding disorder? _____ Yes _____ No

▼ *Appendix 4*

Informed Consent for Colposcopy with Biopsy of Cervix, Endocervix, Vagina, Introitis, Perineum, or Anus

_____ or his/her assistant has explained to me the procedures and local anesthesia necessary to diagnose my condition or my dependent's condition. I understand the nature of the procedure summarized below, and I request and authorize the performance of biopsy of the cervix, endocervix, and possibly the vagina, vulva, perineum, or anus.

I have been informed and understand that the following are possible risks associated with the procedure:
—Light bleeding that may require a sanitary napkin
—Heavy bleeding (rare) that may require a stitch or hospitalization
—Pain during the procedure (usually mild)
—Infection of biopsy site or uterine lining

I have been informed of the following benefits of the procedure:
—Can be done in the office
—Helps diagnose cause of abnormal Pap smear
—Helps plan future therapy

I understand that the procedure to be performed will be done under the guidance of a colposcope (a special microscope). I consent to the administration of such local anesthesia as is considered necessary. I understand that video or photographic equipment may be used during may procedure for later educational purposes.

The procedure of biopsy of the cervix, endocervix, vagina, vulva, perineum, and anus has been explained to me. I have read and understand this information, and I have had all questions answered to my satisfaction. I consent to the procedures outlined in this form.

(Adult patient): _____

Signature: _____ Date: _____

Witness: _____ Time: _____ Date: _____

(Minor patient accompanied by parent or guardian): _____

I, the parent or legal guardian of the above-named minor, an unemancipated minor, do hereby consent to the procedures described above.

Signature (parent/guardian): _____ Date: _____

Witness: _____ Time: _____ Date: _____

Telephone authorization for unaccompanied minors:

Parent/guardian name: _____ Telephone: _____

Caller (clinician) signature: _____ Date: _____

Glossary

• Dennis M. O'Connor
• Gregory L. Brotzman
• Barbara S. Apgar

1. **Portio:** The portion of the cervix that extends into the vagina. The portio incorporates parts of the endocervix and the ectocervix.

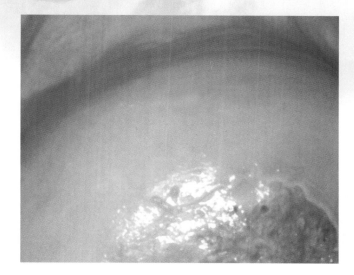

2. **Endocervix:** The portion of the cervical canal covered by columnar epithelium.

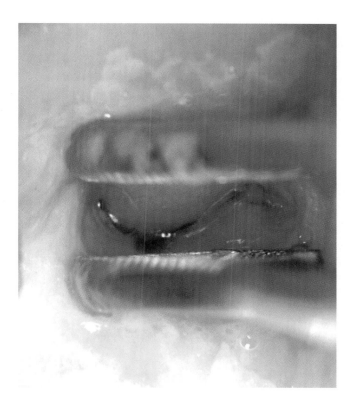

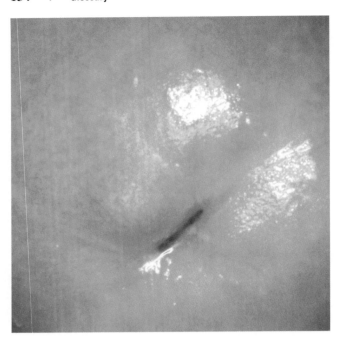

3. **Ectocervix (exocervix):** The portion of the cervix covered by stratified squamous epithelium.

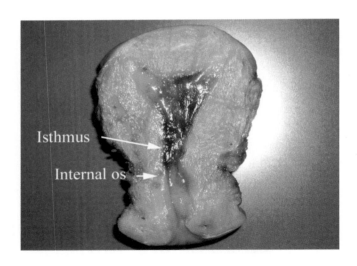

4. **Internal os:** The upper border of the cervical canal. It is adjacent to the isthmus.
5. **Isthmus:** The narrow distal portion of the lower uterine segment.

6. **Fornix:** The recessed vagina that borders the lateral cervix *(arrow)*.

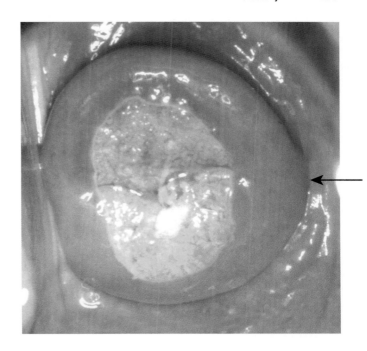

7. **Squamous epithelium:** A multilayered, stratified epithelium that is divided into three zones (basal, parabasal, intermediate, and superficial) and modified by estrogen and progesterone; the superficial layer is the most differentiated layer and periodically undergoes proliferation, maturation, and desquamation; these cells are glycogenated. Colposcopically, the surface has a pink, translucent appearance.

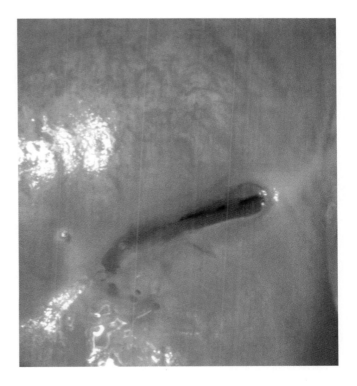

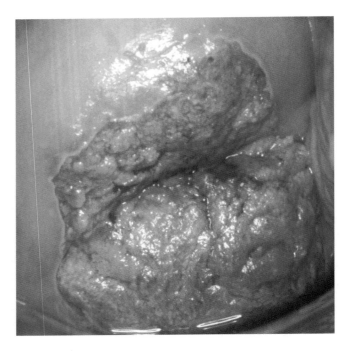

8. **Columnar epithelium:** A singular layer of mucus-secreting tall columnar cells that lines the endocervix and is contiguous with the endometrium; they are arranged in cleftlike infoldings that are not true glands. On colposcopy, there is a grapelike appearance, with the papillary surface reflecting the papillary infolding of the columnar epithelium; the changes become most prominent after the application of 3% to 5% acetic acid. The grapelike clefts diminish in the distal endocervical canal, eventually leading to a flat, salmon-colored surface appearance, which is contiguous with the endometrium at the internal os. The red appearance of the columnar epithelium is due to the close proximity of the underlying stromal blood vessels to the single layer of columnar cells.

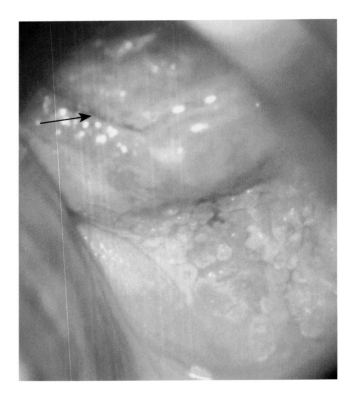

9. **Adenosis:** The presence of columnar epithelium in the vagina, often associated with women exposed to diethylstilbestrol (DES) while in utero. *Arrow* points to the os. Adenosis is present on the posterior vaginal fornix. (Image provided by Dr. Burton Krumholz.)

10. Ectropion: When columnar epithelium everts onto the portio of the cervix.

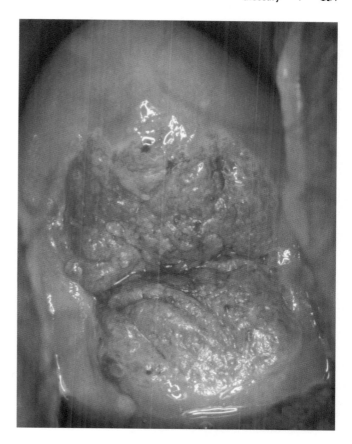

11. The "new" squamocolumnar junction (NSCJ): The current junction where the squamous and columnar cells meet on the surface of the cervix at the time the patient is being evaluated; it demarcates the junction of the endocervical glandular epithelium and the squamous epithelium after squamous metaplasia is completed.

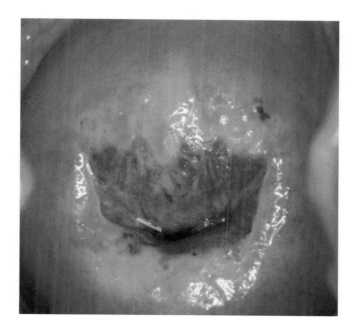

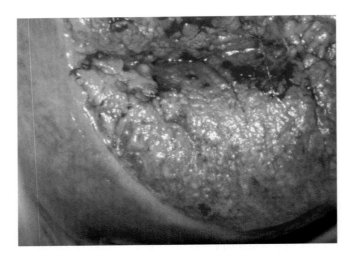

12. **Original (native) squamocolumnar junction (OSCJ):** The location of the squamocolumnar junction at birth where the native squamous epithelium abuts the native columnar epithelium; it later becomes a squamo-squamo junction after the transformation zone undergoes metaplasia.

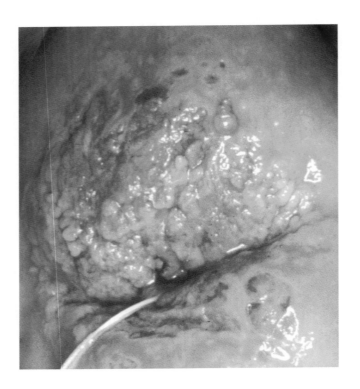

13. **Squamous metaplasia:** The replacement of the columnar epithelium by the stratified squamous epithelium—transformation of one mature epithelial type to another. During transition, the squamous cells show a lack of surface maturation and a lack of glycogen; there is, however, normal cellular cohesion and absent nuclear atypia; a single row of columnar cells overlies the squamous metaplastic cells; there is random distribution and varied stratification depending on maturation. Colposcopically, islands of squamous metaplastic epithelium are present on the tips of the columnar epithelial papillae, which produces a patchy distribution; delicate, translucent bridges or tongues of metaplasia may intersperse with mature columnar epithelium; the metaplastic surface shares features of mature squamous and columnar epithelia.

14. Transformation zone: The geographic area of transformation or metaplasia between the original squamocolumnar junction and the new squamocolumnar junction; nabothian cysts, mature squamous epithelium, squamous metaplasia, mature columnar epithelium, and gland crypts may be present; practically speaking, once the transformation is complete, no remnants of the metaplastic process remain (such as gland openings and nabothian cysts), and the original squamocolumnar junction may be unidentifiable.

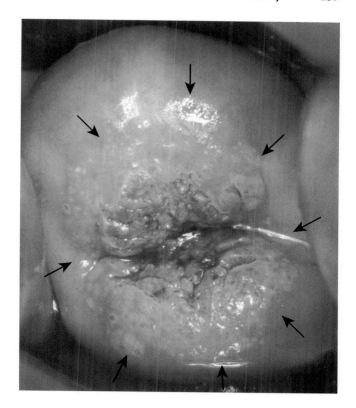

15. Nabothian cysts: Dilated, occluded endocervical gland crypts indicating that squamous metaplasia has occurred. Nabothian cysts may display exaggerated vessels overlying the cyst, but there is usually normal branching distinguishing them from atypical vessels. They provide markers for the transformation zone because they are in squamous areas but are remnants of columnar epithelium.

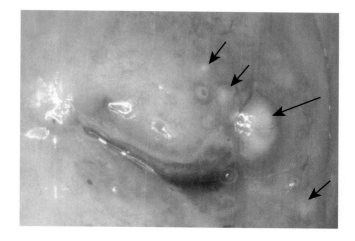

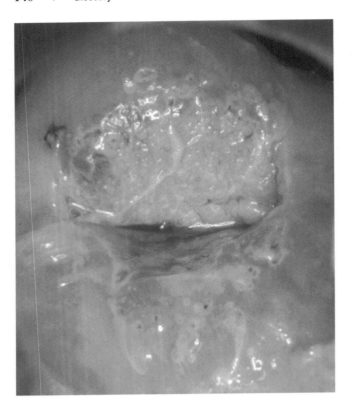

16. Gland openings (ostia): Small endocervical gland crypt openings visible in areas of squamous metaplasia; they represent persistent endocervical gland crypts on the squamous epithelial surface; they are usually surrounded by a rim of metaplasia and often are identified by the mucus extruding from the gland opening; they provide markers for the peripheral extent of the transformation zone.

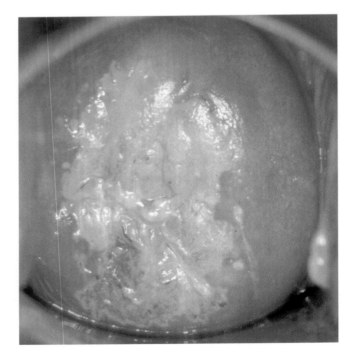

17. Unsatisfactory colposcopy: The entire new squamo-columnar junction is not visualized (360 degrees); the proximal and distal limits of a lesion are not seen if a lesion is present.

18. **Satisfactory colposcopy:** The entire squamocolumnar junction is visualized (360 degrees); the proximal and distal limits of a lesion are seen if a lesion is present.

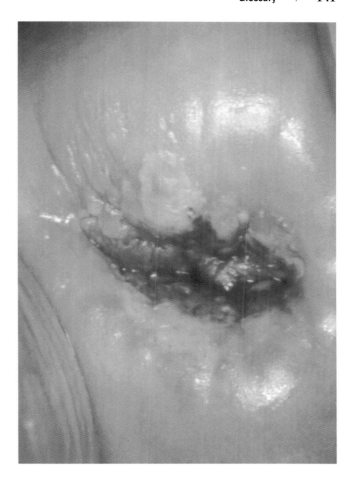

19. **Atypical transformation zone:** The geographic area displaying features of colposcopic abnormalities that can include acetowhite epithelium, punctation, mosaic, leukoplakia, or atypical blood vessels. Each of these terms is described individually, because they are very important features to identify during the colposcopic examination of the cervix; the vast majority of invasive squamous cell cancers of the cervix arise within the transformation zone.

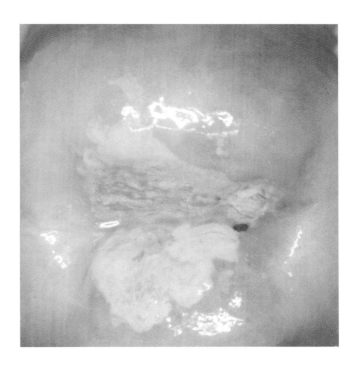

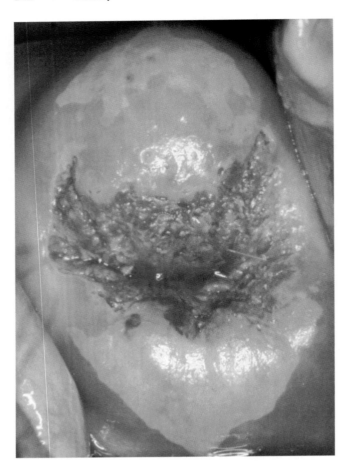

20. **Acetowhite (AW) change or reaction:** Transient white coloration that occurs after the application of 3% to 5% acetic acid to the cervical epithelium; the exact mechanism of how acetic acid produces this whitening is uncertain (either owing to a temporary protein change in cells with enlarged nuclear content or owing to a temporary dehydration of cells); because the reaction is only temporary, 3% to 5% acetic acid may need to be reapplied during colposcopic examination. AW change can be seen in normal or abnormal epithelium, and specific criteria need to be used to distinguish normal from abnormal changes.

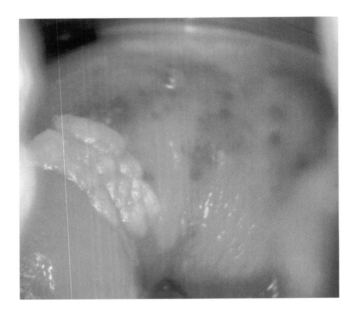

21. **Leukoplakia:** An elevated, white plaque seen before the application of 3% to 5% acetic acid; a nonspecific finding that may represent trauma, infection, or human papillomavirus–related disease, including invasive disease; it usually requires a biopsy for specific diagnosis.

22. Punctation: Small vascular dots that represent the tips of capillary loops located within a field of acetowhite epithelium; punctation may be coarse or fine on colposcopic view.

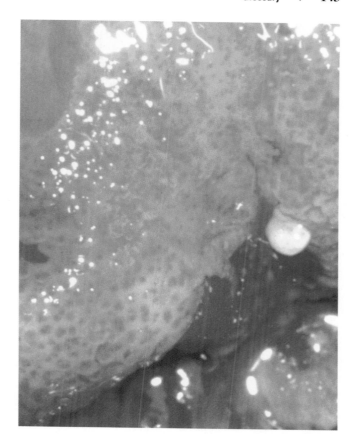

23. Mosaic: Acetowhite tiles bordered by vessels that represent confluent arborizing capillary loops located within a field of acetowhite epithelium; mosaic may be coarse or fine on colposcopic view.

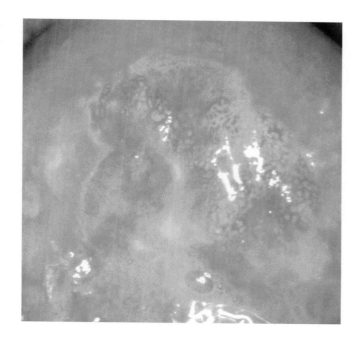

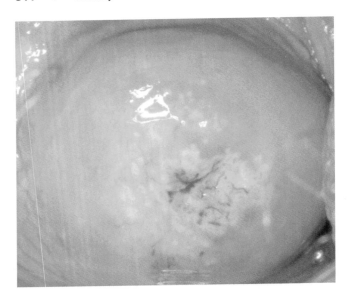

24. Atypical blood vessels: Irregular, nonbranching, superficial vessels with abrupt courses and patterns; they often appear as commas, corkscrews, starbursts, or spaghetti; no specific pattern is universally present; if they are identified, invasive disease must be ruled out.

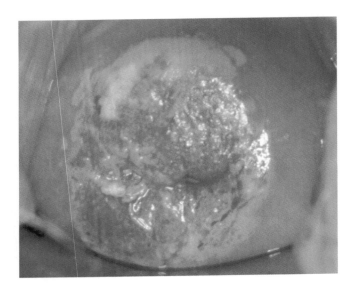

25. Cervical intraepithelial neoplasia (CIN): The histologic description of the three grades of precancerous lesions of the cervix—CIN 1, CIN 2, and CIN 3; the degree of CIN represents the amount of abnormal cellular change in the epithelial layers.

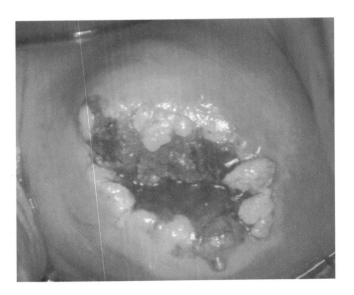

26. Condyloma acuminata: Exophytic, warty lesions caused by human papillomavirus infection; they may display exaggerated vessel patterns; lesions are often multifocal and can be located both within and outside the transformation zone; some are subclinical and are manifested by subtle, minimally raised areas of acetowhite epithelium.

27. Colpitis: Diffuse erythema of the cervix and vagina that is the result of an infection such as trichomoniasis or *Candida* species; underlying stromal vessels are dilated, and the tips are visible through the overlying denuded squamous epithelium, appearing as fine red dots. This is distinguished from punctation, in which the red dots are found within a field of acetowhite epithelium; after the application of Lugol's solution, the denuded, inflamed epithelium exhibits poor iodine uptake, producing a "leopard-skin," blotchy pattern.

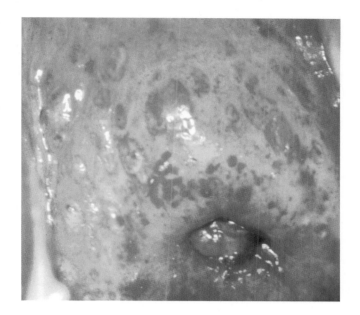

28. Erosion: The overlying epithelium is removed and the underlying stroma is visible; traumatic erosions are most commonly caused by speculum insertion and over-vigorous Papanicolaou test sampling; erosion can also result from irritants such as tampons, diaphragms, and intercourse; it may be a marker for invasive disease, so biopsy may be necessary to confirm diagnosis.

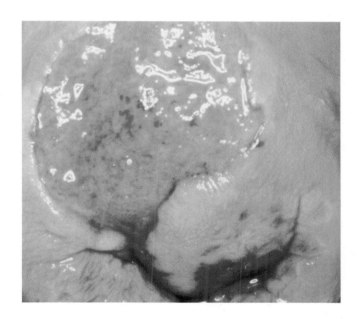

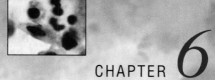

CHAPTER *6*

• Dennis M. O'Connor

Normal Transformation Zone

CHARACTERISTICS AND DEFINITIONS OF THE NORMAL CERVIX

Embryology of the Cervix

The cervix develops from two embryonic sites. The majority of the cervix is derived from the distally fused müllerian ducts, known as the müllerian tubercle. This area is centrally hollow and is lined by the columnar epithelium. At approximately 16 weeks' gestation, the urogenital plate expands upward to the müllerian tubercle and then undergoes cavitation, forming the rudimentary vagina. The surface of this hollow structure is lined by the stratified squamous epithelium. The point where the columnar and squamous cells meet is known as the original, or native, squamocolumnar junction.[1–3] The location of the original squamocolumnar junction probably varies throughout fetal life. From the late second to the early third trimester, the junction is located within the rudimentary endocervical canal. After 8 months of gestation, it is common to find columnar epithelium extending out over the cervical surface.[4] At term, the columnar cells regress into the canal. In some individuals, however, the original squamocolumnar junction may be found extending from the cervix onto the vaginal surface.[1]

Cervical development is probably modulated by the presence or absence of sex steroid hormones, particularly estrogen. Exposure to large amounts of exogenous estrogenic agents in the second trimester can result in cervical deformations such as hood, collar, and coxcomb abnormalities.[3]

Anatomy and Topography of the Cervix

The surface of the cervix extends from the circumferential vaginal fornix to the external cervical os.

The cervix (Latin for neck) is the inferior extension of the uterus. The cervix is divided into two portions. The lower portion extends into the vagina and is the cervix surface that can be visualized using the colposcope. This region of the cervix is known as the vaginal cervix or portio. The upper cervix extends from the upper border of the vaginal fornix to the uterine isthmus and is known as

the supravaginal cervix. The cervix attachment in the vagina is oblique. For this reason, the anterior cervix portio is only one fourth of the total cervix, whereas the posterior cervix portio is one half of the total cervix. In the nulliparous patient, the cervix composes approximately 50% of the total uterine volume and is approximately 3 cm in length. The cervix is cylindrical and measures approximately 2 cm in diameter. The cervix surface extends from the circumferential vaginal fornix to the external cervical os; in the nulliparous patient the os is round and measures 3 to 5 mm in diameter. During pregnancy, the cervix enlarges owing to proliferation of the elastic and smooth muscle fibers and to vascular congestion. After vaginal delivery, the external os enlarges with a linear stellate configuration as a result of scarring from cervical lacerations.[1, 5, 6]

The cervical canal is approximately 3 cm in length and is fusiform in shape.

The cervix is supported by the parametrial soft tissue, the uterosacral ligaments, and the transverse cervical or cardinal ligaments of Mackenrodt. The latter provides the major source of cervical support and is characterized by well-defined fascial ligaments that extend from the lateral cervix through the broad ligament base to the levator ani muscle. The cervical canal is approximately 3 cm in length and is fusiform in shape. The diameter of the canal varies and is approximately 8 mm at its widest point. The cervical canal contains ridges known as plicae palmatae or arbor vitae uteri. The small ridges are lost after vaginal delivery.[1, 2, 6]

Histology of the Normal Cervix

The majority of the portio of the cervix is covered by stratified squamous epithelium.

The majority of the cervix portio is covered by stratified squamous epithelium. The squamous cells have a characteristic basket-weave pattern of maturation identical to that of the squamous mucosa of the vagina. As maturation evolves, the squamous cells enlarge and increase their overall volume, and the amount of nuclear material decreases. Maturation of squamous cells is estrogen dependent. In the premenopausal and postmenopausal states, the less mature cervical cells predominate.[1, 7]

Cervical squamous cells have been arbitrarily divided into four distinct layers. The basal, or germinal, cell layer is composed of a single layer of small cuboidal cells that contain large, darkly staining nuclei. The nuclei are round to oval in shape. Mitotic figures are occasionally seen. The parabasal or prickle-cell layer is composed of irregular polyhedral cells with large, dark, oval nuclei. Nucleoli can be seen in these cells. On electron microscopy, tonofilaments are present, indicating a squamous differentiation. The intermediate or navicular cells are flattened cells with glycogen-rich clear cytoplasm. The nuclei are small, dark, and round. The superficial or stratum corneum layer is composed of flat, elongated cells with small pyknotic nuclei. Collagen is present in the more superficial cells. Scanning electron microscopy of these squamous cells indicates numerous small ridges on the cell surface, which may indicate the presence of keratin filaments.[3] Although these four layers exist, examination of numerous cervical specimens indicates that maturation of the squamous cells varies considerably. The only two layers that can be readily identified are usually the basal and the superficial cells (Fig. 6–1).[7–9]

The only two layers of the squamous epithelium that can be readily identified are usually the basal and the superficial cells.

The basement membrane lies beneath the basal cells. On electron microscopy, it usually measures 3 μm in thickness. The basement membrane is composed of the lamina densa that borders the underlying cervix stroma and the lamina lucida, which borders the basal cell. The basal cells contain foot processes that extend into the basement membrane.[7]

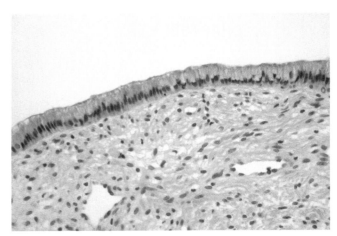

Figure 6–2. Normal endocervical cells. A single layer of tall columnar endocervical cells is shown. The nuclei are generally basal, small, dark, and round (hematoxylin and eosin stain, original magnification ×400).

The basal cells contain numerous cytokeratin filaments, which can be identified immunohistochemically. Cytokeratins 1, 6, 13, 14, 15, 16, 19, and 20 are found in the surface squamous cells of the ectocervix. Cytokeratin 15 predominates in the basal and parabasal cells.[10–13] The basal and parabasal cell layers also contain numerous epidermal growth factor and estrogen receptors; epidermal growth factor stimulates cell mitotic activity and induces keratinization and squamous cell differentiation. Estrogen stimulates DNA synthesis and shortens the cell cycle.[14] A relative lack of estrogen results in minimal proliferation and maturation commonly seen in postmenopausal women who are not using hormone supplemental therapy.

The surface extending from the internal cervical os to the squamous margin is lined by a single layer of tall columnar cells. The nuclei in these cells are round to oval and basal. Most columnar cells are secretory, using apocrine and merocrine systems, but a few are ciliated and may be used for transport (Fig. 6–2). Transmission electron microscopy of these cells demonstrates the presence of cilia, mucin droplets, and secretory granules of varying sizes. The endocervical columnar cells express cytokeratin 16 only.[25, 26]

The endocervical cells invaginate into the cervical stroma to a depth of approximately 5 to 8 mm.

The endocervical cells invaginate into the cervical stroma to a depth of approximately 5 to 8 mm. Although this represents crypt formation, because there are no ductal and acinar structures, by convention the cells have been called endocervical glands owing to their rounded shape on cross-section.[1]

The area where the stratified squamous and columnar cells meet is known as the squamocolumnar junction. This junction is distinctive in only one third of examined specimens (Figs. 6–3 and 6–4). The remainder have evidence of a gradual transformation from one cell type to the other (discussed later).

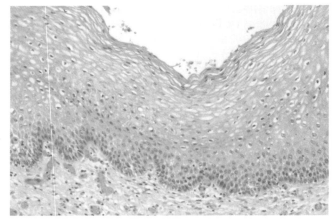

Figure 6–1. Normal ectocervical squamous epithelium. As maturation progresses, the amount of cell cytoplasm increases and the nuclear size decreases. At the basement membrane, the basal and parabasal cells are the most closely approximated. Cytoplasmic clearing in the upper intermediate and superficial layers indicates evidence of glycogenation (hematoxylin and eosin stain, original magnification ×400).

The cervix stroma is composed of fibrous connective tissue, with lesser amounts of smooth muscle and connective tissue fibers. In approximately 1% of cervices, small, rounded structures lined by flattened cuboidal cells can be seen laterally. These represent mesonephric or wolffian remnants.[7, 12]

Cytology of the Normal Cervix

During cytologic sampling, cells removed from the ectocervix are those that have exfoliated from the surface.

Papanicolaou (Pap) smear sampling of the cervix involves scraping of the cervical surface and a portion of the nonvisualized cervical canal using various sampling devices. Stratified squamous cells are markedly cohesive. Therefore, cells removed from the ectocervix are those that have exfoliated from the surface. Under the microscope, they are seen as individual cells. The columnar cells in the cervical canal are less cohesive and can be removed in clumps. Under the microscope, they usually appear as cell groups. In the well-estrogenized patient, the majority of the squamous cells seen under the microscope are from the superficial and intermediate layers. As such, these cells are navicular in shape and contain abundant amounts of cytoplasm. The nuclei are usually small, centrally located, and round. When present, the columnar cells are either linear in arrangement with basal nuclei or grouped in a honeycomb pattern. In the postmenopausal patient, the exfoliated cells are mostly parabasal, with some intermediate forms. These cells are more rounded, with large, centrally located nuclei. The nuclear membranes in all cells are smooth, and the nuclear chromatin is usually granular or finely stippled (Fig. 6−5).[1, 9, 15]

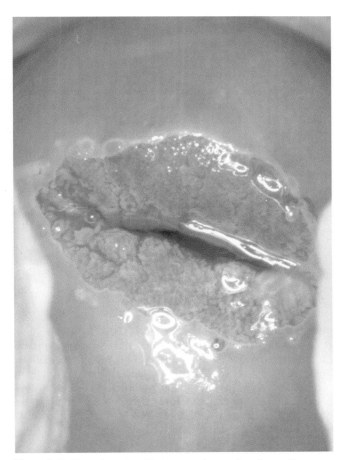

Figure 6−3. Normal cervix with squamocolumnar junction easily seen.

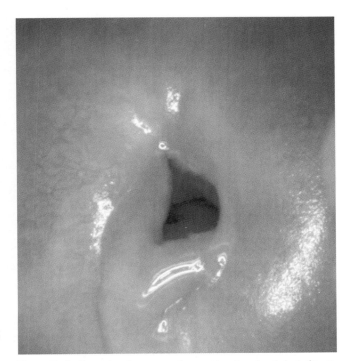

Figure 6−4. Example of squamocolumnar junction located at the os. Clear mucus is present.

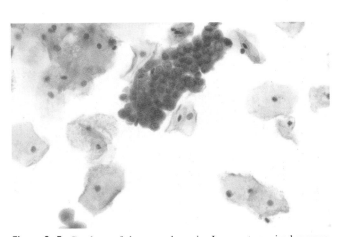

Figure 6−5. Cytology of the normal cervix. In an estrogenized woman, the squamous epithelial cells are large, with polygonal borders. The nuclei are small, round to oval, and dark. Although cell color is laboratory dependent, mature cells tend to be orange or pink. A central cluster of endocervical cells is also present. In cross-section, the cells are arranged in a honeycomb pattern. The endocervical nuclei are slightly larger, with a more open chromatin pattern and micronucleoli (thin-layer preparation, Papanicolaou stain, original magnification ×400).

The amount of cell exfoliation varies with the menstrual cycle. During the proliferative phase, there is increased exfoliation of well-glycogenated superficial cells. In the secretory phase, however, the predominant cell is intermediate in nature, and there is less glycogen.[16]

SQUAMOUS METAPLASIA

Formation of Squamous Metaplasia

Metaplasia is defined as a transformation from one mature cell type to a second mature type.

Metaplasia is defined as a transformation from one mature cell type to a second mature type. This process occurs in different body sites, including the bronchi, stomach, bladder, and salivary glands. The transformation usually involves a conversion from a columnar, secretory type of cell to a stratified, squamous cell. The site of metaplasia that has always generated major interest because of its neoplastic potential is the cervix.[10]

Historically, areas of cervical squamous metaplasia were originally misidentified as either early-differentiated carcinomas or folds in the upper squamous epithelium. German pathologists originally used the terms *epidermidalization* or *epidermoidalization* to describe areas of transformation from columnar to squamous cervical cells. Eventually, this process was reclassified as metaplasia, reserve cell hyperplasia, or squamocolumnar prosoplasia.[17, 18]

Factors that induce squamous metaplasia in the cervix are still poorly understood, but they may include environmental conditions, mechanical irritation, chronic inflammation, pH changes, or changes in sex steroid hormone balance. Metaplasia probably begins with the movement of the original squamocolumnar junction onto the portio, usually as a result of estrogen production or interval vaginal deliveries. The exposure of the delicate columnar cells to an acidic bacteria–laden vaginal environment initiates the process of inflammation and replacement with stratified squamous cells (Fig. 6–6).[2, 15, 17]

It is generally felt that the process of squamous metaplasia begins in the subcolumnar reserve cells.

For decades, it was unclear how this transformation took place. The mechanism of squamous metaplasia has been variously described as continued epithelization with new squamous cells derived from previously formed squamous epithelium, proliferation of subcolumnar nests of squamous basal cells, or development from undifferentiated embryonic rests within the superficial cervix stroma.[13, 19] Presently, it is felt that the process begins in the subcolumnar reserve cells. The origin of reserve cells remains obscure. Suggested parent cells include embryonal urogenital crest cells, fetal squamous cells, and stromal fibroblasts.[19] It is believed that these reserve cells probably arise from the dedifferentiation of overlying columnar cells.[10, 15] The presence of various cytokeratin intermediate filaments in reserve cells (cytokeratins 5, 6, 8, 13, 14, 15, 16, 17, 18, and 19) indicates an epithelial origin of these cells. As the reserve cells proliferate and differentiate into squamous metaplastic cells, there is a decrease in production of cytokeratin 19 and an increase in the cytokeratins commonly seen in mature squamous cells. In contrast, cytokeratins 6 and 16 predominate in metaplastic cells that have the potential to become dysplastic.[10, 12, 13] Other predictors of dysplastic potential in squamous metaplasia include degree of metaplastic proliferation and rate of metaplastic change.[20, 21]

Histology of Squamous Metaplasia

The area of squamous metaplasia is known histopathologically as the transformation zone.

Sixty percent of cervices will have a gradual transformation from columnar to mature squamous epithelium. This area of squamous metaplasia is known histopathologically as the transformation zone. Metaplasia is most commonly seen in the lower third of the endocervical

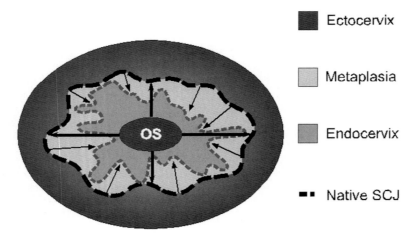

Ectocervix

Metaplasia

Endocervix

■ ▪ Native SCJ

▪ ▪ New SCJ

Figure 6–6. The formation of squamous metaplasia. The original or native squamocolumnar junction (SCJ) migrates onto the portio as the result of changes in the hormonal milieu or of vaginal deliveries *(thick arrows)*. The conversion of the columnar surface into a mature squamous surface (squamous metaplasia) moves the SCJ toward the internal os and, eventually, the endocervical canal. The transformation zone is the area of squamous metaplasia between the original or native SCJ and the new SCJ *(thin arrows)*.

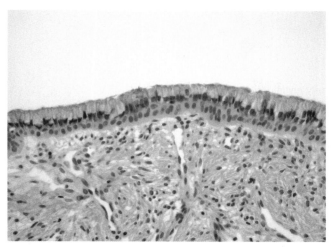

Figure 6–7. Reserve cell hyperplasia. The upper layer consists of tall columnar endocervical cells. Directly underneath is a single layer of cells with scant cytoplasm and uniform round nuclei. Although the term *hyperplasia* is used to indicate the presence of reserve cells, there is only one cell layer, and mitotic figures are absent (hematoxylin and eosin stain, original magnification ×400).

canal.[6] The first evidence of squamous metaplasia is the identification of a single layer of subcolumnar reserve cells, known histologically as reserve cell hyperplasia. The reserve cells are round to cuboidal, with large round to oval nuclei. They can be seen beneath the surface columnar cells and the columnar cells within the endocervical glands (Fig. 6–7). As the reserve cells proliferate, the resultant immature cells gain more cytoplasm, and the nuclei decrease in size. Over time, the surface columnar cells degenerate and are sloughed, and the endocervical glands solidify. The remaining stratified cells develop squamous characteristics and acquire glycogen. Eventually, these cells take on the appearance of mature squamous cells (Fig. 6–8A–C). [1, 7, 9, 22, 23]

The process of metaplasia is highly variable, and it is not uncommon to see areas of well-developed metaplasia interspersed with nonmetaplastic columnar epithelium. Other areas can show well-developed, mature squamous epithelium that overlies endocervical glands with little or no metaplastic proliferation.[9]

Because metaplasia is a process brought about by irritation or inflammation, it is not uncommon to see chronic inflammatory cells. These are usually plasma cells and

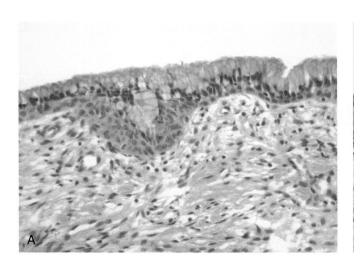

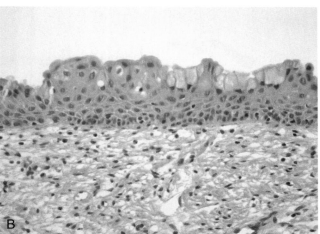

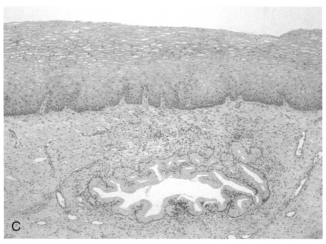

Figure 6–8. Squamous metaplasia. *A,* Early stage of immature metaplasia. The reserve cells have proliferated and created a two- to four-cell layer of uniformly round cells with scant cytoplasm and large nuclei. The endocervical cells are still present at the surface. As metaplasia progresses *(B),* the immature squamous cells continue to proliferate. Maturation results in an increase in cytoplasmic amount, but glycogenation has not yet occurred. The remaining endocervical cells show degeneration and are difficult to recognize. A few acute and chronic inflammatory cells are also seen in the superficial stroma and at the surface. Near completion of the metaplastic process *(C),* the metaplastic cells have matured in glycogenated squamous cells identical to the normal ectocervix. The only evidence of metaplasia is the residual endocervical glands seen under the squamous surface (*A,* hematoxylin and eosin stain, original magnification ×400; *B,* hematoxylin and eosin stain, original magnification ×400, *C,* hematoxylin and eosin stain, original magnification ×40).

Illustration continued on following page

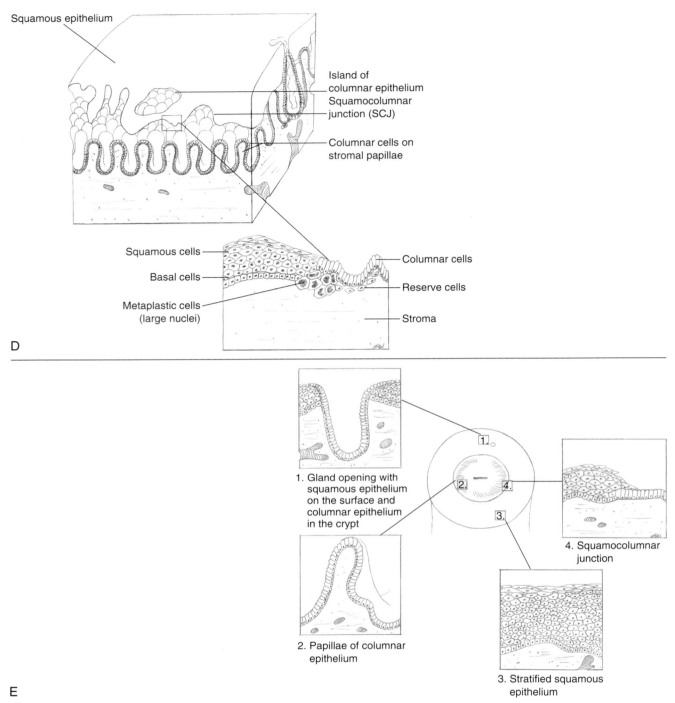

Figure 6-8 *Continued. D,* A graphic representation of a normal transformation zone and a histologic sampling of the squamocolumnar junction. *E,* Graphic representation of histologic sampling of various areas of a normal cervix.

lymphocytes. Occasionally, acute inflammatory cells are present in the underlying stroma and the surface metaplastic cells. As the metaplasia evolves within the endocervical glands, there is squamous bridging across the lumen, resulting in smaller gland structures. In the past, this has been called adenomatous hyperplasia or mucoid degeneration.[18]

Cytology of Squamous Metaplasia

Reserve cells can be seen on a Pap smear. They are commonly found within a mucoid background in linear sheets. The cells are usually round to oval with foamy cytoplasm. The nuclei are round to degenerative in shape and are small and dark. Because of their arrangement and

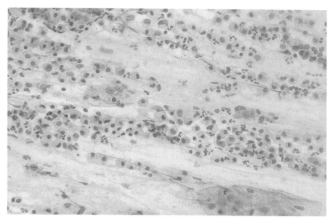

Figure 6—9. Reserve cells seen on Papanicolaou smear. The small, round cells are seen streaming across the field in a mucous background. Mature squamous epithelial cells are seen on the periphery (conventional smear, Papanicolaou stain, original magnification ×400).

size, these cells must be distinguished from a moderate (metaplastic cell) dysplasia (Fig. 6–9).

The presence of metaplastic cells represents cytologic evidence of a transformation zone cellular sample. The cells are typically seen in small groups or sheets. They have cyanophilic cytoplasm and are smaller in size than the mature squamous epithelial cells. The nuclei are slightly larger than intermediate cell nuclei. Their membranes are smooth and round and the chromatin is granular to finely stippled. Micronucleoli may be present (Fig. 6–10).[3]

The appearance of metaplastic cells can be cytologically similar to that of parabasal cells. For this reason, it is difficult to differentiate metaplastic cells from parabasal cells in a postmenopausal woman. Parabasal cells, however, tend to occur in larger numbers in postmenopausal women, whereas they are rarely seen in reproductive-age women. Therefore, the presence of small, oval cells with slightly enlarged nuclei in a background of mature squamous cells represents evidence of squamous metaplasia.

COLPOSCOPY OF THE NORMAL TRANSFORMATION ZONE

The presence of small, oval cells with slightly enlarged nuclei in a background of mature squamous cells represents evidence of squamous metaplasia.

Tissue Basis and Mechanism of Colposcopic Changes in the Normal Cervix

Colposcopy was originally developed by Hinselmann in 1929 as a screening test to identify cervical neoplasia. He noted that small cervical surface abnormalities could be best identified after the application of various contrast agents. Hinselmann used cedar wood oil, iodine solution, and 3% acetic acid, noting that the acetic acid provided the best contrast, with transient development of a white surface coloration.[11] Originally called leukoplakia by Hinselmann, today this coloration is known as acetowhitening of the cervix surface.

Colposcopy uses an external white light source to illuminate the cervix and distal vagina. The color changes represent the ratio of reflected and absorbed light and are related to tissue chromophores and the amount of visualized red blood cell hemoglobin. The amount of reflected light depends on the amount of cellular material that covers a particular tissue surface. Stratified squamous epithelium of the ectocervix has multiple cell layers that form a potential barrier between the light source and the underlying superficial cervical stromal capillaries (Fig. 6–11). On the other hand, a single layer of columnar endocervical cells allows the majority of the light to be absorbed, which illuminates the underlying capillary vessels (Fig. 6–12). Therefore, through the colposcope, the ectocervix has a gray-pink color, whereas the endocervix is more pink-red. Occasionally, individual branching vessels can be identified on the ectocervix. This becomes more prominent in the postmenopausal woman when there are fewer stratified squamous cells to obstruct light absorption.[15, 24]

The application of acetic acid alters the cervix surface. The reasons for this are unclear. Proposed theories include agglutination of nuclear proteins; alterations in cytokeratin filaments, particularly cytokeratins 10 and 19; and cytoplasmic dehydration.[11, 15] The resultant cellular modifications produce more reflected light, and the eye discerns a surface whiteness. The effects are transient, and the acetowhite effect is lost after an interval of approximately 15 seconds to 2 minutes, depending on the number of cells, the amount of individual cell cytoplasm, and the nuclear size.

The acetowhite effect is transient, and the duration of the effect depends on the number of cells, the amount of individual cell cytoplasm, and the nuclear size.

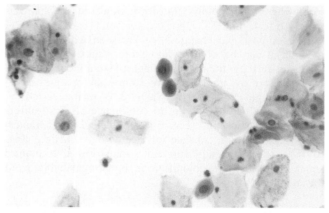

Figure 6—10. Metaplastic cells seen on Papanicolaou smear. The individual metaplastic cells are small and oval. The cytoplasm is a cyan color. The nuclei are slightly increased when compared with the nuclei of the surrounding mature squamous cells. The chromatin is fine and uniformly granular (thin-layer smear, Papanicolaou stain, original magnification ×400).

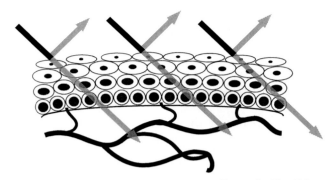

Figure 6–11. The normal ectocervix and the effects of white light exposure after acetic acid application. The surface color is dependent on the amount of light absorption into the underlying stroma, which illuminates the red blood cells in the superficial capillaries. The stratified squamous cells act as a barrier, reflecting some of the light back to the observer. The overall effect is a light pink–to-gray coloration.

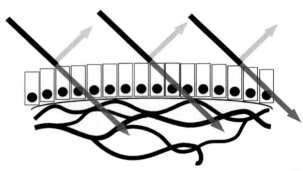

Figure 6–12. The normal endocervix and the effects of white light exposure after acetic acid application. The superficial capillaries are directly beneath the single layer of columnar cells. Most of the light is absorbed, and little is reflected back to the observer. The overall effect is a dark pink–to-red coloration.

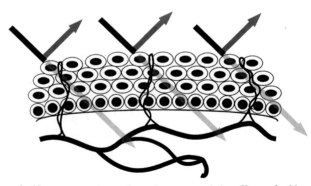

Figure 6–13. The normal transformation zone and the effects of white light exposure, enhanced by acetic acid application. The metaplastic squamous cells have less cytoplasm and more nuclear mass than do their mature counterparts. Most of the light is reflected back to the observer. The overall effect is a translucent-to-flocculent coloration. In addition, thin capillary loops will grow to the surface. When seen on end, they appear as small punctate dots.

Because squamous metaplasia has less cytoplasm and greater nuclear volume per cell, an area of metaplasia will typically appear more white than the surrounding lighter-pigmented ectocervix or darker-pigmented endocervix (Fig. 6–13). Nevertheless, varying degrees of metaplastic cell maturity will require continued reapplication of acetic acid to maintain this acetowhite affect.

Colposcopic Appearance of the Transformation Zone

Hinselmann described the normal cervix using the letters "O," "E" and "U." "O" represented the original mucous membrane. This area was characterized by normal squamous mucosa. "E" represented ectopy, which was the grapelike papillary topography of the endocervix. "U" represented the "umwandlung" zone. This area was felt to be an intermingling of squamous and columnar epithelium.[18] Coppleson modified this terminology to incorporate the terms native squamous epithelium, columnar epithelium, metaplastic epithelium, and undifferentiated metaplastic epithelium. The fourth term was applied to areas of immature metaplasia difficult to distinguish from dysplasia.[24] Today, we use the term transformation zone to identify an area that has the potential to transform into cervical neoplastic abnormalities.

The transformation zone is defined colposcopically as the area bordered by the original and the new squamocolumnar junction.[15, 24, 25] The location of the squamocolumnar junction is variable. During reproductive life, the squamocolumnar junction is commonly located near the external os or on the portio. In approximately 5% of women, it extends beyond the cervix onto the vagina (Figs. 6–14 and 6–15). Twenty-five percent of women have the squamocolumnar junction within the canal. Pregnancy can cause cervical eversion and exposure of the squamocolumnar junction even if it is located within the canal. The transformation zone area is also altered by exposure to oral contraceptive medications, pregnancy, pH changes in the vagina, and vaginal infections. Therefore, the exact size of the transformation zone varies from patient to patient. In children, it averages approximately 3 mm, whereas an adult's transformation zone is approximately 6 to 8 mm.[20, 15, 26]

The colposcopic changes that are seen with squamous metaplasia can be divided into three stages.[15] Stage 1 is characterized by the development of small endocervical papillae and by translucent-to–somewhat opaque acetowhite change (Fig. 6–16). Stage 2 is characterized by fusion of the papillae owing to confluence of the proliferating metaplastic cells (Fig. 6–17). Stage 3 is characterized by a smooth surface of acetowhite change (Fig. 6–18). As the metaplastic cells transform into mature squamous cells, the coloration is indistinguishable from the mature ectocervix.

The interface that is easiest to identify colposcopically after the application of 3% to 5% acetic acid is the new squamocolumnar junction.

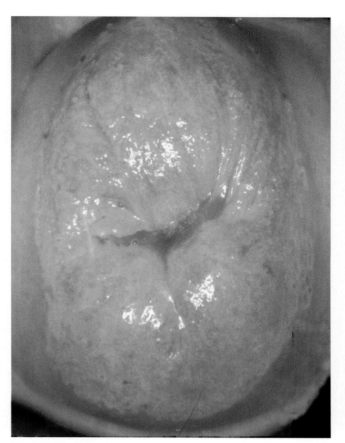

Figure 6–14. A large ectropion.

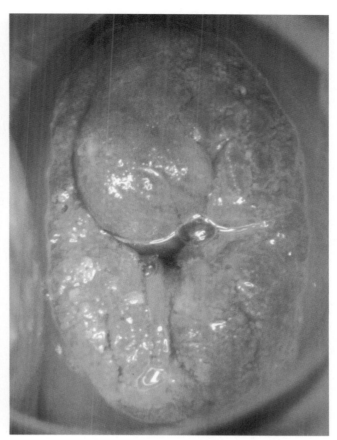

Figure 6–16. A large ectropion with the beginnings of squamous metaplasia.

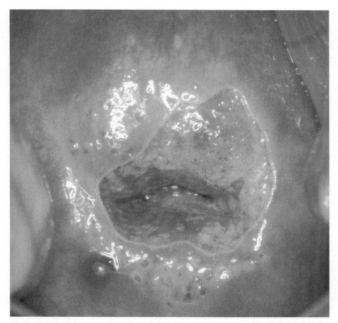

Figure 6–15. Sharp squamocolumnar junction, ectropion, and maturing metaplasia with a few islands of columnar epithelium.

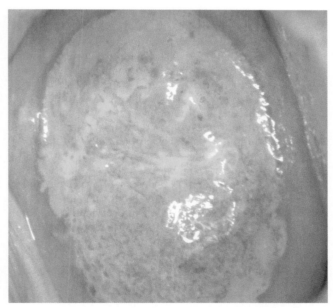

Figure 6–17. Fusion of the papillae and early formation of islands of metaplasia.

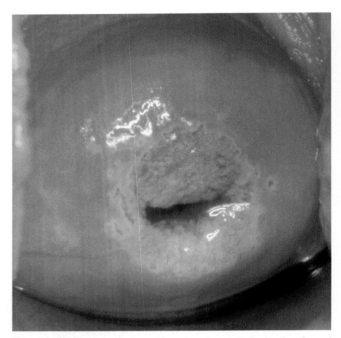

Figure 6–18. Small ectropion with a rim of metaplasia that has formed a smooth, acetowhite surface.

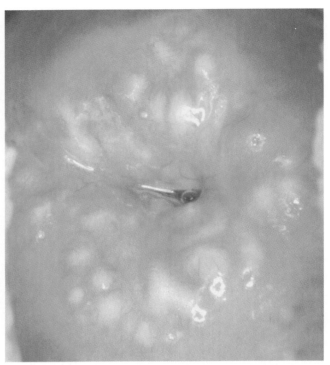

Figure 6–19. An example of multiple nabothian cysts. The most peripheral nabothian cysts mark the colposcopically visible extent of the transformation zone.

The interface that is easiest to identify colposcopically after the application of 3% to 5% acetic acid is the new squamocolumnar junction. This is because of the sharp contrast between the deep red, unaffected endocervix and the white, immature metaplastic area. In contrast, because the squamous cells at the original squamocolumnar junction mature gradually, it is difficult to differentiate colposcopically where metaplasia ends and the mature squamous epithelium of the ectocervix begins. Helpful landmarks include endocervix gland openings, or gland ostia, which are characterized by central reddened residual endocervix encircled by slightly raised whitened metaplasia, and nabothian cysts. The latter are cystic structures covered by a thinned surface and compressed dilated vessels that arborize normally (Fig. 6–19). Because the new squamocolumnar junction represents the area of the most active immature cell proliferation, it is a site that must be completely seen by the colposcopist to accurately access areas where high-grade dysplasia potentially develops.[15, 25]

Although the metaplastic areas are commonly confluent, patches of metaplasia can be seen along the endocervix surface. These patches can occur above a circumferential ring of acetowhite squamous metaplasia. The colposcopist must examine the endocervical canal carefully to identify these patches that still represent areas of the transformation zone (Fig. 6–20).

Vascular changes can be seen in areas of metaplasia. The optimal magnification to identify vascular changes is ×12 to ×16 over the original cervix. The vessels are usually hairpin in shape and 50 to 250 μm apart. Capillary loops extending to the epithelial surface are seen as punctate dots. Because the vessels that proliferate within squamous metaplasia are small, the punctation is fine, and the intracapillary distance between the dots is close. With certain vaginal infections such as trichomoniasis, the vessels will coalesce to form ecchymosis (the strawberry cervix). Mosaic tiles bordered by small-caliber capillaries are less commonly seen but can occur.[15, 24, 25]

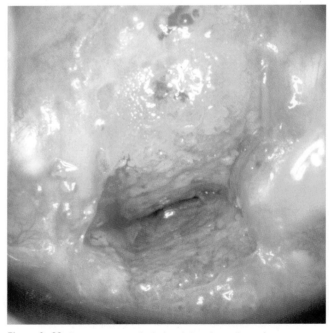

Figure 6–20. Immature metaplasia involving the endocervix.

A satisfactory colposcopic examination is defined by identification of the entire transformation zone. Although it is usually difficult to identify the site of the original or native squamocolumnar junction, it is felt that this site is located in an area that can usually be seen colposcopically. The area of major concern is the location of the new squamocolumnar junction. It is commonly located at the external os or in the endocervical canal, and it has the potential to develop high-grade dysplasias or carcinoma owing to the high rate of cell proliferation at that location. Therefore, by arbitrary definition, a satisfactory colposcopic examination implies circumferential visualization of the entire new squamocolumnar junction. Translucent acetowhite change that occurs on the endocervical papillae represents areas of immature metaplasia and should still be considered part of the colposcopic transformation zone.

WHEN IS A BIOPSY NECESSARY?

Areas of acetowhite change and angioabnormalities represent various degrees of normal and abnormal cell proliferations.

The colposcopic examination is a sensitive procedure. Areas of acetowhite change and angioabnormalities represent various degrees of normal and abnormal cell proliferations and can be easily recognized by the colposcopist in training. The specificity of colposcopy, however, is, at best, fair to good. Although it approaches accuracy rates of 85% or higher for high-grade dysplasias and occult carcinomas, the specificity decreases when one attempts to differentiate between squamous metaplasia and low-grade dysplasias.[27] A biopsy is necessary at any time to establish the origin of acetowhite or angiogenic change. The inexperienced colposcopist will initially biopsy multiple sites in the transformation zone. As his or her experience increases, the colposcopist recognizes that certain surface pattern changes correlate with specific abnormalities. The number of biopsies decreases as the colposcopist becomes more discriminating. Nevertheless, even areas with minimal acetowhite change or fine angiogenic proliferations may harbor a high-grade dysplasia. Therefore, if any question arises, a biopsy is necessary for final diagnosis.

The value of endocervical curettage is highly controversial. Scraping the endocervical canal has been considered useful in the past to evaluate areas that are not visible colposcopically. The question arises as to whether an endocervical curettage is needed in a patient with a satisfactory colposcopic examination. Because it is assumed that squamous abnormalities occur within the transformation zone and because the incidence of glandular abnormalities is infrequent, endocervical curettage in such a patient is probably cost-ineffective. The endocervical curettage may be valuable when the colposcopist is unclear whether she or he sees the entire transformation zone or when patients have cytologic evidence of glandular abnormalities. Evidence indicates that, in some laboratories, an endocervical brush sampling can be used as a substitute for a formal endocervical scraping.[28]

SUMMARY OF KEY POINTS

- At approximately 16 weeks' gestation, the urogenital plate expands upward to the müllerian tubercle, which is lined by columnar epithelium. There it undergoes cavitation and forms the rudimentary vagina lined by stratified squamous epithelium. The point where the columnar and squamous cells meet is known as the original squamocolumnar junction.

- The cervix is divided into two portions. The lower portion extends into the vagina and can be visualized during colposcopy. This region is known as the vaginal cervix or portio. The upper cervix extends from the upper border of the vaginal fornix to the uterine isthmus and is known as the supravaginal cervix.

- The majority of the cervix portio is covered by stratified squamous epithelium. As maturation of the squamous epithelium evolves, the cells enlarge and increase their overall volume as the amount of nuclear material decreases. Maturation of squamous cells is estrogen dependent.

- The squamous epithelium of the cervix is arbitrarily divided into four distinct layers: the basal or germinal cell layer, the parabasal or prickle-cell layer, the intermediate or navicular cell layer, and the superficial or stratum corneum layer. Maturation of the squamous cell varies considerably, and the only two layers that can be readily identified are the basal and the superficial cells.

- A single layer of tall columnar cells lines the surface extending from the internal cervical os to the squamous margin. Most columnar cells are secretory, but a few are ciliated and used for transport. The columnar cells invaginate into the cervical stroma to a depth of approximately 5 to 8 mm. Although this represents crypt formation, because there are no ductal or acinar structures, the cells are called endocervical glands because of their rounded shape on cross-section.

- Stratified squamous cells are markedly cohesive. Therefore, cells removed from the ectocervix during cytologic sampling are those that have exfoliated from the surface. The columnar cells are less cohesive and can be removed in clumps.

- Metaplasia is defined as the transformation from one mature cell type to a second mature cell type. The transformation usually involves a conversion from a columnar, secretory type of cell to a stratified, squamous cell. Factors that are thought to induce squamous metaplasia in the cervix include environmental conditions, mechanical irritation, chronic inflammation, pH changes, or changes in the hormonal environment. Metaplasia usually begins with the movement of the original squamocolumnar junction onto the portio, usually as a result of estrogen production or pregnancy.

Continued on following page

- It is generally felt that the process of squamous metaplasia begins in the subcolumnar reserve cells, which probably arise from the dedifferentiation of overlying columnar cells. The single layer of reserve cells is known histologically as reserve cell hyperplasia.

- As the reserve cells proliferate, the resultant immature cells gain more cytoplasm, the nuclei decrease in size, and stratification occurs. The surface columnar cells eventually slough, while the remaining stratified cells develop squamous characteristics and acquire glycogen. The presence of metaplastic or endocervical cells represents cytologic evidence that the transformation zone has been sampled.

- During colposcopy, the amount of reflected light depends on the amount of cellular material that covers a particular tissue surface. Stratified squamous epithelium has multiple cell layers that form a potential barrier between the light source and the underlying superficial stromal capillaries. A single layer of columnar cells allows the majority of the light to be absorbed, thus illuminating the underlying capillary vessels. Therefore, the ectocervix has a gray-pink color, whereas the endocervix is more pink-red in color. Areas of squamous metaplasia typically appear whiter than the surrounding lighter-pigmented ectocervix or the darker-pigmented endocervix.

- The transformation zone is defined colposcopically as the area bordered by the original and the new squamocolumnar junctions. The location of the transformation zone is variable. The new squamocolumnar junction is identified by the sharp contrast between the deep red endocervix and the white immature metaplastic area. Eventually, it is difficult to differentiate colposcopically where metaplasia ends and where the mature squamous epithelium of the ectocervix begins.

- A satisfactory colposcopic examination is defined by identification of the entire transformation zone. This implies that the entire new squamocolumnar junction is visualized.

References

1. Hendrickson MR, Kempson RL: Uterus and fallopian tubes. In Sternberg SS (ed): Histology for Pathologists. New York, Raven Press, 1992, pp 801–808.
2. Kurman RJ, Norris HJ, Wilkinson E: Tumors of the Cervix, Vagina and Vulva. Atlas of Tumor Pathology, series 3, vol. 4. Bethesda, MD, Armed Forces Institute of Pathology, 1992, pp 1–12.
3. Robboy SJ, Bernhardt PF, Parmley T: Embryology of the female genital tract and disorders of abnormal sexual development. In Kurman RJ (ed): Blaustein's Pathology of the Female Genital Tract, 4th ed. New York, Springer-Verlag, pp 8–10.
4. Linhartova A: Extent of columnar epithelium on the ectocervix between the ages of 1 and 13 years. Obstet Gynecol 1978;52:451.
5. Krantz KE: The anatomy of the human cervix, gross and microscopic. In Blandau RJ, Moghissi K (eds): The Biology of the Cervix. Chicago, University of Chicago Press, 1973, pp 57–69.
6. Singer A: Anatomy of the cervix and physiological changes in cervical epithelium. In Fox H, Well M (eds): Haines and Taylor Obstetrical and Gynaecological Pathology. New York, Churchill Livingstone, 1995, pp 225–248.
7. Lawrence WD, Shingleton HM: Early physiologic squamous metaplasia of the cervix: Light and electron microscopic observation. Am J Obstet Gynecol 1980;137:661.
8. Feldman D, Romney SL, Edgcomb J, Valentine T: Ultrastructure of normal, metaplastic, and abnormal human uterine cervix: Use of montages to study the topographical relationship of epithelial cells. Am J Obstet Gynecol 1984;150:573.
9. Ferenczy A, Wright TC: Anatomy and histology of the cervix. In Kurman RJ (ed): Blaustein's Pathology of the Female Genital Tract, 4th ed. New York, Springer-Verlag, pp 185–199.
10. Gigi-Leiter O, Geiger B, Levy R, Czernobilsky B: Cytokeratin expression in squamous metaplasia of the human uterine cervix. Differentiation 1986;31:191.
11. Maddox P, Szarewski A, Dyson J, Cuzick J: Cytokeratin expression and acetowhite change in cervical epithelium. J Clin Pathol 1994;47:15.
12. Smedts F, Ramaekers F, Leube RE, et al: Expression of keratins 1, 6, 15, 16 and 20 in normal cervical epithelium, squamous metaplasia, cervical intraepithelial neoplasia and cervical carcinoma. Am J Pathol 1993;142:403.
13. Smedts F, Ramaekers F, Troyanovsky S, et al: Basal-cell keratins in cervical reserve cells and a comparison to their expression in cervical intraepithelial neoplasia. Am J Pathol 1992;140:601.
14. Kupryjanczyk J: Epidermal growth factor receptor expression in the normal and inflamed cervix uteri: A comparison with estrogen receptor expression. Int J Gynecol Pathol 1990;9:263.
15. Burke L, Antonioli DA, Ducatman BS: Colposcopy: Text and Atlas. Norwalk, CT, Appleton & Lange, 1991, pp 29–59.
16. Papanicolaou GN, Traut HF, Marchetti AA: The Epithelia of Woman's Reproductive Organs. New York, The Commonwealth Fund, 1948, pp 30–36.
17. Cullen TS: Cancer of the Uterus. New York, D Appleton, 1900, pp 180–187.
18. Fluhmann CF: The Cervix Uteri and Its Diseases. Philadelphia, WB Saunders, 1961, pp 56–78.
19. Szamborski J, Liebhart M: The ultrastructure of squamous metaplasia in endocervix. Path Europ 1973;1:13.
20. Autier P, Coibion M, Huet F, Grivegnee AR: Transformation zone location and intraepithelial neoplasia of the cervix uteri. Br J Cancer 1996;74:488.
21. Moscicki AB, Burt VG, Kanowitz S, et al: The significance of squamous metaplasia in the development of low grade squamous intraepithelial lesions in young women. Cancer 1999;85:1139.
22. Gould PR, Barter RA, Papadimitriou JM: An ultrastructural, cytochemical and autoradiographic study of the mucous membrane of the human cervical canal with reference to subcolumnar basal cells. Am J Pathol 1979;95:1.
23. Tsutsumi K, Sun Q, Yasumoto S, et al: In vitro and in vivo analysis of cellular origin of cervical squamous metaplasia. Am J Pathol 1993;143:1150.
24. Coppleson M, Pixley E, Reid B: Colposcopy. Springfield, IL, Charles C Thomas, 1971, pp 14–16, 53–110, 155–192.
25. Kolstad P, Stafl A: Atlas of Colposcopy. Baltimore, University Park Press, 1972, pp 35–56.
26. Gilmour E, Ellerbrock TV, Koulos JP, et al: Measuring cervical ectopy: Direct visual assessment of the verses computerized planimetry. Am J Obstet Gynecol 1997;176:108.
27. Sheshadri V, O'Connor DM: The agreement of colposcopic grading as compared to directed biopsy results. J Lower Genital Tract Dis 1999;3:150.
28. Anderson W, Frierson H, Barber S, et al: Sensitivity and specificity of endocervical curettage and the endocervical brush for the evaluation of the endocervical canal. Am J Obstet Gynecol 1988;159:702.

Cytology, Colposcopy, and Histology of the Normal Transformation Zone

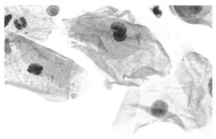

Features suggestive of a normal transformation zone:
- Nabothian cysts
- Glycogenated epithelium
- Faint acetowhite epithelium suggestive of squamous metaplasia
- Gland openings

A.

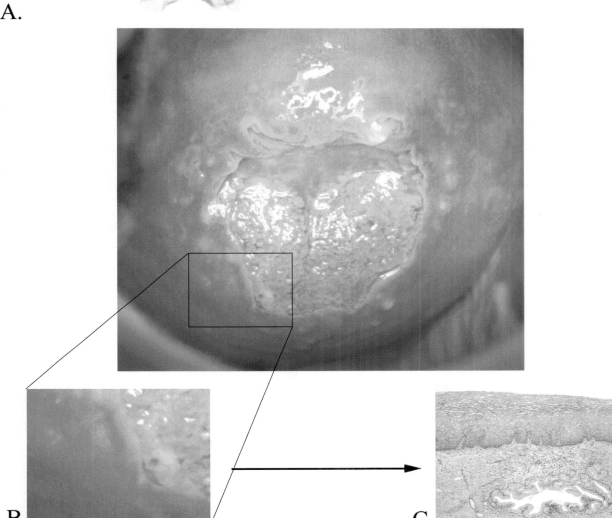

B.

C.

A. Cytology reveals normal, superficial, and intermediate squamous epithelial cells. Note that the superficial cells have a somewhat pink cytoplasm and a relatively small nucleus, approximately the size of an erythrocyte. The intermediate squamous cells have larger nuclei and, with this stain, have a slightly blue cytoplasm.

B. Area of biopsy representing mature, stratified squamous epithelium.

C. Histology reveals normal stratified squamous epithelium. Note the residual gland cleft, a remnant of the transformation process, just beneath the epithelium.

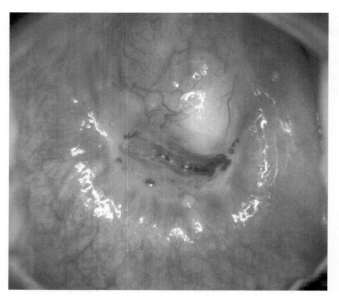

Plate 6-1. Large nabothian cyst and distinct, fine, normal, branching vessels of the cervical squamous epithelium.

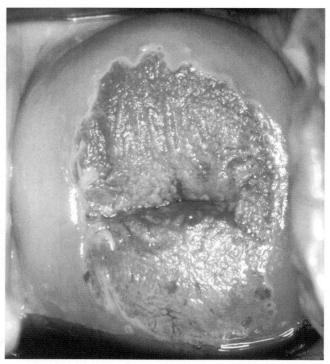

Plate 6-2. Ectropion with clearly visualized squamocolumnar junction.

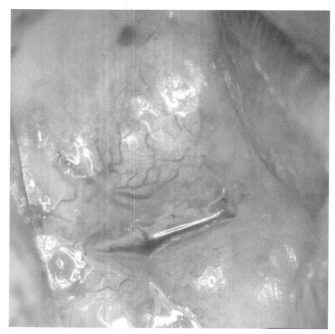

Plate 6-3. Close-up of prominent normal arborizing vessels.

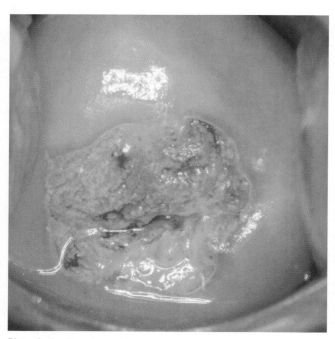

Plate 6-4. Ectropion with immature metaplasia on the anterior and posterior lips of the cervix.

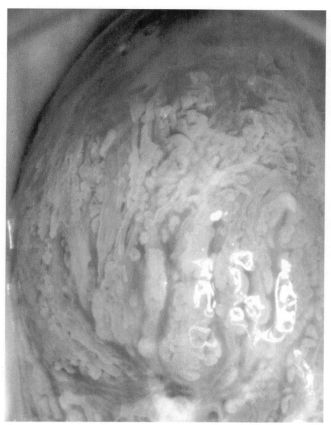

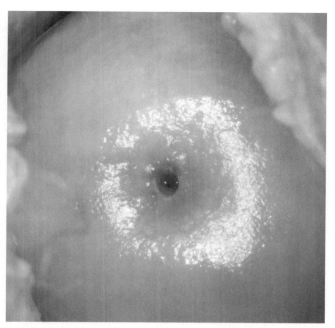

Plate 6–6. Featureless mature transformation zone with squamocolumnar junction at the narrow os.

Plate 6–5. Close-up of immature metaplasia after the application of acetic acid.

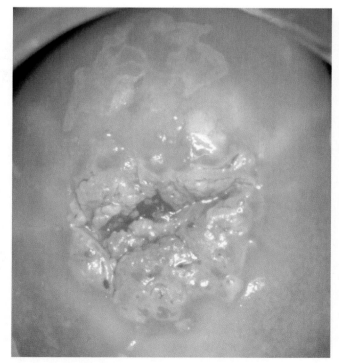

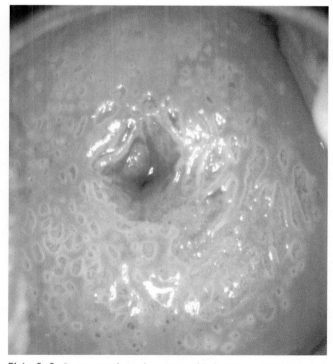

Plate 6–7. Peripheral islands of immature metaplasia along with central metaplasia.

Plate 6–8. Large transformation zone with immature metaplasia and multiple islands of columnar epithelium.

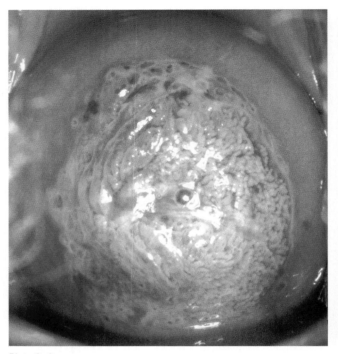

Plate 6–9. Large ectropion with very active squamous metaplasia.

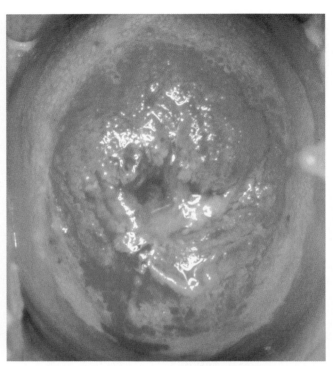

Plate 6–10. Congenitally large transformation zone with a wide rim of immature metaplasia. There is an ill-defined fine mosaic pattern present and mucus present centrally.

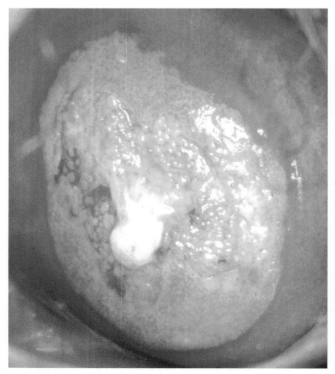

Plate 6–11. Field of immature metaplasia with a fine mosaic pattern.

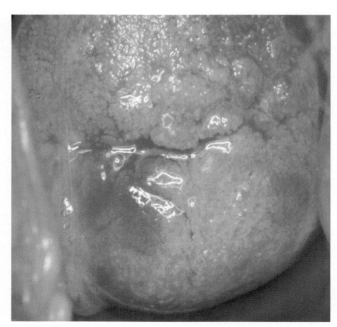

Plate 6–12. Close-up view of columnar epithelium and metaplasia.

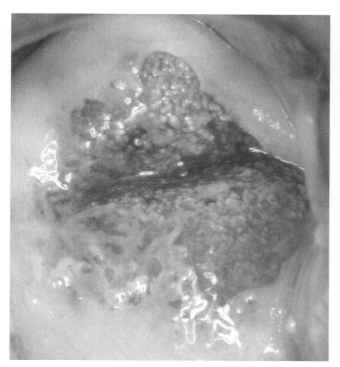

Plate 6–13. Ectropion with tongues of squamous metaplasia.

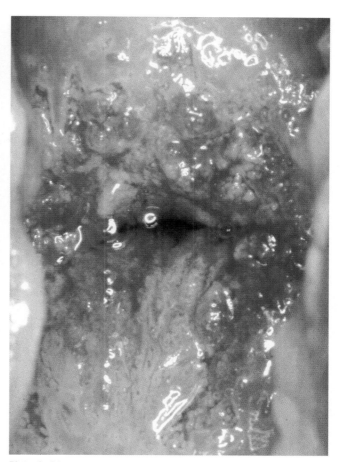

Plate 6–14. Immature metaplasia after the application of acetic acid. The new squamocolumnar junction is jagged.

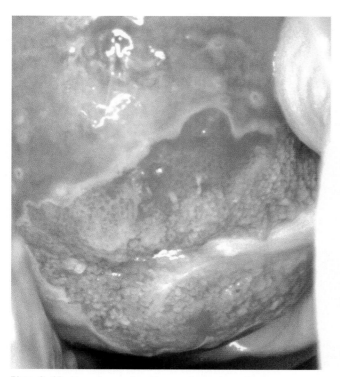

Plate 6–15. Ectropion and evidence of transformation zone remnants superiorly with several gland openings.

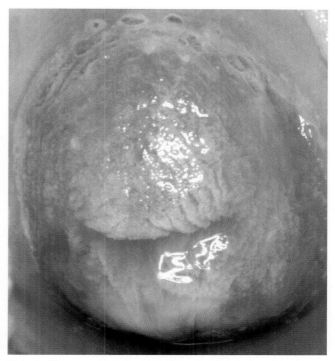

Plate 6–16. Large ectropion with islands of columnar epithelium superiorly and mucus inferiorly.

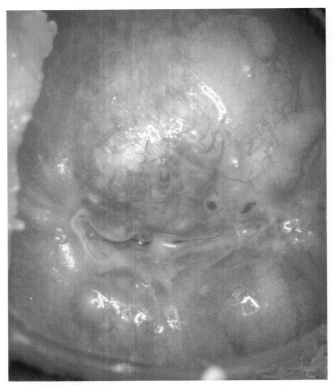

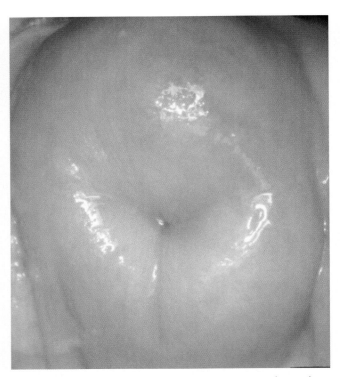

Plate 6-17. Multiple large nabothian cysts and prominent normal vessels. The squamocolumnar junction is at the os.

Plate 6-18. Mature transformation zone with the squamocolumnar junction recessed inside the os. There are no visible remnants of the transformation zone on the exocervix.

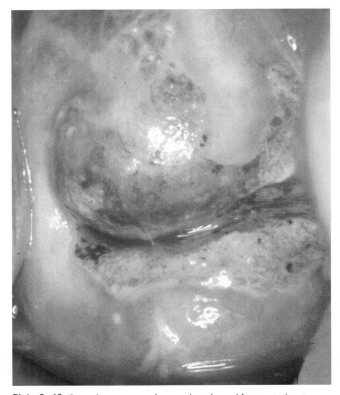

Plate 6-19. Irregular squamocolumnar junction with a maturing tongue of metaplasia on the anterior lip of the cervix.

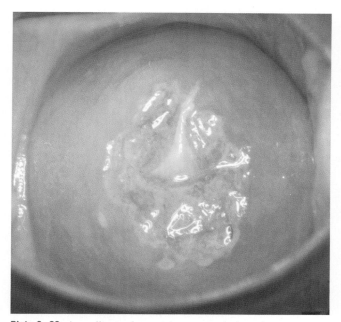

Plate 6-20. A small ectropion, squamous metaplasia, and mucus.

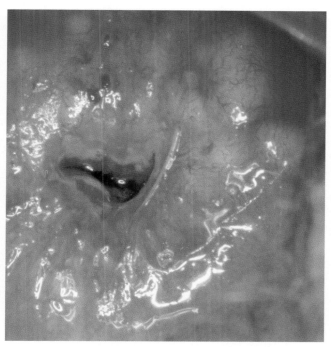

Plate 6-21. Nabothian cysts with dilated overlying blood vessels. There is a rim of metaplasia at the cervical os, and a portion has been disrupted at 6 o'clock by insertion of the speculum.

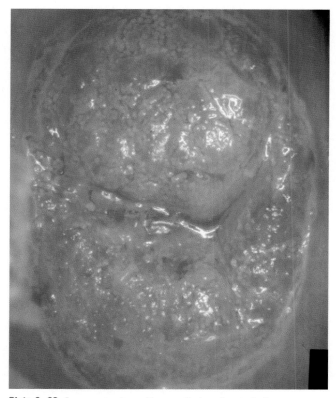

Plate 6-22. Large ectropion with a small rim of metaplasia.

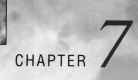

CHAPTER 7

• Adolf Stafl

Angiogenesis of Cervical Neoplasia

Of all the diagnostic methods for detection of cervical neoplasia, colposcopy is the only one that allows the study of the terminal vascular network of the cervix. By comparing the colposcopic, histologic, and vascular findings, it is possible to evaluate the pathogenesis of cervical neoplasia from normal cervix to invasive carcinoma.

NORMAL COLPOSCOPIC FINDINGS

The vasculature of the original squamous epithelium is seen as a network of fine branching capillaries.

In 70% of all prepubertal girls, there is an eversion of columnar epithelium to the ectocervix.[1, 2] There are no changes in the epithelium when this congenital eversion of the columnar epithelium is exposed to the alkaline vaginal environment before puberty. On colposcopic examination, the grape-like structures of the columnar epithelium are visible (Fig. 7–1). There is a sharp squamocolumnar junction without any metaplastic changes. The vessels below the original epithelium (columnar or squamous) are not clearly visible (Fig. 7–2). Using a special photographic technique developed by Kolstad, it is possible to increase the contrast of these vessels (Fig. 7–3).

In each of these grapelike structures of the columnar epithelium, there is a quite complicated bundle of capillaries that are separated from the observer by just one layer of columnar cells. This explains why the columnar epithelium looks intensely red to the naked eye.

However, the morphology of the vessels still cannot be sufficiently evaluated. Stafl developed a special histochemical technique for alkaline phosphatase that allows us to study the morphology of the vessels even in small biopsies from the cervix.[3] Using this technique, the vasculature of the original squamous epithelium is seen as a network of fine branching capillaries. Under the original squamous epithelium, there is a flat capillary network on the border between the stroma and the epithelium (Fig. 7–4). In the columnar epithelium, the vascular picture is completely different. In each of these grapelike structures of the columnar epithelium, there is a quite complicated bundle of capillaries that are separated from the observer

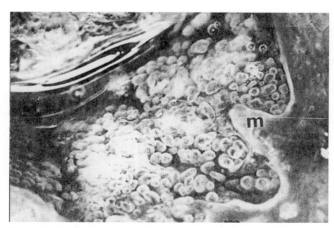

Figure 7–1. Junction between the columnar epithelium (grapelike structures) and the metaplastic (m) epithelium. (Reprinted with permission from Kolstad P, Stafl A: Atlas of Colposcopy. Oslo, Universitetsforlaget, 1982, p 55.)

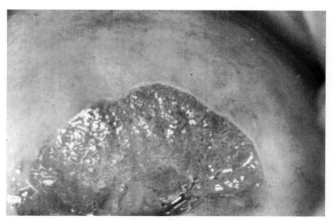

Figure 7–2. Colpophotograph of 11-year-old prepubertal girl. A sharp squamocolumnar junction without any metaplastic changes is visible. The vessels below the original squamous epithelium and the columnar epithelium are not clearly visible.

167

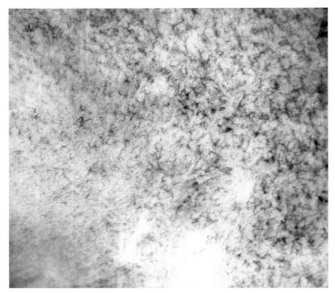

Figure 7–3. Colpophotograph of the vessels below the original squamous epithelium. A network of fine capillaries is visible.

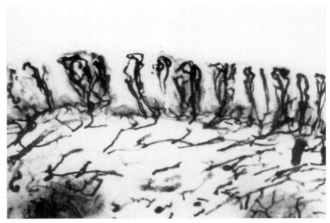

Figure 7–5. Capillaries in the grapelike structures of the columnar epithelium.

by just one layer of columnar cells (Fig. 7–5). This explains why the columnar epithelium looks intensely red to the naked eye. Although this epithelium is often described as inflamed or as an erosion, this redness has nothing to do with inflammation or erosion but reflects that these vessels are separated from the examiner's view by just a single layer of columnar cells.

The low pH of the vagina is the main stimulus to squamous metaplasia.

In puberty, because of the stimulation of estrogen, there is more glycogen in the epithelial cells. The glycogen is transformed by lactobacilli into lactic acid, and the

pH of the vagina decreases. The low pH of the vagina is the main stimulus for the initiation of squamous metaplasia. In Figure 7–6, it is possible to recognize the grapelike structures of the columnar epithelium. In between the arrows, the picture is different. Individual grapelike structures are not visible owing to a coalescence of these structures, and a flat surface develops that is still covered with columnar epithelium. When squamous metaplasia begins, it starts on the top of connected papillae—a suprapapillary metaplasia. It is possible to identify the vascular structures of the columnar epithelium, which are partially connected (Fig. 7–7). When the connection of the grapelike structures is not completed, two possible outcomes result. Either there is a connection with the surface or there is not. When these connections are visible, they are called *gland openings*. When the connection with the surface is lost, a retention cyst may develop.

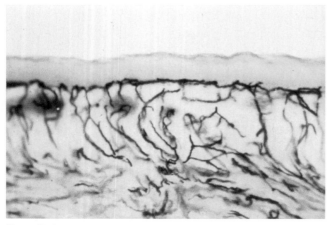

Figure 7–4. Histochemical demonstration of capillaries below the original squamous epithelium. There is a flat capillary network on the border between the squamous epithelium and stroma.

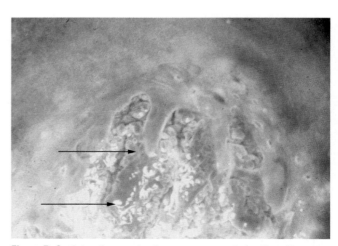

Figure 7–6. Colpophotograph of squamous metaplasia. Grapelike structures of the columnar epithelium are visible. Between the arrows, there is a coalescence of the papillae, and a flat surface has developed that is still covered with columnar epithelia. (Reprinted with permission from Kolstad P, Stafl A: Atlas of Colposcopy. Oslo, Universitetsforlaget, 1982, p 55.)

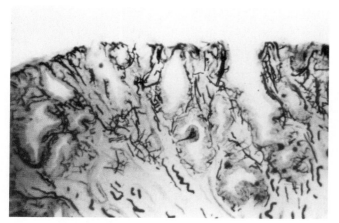

Figure 7–7. On vascular preparation, we can see coalescence of vascular structures of the original grapelike structures of the columnar epithelium.

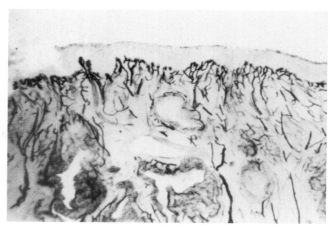

Figure 7–9. In well-differentiated metaplastic squamous epithelium, the vascular pattern is similar to that of original squamous epithelium.

These retention cysts are called *nabothian follicles.* In Figure 7–8, connected papillae are visible on the right side. Squamous metaplasia from the left side is on the top of connected papillae. The vascular pattern under a well-differentiated squamous epithelium is similar to the vascular pattern under the original squamous epithelium. There is just a flat capillary network on the border between the stroma and the epithelium. Only the remnants of the columnar epithelium in the stroma signify that this is, in fact, a well-differentiated squamous epithelium (Fig. 7–9).

VASCULAR NETWORK IN CERVICAL INTRAEPITHELIAL NEOPLASIA

The metaplastic epithelium fills all the clefts and folds of the columnar epithelium. By symmetrical compression of these vascular structures, punctation develops. In some lesions, the structures of the columnar epithelium are so compressed that they even disappear, and therefore the intercapillary distance is increased.

In the lesions of cervical intraepithelial neoplasia (CIN), the coalescence of vascular structures of the columnar epithelium is not present, and the metaplastic epithelium completely fills the folds and clefts of the columnar epithelium. The original vascular structures of the columnar epithelium are remodeled to vessels either of punctation or of mosaic. Figure 7–10 shows the beginning of atypical squamous metaplasia. The vascular structures are not connected, and the metaplastic epithelium completely fills the folds and clefts of the columnar epithelium. Colposcopically, we see reddish fields separated by whitish borders; this colposcopic finding is called *reverse mosaic.* In vascular preparations (Fig. 7–11), vascular structures of the original columnar epithelium can be recognized. They are not connected, and the metaplastic epithelium fills all the clefts and folds of the columnar epithelium. By symmetrical compression of these vascular

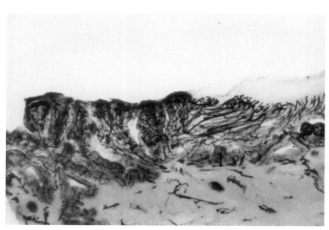

Figure 7–8. Squamous metaplasia *(right)* on the top of connected papillae.

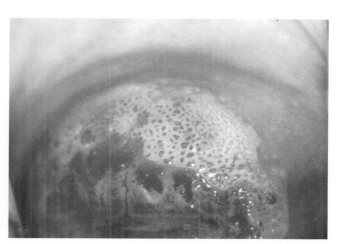

Figure 7–10. Reverse mosaic. The beginning of atypical squamous metaplasia.

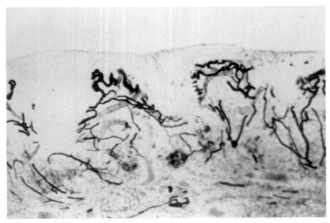

Figure 7–11. Vascular structures of the columnar epithelium are not connected, and the metaplastic epithelium completely fills the clefts of the columnar epithelium.

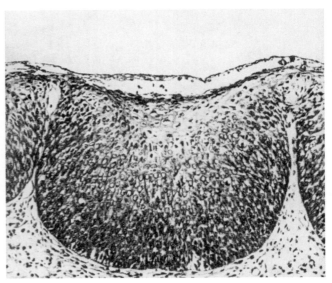

Figure 7–13. Histology in mosaic. The epithelium grows in blocks, and the vessels in the stroma papillae are compressed.

structures, punctation develops. In the vascular preparation of punctation (Fig. 7–12), some structures of the columnar epithelium are so compressed that they even disappear, and therefore the intercapillary distance (the distance in between the reddish points of punctation) is increased. The increased intercapillary distance relates to the degree of histopathologic changes.

In mosaic, the vessels surround the blocks of pathologic epithelium in basket-like structures, and the branching of these vessels in these structures is completely irregular. The corresponding histologic picture (Fig. 7–13) shows complete loss of stratification and is described as CIN 3, or carcinoma in situ in older terminology. When the nuclei are observed in high magnification, their morphology is practically identical to that of invasive cancer (Fig. 7–14).

CIN 3 is a precancerous lesion because if it is not treated, some cases may progress to invasive cancer. Our understanding of how many cases will progress in what period of time is very limited. Most of our knowledge is based on the papers of Petersen[4] and Lange[5] from Scandinavia. They followed, without treatment, a group of 67 patients with preinvasive cancers confirmed by two separate biopsies. In 1 year, 5% of them progressed to invasive carcinoma. After 8 years, 50% progressed to invasion. The study was criticized because the biopsies were taken without colposcopic guidance. Therefore, there exists a possibility either that the entire lesion was removed in the biopsy or, more likely, that the invasive carcinoma was already present but the biopsy was taken from a different area on the cervix. In spite of this criticism, the paper demonstrated that in patients with CIN 3, there exists a potential for invasion, and for ethical reasons no further follow-up studies of untreated CIN 3 were done.

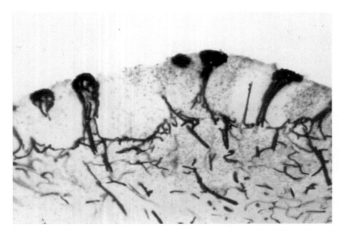

Figure 7–12. Vascular structures in an area of punctation. The original vessels of the columnar epithelium are restructured and compressed. Some are so compressed that they disappear.

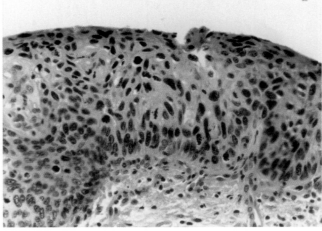

Figure 7–14. Histology of a cervical intraepithelial lesion (CIN), grade 3.

Another study was performed by Green in New Zealand in 1969.[6] He reported on 539 patients with CIN 3 who were followed up without treatment for 3 to 9 years, and only one invasive carcinoma developed. This was exactly the same expected number of invasive carcinomas in 539 cytologically normal women followed for the same time. In this study, there was a very careful exclusion of invasive carcinoma at the onset by clinical examination, cytology, colposcopy, and histology. In 1984, Indoe[7] reported that of the 948 patients in the Green study—those with histologically proven CIN 3 who were followed for 5 to 28 years—invasive cancer developed in 41 (4.3%). This unfortunate study showed that CIN 3 is a precursor of invasive carcinoma. However, the possibility of invasion may take years to develop and may not develop in all patients.

The pathologic epithelium has high metabolic needs, but its own growth compresses the vessels that supply it.

Figure 7–13 shows the histologic findings of mosaic. Blocks of pathologic epithelium are visible, and they are separated by stromal papillae. There are vessels in the stromal papillae. If the epithelium proliferates, it will compress the vessels in the stromal papillae. The pathologic epithelium has high metabolic needs, but its own growth compresses the vessels that supply it. The metabolism is diminished, and a biologic equilibrium develops. The epithelium cannot further proliferate unless new vessels develop.

In summary, the capillaries in stromal papillae of a CIN 3 lesion are compressed. The metabolic supply of the epithelium is compromised. The epithelium cannot further proliferate unless new vascularization evolves. Biologic equilibrium develops, and CIN 3 can persist for years in the absence of treatment.

ANGIOGENESIS OF INVASION

Tumors cannot grow beyond a few hundred thousand cells unless new capillaries develop. Tumors must send out chemical signals that induce capillaries to grow.

In 1971, Folkman[8] wrote that tumors cannot grow beyond a few hundred thousand cells unless new capillaries develop. Tumors must send out chemical signals that induce capillaries to grow. This process is called *angiogenesis*. He demonstrated that, in mice, a small tumor could cause the proliferation of new vessels, which, in turn, supply the metabolic needs of the tumor, so the tumor can grow. Folkman suggested that this neovascularization might be caused by a hypothetical tumor angiogenesis factor.

It is possible to shrink tumors in animals or even to make them disappear with use of angiostatin or endostatin.

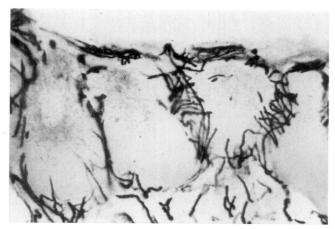

Figure 7–15. Neovascularization in a case of microinvasive carcinoma. The newly developed vessels run parallel to and just below the epithelium surface.

Similar vascular findings are found in different women. In some cases of mosaic, it is possible to see new vessels growing from the top of the basket-like structure, and these vessels run parallel with the surface and are just covered with a few layers of cells (Fig. 7–15). These vessels can be visible very clearly colposcopically as "atypical vessels" (Fig. 7–16). Based on these findings, Stafl[9] in 1975 stated that "when it will be possible to prevent angiogenesis then it will be possible to prevent invasion." Folkman and Cao et al continued with their animal research, and in 1983[10] they isolated tumor angiogenesis factors. In 1998,[11] they isolated the angiogenesis blocking factors angiostatin and endostatin. In animal experiments, they demonstrated that with angiostatin or endostatin it is possible to shrink tumors or even to make them disappear. The potential of angiostatin cancer therapy is significant because the therapy is noninvasive, there is no radiation effect, and the tumor does not develop resistance as in chemotherapy.

There is a positive outlook for the future. Drugs have already been tested in humans to block angiogenesis.

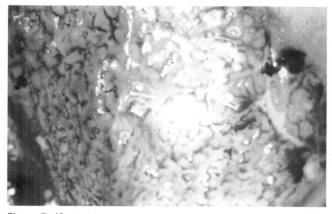

Figure 7–16. Atypical vessels in a case of microinvasive carcinoma. The vessels run parallel to the surface and are winding and small.

Presently, there are 17 active human trials with angiostatin treatment in the United States. The National Cancer Institute has put a high priority on angiogenesis research, and several pharmaceutical companies are developing industrial methods to produce angiostatin.

In conclusion, what started as a pure colposcopic and morphologic research of vessels during the development of cervical neoplasia could result in a new modality of treatment of cancer in the new millenium.

SUMMARY OF KEY POINTS

- In 70% of all prepubertal girls, there is an eversion of the columnar epithelium to the ectocervix.

- In puberty, the stimulation of estrogen increases glycogen in vaginal epithelial cells. The glycogen is transformed by lactobacilli into lactic acid, reducing the pH of the vagina. The low pH of the vagina is the main stimulus to formation of squamous metaplasia.

- The vasculature of the original squamous epithelium is seen as a network of fine, branching capillaries.

- The capillaries in each of the grapelike structures of the columnar epithelium are separated from the observer by just one layer of columnar cells. This explains why the columnar epithelium looks intensely red to the naked eye.

- The metaplastic epithelium fills all the clefts and folds of the columnar epithelium. By symmetrical compression of these vascular structures, punctation develops.

- In some lesions, the structures of the columnar epithelium are so compressed that they even disappear, and therefore the intercapillary distance is increased.

- In mosaic, the vessels surround the blocks of pathologic epithelium in basket-like structures, and the branching of the vessels in these structures is completely irregular.

- Intraepithelial neoplasia has high metabolic needs, but its own growth compresses the vessels that supply it. The epithelium cannot further proliferate unless new vessels develop.

- Tumors cannot grow beyond a few hundred thousand cells unless new capillaries develop. Tumors must send out chemical signals that induce capillaries to grow.

- Tumors cause the proliferation of new vessels in a process called angiogenesis. This neovascularization is caused by tumor angiogenesis factor.

- Neovascularization can be visible through the colposcope as so-called atypical vessels. Drugs have already been tested in humans to block angiogenesis.

References

1. Pixley E: Morphology of the fetal and prepubertal cervical vaginal epithelium. In Jordan JA, Singer A (eds): The Cervix. Philadelphia, WB Saunders, 1976, pp 75–87.
2. Linhartova A: Congenital ectopy of the uterine cervix. Int J Gynec Obstet 1970;8:653.
3. Stafl A: Histochemical technique for visualization of capillaries of the uterine cervix. Cesk Morf 1962;10:336.
4. Petersen O: Precancerous changes of the cervical epithelium in relation to manifest cervical carcinoma. Acta Radiol 1955;(suppl 127):74.
5. Lange P: Clinical and histological studies of cervical carcinoma. Acta Path Microbiol Scand 1960;143:37.
6. Green GH: Invasive potentiality of cervical carcinoma in situ. Int J Gynaec Obstet 1969;7:157.
7. Indoe WA, McLean MR, Jones RW, Mullins PR: The invasive potential of carcinoma in situ of the cervix. Obstet Gynecol 1984;64:451.
8. Folkman J: Anti-angiogenesis. Ann Surgery 1972;175:409.
9. Stafl A, Mattingly RF: Angiogenesis of cervical neoplasia. Am J Obstet Gynecol 1975;121:845.
10. Folkman J: Angiogenesis: Initiation and modulation. Symp Fundam Cancer Res 1983;36:201.
11. Cao Y, O'Reilly M, Marshall B, et al: Expression of angiostatin cDNA in a murine fibrosarcoma suppresses primary growth and produces long-term dormancy of metastases. J Clin Invest 1998;101:1055.

• Gregory L. Brotzman
• Barbara S. Apgar

CHAPTER *8*

Abnormal Transformation Zone

The process of transformation from normal meta-plastic cells to atypical cells occurs under the influence of human papillomavirus and cofactors.

The normal transformation zone (TZ) contains mature stratified squamous epithelium, squamous metaplasia, nabothian cysts, gland openings, and normal arborizing or fine reticular blood vessels. Normal squamous cells are well glycogenated and contain very little protein.[1] Under the influence of human papillomavirus (HPV) and oncogenic cofactors, the normal metaplastic epithelial cells are transformed to atypical metaplastic cells, and the process is initiated to convert the normal TZ to an abnormal transformation zone (ATZ).

The hallmark of the ATZ is the transition to a dedifferentiated cellular state that is characterized by an increased nuclear-cytoplasmic ratio.

The ATZ occurs as a result of one or more oncogenic factors that stimulate metaplastic cells to become atypical metaplastic cells, thus developing into blocks of epithelium that exhibit pleomorphism, nuclear atypia, and disorganization rather than the normal pattern of stratification of the squamous epithelial cells. These abnormal cells stimulate the capillary endothelial cells of adjacent capillaries, thus initiating an alteration of the vascular network. The blood vessels become compressed and tortuous and extend up to the surface of the epithelium, where they can be recognized by their characteristic colposcopic appearance. The abnormal cells expand centripetally by mechanically displacing and eventually replacing the normal squamous and columnar epithelium.[2] The cellular hallmark of the ATZ is the transition to a dedifferentiated cellular state and the evolution of dedifferentiated cells, called basaloid cells, which are characterized by nuclear atypia and enlargement and reduction of cytoplasm (increased nuclear-cytoplasmic ratio). On an ultrastructural level, the abnormal epithelial cells exhibit decreased glycogen and disruption of desmosomes (cellular bridges).[3, 4]

The primary responsibility of the colposcopist is to rule out the presence of invasive cancer in each ATZ. Because invasive cervical cancer is rare compared with cervical intraepithelial neoplasia (CIN), the colposcopist must look for signs of invasive disease each time the ATZ is examined. The early warning signs of cervical cancer may not be obvious to the colposcopist unless a high index of suspicion is present. Each patient must be presumed to have invasive carcinoma until the absence of an invasive lesion is verified colposcopically. Accurate identification of the entire TZ and appropriate recognition of the colposcopic signs of CIN and invasive cancer are essential steps in the colposcopic examination. Understanding the development of the normal TZ will lead to an appreciation of why CIN and invasion occur within the confines of the TZ in the vast majority of cases.

The ATZ is manifested as a wide spectrum of epithelial and vascular findings.

The colposcopic patterns of the ATZ reflect disorganization or derangement of the normal epithelial and stromal architecture. The visual expression of abnormal cellular changes in the squamous and columnar epithelium is the hallmark of the abnormal TZ. These changes may be manifested colposcopically as a wide spectrum of epithelial and vascular findings that are discussed in more detail in the following chapters. It appears that in the majority of cases, cervical neoplasia progresses through various stages of CIN to invasion over an extended period of time.[5] Colposcopically, the cellular transformation from metaplasia to atypia, then to intraepithelial neoplasia and invasion, results in characteristic features of the ATZ including leukoplakia, acetowhite epithelium, abnormal blood vessels (mosaic and punctation), atypical blood vessels, and ulcerations (Figs. 8–1 and 8–2). The colposcopically visible epithelial and vascular abnormalities of the ATZ may vary in appearance from one examination to the next. The ATZ may appear normal to the naked eye, but characteristic abnormal findings may become evident on colposcopic examination.

Misinterpretation of trivial TZ changes as ATZ findings can lead to mismanagement and overtreatment of the patient.

The hallmark features of the ATZ associated with preinvasive disease include acetowhite epithelium and the presence of vascular abnormalities referred to as mosaic

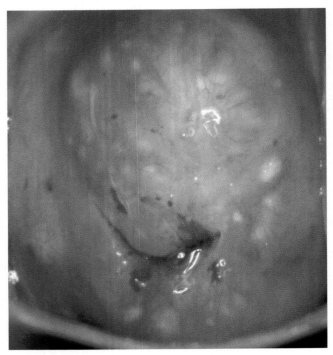

Figure 8–1. Normal, large transformation zone with multiple nabothian cysts present.

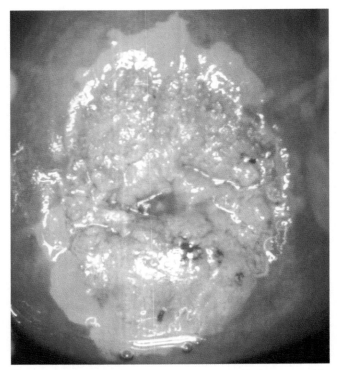

Figure 8–2. Abnormal, large transformation zone with dense acetowhite epithelium.

estrogen deficiency and pregnancy can produce an abnormal-appearing TZ. Distinguishing physiologic changes associated with pregnancy, such as decidualization and squamous metaplasia, from CIN can prove to be a formidable challenge to the colposcopist. Beginning colposcopists may be inclined to biopsy all acetowhite epithelium before developing the ability to differentiate normal TZ variants from ATZ findings. Misinterpretation of trivial TZ changes as ATZ findings can lead to mismanagement and overtreatment of the patient. The goals of the colposcopist should be to develop accurate skills for recognition of the ATZ, including warning signs of cervical cancer, and to appropriately identify the spectrum of normal colposcopic findings, including variations that have no clinical significance.

Because recognition of the findings of the ATZ is of critical importance, various techniques are used to highlight the abnormal epithelial and vascular components and to allow the colposcopist to perform appropriate biopsies. Features that can help distinguish the ATZ from a normal TZ are discussed more specifically in later chapters but include the following general guidelines[6]:

- Color of the lesion before and after the application of 3% to 5% acetic acid
- Sharpness of the margins separating the lesion from the surrounding normal epithelium
- Presence and characteristics of blood vessels
- Uptake or rejection of iodine solution

LEUKOPLAKIA

Leukoplakia or white plaque is visible grossly as a white, often raised, area that is not necessarily confined to the TZ.

Leukoplakia (white plaque) is visible grossly as a white, often raised, area that is not necessarily confined to the TZ. Because leukoplakia appears white before the application of 3% to 5% acetic acid, it is differentiated from epithelium that appears white only after the application of acetic acid (acetowhite epithelium) (Fig. 8–3A). Cytologically, leukoplakia is represented by hyperkeratosis (squamous cells without the presence of nuclei) or parakeratosis (squamous cells with pyknotic or degenerating nuclei). Histologically, leukoplakia may be represented as thickened, keratinized squamous epithelium. Normal glycogen-producing squamous epithelium of the cervix does not exhibit keratin. When the epithelium is keratinized and light cannot effectively pass thorough the epithelial layers, the light rays are reflected back, giving the tissue a whitish appearance. Depending on its adherence to the underlying epithelium, leukoplakia may be dislodged during cytologic sampling or after wiping the cervix with a cotton swab.

Leukoplakia usually occurs as a result of irritation to the epithelium, such as trauma, chronic infection, or neoplasia. Leukoplakia can result from diaphragm or cervical cap use; from developmental variants, such as benign acanthotic nonglycogenated epithelium; and, less often, from CIN or invasive carcinoma.[7] Leukoplakia is often a

and punctation. In more advanced lesions, particularly invasion, atypical blood vessels may be present, and the full extent of the ATZ may not be visible. At times, normal epithelial and vessel variations that occur with

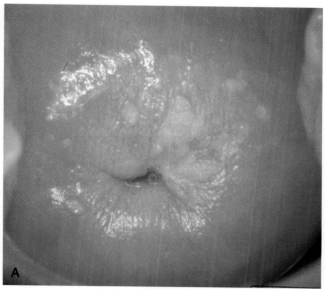

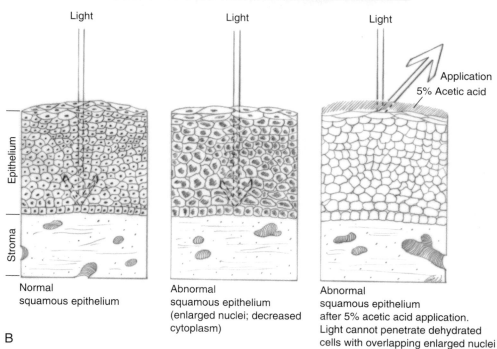

Figure 8–3. *A,* Example of leuko-plakia extending from the 12-o'clock to the 4-o'clock position. *B,* Light is absorbed by normal squamous epithelium but is reflected back with abnormal epithelium. This produces the acetowhite appearance of cervical intraepithelial neoplasia.

Light

Light

Light

Application 5% Acetic acid

Epithelium

Stroma

Normal squamous epithelium

Abnormal squamous epithelium (enlarged nuclei; decreased cytoplasm)

Abnormal squamous epithelium after 5% acetic acid application. Light cannot penetrate dehydrated cells with overlapping enlarged nuclei

B

benign finding, but histologic sampling must be performed to distinguish between benign hyperkeratosis and neoplasia.[2, 8] Growth of a significant lesion, such as keratinizing carcinoma, may produce a dense, irregular surface contour, but the most apparent colposcopic finding may be leukoplakia. Biopsy is necessary to distinguish between normal and abnormal epithelium.

ACETOWHITE EPITHELIUM

Epithelium that appears grossly normal but turns white after application of 3% to 5% acetic acid is called acetowhite epithelium.

In contrast to leukoplakia, epithelium that appears grossly normal but turns white after the application of 3% to 5% acetic acid is referred to as acetowhite epithelium. The exact mechanism of the acetowhite reaction change is not completely understood. When dilute acetic acid is applied to normal, mature squamous epithelium, it has no effect. However, in other situations, the acetowhite reaction is represented by varying degrees of whiteness depending on whether metaplastic cells or abnormal cells are present. Because abnormal epithelial cells contain an increased amount of protein, varying degrees of acetowhiteness or white epithelium will result. Immature metaplastic epithelium exhibits a distinctive acetowhite reaction. Application of 3% to 5% acetic acid produces accentuation of the clefts or infoldings of the columnar epithelium as they enlarge and swell with the application of the solution (Fig. 8–3B).

Colposcopists evaluate the color and density of the acetowhite reaction to assess the severity of the lesion. Abnormal acetowhite epithelium varies from a faint or a bright white (low-grade changes) (Fig. 8–4) to a dense gray-white (high-grade lesions) (Fig. 8–5). It is believed that when 3% to 5% acetic acid is applied to cells with enlarged nuclei and decreased cytoplasm, as in CIN, there is a temporary dehydration of the cells. This dehydration causes the nuclei to overlap, making it difficult for light to pass though the epithelium, thus creating a whitish appearance on colposcopic examination. Unlike metaplastic cells that progress from immature to well-differentiated, the ATZ cells remain immature or dedifferentiated to varying degrees, depending on the severity of the abnormality, and undergo an acetowhite reaction.[5]

Any cells with an enlarged nucleus, such as metaplastic cells or cells traumatized by infection or friction, may exhibit varying degrees of acetowhiteness.

Not all epithelium that turns acetowhite is abnormal. Any cell with an enlarged nucleus, such as metaplastic cells or cells traumatized by infection or friction, may exhibit varying degrees of acetowhiteness. For this reason, further colposcopic assessment of acetowhite epithelium is important. Gross visual inspection of the cervix after 3% to 5% acetic acid application without magnification and illumination has limitations. The magnified, illu-

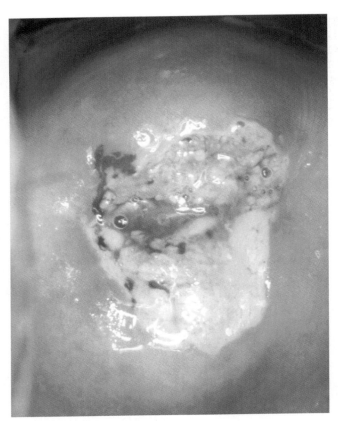

Figure 8–5. Dense acetowhite epithelium of high-grade cervical intraepithelial neoplasia on the posterior lip of the cervix.

minated examination can help differentiate abnormal epithelium from normal variants such as immature metaplasia and reparative changes. At times, it may be impossible to differentiate between benign and neoplastic findings, and biopsy is the only solution.

It is possible to have varying degrees of acetowhiteness within the same lesion, with peripheral faint acetowhite change accompanied by a central dense acetowhite reaction. This finding is known as an internal margin, and it may be associated with significant high-grade lesions (Figs. 8–6 and 8–7). Histologically, an internal border is represented by a sharp demarcation between the two intraepithelial grades of severity. It is important to recognize an internal margin. If the colposcopist performs a biopsy of only the peripheral component of the acetowhite lesion, the histology will not be reflective of the true severity of the lesion because the most abnormal area is often adjacent to the squamocolumnar junction. It is therefore important to sample the central lesion, because the central and peripheral lesions likely represent two significantly different pathologic processes in the same lesion.

It is important to determine whether the acetowhite reaction is present on the squamous or columnar epithelium. If the columnar epithelium exhibits an acetowhite reaction, it may represent metaplastic epithelium or a glandular epithelial abnormality. If there is cytologic evidence of a glandular lesion, the columnar epithelium

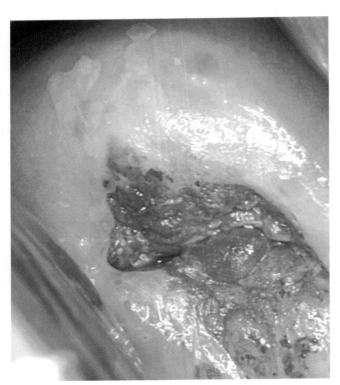

Figure 8–4. Peripheral, mild acetowhite epithelium of a low-grade lesion.

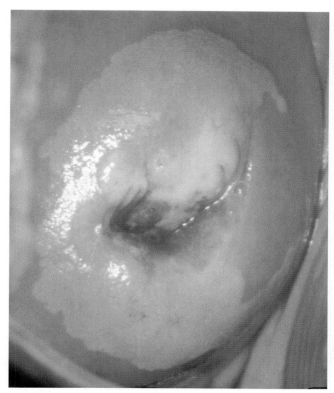

Figure 8–6. Peripheral low-grade lesion and a central denser acetowhite epithelium of a high-grade lesion at 12 o'clock, with an internal margin noted.

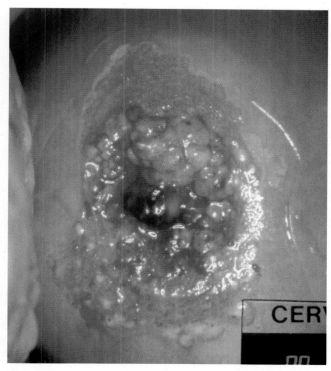

Figure 8–8. Irregular contour of the endocervical tissue at 12 o'clock may represent a glandular lesion.

should be carefully visualized (Fig. 8–8). If intraepithelial neoplasia is present at the mouth of a glandular crypt, it may appear as a white-cuffed gland opening (Fig. 8–9). These cuffed gland openings should be easily distinguished from the faint rim of metaplastic epithelium surrounding normal gland openings.

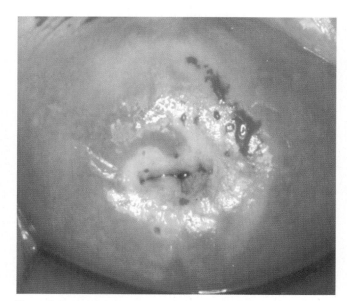

Figure 8–7. Peripheral low-grade lesion and a central denser acetowhite epithelium of a high-grade lesion. The internal margin is noted at 12 o'clock. Some background blood is present at 2 o'clock.

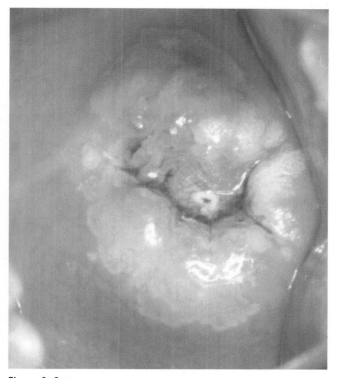

Figure 8–9. Large lesion, with peripheral low grade and central high grade, and a cuffed gland at 12 o'clock.

UPTAKE OR REJECTION OF IODINE

In addition to the use of dilute acetic acid to define the ATZ, dilute Lugol's solution is used to more precisely define the lesion tissue. Normal squamous epithelium is well glycogenated, and when a dilute iodine solution is applied, a mahogany-brown stain of the epithelium is produced (Fig. 8–10). Normal columnar epithelium, condylomata acuminata, high-grade lesions, and many low-grade lesions do not contain glycogen and will "reject" iodine when it is applied. Either a mustard-yellow or a variegate uptake pattern is produced, indicating the lack of cellular glycogen.

PUNCTATION AND MOSAIC

Punctation is a colposcopic finding reflecting the capillaries in the stromal papillae that are seen end-on and penetrate the epithelium.

The arrangement of the terminal vessels in the stroma underlying the squamous epithelium leads to the colposcopic vascular findings, which can be normal, arborizing vessels or abnormal vessels called punctation or mosaic.[5] If the abnormal epithelium does not contain any stromal papillae, it will appear white only after the application of 3% to 5% acetic acid and will lack colposcopically apparent vessels (Fig. 8–11).[4] Punctation is a colposcopic finding reflecting the capillaries in the stromal papillae that are seen end-on and penetrate the epithelium (Figs. 8–12A and 8–12B). When the stroma and accompanying

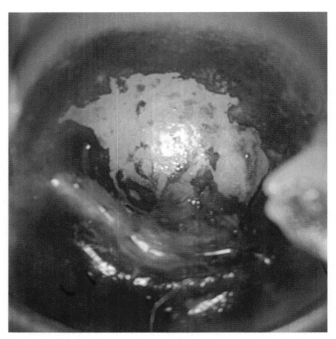

Figure 8–10. Example of rejection of iodine with cervical intraepithelial neoplasia.

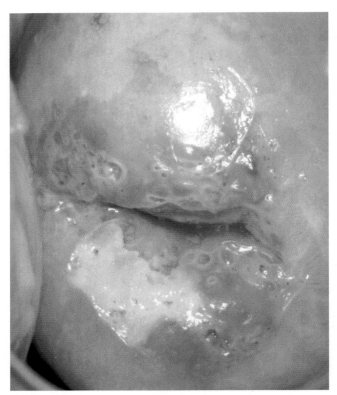

Figure 8–11. Example of a high-grade lesion with dense acetowhite epithelium on the posterior lip of the cervix and no abnormal vessels present.

capillaries are "pressed" between islands of squamous epithelium in a continuous fashion, a cobblestone or chicken-wire pattern called mosaic is produced (Figs. 8–12C and 8–13).[4, 9]

If the punctation or mosaic is not located in a field of acetowhite epithelium, it is unlikely to be associated with CIN.

Punctation and mosaic can be seen in both normal and abnormal cervical epithelium. Abnormal vessels can be visualized with a red-free (green-filtered) light. Examples of nonneoplastic epithelium exhibiting punctation, mosaic, or both include inflammatory conditions such as trichomoniasis (Fig. 8–14), gonorrhea, or chlamydial infection or very active immature squamous metaplasia. If the punctation or mosaic is not located in a field of acetowhite epithelium, it is unlikely to be associated with CIN. The punctation or mosaic pattern is described as fine or coarse. If the vessels are fine in caliber, regular, and located close together, it is more likely that the patterns represents a benign process or low-grade CIN (Figs. 8–15 and 8–16). If the intercapillary distance of the vessels is increased and they are coarser in appearance, the grade of the lesion is usually more severe, and it is unlikely that a benign process is present (Figs. 8–17 and 8–18). It should be emphasized that many preinvasive lesions lack abnormal vessels and are identified only by the presence of acetowhite epithelium.

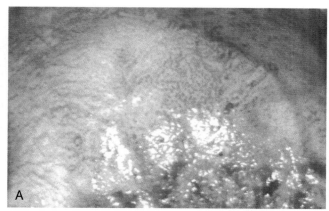

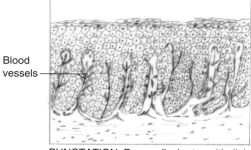

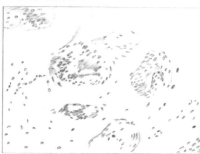

Figure 8–12. *A,* High-power view of a fine punctation vessel pattern. *B,* Perpendicular and cross-sectional graphic of punctation. *C,* Perpendicular and cross-sectional graphic of mosaic.

Blood vessels

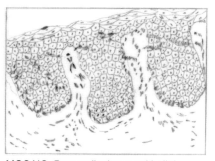

A

B

PUNCTATION: Perpendicular to epithelial surface shows blood vessels between rete pegs.

PUNCTATION: Cross-section of blood vessels between rete pegs.

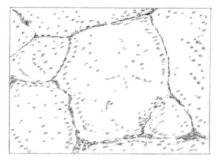

C

MOSAIC: Perpendicular to epithelial surface reveals broader rete pegs which blood vessels encircle in a basket-like arrangement.

MOSAIC: Cross-section—rete pegs evident.

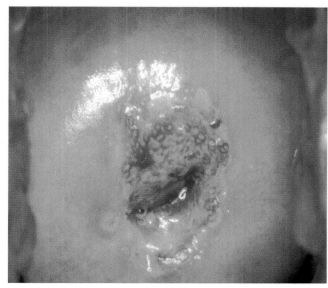

Figure 8–13. Example of cobblestone appearance of mosaic in a high-grade lesion.

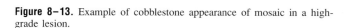

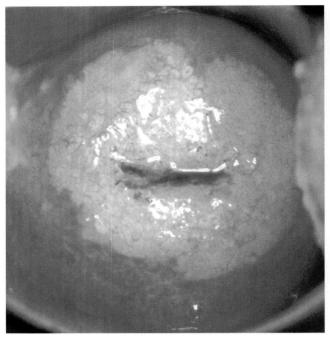

Figure 8–14. Fine mosaic in a field of immature metaplasia.

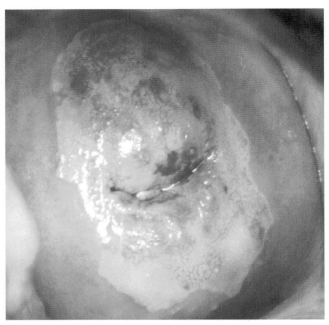

Figure 8–16. Peripheral, fine mosaic in a large, low-grade lesion.

ATYPICAL VESSELS

Although atypical vessels are the hallmark of invasion, they can be associated with other conditions such as inflammation, postradiation effect, condyloma, or normal epithelium.

When an intraepithelial lesion progresses to a microinvasive or frankly invasive lesion, there may be release of tumor angiogenic factor, leading to the development of aberrant vessels, known as atypical vessels.[5] These vessels do not display the normal arborizing vessel patterns. Rather, they are described as nonarborizing, atypical ves-

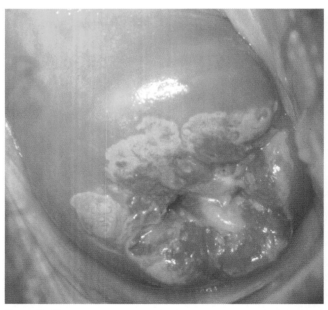

Figure 8–15. Low-grade lesion with fine punctation at 12 o'clock and mosaic at 9 o'clock.

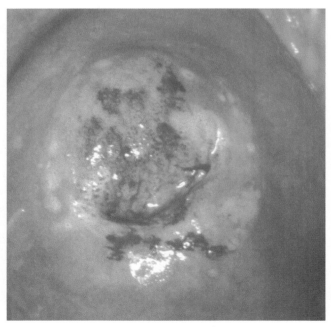

Figure 8–17. Coarse punctation at the 9-o'clock position.

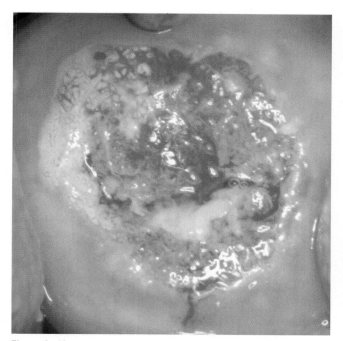

Figure 8–18. Coarse mosaic in a field of acetowhite epithelium at the 10- to 12-o'clock position.

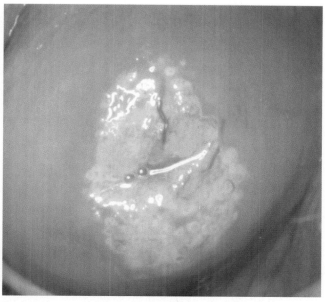

Figure 8–20. Large, sausage-shaped, atypical blood vessel.

postradiation changes, inflammatory conditions, and exophytic condylomata acuminata.

ULCERATIONS

When a breach of the epithelium occurs, the underlying stromal vessels are revealed, leading to a reddish appearance of the epithelium.

In addition to acetowhite epithelium, red areas such as ulcerations and erosions may be apparent in the ATZ.

sels with corkscrew, comma, or hairpin patterns (Figs. 8–19 and 8–20). Atypical vessels are a hallmark sign of microinvasive or frankly invasive cervical cancer. They may also be seen in other conditions where there may be aberrant vessel growth, such as healing granulation tissue,

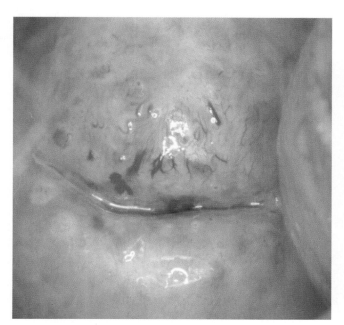

Figure 8–19. Atypical vessels on the anterior aspect of the cervix.

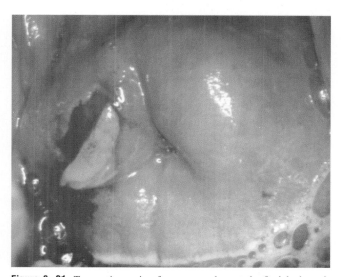

Figure 8–21. Traumatic erosion from a speculum at the 9-o'clock position.

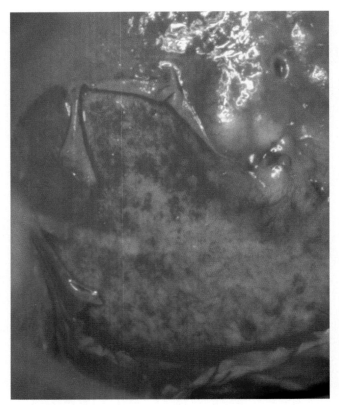

Figure 8–22. Example of how epithelial edges can roll up by detaching from the underlying basement membrane.

When the overlying squamous epithelium is interrupted for some reason and there is a breach of the epithelium, the underlying stromal vessels are revealed, leading to a reddish appearance of the epithelium (Fig. 8–21). Although these red areas may be traumatic in origin and not portend any neoplastic process, careful colposcopic evaluation and directed biopsy are essential. Ulcerations can also result from infections such as herpes simplex virus. Benign ulcerations can occur as a result of speculum or tampon trauma or pessary use.

The cellular debris present in the ulcer imparts a whitish or gray appearance to the ulcer base. Whenever there is suspicion that an ulcer is associated with a neoplastic process, it should be biopsied. Even when the suspicion of neoplasia is low, any ulcer that has not resolved over a period of a few weeks should be biopsied. Scrutiny of the ulcer margins can help distinguish a true ulcer from a traumatic epithelial lesion. Following a traumatic event, the edges of the ulcer are usually normal in appearance.[5] With high-grade CIN, there is a decreased number of desmosomes present, thus accounting for the finding of peeling edges and true erosions.[10] The epithelium is actually peeling off the underlying basement membrane, producing an erosion or rolled lesion margin (Fig. 8–22).

References

1. Cartier R: Dysplasias of squamous epithelium. In Practical Colposcopy. Paris, France, Laboratorie Cartier, 1984, pp 21–23.
2. Ferency A, Wright T: Anatomy and histology of the cervix. In Kurman R (ed): Blaustein's Pathology of the Female Genital Tract, 4th ed. New York, Springer-Verlag, 1994.
3. Feldman D, Romney S, Edgcomb J, Valentine T: Ultrastructure of normal, metaplastic, and abnormal human uterine cervix: Use of montages to study the topographical relationship of epithelial cells. Am J Obstet Gynecol 1984;150:573.
4. Coppleson M, Pixley E, Reid B: Colposcopy. A Scientific and Practical Approach to the Cervix, Vagina and Vulva in Health and Disease, 3rd ed. Springfield, IL, Charles C Thomas, 1987.
5. Coppleson M, Dalrymple J, Atkinson K: Colposcopic differentiation of abnormalities arising in the transformation zone. Obstet Gynecol Clin North Am 1993;20:83.
6. Burghardt E, Pickel H, Girardi F (eds): Colposcopy Cervical Pathology Textbook and Atlas, 3rd ed. New York, Thieme, 1998.
7. Wespi H: Colposcopic-histologic correlations in the benign acanthotic nonglycogenated squamous epithelium of the uterine cervix. Colp Gynecol Laser Surg 1986;2:147.
8. Gray LA: Colposcopy. In Dysplasia, Carcinoma-in-Situ and Microinvasive Cancer of the Cervix Uteri. Springfield, IL, Charles C Thomas, 1964, pp 246–249.
9. Burghardt E: Premalignant conditions of the cervix. Clin Obstet Gynaecol 1976;3:257.
10. Richart R: Cervical intraepithelial neoplasia. Pathol Ann 1973;8: 301.

Cytology, Colposcopy, and Histology of the Abnormal Transformation Zone

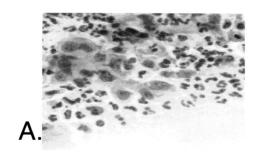

A.

Features suggestive of an ATZ:
- Acetowhite epithelium
- Erosion/ulceration
- Internal margins
- Abnormal/atypical blood vessels
- Leukoplakia

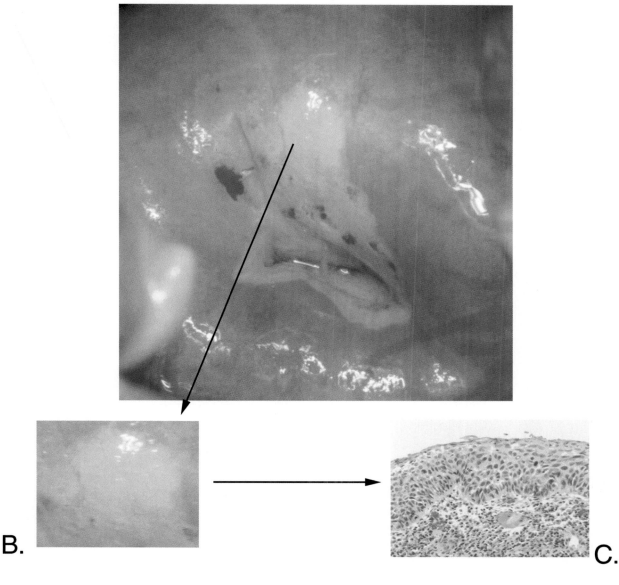

B.

C.

A. HSIL cytologic smear. The epithelial cells show coarse nuclear chromatin and irregular nuclear outlines with increased nuclear-cytoplasmic ratio.

B. Area of biopsy. Dense acetowhite epithelium.

C. In this lesion, CIN 2 and CIN 3 are present. There is basal epithelial crowding with lack of maturation. Basement membrane is intact.

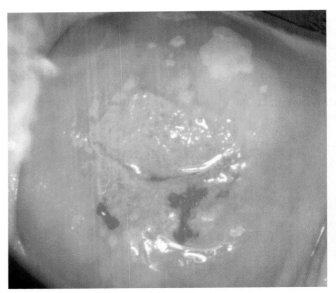

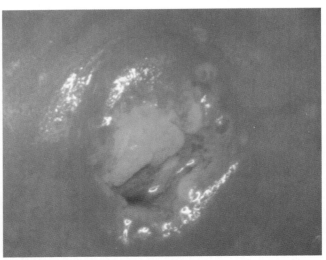

Plate 8-2. High-grade lesion with dense acetowhite epithelium on the anterior lip of the cervix.

Plate 8-1. Peripheral geographic acetowhite epithelium of a low-grade cervical intraepithelial lesion.

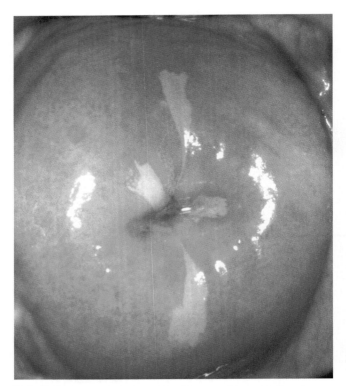

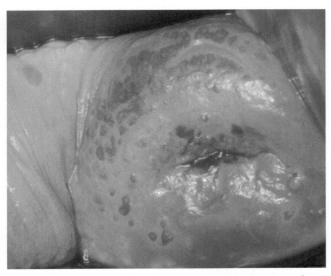

Plate 8-3. Low-grade lesion with mild acetowhite epithelium in geographic patterns.

Plate 8-4. Abnormal transformation zone with blotchy areas of erythema (so-called strawberry spots) from *Trichomonas vaginalis*.

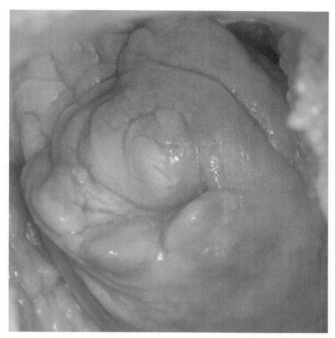

Plate 8–5. Cervix distorted from prior treatment exhibiting leukoplakia from 9 to 12 o'clock.

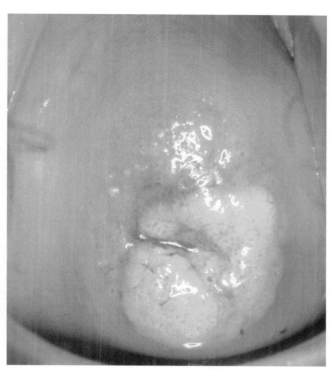

Plate 8–6. High-grade lesion with dense acetowhite epithelium and an irregular surface contour.

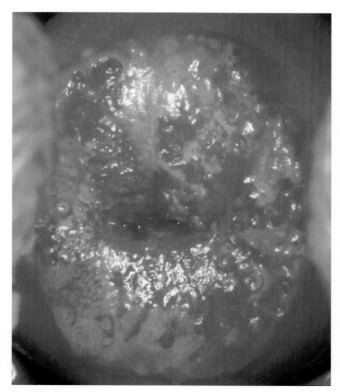

Plate 8–7. High-grade lesion with acetowhite epithelium and coarse mosaic at the 1-o'clock position.

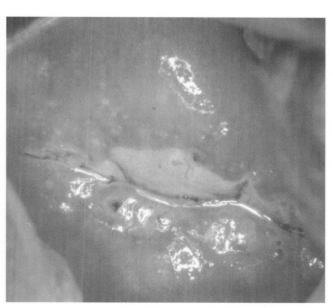

Plate 8–8. Acetowhite epithelium on the anterior lip of cervix with inadequate view of squamocolumnar junction.

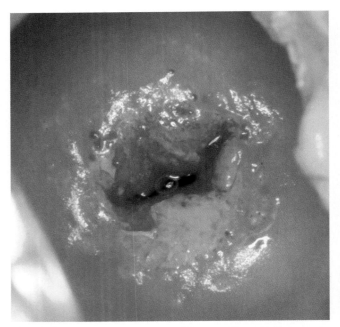

Plate 8-9. Low-grade lesion with mild acetowhite epithelium on the posterior lip of the cervix.

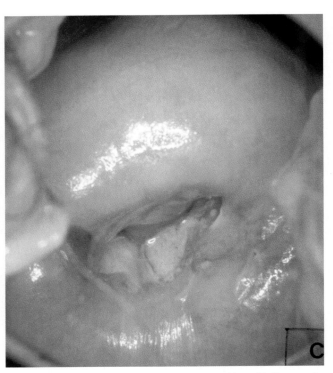

Plate 8-10. High-grade lesion with dense acetowhite epithelium on the posterior lip of the cervix near the os.

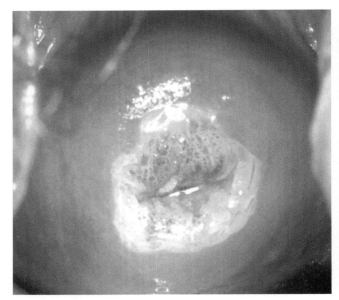

Plate 8-11. High-grade lesion with coarse punctation on the anterior lip of the cervix.

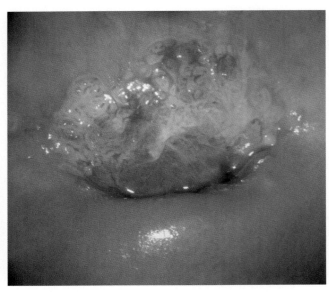

Plate 8-12. Acetowhite epithelium with mosaic that was high-grade cervical intraepithelial lesion on biopsy.

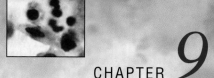

CHAPTER *9*

Colposcopic Assessment System

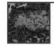

A

- Mary M. Rubin
- Dorothy M. Barbo

Rubin and Barbo Colposcopic Assessment System

COLPOSCOPIC GRADING HISTORY

The purpose of a thorough and systematic colposcopic assessment is to assist the colposcopist in selecting the most abnormal lesions to biopsy and to rule out the presence of invasive cancer.

The purpose of a colposcopic assessment method is to assist the colposcopist in selecting the most abnormal lesions to biopsy and to rule out the presence of invasive cancer. Using a systematic approach to colposcopic assessment is not a new exercise, although there is currently much more discussion about the approach as colposcopists attempt to accurately determine the presence or absence of cervical disease. In the early days of colposcopic evaluation, pioneers of the art and science of colposcopy, such as Burghardt, Coppelson, and Kolstadt and Stafl, defined certain colposcopic criteria that were thought to be associated with abnormalities, especially higher-grade lesions.[1-3] These abnormal findings included leukoplakia, acetowhite epithelium, punctation, mosaic, and atypical vessels. Squamous metaplasia, gland openings, islands of columnar epithelium, and nabothian cysts were considered normal findings. More recently, others have used modifications of these same colposcopic descriptors and have developed grading systems for normal and abnormal findings.[4]

When complex squamous lesions occupying the majority of the transformation zone are present, the task of selecting the most abnormal sites for biopsy can be challenging.

The presence of any abnormal findings during colposcopic examination usually initiates performance of a colposcopically directed biopsy. When a focal lesion is present or when several similar lesions are observed, the choice of a biopsy site is relatively clear. However, when complex squamous lesions that occupy the majority of the transformation zone are present, the task of selecting the biopsy sites that best represent the most abnormal lesion can be challenging, especially for the novice colposcopist. Attempts to clarify the abnormal findings by adding descriptors to these entities and by creating a quantifiable grading system are described later in this chapter.[5] Clinician educators such as Wright and Burke and their colleagues have also developed modified versions of a quantifiable system.[6, 7]

The Rubin and Barbo assessment method retains the descriptors of some of the previous grading systems but eliminates the numbers, adds descriptors for normal findings, and focuses on the possibility of microinvasive or invasive disease.

In an attempt to provide the practitioner of colposcopy with an organized framework for critically assessing the health of the cervix, Rubin and Barbo[8] developed an assessment method that retains the best descriptors of some of the previous colposcopic grading systems, but eliminates the numbers, which can be confusing. In addition, it expands the systems to include descriptors for normal findings. More importantly, it includes descriptors that focus the clinician's pattern recognition process on the possibility of microinvasive or frankly invasive disease. The Rubin and Barbo colposcopic assessment method evolved from the authors' many years of experience performing colposcopic examinations and from their collaborative colposcopic teaching efforts. The system was initially pilot-tested on new learners of colposcopy, allowing subsequent revisions to be made. All clinicians (physicians and advanced practice professionals alike) can benefit from a systematic method that points out the key features of the normal and abnormal transformation zones and assists in selecting the most severe findings for biopsy.

RUBIN AND BARBO COLPOSCOPIC ASSESSMENT CONCEPTS

The key concepts of the Rubin and Barbo assessment method include the dimensions of color, vessel, border, and surface pattern.

The key concepts of the system include the dimensions of color, vessel, border, and surface pattern. Descriptors of cervical findings in each category (normal, preinvasive disease, and invasive disease) are presented in a grid format summarized in Table 9–1. Appropriate application of the descriptors in each category enables the colposcopist to accurately determine the most severe lesion for colposcopic biopsy.

Color

As the nuclear-to-cytoplasmic ratio of the cells increases in cervical intraepithelial neoplasia grade 2, the intensity of the acetowhiteness also increases, resulting in a whiter color or in a gray-white tone.

It is also important to observe the speed at which acetowhite changes occur as well as the duration and the rapidity of disappearance, which often correlate with the severity of the histopathology.

The first category is color, and it begins with the pink hue of normal mature squamous epithelium (Fig. 9–1) and the translucent appearance of squamous metaplasia (Fig. 9–2). As abnormal epithelium evolves, it initially takes on an acetowhite characteristic, sometimes appearing shiny white (Fig. 9–3) or snow white (Fig. 9–4). As the nuclear-to-cytoplasmic ratio of the cells increases in cervical intraepithelial neoplasia (CIN) grade 2, the intensity of the acetowhiteness also increases, resulting in a whiter color or in a gray-white tone (Fig. 9–5). When the cellular abnormality progresses to a CIN 3, the acetowhiteness becomes very intense, the whitest of any category.

▼ Table 9–1

Colposcopic Abnormality: Rubin and Barbo Colposcopic Assessment System

Grade	Color	Vessels	Border	Surface
Normal	Pink Translucent	Fine Lacy Normal branching	Normal transformation zone	Flat
Grade 1 HPV/mild dysplasia CIN 1 LSIL	White Shiny white Snow white	None Fine punctation Fine mosaic	Diffuse Feathery Flocculated Geographic	Flat Micropapillary Macropapillary
Grade 2 Moderate dysplasia CIN 2 HSIL	Whiter Shiny gray White	None Punctation Mosaic	Clearly demarcated	Flat Slightly raised
Grade 3 Severe dysplasia/CIS CIN 3 HSIL	Whitest Dull white Oyster white	None Coarse punctation Coarse mosaic Dilated ↑ Intercapillary distance	Sharp Demarcated Straight Internal border	Raised
Microinvasion Frank invasion	Red Yellow Dull gray	Atypical Irregular Bizarre	Clearly demarcated Peeling Rolled edges	Nodular Ulcerated Necrotic Exophytic

CIN, cervical intraepithelial neoplasia; CIS, carcinoma in situ; HPV, human papilloma virus; HSIL, high-grade squamous intraepithelial lesion; LSIL, low-grade squamous intraepithelial lesion.

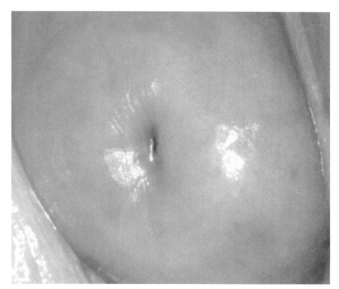

Figure 9–1. Normal cervix covered with mature, featureless squamous epithelium.

The epithelium can also appear dull, opaque, or pearly-oyster white in this grade of abnormality (Fig. 9–6). With microinvasion or frank invasion, the color tone becomes a dull yellow or red, consistent with the increased nuclear density of the cells and the increased vascularity.

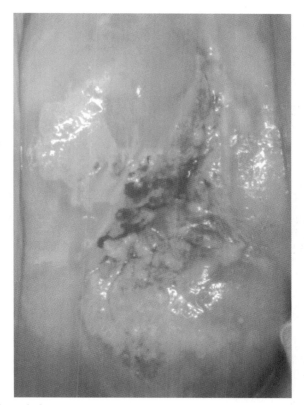

Figure 9–3. Shiny white epithelium with geographic borders typical of low-grade lesions.

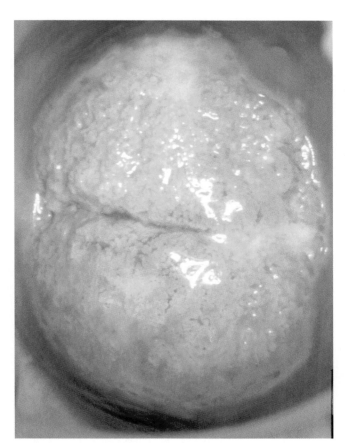

Figure 9–2. Large ectropion with immature metaplasia.

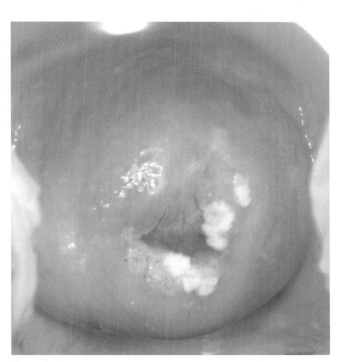

Figure 9–4. Bright white epithelium on the posterior lip of the cervix associated with condyloma. There is also some faint white epithelium from 6 o'clock to 9 o'clock, associated with cervical intraepithelial neoplasia, grade 1.

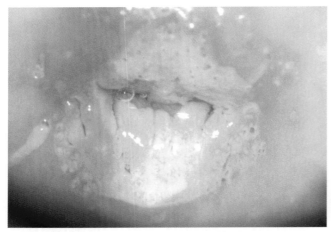

Figure 9–5. High-grade lesion with dense white epithelium on the posterior lip of the cervix.

As ulceration of the epithelium occurs, a yellow tone appears first, followed by a dull gray tone indicating cell death and necrosis (Figs. 9–7 and 9–8). It is important to observe not only the intensity of the color tone changes but also the speed at which acetowhite changes occur, as well as the duration and the rapidity of disappearance. This often correlates with the severity of the histopathology.

Vessel

Vessel patterns can range from the lacy network of vessels associated with normal mature squamous epithelium to the neovascular proliferation associated with high-grade and invasive lesions.

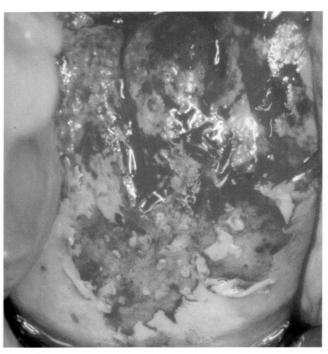

Figure 9–7. Example of an invasive cancer with yellow color, peeling epithelium, resultant ulcerations, and bleeding.

The second category is vessel pattern. Experts in the field of colposcopy, such as Kolstadt and Stafl, provide in-depth explanations for the progression of vascular abnormalities.[3] Vascular patterns associated with normal mature or maturing squamous epithelium can range from

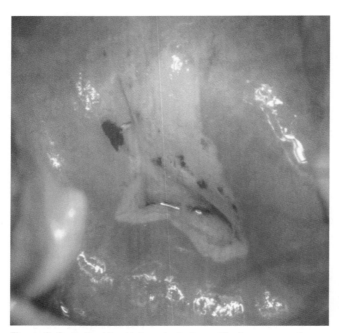

Figure 9–6. Dull-white high-grade lesion with the squamocolumnar junction not seen.

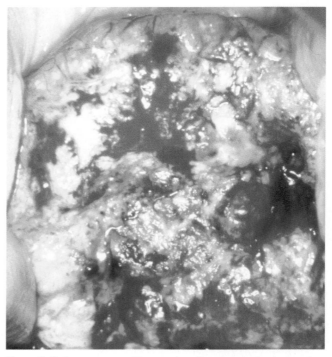

Figure 9–8. Large cancer with necrotic yellow base and raised surface contour.

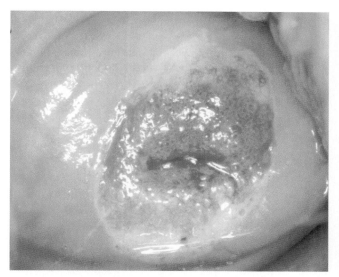

Figure 9–9. Ectropion with a rim of metaplasia and a fine, irregular mosaic pattern anteriorly.

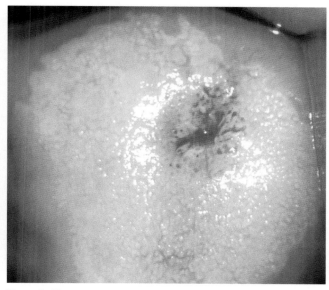

Figure 9–12. Dense white epithelium with coarse mosaic pattern.

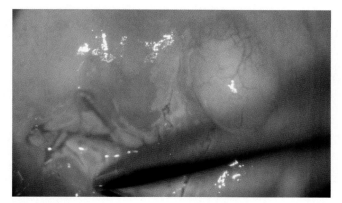

Figure 9–10. Large nabothian cyst with prominent normal branching blood vessels.

a lacy network of fine vessels (Fig. 9–9) to a dilated but branching configuration that overlies nabothian cysts (Fig. 9–10). When the first changes of abnormal cellular development occur, there may be no apparent vessels, or only very fine mosaic and punctation may be present (Fig. 9–11). As cells progress to the CIN 2 category, there are either no vessels or abnormal vessels of punctation or mosaic (Fig. 9–12). When preinvasive cellular change reaches the CIN 3 category, the neovascular proliferation may not have kept pace with the cellular growth, and the lesions may be devoid of vessel patterns. However, if vessel patterns are present, the punctation and mosaic patterns usually appear coarse or dilated, with an increasing intercapillary distance. At this stage, the vessel patterns may exhibit variation in size (Fig. 9–13).

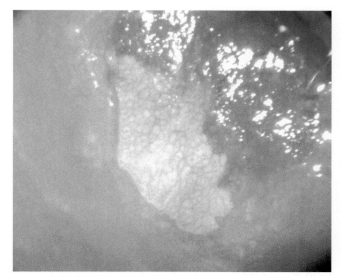

Figure 9–11. Example of fine mosaic and punctation on the lateral aspect of the cervix.

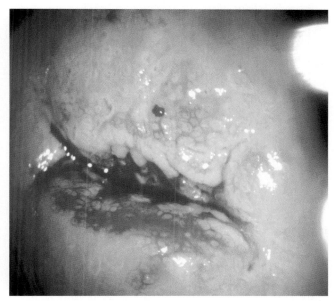

Figure 9–13. Very coarse, irregular mosaic vessels.

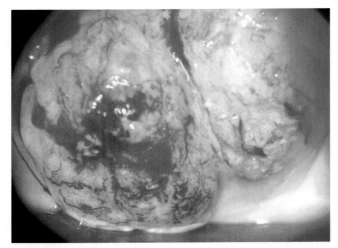

Figure 9–14. Example of atypical vessels with irregular, nonbranching patterns.

As the basal cells breach the basement membrane in microinvasive or frankly invasive disease, the vascular network becomes disorganized in its attempt to nourish the rapidly proliferating cellular growth. Changes in vessel size, caliber, shape, and mutual arrangement produce the bizarre atypical vessels often viewed as "hockey sticks," "commas," or "corkscrews" (Fig. 9–14). As the cancer progresses, the thin-walled, dilated vessels can break through the epithelial surface, creating lakes and pools easily seen on colposcopic examination (Fig. 9–15). Atypical vessels are best viewed with a red-free (green) filter before application of acetic acid. Some coarse, abnormal vessels such as punctation and mosaic may be more pronounced when viewed through the green filter after the application of acetic acid.

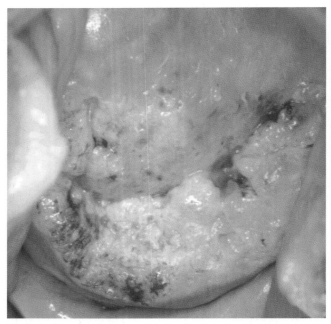

Figure 9–15. Example of a vascular pool on the posterior lip of the cervix in a patient with invasive cancer.

Border

Lesion borders may be the feathered margins of low-grade lesions or the straight and often peeling margins of high-grade disease.

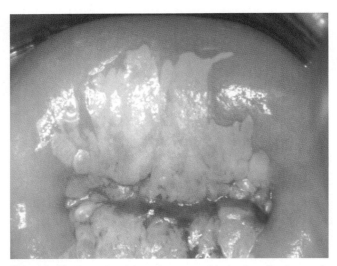

Figure 9–16. Example of irregular geographic border of a low-grade lesion.

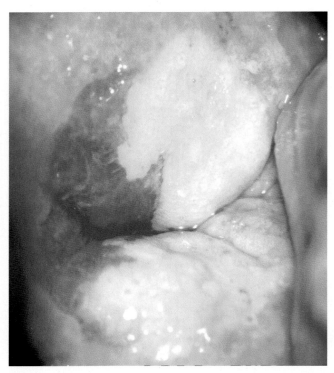

Figure 9–17. Example of a high-grade lesion (cervical intraepithelial lesion, grade 3) at 12 o'clock, with sharper borders as compared with a low-grade lesion. A CIN2 lesion is present on the posterior lip.

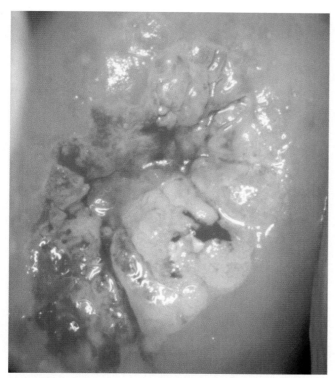

Figure 9–18. Example of high-grade cervical intraepithelial lesion with dense white epithelium and sharp margins, lower left quadrant of the cervix.

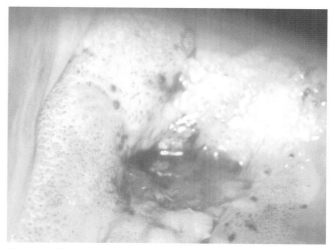

Figure 9–20. Dense white epithelium with very coarse mosaic and peeling edges at 5 o'clock and 12 o'clock.

The third category, border, refers to the edges of the lesions. Normal squamous epithelium will not have borders other than the edges of squamous metaplasia seen as the limits of the transformation zone (see Fig. 9–2).

The borders of low-grade disease will often be indistinct or have a flocculated, feathered appearance (Fig. 9–16). The borders become more demarcated and occasionally geographic as abnormalities progress to CIN 2 (Fig. 9–17). The characteristics of CIN 3 lesions include sharply demarcated, smoother, straighter borders (Fig. 9–18). High-grade lesions are often closest to the squamocolumnar junction (SCJ), where cells have the greatest mitotic activity. A lesion within a lesion, as first discussed by Reid, creates an internal border outlining the greater abnormality (Fig. 9–19). When cellular proliferation reaches a microinvasive or frankly invasive degree of abnormality, the borders are often peeling or rolled (Fig. 9–20).

Surface

The surface contour may be the flat or micropapillary surface of low-grade disease or the raised or ulcerated surface pattern of invasive disease.

The final category, surface, completes the descriptors for squamous cellular growth. Normal epithelium is usually flat (Fig. 9–21). As minor-grade cellular changes occur, the epithelium remains relatively flat (see Fig. 9–11). However, integration of human papillomavirus (HPV) can produce a micropapillary or a macropapillary (exophytic, condylomatous) surface (Fig. 9–22). As preinvasive disease progresses to CIN 2, the lesions are still relatively flat or only slightly raised (Fig. 9–23). CIN 3 lesions are most often raised, intensifying the demarcation of the borders (Figure 9–24). As cellular proliferation breaches the basement membrane, microinvasive and frankly invasive lesions can appear ulcerated. As tumor diathesis oc-

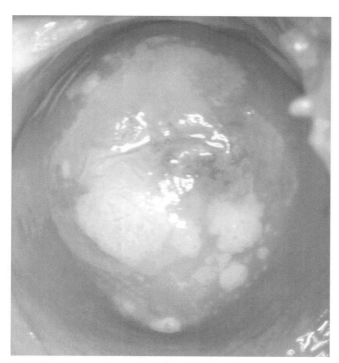

Figure 9–19. Large, low-grade lesion with central, denser, white, high-grade lesion.

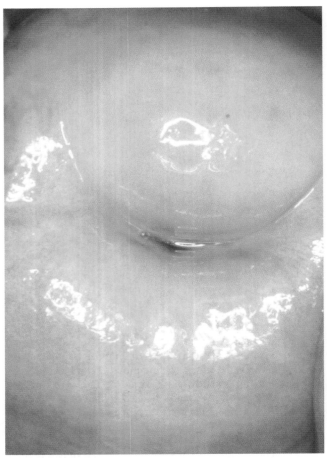

Figure 9-21. Example of flat, featureless, normal squamous epithelium.

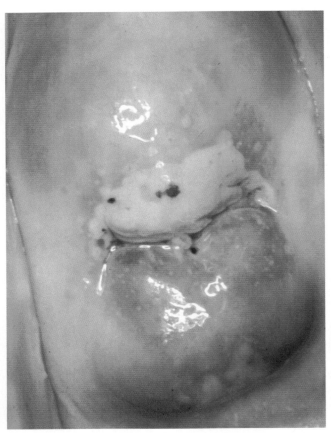

Figure 9-23. High-grade lesion with white epithelium and a relatively flat surface contour.

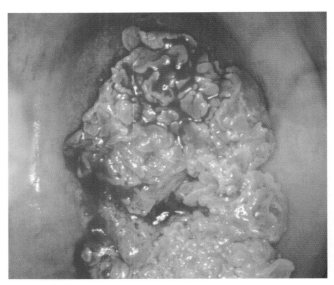

Figure 9-22. Example of micropapillary surface typical for exophytic condyloma.

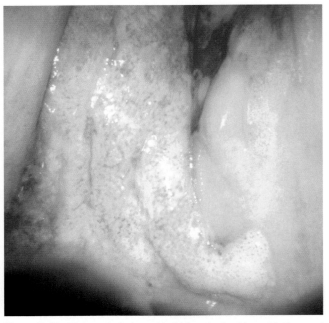

Figure 9-24. High-grade lesion with thick, raised, white epithelium and sharp border and coarse punctation.

curs, lesions may present as ulcerated, nodular, or exophytic growths (see Figs. 9–8 and 9–15).

SUMMARY

The Rubin and Barbo colposcopic assessment system is a systematic review of the chief features of the transformation zone—color, vessel, border, and surface. It helps the novice or occasional colposcopist develop colposcopic skills and locate small, early, and most severe changes in the atypical transformation zone for directed biopsies. This methodology is most applicable to squamous lesions, although adenocarcinoma or adenosquamous lesions will show some of these features, especially surface and vascular changes.

No assessment system is perfect, because squamous lesions do not always fit neatly into one line of descriptors. However, this system assists the colposcopist in a more thoughtful assessment of the epithelial and vascular features of a lesion, resulting in a more precise biopsy-site selection. The pathologist thus receives the most appropriate tissue specimen. This process enables the clinician to make accurate treatment and management decisions. Ultimately, both the colposcopist and the patient benefit from this reasoned approach to colposcopic evaluation.

correlate more with the presence of invasive cancer.

- When the first changes of abnormal cellular development occur, there may be no apparent vessel pattern, or a very fine mosaic and punctation may be present.

- As the vascular network becomes more disorganized as a result of increasing disease severity and neovascularization, the caliber, shape, and arrangement of the vessels produce the bizarre patterns of atypical vessels.

- The borders of low-grade lesions are described as indistinct or feathered, whereas the borders of high-grade lesions are sharply demarcated and may even exhibit peeling or separation from the underlying stroma.

- The surface epithelium can range from the relatively flat micropapillary surface of low-grade lesions to the markedly raised or even exophytic lesions of invasive disease.

SUMMARY OF KEY POINTS

- The purpose of a thorough and systematic colposcopic assessment is to assist the colposcopist in selecting the most abnormal lesions to biopsy to rule out the presence of invasive disease.

- The task of selecting the most appropriate site for biopsy can be challenging if the lesion is complex and occupies the majority of the transformation zone.

- The Rubin and Barbo assessment method includes some of the common descriptors of abnormal colposcopic findings and also includes descriptors for normal cervical findings.

- The Rubin and Barbo assessment method not only measures the intensity of the acetowhite epithelial changes but also addresses other color-tone changes, such as red, yellow, and dull gray, that

References

1. Burghardt E: Histopathologic basis of colposcopy. In Colposcopy-Cervical Pathology Textbook and Atlas, 2nd ed. New York, Georg Thieme Verlag, 1991, p 61.
2. Coppleson M, Pixley E, Reid B: The tissue basis of colposcopic appearances. In Colposcopy: A Scientific and Practical Approach to the Cervix, Vagina, and Vulva in Heath and Disease, 3rd ed. Springfield, IL, Charles C Thomas, 1986, p 114.
3. Kolstadt P, Stafl A: Diagnostic criteria. In Atlas of Colposcopy, 2nd ed. Baltimore, University Park Press, 1977, p 23.
4. Anderson M, Jordan J, Morse A, et al: Colposcopic appearances of cervical intraepithelial neoplasia. In A Text and Atlas of Integrated Colposcopy, 2nd ed. London, Chapman & Hall Medical, 1996, p 87.
5. Campion M, Ferris D, diPaola F, et al: The abnormal cervix. In Modern Colposcopy: A Practical Approach. Augusta, GA: Educational Systems, 1991, pp 7-17–7-27.
6. Wright C, Lickrish G, Shier, M: The abnormal transformation zone. In Basic and Advanced Colposcopy, 2nd ed. Komoka, ON, Biomedical Communications, 1995, pp 9–12.
7. Burke L, Antonioli D, Ducatman B: Atypical transformation zone. In Colposcopy Text and Atlas. Norwalk, CT, Appleton & Lange, 1991, p 61.
8. Rubin M: Follow-up of an abnormal Pap test and colposcopy. In Wallis LA (ed): Textbook of Women's Health. New York, Little, Brown, 1997, p 901.

B

• Frank Girardi
• Karl Tamussino

Burghardt's System

Hinselmann introduced colposcopy as a method for the early detection of cervical cancer in 1925, long before cervical cytology was developed.[1] The goal of both colposcopy and cytology is to predict the histologic status of the cervix. A number of studies have shown that using colposcopy and cytology together increases diagnostic accuracy.[2] However, colposcopy has not achieved worldwide acceptance as a screening modality. It is most often used to evaluate patients with abnormal cervical cytology. In this setting, the goal of colposcopy is to visualize abnormal areas on the cervix, to evaluate these lesions, to estimate the underlying histology, and to identify the most severe area so directed biopsy can be performed. Every colposcopist tries to predict the histology based on the colposcopic findings, even though a histologic diagnosis requires microscopic evaluation of a tissue specimen.

> **Predicting the histology of original squamous epithelium, ectopy, or completely normal transformation zones is relatively easy. It becomes more difficult when the colposcopic findings are abnormal.**

Predicting the histology of original squamous epithelium, ectopy, or completely normal transformation zones is relatively easy. It becomes more difficult when the colposcopic findings are abnormal. Predicting histology becomes even more challenging when benign and atypical colposcopic findings are similar, differing in only subtle features. If these diagnostic features were added to the list of colposcopic findings, the terminology of colposcopy would be expanded and would become the basis for a kind of predictive colposcopy. For such a system to be useful, the diagnostic features must be well known. Unfortunately, none of these colposcopic features are pathognomonic of malignancy. They are expressed to a variable degree and only facilitate the colposcopic assessment.

> **It is important to remember that Burghardt's system was meant to apply to colposcopy used as a screening test in all women, not just to evaluate those with an abnormal cervical cytology report.**

We use the colposcopic terminology presented at the World Congress for Colposcopy and Cervical Pathology in Rome in 1990.[1, 3] This terminology takes into account the fact that identical colposcopic lesions can be found both within and outside the transformation zone. Also, the subclassification of white epithelium, mosaic, punctation, and leukoplakia into major and minor categories implies a certain qualitative assessment. To better present Burghardt's system, we modified the 1990 nomenclature to include grading (Table 9–2). We use the term *atypical transformation zone* interchangeably with *white epithelium*. It is also important to remember that Burghardt's system was meant to apply to colposcopy used as a screening test in all women, not just to evaluate those with abnormal cervical cytology reports.

In practice, the colposcopist has to distinguish between nonsuspicious and suspicious findings and is increasingly able to do so once experience is gained. Suspicious findings are not always synonymous with abnormal findings because the latter are not always due to premalignant or invasive lesions.

DIFFERENTIAL COLPOSCOPY USING THE 1990 ROME NOMENCLATURE

Normal Colposcopic Findings

Original Squamous Epithelium and Squamous Epithelium of Metaplastic Origin

The original squamous epithelium on the outer aspect of the cervix has a continuous smooth surface (Fig. 9–25A). During the reproductive period it displays a reddish color that can vary from pale pink to intense pink during the phases of the menstrual cycle. The deep-brown staining resulting from the application of iodine reflects its glycogen content (Fig. 9–25B).

> **Squamous epithelium of metaplastic origin shows gland openings or nabothian cysts, reflecting that this area was originally covered by columnar epithelium.**

At first glance, original squamous epithelium does not differ from secondary squamous epithelium (i.e., that of metaplastic origin). Squamous epithelium of metaplastic origin shows gland openings or nabothian cysts (also called nabothian follicles or ovula), reflecting that this area was originally covered by columnar epithelium (Fig. 9–26).

▼ Table 9–2

Colposcopic Terminology

Normal Findings

Inside the TZ	Outside the TZ
Original squamous epithelium	Original squamous epithelium
Columnar epithelium (ectopy)	Adenosis
Normal TZ	

Abnormal Findings

Inside the TZ	Outside the TZ
Nonsuspicious (Acetonegative)	**Nonsuspicious (Acetonegative)**
Nonsuspicious iodine-yellow area	Nonsuspicious iodine-yellow area
Doubtful (Acetowhite)	**Doubtful (Acetowhite)**
Atypical TZ, white epithelium	
Fine mosaic	Fine mosaic
Fine punctation	Fine punctation
Thin leukoplakia	Thin leukoplakia
Erosion	Erosion
Suspicious (Dense Acetowhite)	**Suspicious (Dense Acetowhite)**
Atypical TZ, white epithelium	
Coarse mosaic	Coarse mosaic
Coarse punctation	Coarse punctation
Thick leukoplakia	Thick leukoplakia
Ulcer	Ulcer
Atypical vessels	Atypical vessels

Colposcopically Suspect Invasive Carcinoma

Microinvasive carcinoma
Frankly invasive carcinoma

Unsatisfactory Colposcopy

Squamocolumnar junction not visible
Severe inflammation or atrophy
Cervix not visible

Miscellaneous Findings

Condylomatous lesions
Inflammation
Atrophy
Ulcer
Endometriosis
Other

TZ, transformation zone.

Atrophic Squamous Epithelium

After menopause, the squamous epithelium becomes thin and devoid of glycogen. The epithelial thinning and glycogen loss are patchy, resulting in irregular iodine uptake and a stippled colposcopic appearance.

After menopause, in the absence of estrogen replacement, the squamous epithelium becomes thin and devoid of glycogen and the stromal blood supply diminishes. The epithelium becomes pale and can show a fine network of capillaries. The epithelial thinning and glycogen loss are

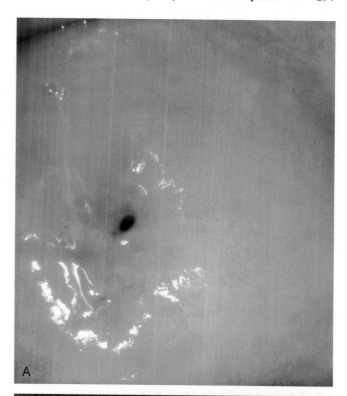

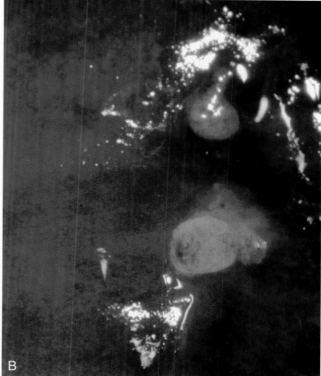

Figure 9–25. Original squamous epithelium in a woman of reproductive age. *A,* The surface is completely smooth and has a fresh reddish color. *B,* After application of iodine, the original squamous epithelium stains uniformly dark brown. Note the small, poorly demarcated iodine-yellow area that indicates metaplastic epithelium covering a nabothian cyst.

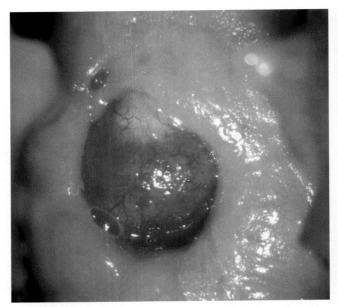

Figure 9–26. Broad-based nabothian follicle. Note the typical long, regularly branching blood vessels shining through the attenuated epithelium.

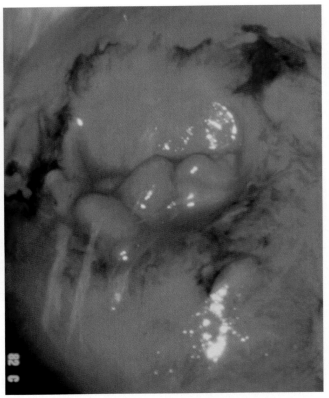

Figure 9–27. Atrophic squamous epithelium after application of iodine. The irregular, patchy uptake owing to focal glycogen retention is characteristic. Note the retention cysts at the external os, which are covered with atrophic epithelium.

patchy, resulting in irregular iodine uptake and a stippled colposcopic appearance (Fig. 9–27). In the elderly patient, the epithelium assumes a uniform light brown to yellow color as a result of complete loss of glycogen. The thin epithelial covering is fragile and makes the terminal vessels vulnerable to minor degrees of trauma, which can result in erosions and subepithelial bleeding.

Ectopy

> **Because ectopy is formed by columnar epithelium, which does not contain glycogen, it is always iodine negative.**

Columnar epithelium situated on the ectocervix some distance from the external os is called *ectopy*. The columnar epithelium of the endocervical canal is everted onto the outer aspect of the cervix (hence the old term, ectropion). The SCJ is on the outer aspect of the cervix, not in the endocervical canal.

Ectopy appears classically as a red patch. Because ectopy is formed by columnar epithelium, which does not contain glycogen, it is always iodine negative. Ectopy is usually covered by mucus secreted by the columnar epithelium. Dilute acetic acid (3%) helps remove the mucus, revealing a distinctive papillary structure, and causes the tissue to swell. This throws the mucosal architecture into sharp relief and gives the papillae a grapelike appearance. After the application of diluted acetic acid, the intense red of the red patch of ectopy changes to a pink or whitish color (Fig. 9–28).

The SCJ is the border between the squamous epithelium on the ectocervix and the columnar epithelium of the endocervical canal. Normally, it lies on the ectocervix and is sharp and steplike (see Fig. 9–28*B*). But careful examination of the margin of the SCJ often reveals a slender seam, a white color, and gland openings indicat-

ing the initiation of the transformation of columnar epithelium to squamous epithelium. This process of transformation is called *metaplasia*. It is important to pay close attention to the margins of ectopy so that significant lesions are not overlooked.

Transformation Zone

> **Fields of metaplastic epithelium within the transformation zone can vary widely in their maturation and are easily verifiable with Schiller's test, a selective indicator of epithelial maturity.**

The process of transformation characteristically begins at the SCJ. The flat epithelial seam around the periphery of an ectopy can be distinguished from the original squamous epithelium and from the columnar epithelium by its variable color and by the presence of gland openings (Fig. 9–29). It is impossible to tell colposcopically whether the transformation process at this site is due to ascending healing or to squamous metaplasia. Fields of metaplastic epithelium within a transformation zone can vary widely in their maturation and are easily verifiable with Schiller's test, which is a sensitive indicator of epithelial maturity (see Fig. 9–28*C*). The topographic progress of transformation may be haphazard. Islands of squamous epithelium can appear in a sea of columnar epithelium. The metaplastic epithelium can form finger-like processes that interdigitate with columnar epithelium.

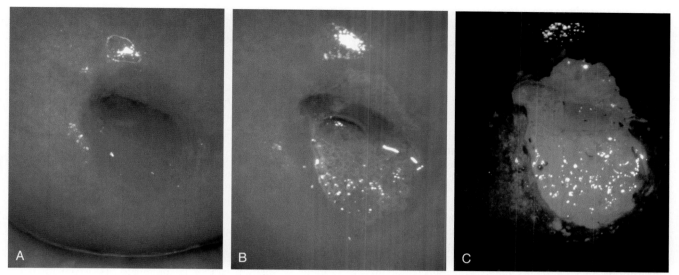

Figure 9–28. Ectopy. *A,* Before application of acetic acid, there is a small red area on the anterior and posterior lips of the external os. *B,* After application of 3% acetic acid, the grapelike structure is unmistakable. A thin rim of transformation zone is visible at the periphery. *C,* After application of iodine, the columnar epithelium is unstained (iodine negative). The transformation zone at the margin is identifiable by the incomplete staining of the new squamous epithelium.

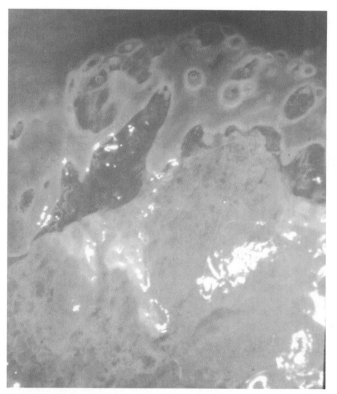

Figure 9–29. Transformation zone with residual foci of columnar epithelium after application of acetic acid.

Small islands of columnar epithelium can persist even when most of the ectopy is fully transformed. The transformation of an ectopy may not always proceed to completion, and areas of columnar epithelium can remain in the native state. The transformation zone can be distinguished from original epithelium only by the presence of

gland openings, more prominent vessels, and nabothian cysts.

Abnormal Colposcopic Findings

Nonsuspicious Iodine-Yellow Areas

European colposcopists have recognized that the majority of abnormal colposcopic findings are due to acanthotic epithelium. In the United States, acanthotic epithelium is referred to by a large number of confusing terms. An appreciation of the significance of acanthotic epithelium is important in understanding the features of the transformation zone.

Acanthotic epithelium is a great imitator. It can arise in the transformation zone and be associated with both benign and malignant conditions. The metaplastic process can result in normal epithelium, atypical epithelium, or acanthotic epithelium. Normal squamous epithelium can also change to keratinizing acanthotic epithelium, as in the case of prolapse.

Significantly for colposcopic diagnosis, acanthotic epithelium can develop in clearly demarcated fields. Colposcopic features of acanthosis include the decreased transmission of light into the underlying stroma and the presence of white epithelium. To the colposcopist, the epithelium appears as thicker than normal squamous epithelium. If the acanthotic epithelium is focal, the individual areas have sharp borders.

Acanthotic epithelium often forms rete pegs and is subdivided by tall stromal papillae that contain blood vessels and nerve endings. Acanthosis is a histologic term that denotes elongation and fusion of the rete pegs. Acanthotic epithelium is composed mostly of prickle cells, and the surface cells usually exhibit parakeratosis or hyperkeratosis. With this condition, there is hyperplasia of all layers of the epithelium composing the rete pegs. The pegs can appear as isolated columns or can be arranged in interlacing netlike ridges, therefore appearing in the transformation zone as leukoplakia, punctation, mosaic, or even white epithelium. These changes are usually induced by HPV and can also occur outside the transformation zone.

> **If the Schiller's (iodine) test is used at every colposcopic examination, one will encounter sharply circumscribed iodine-yellow areas that are otherwise not visible or are overlooked because they are so subtle.**

Colposcopically, inconspicuous iodine-yellow areas are usually caused by benign acanthotic epithelium. If one uses the Schiller's (iodine) test at every colposcopic examination, one will encounter sharply circumscribed iodine-yellow areas that are otherwise not visible or are overlooked. Such areas are especially striking if the cervix at first appears completely normal (Fig. 9–30A, B). Besides such nonsuspicious and isolated foci, iodine-yellow areas are also found in combination with other colposcopic lesions; the latter are therefore bigger and have different outlines than first suspected (Fig. 9–31).

Atypical Transformation Zone, White Epithelium

We do not use the term atypical transformation zone as an umbrella designation for practically all abnormal colposcopic appearances such as leukoplakia, punctation, and mosaic, because these findings can also occur outside the transformation zone. Naturally, it would be possible to expand the concept of transformation to every type of colposcopic lesion because, in the end, all atypical epithelia are the result of transformation, whether of columnar or of original squamous epithelium. However, it appears more reasonable to confine the use of the term *transformation zone* to its original context—that is, the area where columnar epithelium is transformed to squamous epithelium. This area is characterized by the presence of ectopy.[4-6]

In contrast, areas of potential change within the squamous epithelium cannot be predicted. To avoid misinterpretation, we continue to use the term atypical transformation zone interchangeably with white epithelium. White epithelium does not always demonstrate the patterns of mosaic, punctation, or leukoplakia. It does, however, usually contain gland openings and even retention cysts. The atypical transformation zone (white epithelium)

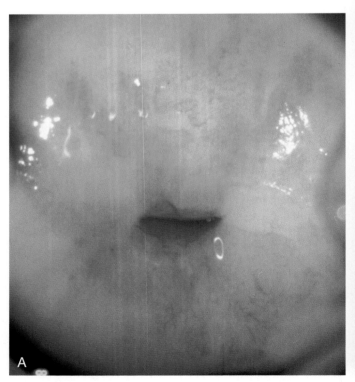 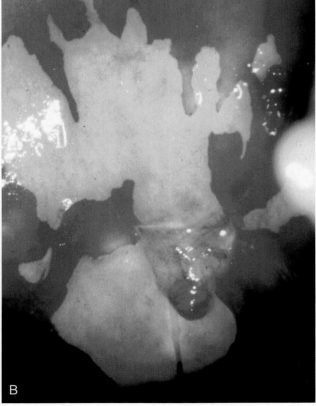

Figure 9–30. *A,* After application of acetic acid, only nuances in color suggest a lesion in original squamous epithelium. *B,* Application of iodine reveals bizarrely shaped, iodine-yellow areas. The contours remained unchanged over a 5-year period. Histology showed benign acanthotic epithelium.

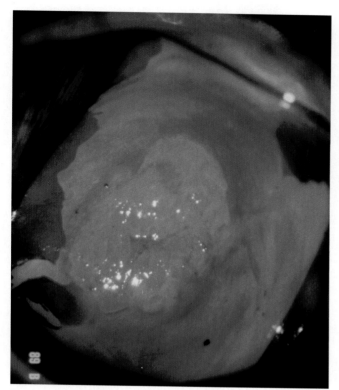

Figure 9–31. Atypical transformation zone after application of iodine. Note the borders between the smooth, iodine-yellow lesion in the periphery, which corresponds to benign acanthotic epithelium, and the more intensive yellow lesion around the external os, which corresponds to cervical intraepithelial lesion, grade 3 (high-grade squamous intraepithelial lesion).

is characterized by the hallmarks of transformation but differs from the normal transformation zone in one or more of the following features:

Color
Borders
Response to acetic acid
Appearance of gland openings
Surface contour, extent, or size
Iodine uptake
Appearance of blood vessels
Keratinization
Erosions and ulcers

These criteria do not always signify the development of atypical epithelium. Transformation can also result in an acanthotic epithelium with only slight keratinization and no elongated stromal papillae, and thus it will not appear colposcopically as leukoplakia, punctation, or mosaic. When compared with normal epithelium, acanthotic epithelium undergoes a more distinct color change with acetic acid, and its junction with the original squamous epithelium is sharp (see Fig. 9–31). In spite of these differences, it is not always possible to distinguish colposcopically between acanthotic epithelium and CIN.

Even the white epithelium of CIN may lack vessel patterns, making it difficult to distinguish from a normal transformation zone (Fig. 9–32).

Almost all colposcopically significant lesions have sharp borders.

In most cases, one can distinguish between significant and nonspecific colposcopic lesions on the basis of sharp borders. However, this feature cannot be used to distinguish between acanthotic and atypical epithelia because both have sharp borders.

Borders. Borders are one of the most important colposcopic findings. Almost all colposcopically significant lesions have sharp borders. Any sharply circumscribed epithelium must have been formed by metaplasia. If the acanthotic epithelium is focal, the individual areas have sharp borders, often recognizable by colposcopy. In any case, the borders become distinct with the application of iodine. In most cases, one can distinguish between significant and nonspecific colposcopic lesions on the basis of sharp borders. However, this feature cannot be used to distinguish between acanthotic and atypical epithelia because both have sharp borders.

Grayish-red tones, which give the transformation zone an opaque appearance, and yellow shades that are probably due to marked inflammatory infiltration of the stroma, are worrisome.

Color. Color tones can be difficult to evaluate. With the exception of the fresh red of the normal transformation zone before the application of diluted acetic acid, any other shade of red should be viewed with suspicion. Grayish-red tones, which give the transformation zone an opaque appearance, and yellow shades, which are probably due to marked inflammatory infiltration of the stroma (Fig. 9–33), are worrisome. In such cases, 3% acetic acid usually induces a distinct white color change and reveals the sharp borders (Fig. 9–34).

Response to Acetic Acid. The best criterion is the acetic acid test. Application of 3% acetic acid clarifies the colposcopic appearance by removing the cervical mucus. It also induces swelling of the atypical epithelium because of its poor cellular cohesiveness. The more marked the acetowhite change and the greater the swelling, the higher the likelihood of epithelial atypia (Fig. 9–35). However, the spectrum of color change is wide. Acetic acid slightly changes the color of the ectocervix from reddish to gray. The gray color is in proportion to the degree of keratinization of the abnormally differentiated epithelium.

The atypical transformation zone remains unstructured except for the gland openings and thus displays a white surface (Fig. 9–36). This feature is called white epithelium if neither mosaic nor punctation is present. The cohesiveness of the epithelium is directly proportional to

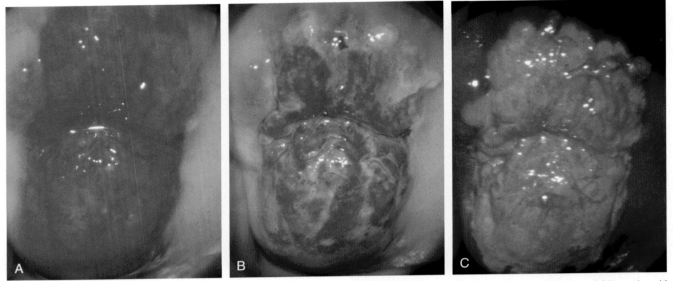

Figure 9-32. *A,* Red area demarcated from the original squamous epithelium before application of acetic acid. *B,* Application of 3% acetic acid reveals an atypical transformation zone (white epithelium). Some gland openings are cuffed. Histology showed cervical intraepithelial neoplasia, grade 3 (high-grade squamous intraepithelial lesion). *C,* After application of iodine, the pathologic epithelium is typically iodine yellow.

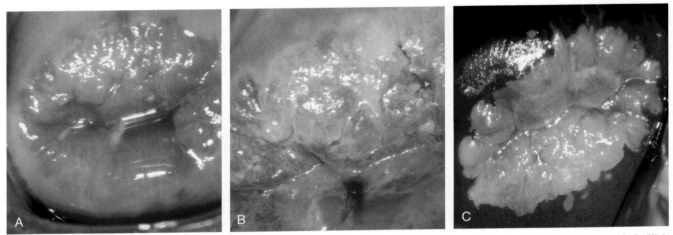

Figure 9-33. Atypical transformation zone (acetowhite epithelium). *A,* Indistinct grayish-red epithelium before application of acetic acid. *B,* High magnification of the atypical transformation zone (acetowhite epithelium). The entire squamocolumnar junction is visible. *C,* The iodine-yellow areas between 12 o'clock and 3 o'clock on the anterior lip and near the external os on the posterior lip showed cervical intraepithelial neoplasia, grade 2 (high-grade squamous intraepithelial lesion).

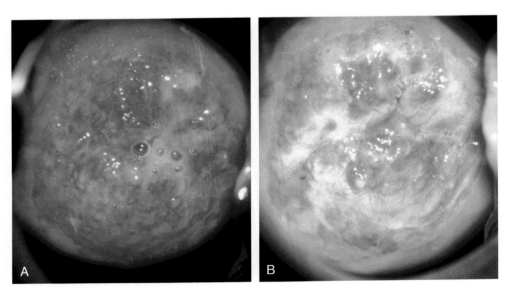

Figure 9-34. Transformation zone. *A,* The red area is a markedly vascular transformation zone before application of acetic acid. *B,* Application of 3% acetic acid reveals an atypical transformation zone (acetowhite epithelium) with cuffed gland openings on the anterior lip. Histologically, the acetowhite epithelium corresponded to cervical intraepithelial neoplasia, grade 3 (high-grade squamous intraepithelial lesion), and the pale pink area at 12 o'clock to thin metaplastic epithelium.

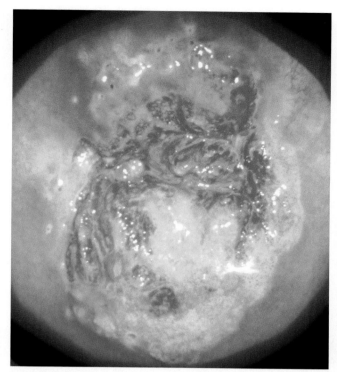

Figure 9-35. Patchy appearance after application of acetic acid. Some reddish areas and cuffed gland openings lie between the coarse and irregular acetowhite patches. Histology showed cervical intraepithelial neoplasia, grade 3 (high-grade squamous intraepithelial lesion).

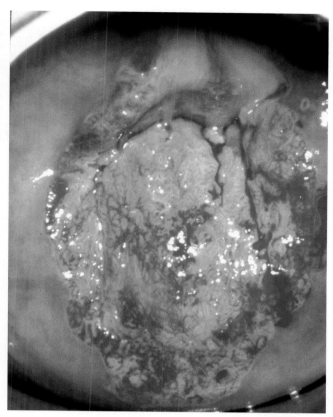

Figure 9-37. Atypical transformation zone (acetowhite epithelium) after application of 3% acetic acid. Note the friability of the large lesion. Histology showed cervical intraepithelial neoplasia, grade 3 (high-grade squamous intraepithelial lesion) with early stromal invasion.

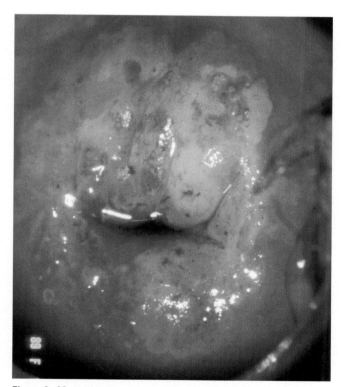

Figure 9-36. Atypical transformation zone (acetowhite epithelium) with cuffed gland openings. Histology showed cervical intraepithelial neoplasia, grade 3 (high-grade squamous intraepithelial lesion).

its differentiation. The effect of acetic acid is thus greatest on undifferentiated epithelium (Fig. 9-37). Its effect on mildly dysplastic epithelium is considerably less than its effect on high-grade CIN (Fig. 9-38).

> **Metaplasia can also involve the glandular crypts. In such cases, the gland openings will be completely lined by squamous epithelium. Colposcopically, such events are evidenced by the development of white rings after application of 3% acetic acid. The ring is wider and more pronounced with atypical epithelium than with normal or acanthotic epithelium.**

Appearance of Gland Openings. Gland openings are a characteristic feature of the transformation zone. They are visible proof that columnar epithelium has been replaced by squamous epithelium. The metaplasia is often restricted to the rims of the gland outlets, leaving the gland mouths open. The metaplasia can also involve the glandular crypts. In such cases, the gland openings will be completely lined by squamous epithelium. Colposcopically, such events are evidenced by the appearance of white rings after application of acetic acid (Fig. 9-39). The ring will be wider and more pronounced with atypical epithelium than with normal or acanthotic epithelium

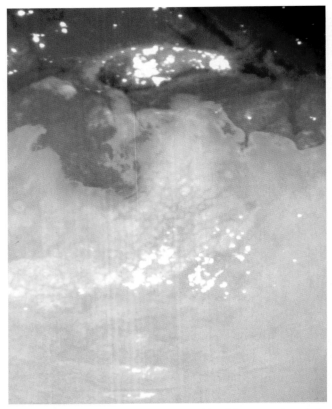

Figure 9–38. Moderately coarse mosaic with mild accentuation of the surface contour after application of acetic acid. Histology showed cervical intraepithelial neoplasia, grade 2 (high-grade squamous intraepithelial lesion).

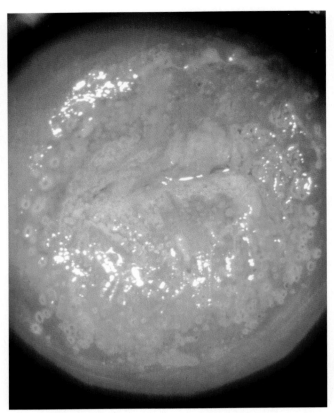

Figure 9–39. Atypical transformation zone with numerous cuffed gland openings. Histology showed cervical intraepithelial neoplasia, grade 1 (low-grade squamous intraepithelial lesion).

(Fig. 9–40). Such an appearance is referred to as a *cuffed gland opening.*

Surface Extent (Size of Lesion). Morphometric studies of conization specimens have shown that the surface extent of atypical epithelium is associated with the degree of atypia. Lesions owing to early stromal invasion are larger than those owing to high-grade cancer precursors. The marked increased in the surface extent of early invasion is due to coalescence of fields of CIN. There is a direct relationship between size and likelihood of invasion. Colposcopically suspicious but small lesions are rarely of histologic significance, whereas highly suspicious lesions are usually extensive. Small lesions are more likely to be CIN than invasive cancer.

These size considerations do not apply to acanthotic epithelium, which can cover the entire cervix or parts of the vagina. Size alone is not a diagnostic criterion but should be considered in concert with other criteria. If the latter indicate atypia, large size should raise the index of suspicion.

Iodine Uptake. Iodine staining of colposcopic lesions is variable. Brownish or brown staining owing to glycogen usually indicates benign squamous epithelium (see Fig. 9–25B). Well-developed acanthotic epithelium characteristically stains a uniform canary yellow and remains flat (see Figs. 9–30B and 9–31). Atypical epithelium also stains canary yellow but becomes mottled, and the surface is not as smooth. Staining with iodine also enhances the abruptness and morphology of epithelial borders.

Appearance of Blood Vessels. The nature of blood vessels provides an important diagnostic clue. The vascular pattern is enhanced by inflammation and by attenuation of the surface epithelium and is a prominent feature of well-circumscribed lesions.

A rich vascular bed suggests unusual transformation but is not pathognomonic of epithelial atypia. The individual vessels of the normal transformation zone tend to be long and regularly arborizing, with no abrupt change in direction or in caliber. The vessels decrease in caliber as they progress distally. Epithelial atypia is only likely in the presence of atypical vessels arranged in a haphazard manner.

Mosaic

Mosaic and punctation patterns within the transformation zone are more likely to represent CIN than are the same lesions outside the transformation zone.

The appearances of mosaic are determined by epithelial changes that usually allow a distinction between fine mosaic and coarse mosaic patterns. It can be difficult,

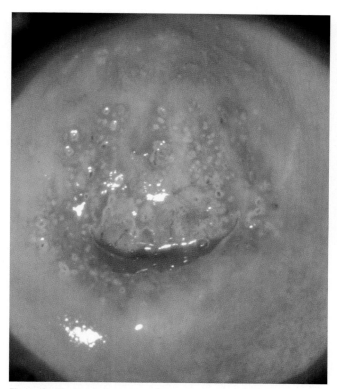

Figure 9–40. Atypical transformation zone with numerous cuffed gland openings. Histology showed benign acanthotic epithelium.

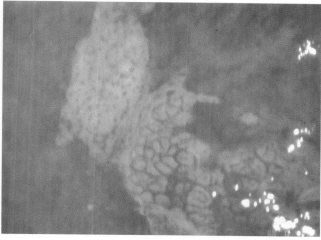

Figure 9–42. Mosaic and punctation entirely outside the transformation zone. Histology showed cervical intraepithelial neoplasia, grade 2 (high-grade squamous intraepithelial lesion).

of punctation and mosaic and epithelial atypia. Punctation and mosaic can occur in isolated fields and can coexist with other lesions (Fig. 9–43). In the latter case, the more peripherally located lesions usually represent lower-grade lesions (CIN 1, low-grade squamous intraepithelial

however, to classify a mosaic as fine or coarse (Fig. 9–41). Intermediate forms are usually caused by lower-grade squamous intraepithelial lesions, which may also produce various forms of mosaic, depending on the degree of atypia and epithelial architecture.

Gland openings and nabothian follicles are not usually found within areas of punctation or mosaic. Mosaic and punctation can also be found outside the transformation zone, in original squamous epithelium (Fig. 9–42). This is fundamental to the understanding of the morphogenesis

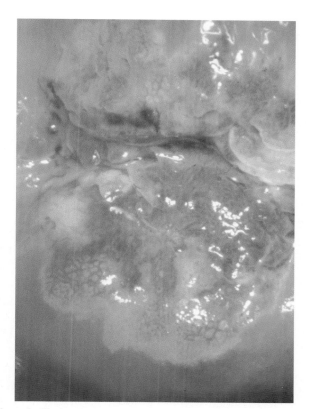

Figure 9–43. Atypical transformation zone (acetowhite epithelium) and fine mosaic and punctation at the edge of the lesion on the posterior lip between 5 o'clock and 8 o'clock. Histology showed cervical intraepithelial neoplasia, grade 3 (high-grade squamous intraepithelial lesion), and cervical intraepithelial neoplasia, grade 1 (low-grade squamous intraepithelial lesion), respectively.

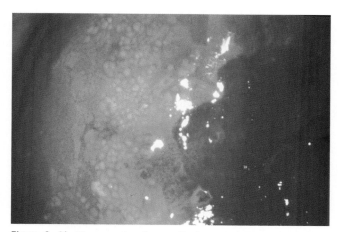

Figure 9–41. Fine mosaic after application of acetic acid. Histology showed cervical intraepithelial neoplasia, grade 3 (high-grade squamous intraepithelial lesion).

lesions) or acanthotic epithelium. This has been confirmed by topographic studies showing that mosaic and punctation occur more commonly outside than inside the transformation zone (84% versus 16%, respectively). Histologically, mosaic and punctation outside the transformation zone corresponded to benign acanthotic epithelium in 70% of treated cases and to CIN in only 30% of cases. Within the transformation zone, the respective rates were 20% and 80%.[7] In other words, mosaic and punctation patterns within the transformation zone are more likely to represent CIN than are the same lesions outside the transformation zone.

Surface Structure. Fine and coarse mosaics occur in sharply demarcated areas in the plane of the surface epithelium. Fine mosaic shows a fine network of pale red lines. Such an area may not display the mosaic pattern throughout its entirety; in places, the surface may be uniform and flat because the epithelium is not supported by elongated stromal papillae. The whole area remains in the same plane as before. Coarse mosaic is characterized by greater irregularity of the mosaic pattern. The network of fissures is more pronounced and is intensely red (Fig. 9–44). The furrows are more widely spaced, and the epithelial cobbles between them are bigger and more variable in shape than they are in fine mosaic.

The effect of acetic acid on a coarse mosaic is almost immediate. The effect of acetic acid on a fine mosaic may take a minute to develop.

Response to Acetic Acid. Before application of acetic acid, an area of fine mosaic can look quite nonspecific and may remind one of a relatively vascular transforma-

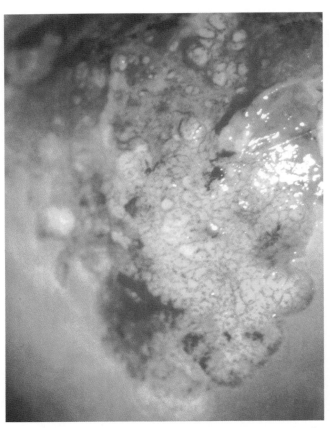

Figure 9–45. Coarse mosaic near the external os of the posterior lip. Histology showed cervical intraepithelial neoplasia, grade 3 (high-grade squamous intraepithelial lesion). There is also a fine mosaic with dense vascular network. Histology showed benign acanthotic epithelium.

tion zone that is usually devoid of gland openings or cysts. A distinct color change to gray-white occurs with acetic acid application, and the margins become sharp. The blood vessel patterns may become less conspicuous. The whole area remains in the same plane. With coarse mosaic, the swelling from acetic acid makes the coarse pattern stand out in sharp contrast to the surrounding epithelium. The gradual appearance of the coarse mosaic following acetic acid application is in contrast to the delayed effect of the acetic acid on the fine mosaic pattern.

Vessel Pattern of Mosaic. The first hint of atypia is the confinement of blood vessels to sharply circumscribed areas (especially with iodine). Small, evenly distributed epithelial fields subdivided by thin red ridges (Fig. 9–45) produce the delicate mosaic pattern associated with acanthotic epithelium. In coarse mosaic, the dividing lines are more definite, and the resulting fields are larger and more irregular. Even relatively regular and more or less parallel vessels can appear suspicious when they are wider and show an abrupt change in caliber. The vascular pattern can, on occasion, mimic the appearance of mosaic. Closer inspection, however, shows vessels with treelike branching and uniform reduction in caliber in a poorly circumscribed area.

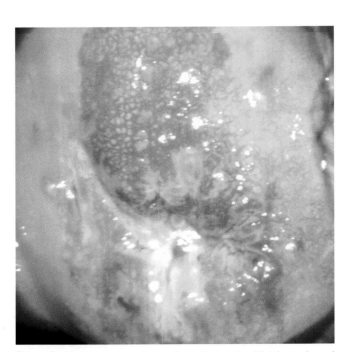

Figure 9–44. Coarse mosaic on the anterior lip. Histology showed cervical intraepithelial neoplasia, grade 3 (high-grade squamous intraepithelial lesion).

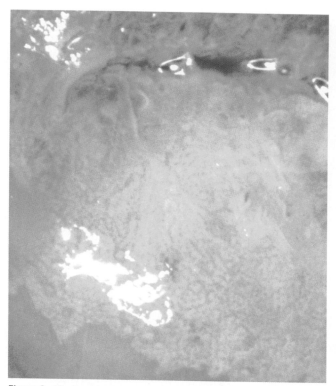

Figure 9–46. Combination of fine mosaic and fine punctation. Histologically, the mosaic corresponded to benign acanthotic epithelium and the punctation to cervical intraepithelial neoplasia, grade 1 (low-grade squamous intraepithelial lesion).

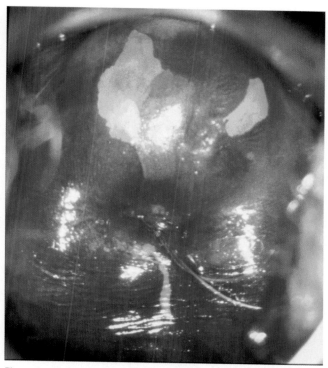

Figure 9–47. Application of iodine (Schiller's test) reveals three distinct areas outside the transformation zone: At 12 o'clock, iodine-positive punctation. Histology showed cervical intraepithelial neoplasia, grade 1 (low-grade squamous intraepithelial lesion) with koilocytosis. At 11 o'clock and 1 o'clock, unsuspected iodine-yellow areas. Histology showed benign acanthotic epithelium.

Punctation

There are two types of punctation of diagnostic importance: fine and coarse punctation. The examiner should be aware that similar colposcopic appearances could be due either to benign acanthotic epithelium or to atypical epithelium that differs only in arrangement and degree of expression. Although there are good diagnostic criteria to distinguish between fine and coarse punctation, some punctations cannot be classified unequivocally.

Color. Fine punctation characteristically imparts delicate stippling to an otherwise circumscribed grayish-white to reddish area. When the epithelium is keratinized, the dots may appear white, but they are usually red and remain in the same plane as the surface epithelium, even after the application of acetic acid. The dots in fine punctation are close together. Fine punctation is often combined with equally fine mosaic (Fig. 9–46). Fine focal punctation may be due to inflammation, in which case the margins of the inflamed area appear indistinct after application of iodine. Fine, regular punctation can also be caused by HPV infection. With Schiller's iodine test, the punctations become yellow to ochre, whereas the adjacent epithelium stains brown. This is known as iodine-positive punctation (Fig. 9–47).

Surface Structure. Usually, punctations are imprinted on a uniform surface that is undisturbed by gland openings, nabothian follicles, or any other signs of a transformation zone. The degree to which punctation is expressed depends on the underlying epithelial abnormality.

Fine punctation is characterized by small, closely placed petechiae. In coarse punctation, the petechiae are more pronounced, larger, and farther apart. In extreme cases, punctation appears in the form of papillae. This is called *papillary punctation* (Fig. 9–48). With higher magnification, corkscrew capillaries can be seen in the papillae.

Response to Acetic Acid. After application of acetic acid, coarse punctation stands out from the plane of the surrounding surface epithelium. Coarse and fine punctation may be combined with coarse and fine mosaic. The two patterns may overlap, with intermingling of dots and fissures (Fig. 9–49).

Vessel Pattern of Punctation. The blood vessels in punctation are fine to coarse and are hairpin, comma, or tortuous (corkscrew) in shape but are still regularly arranged. Within this pattern, the appearances show wide variation. The capillary loops in punctation owing to acanthotic epithelium are delicate and regular, with no increase in the intercapillary distance. The corkscrew- and comma-shaped vessels associated with atypical epithelium are coarser and show haphazard branching and great variation in caliber; the intercapillary distance is increased (Fig. 9–50).

Histologically, leukoplakia corresponds to parakeratosis or true keratinization, which cannot be distinguished colposcopically.

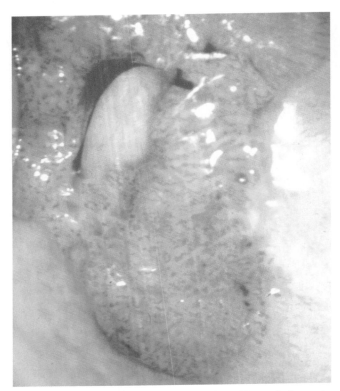

Figure 9–48. Pronounced papillary punctation with atypical vessels. Histology showed microinvasive cancer.

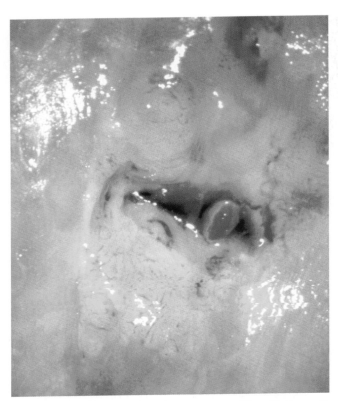

Figure 9–50. Atypical transformation zone, acetowhite epithelium with various types of suspicious vessels. Histology showed cervical intraepithelial neoplasia, grade 3 (high-grade squamous intraepithelial lesion). There is a cervical polyp covered with metaplastic epithelium.

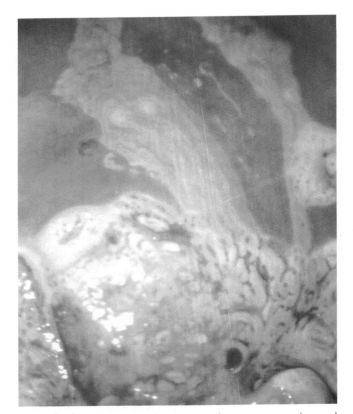

Figure 9–49. Combination of coarse mosaic, coarse punctation, and acetowhite epithelium with cuffed gland openings. Note the small erosion within the acetowhite epithelium. Histology showed cervical intraepithelial neoplasia, grade 3 (high-grade squamous intraepithelial lesion).

Keratinization. Leukoplakia can usually be seen with the naked eye, but sometimes the colposcope is necessary (Fig. 9–51). Histologically, leukoplakia corresponds to parakeratosis or true keratinization, which cannot be distinguished colposcopically. However, keratinization is not a particularly useful diagnostic criterion. All grades of keratinization, from mild parakeratosis to pronounced hyperkeratosis, can occur with acanthotic and atypical epithelia, both of which appear colposcopically as leukoplakia. A mild degree of keratinization often corresponds to acanthotic epithelium (Fig. 9–52), whereas "flaky keratin" suggests epithelial atypia (Fig. 9–53).

A colposcopically delicate white patch usually corresponds to parakeratosis, whereas hyperkeratosis usually produces a thick, rough-surfaced plaque.

Surface Contour. It is important to appreciate that the type of epithelium underlying leukoplakia cannot be predicted colposcopically. The keratinized layer obscures the underlying epithelium and epithelial borders. The epithelium may be acanthotic, especially when the leukoplakia is fine. A colposcopically delicate white patch, however, usually corresponds to parakeratosis, whereas hyperkeratosis usually produces a thick, rough-surfaced plaque. Fine leukoplakias are well circumscribed, their surface either flat or finely pitted. When keratinization is marked, the overlapping keratinized layer obscures the margins. The surface may be smooth, but it is usually pitted, and it may even have a mosaic appearance. Partial shedding or

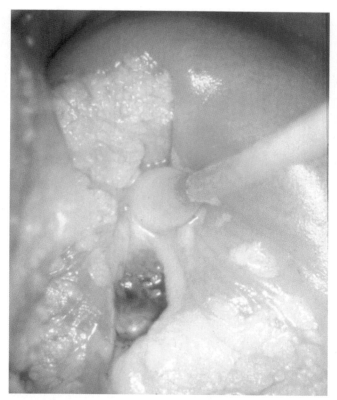

Figure 9–51. Atypical transformation zone with keratosis before acetic acid. Histology showed cervical intraepithelial neoplasia, grade 3 (high-grade squamous intraepithelial lesion).

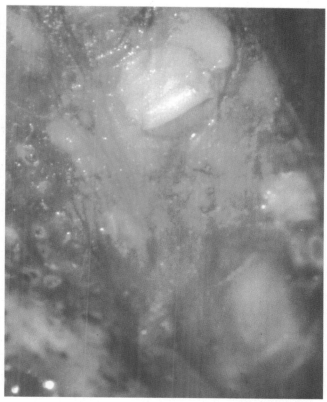

Figure 9–53. Flaky keratosis at the edge of an atypical transformation zone with cuffed gland openings. Histology showed cervical intraepithelial neoplasia, grade 3 (high-grade squamous intraepithelial lesion).

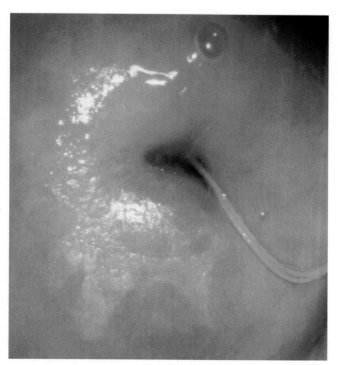

Figure 9–52. Sharply demarcated but only slightly keratotic area on the posterior lip of the cervix. Histology showed benign acanthotic epithelium with parakeratosis.

removal of the keratin can result in a plaquelike appearance, referred to as *plaquelike leukoplakia* or *thick leukoplakia.*

If the keratin layer is completely removed, the underlying epithelium can display a pattern, often punctation, that Hinselmann called the ground (base) of leukoplakia.[8] When cornification is more pronounced, the underlying epithelium can show features of CIN 3, early stromal invasion, deeper invasion, or only acanthosis. Even Schiller's test cannot provide further diagnostic clues. Moderate-sized leukoplakias typically stain canary yellow with iodine, which also enhances their sharp demarcation.

> **Atypical epithelium lacks cohesiveness and is more loosely structured than is normal squamous epithelium. It is also less firmly attached to the underlying stroma, from which it can easily detach to produce an erosion.**

Erosion and Ulcer. The old colposcopic literature called all grossly visible lesions erosions and used the term true erosions for epithelial defects. Today, the term *erosion* is restricted to epithelial defects. Deep defects with exposure of the stroma are called *ulcers.*

To regard erosion as an abnormal colposcopic finding is correct insofar as it does not normally occur in women of childbearing age. In contrast, the atrophic epithelium of postmenopausal women is prone to erosions, even as a

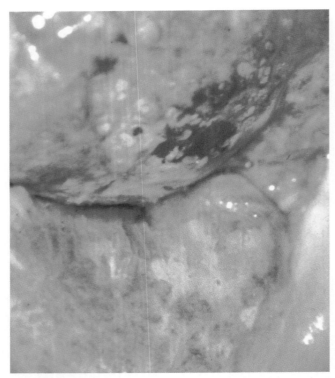

Figure 9–54. Atypical transformation zone (white epithelium) with an erosion on the anterior lip. The denudation of the epithelium has revealed the intensely red stroma. Histology of the acetowhite epithelium showed cervical intraepithelial neoplasia, grade 3 (high-grade squamous intraepithelial lesion).

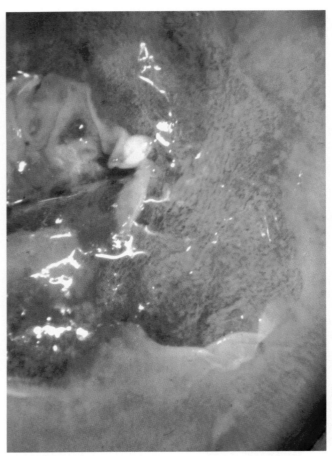

Figure 9–55. Extensive erosion. There are islands of cervical intraepithelial neoplasia, grade 3 (high-grade squamous intraepithelial lesion), both toward the end of the cervical canal and bordering the peripheral normal squamous epithelium. The texture of the exposed stroma is apparent.

result of a pelvic examination. Atypical epithelium is particularly vulnerable because it lacks cohesiveness and is more loosely structured than is normal squamous epithelium. This accounts for the exfoliation of cells detected in smears and for the swelling induced by diluted acetic acid. The epithelium is also less firmly attached to the underlying stroma, from which it can detach with ease to produce an erosion. Erosions and ulcers receive less attention if they occur within a colposcopic lesion (Fig. 9–54).

Color. An ulcer can be recognized by its intense red color, its granular floor, and its punched-out margin (Fig. 9–55). It is important not to miss larger ulcers that result from detachment of whole epithelial fields. Careful examination of the edges of such defects will reveal residual epithelium, which differs from the surrounding normal epithelium in color and in its reaction with diluted acetic acid. Such residual epithelial margins should be biopsied.

Iodine Uptake. Erosions and ulcers are seen better with iodine than in their native state, because the exposed stroma contains no glycogen and thus does not stain.

COLPOSCOPIC SIGNS OF INVASIVE CERVICAL CANCER

Signs of Early Invasive Carcinoma

Foci of early stromal invasion that reach only a fraction of a millimeter into the cervical stroma cannot be seen directly with the colposcope. Also, such foci arise more often from glands involved by CIN than from atypical surface epithelium. In the latter case, the colposcopic appearance is that of the parent surface epithelium. The colposcopic signs of early stromal invasion are indirect.

There is a direct relationship between the size of a lesion and the likelihood of invasion.

Early stromal invasion is more common when there are different types of epithelia.

Size. There is a direct relationship between the size of a lesion and the likelihood of invasion.[5] The coexistence of different epithelia shows that invasive potential is acquired by their coalescence and not by progression of one type to another. Also, early stromal invasion is more common when there are different types of epithelia. Some cases show all these features.

Microinvasion should be suspected when relatively flat lesions display focal collections of atypical vessels.

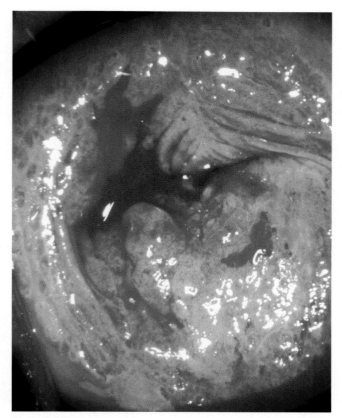

Figure 9–56. Atypical transformation zone (acetowhite epithelium) with a strikingly coarse surface. In the entire area there are irregularly located comma-shaped vessels. The conization specimen showed cervical intraepithelial neoplasia, grade 3 (high-grade squamous intraepithelial lesion) with early stromal invasion.

Vessels. The first hint of atypia is the confinement of blood vessels to sharply circumscribed areas. The vessels may display bizarre shapes and exhibit abrupt changes in caliber. The corkscrew- and comma-shaped vessels associated with atypical epithelium are coarser and show haphazard branching and great variation in caliber. The intercapillary distance is increased.

Increased vascularity also suggests invasion (Fig. 9–56). Although the likelihood of early stromal invasion increases with the size of a lesion, quite small or poorly vascularized lesions can be invasive. Some cases of early stromal invasion show only minimal colposcopic changes. Microinvasion should be suspected when relatively flat lesions display focal collections of atypical vessels.

The diagnosis of an invasive lesion arising within a vascular transformation zone is difficult, if not impossible. Hints of invasion in such cases can be sought only retrospectively by carefully correlating the colposcopic findings with the histology of the conization specimen.

Colposcopic Signs of Microinvasive Carcinoma

Colposcopic detection of small microinvasive lesions depends on their volume.

Surface Contour. Colposcopic detection of microinvasive carcinomas depends on their size and location. A microinvasive carcinoma entirely within the cervical canal will be missed by inspection of the ectocervix. Somewhat larger tumors can produce a slight bump on the surface that gives away their location, or they can form a confined polypoid lesion (Fig. 9–57).

Atypical vessels show a completely irregular and haphazard disposition, great variation in caliber, and abrupt changes in direction, often forming acute angles. The intercapillary distance is increased and tends to be variable. The vessels are often drawn out, have an irregular course, and are prone to bleeding.

Vessels. Ectocervical lesions characterized by focal collections of atypical vessels are highly suspicious for microinvasive carcinoma. Atypical vessels are invariably restricted to the invasive focus (Fig. 9–58). Atypical vessels show a completely irregular and haphazard disposition, great variation in caliber, and abrupt changes in direction, often forming acute angles. The intercapillary distance is increased and tends to be variable. The vessels are often drawn out, have an irregular course, and are prone to bleeding.

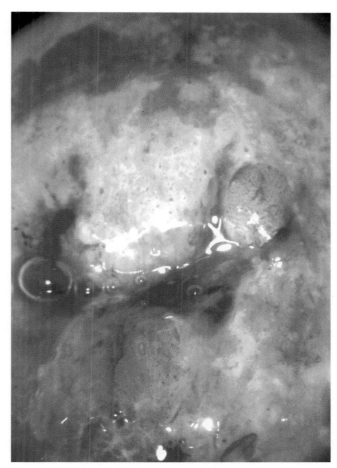

Figure 9–57. Small invasive carcinoma at 12 o'clock.

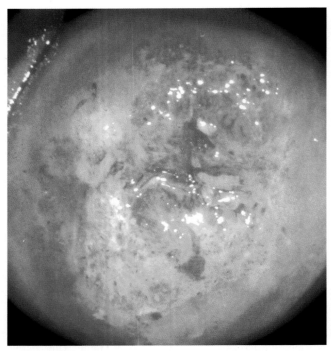

Figure 9–58. Atypical transformation zone (acetowhite epithelium). Note the small invasive lesion with atypical vessels at 9 o'clock. Histology showed cervical intraepithelial neoplasia, grade 3 (high-grade squamous intraepithelial lesion) and microinvasive carcinoma.

SUMMARY OF KEY POINTS

- Predicting the histology of original squamous epithelium, ectopy, or completely normal transformation zones is relatively easy. It becomes more difficult when the colposcopic findings are abnormal.

- Burghardt's system was meant to apply to colposcopy used as a screening test in all women, not just to evaluate those with an abnormal cytology report.

- Mature metaplastic epithelium shows gland openings or nabothian cysts, which demonstrate that this area was originally covered by columnar epithelium.

- After menopause the squamous epithelium becomes thin and devoid of glycogen. The epithelial thinning and glycogen loss are patchy, resulting in irregular iodine uptake and a stippled colposcopic appearance.

- Because ectopy is formed by columnar epithelium, which does not contain glycogen, it is always iodine negative.

- If one uses Schiller's (iodine) test at every colposcopic examination, one will encounter sharply circumscribed iodine-yellow areas that are otherwise not visible or are overlooked because they are subtle.

- In most cases, it is possible to distinguish between significant and nonspecific colposcopic lesions on the basis of sharp borders. However, this feature cannot be used to distinguish between acanthotic epithelium and CIN because both have sharp borders.

- The size of a lesion has nothing to do with its histologic status and cannot be used as a differential diagnostic criterion.

- Worrisome findings include grayish-red tones, which give the transformation zone an opaque appearance, and yellow shades, which are probably due to marked inflammatory infiltration of the stroma.

- Metaplasia involving the glandular crypts appears colposcopically as a white ring after application of acetic acid. The ring will be wider and more pronounced with atypical epithelium than with normal or acanthotic epithelium.

- Mosaic and punctation patterns within the transformation zone are more likely to represent CIN than are the same lesions outside the transformation zone.

- The effect of acetic acid on coarse mosaic is almost immediate. The effect of acetic acid on fine mosaic may take a minute to develop.

- Histologically, leukoplakia corresponds to either parakeratosis or true keratinization. It cannot be distinguished colposcopically.

- Atypical epithelium lacks cohesiveness and is more loosely structured than is normal squamous epithelium. It is also less firmly attached to the underlying stroma, from which it can easily detach to produce an erosion.

- There is a direct relationship between the size of a lesion and the likelihood of invasion. Invasive potential is acquired by the coalescence of lesions.

- Early stromal invasion is more common when there are different types of epithelia.

- Microinvasion should be suspected when relatively flat lesions display focal collections of atypical vessels.

- Atypical vessels show a completely irregular and haphazard disposition, great variation in caliber, and abrupt changes in direction, often forming acute angles. The intercapillary distance is increased and tends to be variable. The vessels are often drawn out, have an irregular course, and are prone to bleeding.

References

1. Hinselmann H: Introduction to Colposcopy. Hamburg, Hartung, 1933.
2. Burghardt E, Pickel H, Girardi F: Colposcopy—Cervical Pathology: Textbook and Atlas, 3rd ed. New York, Thieme, 1998.
3. Stafl A, Wilbanks G: An international terminology of colposcopy. Report of the Nomenclature Committee of the International Federation of Cervical Pathology and Colposcopy. Obstet Gynecol 1991;77: 313.
4. Burghardt E: On the atypical transformation zone. Geburtshilfe Frauenheilkd 1959;19:676.
5. Glatthaar E: The Morphogenesis of Squamous Cell Carcinoma of Cervical Cancer. Basel, Karger, 1950.
6. Treite P: The Early Diagnosis of Squamous Cell Carcinoma of the Uterine Cervix. Stuttgart, Enke, 1944.
7. Girardi F: The topography of abnormal colposcopy findings. Cervix 1993;11:45.
8. Hinselmann H: The etiology, symptoms and diagnosis of uterine cancer. In Veit J, Stöckel W (eds): Handbuch der Gynäkologie, vol. 6.1. Munich, Bergmann, 1930, p 854.

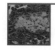

• Mitchell D. Greenberg

C
Reid's Colposcopic Index

Attempts to grade the severity of cervical lesions by the prominence of the acetowhite reaction or by the mere presence of aberrant vessels are unsuccessful.

Attempts to grade the severity of cervical lesions by the prominence of the acetowhite reaction or by the mere presence of aberrant vessels are unsuccessful. In contrast, each of four colposcopic criteria described in this chapter is significantly correlated with histologic severity. The colposcopic signs (margins, color, vascular patterns, and iodine staining) are graded into two objective categories: low-grade CIN 1 or high-grade CIN 2 to CIN 3. Combined into a weighted index called Reid's Colposcopic Index (RCI), these colposcopic features are more than 90% accurate in predicting histologic findings. Because this method relies on critical analysis rather than on pattern recall, the use of this grading system greatly simplifies the learning and practice of colposcopy and ensures that serious disease will not be missed and that trivial findings will not be overinterpreted.

It is critically important that the colposcopist be able to differentiate among normal, minimally abnormal, and significantly abnormal colposcopic patterns.

The primary objective for the colposcopist is to identify the most severe lesion on the cervix and perform a colposcopically directed biopsy. It is critically important that the examiner be able to differentiate among normal, minimally abnormal, and significantly abnormal colposcopic patterns. Other objectives of colposcopy include ruling out invasive cancer and determining whether the colposcopy is satisfactory or unsatisfactory.

DEFINING THE PROBLEM

Less-experienced colposcopists may tend to accept all areas that demonstrate either acetowhite change or abnormal surface vessels as foci of preinvasive or invasive disease.

Learning to differentiate benign features from low-grade and high-grade CIN has been shown to be a challenge.[1-3] More experienced colposcopists recognize that normal squamous metaplasia, various grades of CIN, and some cervical cancers exhibit varying degrees of acetowhite changes, with or without abnormal vessel patterns. However, less-expert colposcopists may (incorrectly) tend to accept all areas that demonstrate either acetowhite change or abnormal surface vessels as foci of preinvasive or invasive disease.

There appear to be different mechanisms for formation of the acetowhite reaction at opposite ends of the neoplastic spectrum. The acetowhite change seen in high-grade lesions is thought to occur because osmotic dehydration accentuates the high content of optically dense chromatin in CIN 3. On the other hand, the acetowhite change of minor lesions is thought to be more than likely attributable to a transient reaction between acetic acid and abnormal envelope proteins in HPV-infected keratinocytes. The acetowhite change of intermediate-grade lesions appears to reflect a combination of both events. Although similarities exceed differences, it is usually possible for the skilled colposcopist to differentiate one end of the morphologic spectrum from the other. However, such distinction depends on the use of objective colposcopic criteria. Colposcopic impressions based on whimsical grading of the "degree of acetowhiteness" or the "prominence" of any vascular atypia are not reliable.

Colposcopic impressions based on whimsical grading of the "degree of acetowhiteness" or the "prominence" of any vascular atypia are not reliable.

Histologic examination is the current "gold standard" for diagnosis of cervical disease. Histologic specimens are obtained by a colposcopically directed biopsy and/or an excisional procedure such as conization or loop excision. Predicting histology from the colposcopic impression has never been a formal requirement of the triage process. Some believe that it is unnecessary and that rigid adherence to the triage rules is merely intended to protect the physician from error. Unfortunately, the prominent areas of colposcopic change do not necessarily coincide with the areas of greatest histologic severity. Large areas of minor-grade lesions or squamous metaplasia are often overinterpreted, and subtle avascular patches of CIN 3 are easily overlooked. This fact may lead to the selection of the wrong sites for colposcopically directed biopsies, even when multiple samples are obtained.

Modern colposcopy is more than a simple intermediate link between cytologic screening and histologic diagnosis. The method provides information about a cervical lesion that is of diagnostic, prognostic, therapeutic, and scientific value. It provides a means for the clinician to supervise and control the triage and diagnostic process, permitting the clinician and the patient to make well-informed and mutual treatment decisions.

To avoid overtreatment of low-grade lesions using a "see and treat" approach, accurate colposcopic assessment of the histologic grade of the lesion is essential before excision of the transformation zone.

An evolving school of colposcopic practice recommends a somewhat static and inflexible diagnostic and therapeutic approach to cytologic abnormalities based on clinical application of modern electrosurgical excision techniques. It is suggested by some that the response to abnormal cervical cytology should be colposcopic identification of an acetowhite lesion, followed by electrosurgical excision of the complete lesion. Thus, the histology of the excised specimen provides the final diagnosis. Colposcopic assessment serves the limited purpose of lesion identification and excision margin identification. This approach is based on the reality that colposcopic errors do occur. By treating all women with excision of the transformation zone, one can avoid inappropriate treatment of a misdiagnosed cancer with ablative therapy chosen on the basis of colposcopy and histology of colposcopically directed biopsy. However, to avoid overtreatment of low-grade lesions using a "see and treat" approach, accurate colposcopic assessment of the histologic grade of the lesion is essential before excision of the transformation zone.

When the see and treat approach is not used, the colposcopic impression is a necessary safeguard against inaccurate or confusing histologic diagnoses resulting from misdirected biopsies.

When the see and treat approach is not used, the colposcopic impression is a necessary safeguard against inaccurate or confusing histologic diagnoses resulting from misdirected biopsies and is an aid in rendering treatment decisions. Despite this, much subjectivity remains as to the colposcopic impression of probable histologic diagnosis. To compensate for the myriad of colposcopic features and the degrees of variation of normal and abnormal, experienced colposcopists have endeavored to develop colposcopic grading systems. The aim of colposcopic grading is to provide an objective, reproducible, and meaningful guide to histologic severity and potential for neoplastic progression.

The RCI is a scoring system that correlates colposcopic impression with histologic severity.

From a practical point of view, the RCI provides a scored, less subjective measurement of lesion severity based on colposcopic signs and provides the examiner with direction for the targeted biopsy. This scoring system developed, by Reid et al in 1984,[3] uses four colposcopic signs to differentiate minor-grade cervical abnormalities from areas of high-grade colposcopic change. This index correlates colposcopic impression and histologic severity. Originally, five colposcopic signs (thickness, color, contour, vascular atypia, and iodine staining) were graded, but eventually the RCI was changed to include only four categories; thickness was moved into the contour category. Summing the aggregate for all the signs produced the colposcopic index.

DEFINITIONS OF COLPOSCOPIC CRITERIA

Under the RCI, the colposcopic signs are scored in the following categories:

1. Sharpness of the margins
2. Epithelial color
3. Vascular patterns
4. Iodine staining

All colposcopic signs except for iodine staining are scored after the application of copious amounts of 3% to 5% acetic acid. Once an area of acetowhite change appears, the lesion is assessed and then scored. One-quarter strength Lugol's iodine (¼ iodine, ¾ water) is then applied sparingly with a soaked cotton ball, and the iodine staining reaction is assessed and scored.

The predictive accuracy of the RCI is maximized only when exact colposcopic criteria are used.

The predictive accuracy of the RCI is maximized only when exact colposcopic criteria are used. These four categories were initially developed in a series of pilot studies and tested by a prospective computer analysis. For each criterion, there is a category typical of low-grade intraepithelial changes (HPV/CIN 1, mild dysplasia) and a category indicative of high-grade intraepithelial changes (CIN 2 to CIN 3, moderate to severe dysplasia). Definitions of

▼ Table 9–3

Reid's Colposcopic Index

Colposcopic Sign	0 Points	1 Point	2 Points
Margin	Condylomatous or micropapillary contour	Regular lesions with smooth, straight outlines	Rolled, peeling edges
	Indistinct borders	Sharp peripheral margins	Internal borders between areas of differing appearance
	Flocculated or feathered margins		
	Jagged, angular lesions		
	Satellite lesions, acetowhite change that extends beyond the transformation zone		
Color	Shiny, snow-white color	Shiny, gray-white	Dull, oyster gray
	Indistinct acetowhite change, semitransparent rather than completely opaque	Intermediate white	
Vessels	Uniform, fine caliber	Absence of surface vessels	Definite punctation or mosaic
	Randomly arranged patterns		Individual vessels dilated, arranged in sharply demarcated, well-defined patterns
	Nondilated capillary loops		
	Ill-defined areas of fine punctation or mosaic		
Iodine staining	Positive iodine uptake, producing a mahogany-brown color	Partial iodine uptake (variegated and tortoiseshell)	Yellow staining of a lesion, which is scored 3/6
	Yellow staining by an area that is recognizable as a low-grade lesion by above criteria (<2/6)		Mustard-yellow appearance
Colposcopic score	0–2 = HPV or CIN 1 (low-grade disease)	3–4 = CIN 1 or CIN 2 (intermediate-grade disease)	5–8 = CIN 2 or CIN 3 (high-grade disease)

CIN, cervical intraepithelial neoplasia; HPV, human papilloma virus.

these gradations follow and are summarized in Table 9–3.

COLPOSCOPIC SIGNS

Sharpness of Peripheral Margins

The following types of lesions indicate a score of 0:

- Lesions with feathered, finely scalloped margins (resembling "beat to beat" variation on an electronic fetal monitoring tracing) (Fig. 9–59)
- Angular, irregular, or geographic map–like peripheral lesions (even if a portion of the lesion demonstrates a straight regular area, the lesion itself is assessed as irregular) (Fig. 9–60)
- Flat lesions with indistinct borders (Fig. 9–61)
- "Satellite" lesions not contiguous with the new SCJ
- Any lesion showing an irregular surface contour that appears condylomatous, micropapilliferous, or microconvoluted (Figs. 9–62 and 9–63)

The following type of lesions indicates a score of 1:

- Lesions that are biologically regular, with smooth, straight margins (Fig. 9–64)

The following types of lesions indicate a score of 2:

- Lesions in which cell-to-cell cohesiveness is so fragile that the epithelial edges tend to detach from the underlying stroma and curl back on themselves or roll over. This may be caused by insertion and opening of the speculum that "scrapes" the tissue, or it

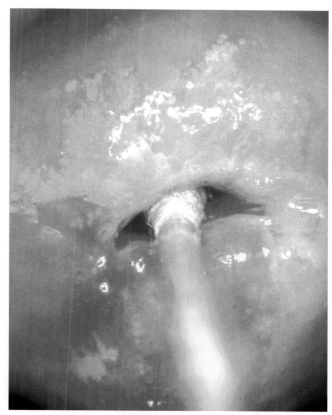

Figure 9–59. The acetowhite lesion found on the anterior cervix has peripheral margins that are irregular and feathered. This is a biopsy-proven cervical intraepithelial neoplasia, grade 1 (low-grade squamous intraepithelial lesion), and the colposcopy was unsatisfactory.

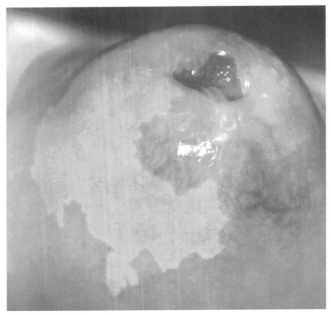

Figure 9–60. This lesion represents a geographic map–like, low-grade dysplasia. The lesion itself is irregular, and it extends to the posterior cervical portio.

may be produced by the colposcopist's gently pushing away the lesion tissue with a cotton swab. Rolling or peeling edges are found almost exclusively at the new SCJ, and such lesions are scored 2, regardless of the appearance of the peripheral margins (Fig. 9–65).

- Lesions that demonstrate an internal demarcation (internal margin) between two different colposcopic patterns, or "two lesions in one" (the peripheral area

represents an early minor-grade change and the central area represents the subsequent evolution of a high-grade dysplasia at the advancing edge of the NSCJ) (Fig. 9–66)

Note: The colposcopic sign of two lesions in one is confirmed when the colposcopist examines the peripheral tissue first, then moves the inspection centrally on any radius. If there is a different colposcopic pattern as described, the central lesion is invariably of higher grade than the peripheral lesion, and the examiner should then target the biopsies to that central area. Colposcopists should always look carefully for internal margins. Often, the central higher-grade lesion is subtle, and it is the colposcopist's responsibility to identify what is often a "needle in a haystack" lesion.

Note: Iodine staining is particularly useful in assisting in the identification of subtle CINs that were missed when assessment was performed with 3% to 5% acetic acid alone.

Epithelial Color

The following types of lesions indicate a score of 0:

- Less intense degrees of acetowhite change, seen as semitransparent (rather than completely opaque) (Fig. 9–67)
- Lesions that show a snow-white color (typical of an exophytic condyloma) or those that demonstrate an intense surface shine (Fig. 9–68)

Note: Minor-grade lesions are transient in that they appear and disappear quickly.

The following type of lesions indicates a score of 1:

- Intermediate lesions that are distinguished by a gray-white color. It is believed that the gray-white discoloration reflects light absorption within the atypical nuclei at the epithelial base, whereas the preservation

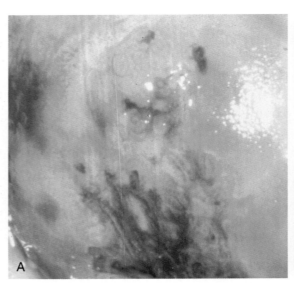

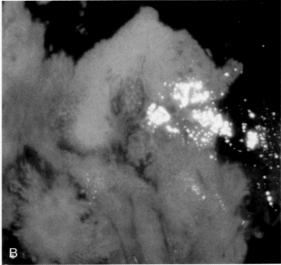

Figure 9–61. *A,* This is the same cervix that contains a cervical intraepithelial neoplasia grade 3 lesion. The peripheral margin is indistinct at 12 o'clock. *B,* Peripheral margin becomes distinct only after the application of diluted Lugol's iodine.

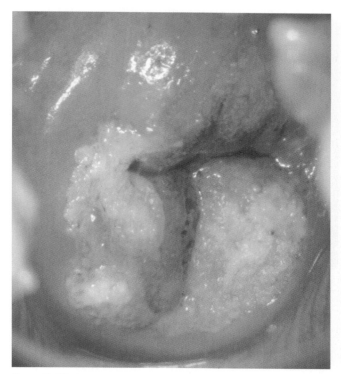

Figure 9–62. Example of a nonexophytic condylomatous lesion, micro-papilliferous in appearance.

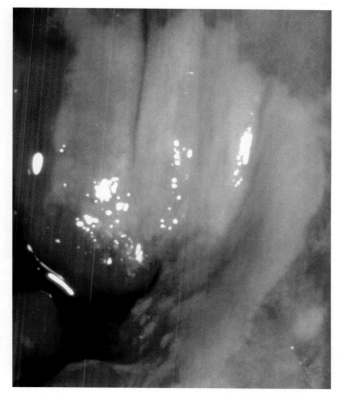

Figure 9–64. A small, focal cervical intraepithelial neoplasia, grade 3 at 12 o'clock demonstrates the biologically regular lesion. These thickened and smooth types of lesions that do not have surface blood vessels are commonly high grade.

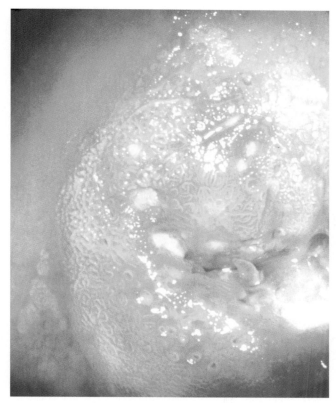

Figure 9–63. A microconvoluted, condylomatous lesion with an irregular and inconsistent surface contour.

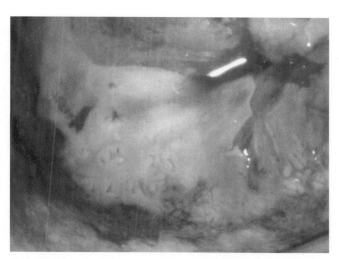

Figure 9–65. This high-grade cervical intraepithelial neoplasia demonstrates a rolled, peeling margin at 6 o'clock. The epithelium that is peeling is a result of a lack of desmosomes, which adheres the surface epithelium to the underlying stroma.

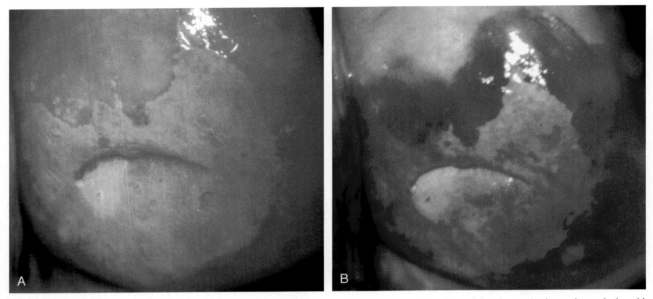

Figure 9–66. *A,* Example of two lesions in one, in which the central lesion is of higher grade than the peripheral one. An internal margin is evident when the colposcopist inspects, moving from the periphery, centrally on any radius. *B,* Demonstrates the value of iodine in further identifying different lesions.

of surface reflectivity is probably due to keratin formation within areas of cellular maturation in the upper layers (Fig. 9–69).

Note: In practice, most lesions are scored in the intermediate category.

The following types of lesions indicate a score of 2:

- Dull, oyster shell–white, thickened epithelium (it is

believed that this is due to intense light absorption within chromatin dense nuclei)
- Loss of surface reflectivity (it is believed that this is due to the paucity of cytoplasm in the superficial epithelial cells) (Fig. 9–70)

Note: Major-grade lesions take longer to materialize because of the nuclear density, and when they do appear, they remain visible longer than minor-grade lesions.

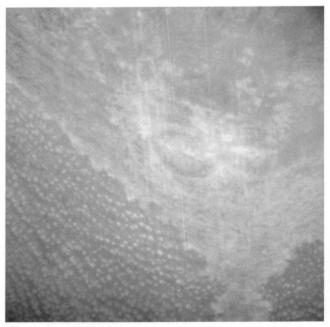

Figure 9–67. The color in this example is indistinct, and the lesion is semitransparent. This type of surface acetowhitening is indicative of cervical intraepithelial neoplasia, grade 1 or physiologic metaplasia.

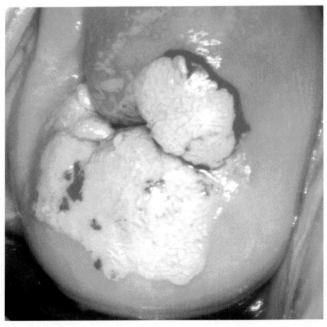

Figure 9–68. This exophytic condyloma exhibits a shiny, snow-white color, whereas condylomatous-looking invasive cancers are typically dull yellowish-white lesions.

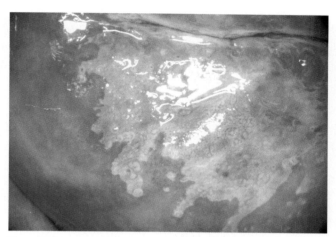

Figure 9–69. This cervical intraepithelial neoplasia, grade 1 is typical in that it exhibits an irregular margin and a shiny gray color, with a fine mosaic pattern. Most low-grade lesions are gray-white in color.

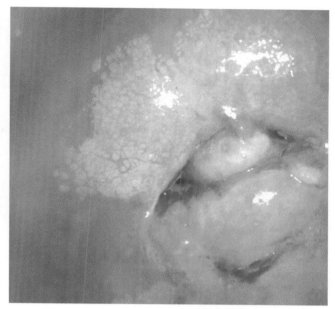

Figure 9–71. Low-grade lesions often exhibit a fine mosaic and punctate pattern. This example reveals loose arcades of haphazardly oriented surface vessels that represent an exaggeration of the normal loop cervical capillaries.

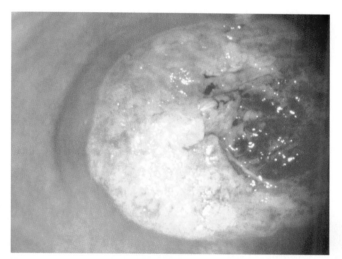

Figure 9–70. Most high-grade lesions are dull oyster white in color. This lesion has smooth and regular margins and is devoid of surface vessels.

Vascular Patterns

The following type of lesions indicates a score of 0:

- Ill-defined, yet obvious, areas of fine punctation or fine mosaic formed by loose aggregations of nondilated capillaries with uniform caliber. These vessels are normal looped cervical capillaries that are exaggerated because of a proliferative effect secondary to HPV infection (Fig. 9–71).

Note: Minor-grade lesions often reveal prominent vascular change; occasionally, normal congenital metaplasia may be mistaken for a low-grade lesion (Fig. 9–72).

The following type of lesions indicates a score of 1:

- A lesion devoid of surface vessels. Most high-grade lesions have absent vessels. It is believed that this is due to the gradual compression and depression of the normal capillary looped vessels within a nuclear-

dense lesion, preventing them from being visualized (Fig. 9–73).

The following type of lesions indicates a score of 2:

- Coarse, dilated punctation or significant mosaic vascular patterns. These vessels are confined to signifi-

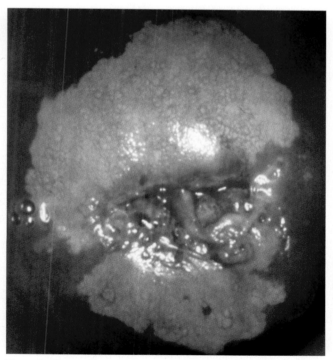

Figure 9–72. Although the vessels in this example are prominent, they are nondilated and irregular.

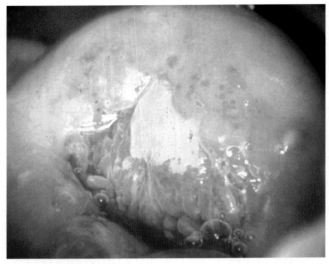

Figure 9–73. This cervical intraepithelial neoplasia, grade 3 does not exhibit surface blood vessels owing to the thickened epithelium. Most cervical intraepithelial neoplasia grade 2 and grade 3 lesions do not have surface vessels apparent.

cant plaques of acetowhite change, are dilated, and are arranged in sharply demarcated, well-defined patterns.

Note: These vessels are formed because of angiogenesis (e.g., new vessels feeding a neoplasia), as distinct from the vessels found in low-grade disease (Fig. 9–74).

Iodine-Staining Reaction

The following types of lesions indicate a score of 0:

- Positive iodine staining, producing a mahogany brown color (Fig. 9–75)
- Negative iodine uptake by an area that is recognizable as a minor-grade lesion with the three acetic acid criteria (e.g., a lesion that stains yellow and scores less than three points on the first three criteria) (Fig. 9–76)

The following type of lesions indicates a score of 1:

- Partial iodine staining, differing degrees of iodine uptake, or rejection imparts a variegated, "tortoise-shell" appearance (Fig. 9–77).

The following type of lesions indicates a score of 2:

- Mustard-yellow staining in an area that was already recognized as significant by the three acetic acid criteria. It is important to understand that iodine staining of both trivial and significant lesions is characterized by the same yellow discoloration. Hence, differentiation of the number of points assigned for iodine staining depends on the application of other colposcopic features, not on the shade of the iodine stain (Fig. 9–78).

Note: Normal columnar epithelium, biopsy sites, and other epithelial altering conditions (e.g., vaginitis, atrophy) result in yellowish discoloration as well, but because these are not lesions, they are not to be scored.

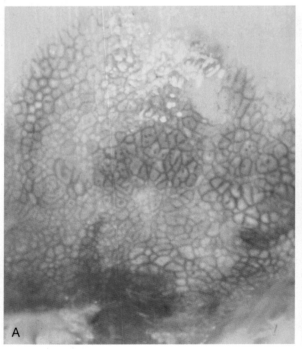
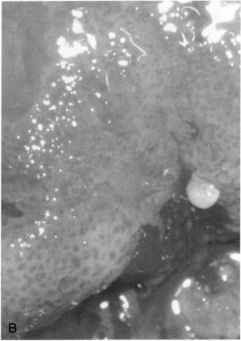

Figure 9–74. *A,* The vessels depicted here and in *B* represent neovascularization or an angiogenic response to a significant neoplasia. This figure reveals a classic mosaic pattern typical of late-stage lesions on the verge of malignant transformation. *B,* Dilated, coarse punctation is evident.

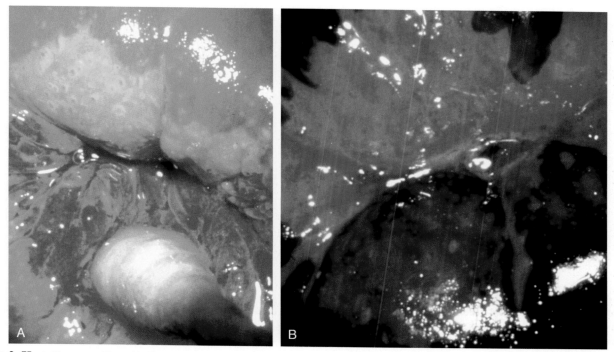

Figure 9–75. *A,* The acetowhite epithelium represents an equivocal cervical intraepithelial neoplasia, grade 1 at 12 o'clock. *B,* Mahogany brown color or complete uptake of the iodine is consistent with normal epithelium.

Figure 9–76. *A,* Example of a minor-grade lesion with respect to the margins, color, and vessels. *B,* Lesion is mustard yellow when iodine is applied.

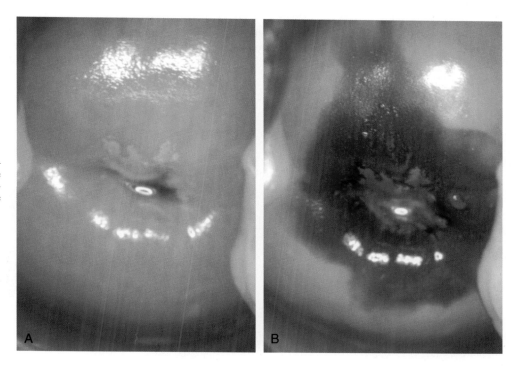

How the Scoring System Is Applied

Typically, a score of zero is indicative of low-grade disease and a score of two is consistent with high-grade disease.

The colposcopic signs are scored in each category. The minimum score in each category is zero and the maximum is two. Typically, in any given category, a score of zero is indicative of low-grade colposcopic disease patterns, and a score of two is consistent with high-grade disease. From time to time, the examiner will notice

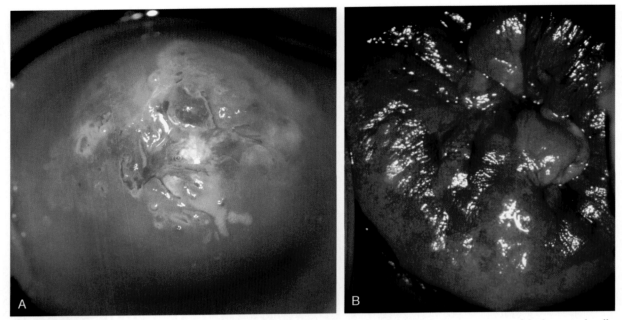

Figure 9–77. *A,* Lesion in evolution. *B,* Iodine staining shows a tortoiseshell-like pattern, in that there are areas of both mustard yellow and mahogany brown.

when scoring lesions that the signs are commingled. When this occurs, it may suggest that there is a lesion in evolution (e.g., CIN 1 to CIN 2, CIN 2 to CIN 3), or it may represent a CIN 3 that is early in the neoplastic process (e.g., a thickened, dull-white lesion devoid of surface blood vessels).

The calculation of the scoring is cumulative in that each of the four categories is assigned a score; therefore, the numerator fluctuates and the denominator is fixed at eight. If the lesions score five or greater, these are typically high-grade lesions (e.g., CIN 2 to CIN 3). A score of two or lower usually indicates low-grade lesions (e.g.,

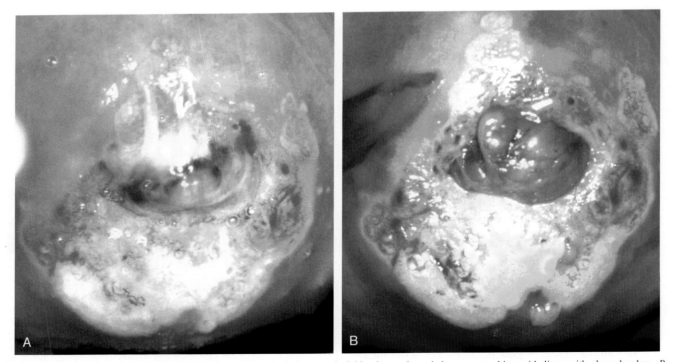

Figure 9–78. *A,* This lesion has significant abnormalities, including atypical blood vessels and dense acetowhite epithelium with sharp borders. *B,* This image shows how the lesion rejects the iodine, giving a mustard-yellow appearance to the areas of acetowhite epithelium.

HPV effect/CIN 1). There may be overlapping scores and lesions, whereas a lesion that scores three to four may represent a CIN 1 to CIN 2 or a CIN 2.

> Points on the RCI are scored for each individual criterion and are then added together to generate the colposcopic index.

The easiest way to learn the method is to draw a simple diagram that defines any areas of variable colposcopic appearance. Points on the RCI are scored for each individual criterion and are then added together to generate the colposcopic index (see Table 9–3). At first, this is a tedious exercise. However, practice makes the scoring of the four criteria intuitive. When a colposcopist reaches this stage, a marked improvement in diagnostic accuracy is usually obtained.

Can the RCI Assist in Differentiating "Mimics" from "Real Disease"?

Often, the colposcopist is performing a colposcopy in response to equivocal or minimally abnormal cervical cytology. Owing to the lack of specificity for disease in this clinical situation, colposcopists are faced with the challenge of differentiating between the acetowhite change of metaplasia and the acetowhite change of minor CIN. This becomes a dilemma in that there is pressure on the colposcopist to perform a cervical biopsy and then resulting

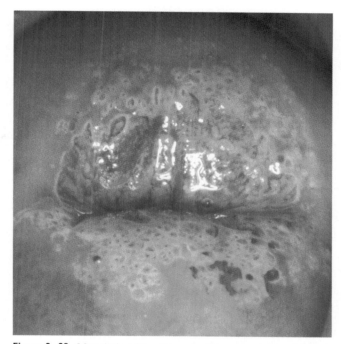

Figure 9–80. Metaplasia with mild acetowhiteness and several islands of columnar epithelium present.

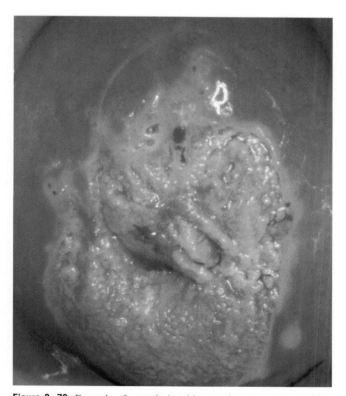

Figure 9–79. Example of metaplasia with a semitransparent acetowhiteness.

pressure on the pathologist to make a diagnosis. When the cytology is inconclusive, the pathologist may report with ambiguous language such as "suggestive of," "equivocal with," or "minimal signs of" low-grade disease. Therefore, in these instances, the pressure remains on the clinician to have the confidence either to not take a biopsy or to notify the pathologist that nothing was unduly alarming relative to the colposcopic signs. In such cases, the clinician performs a biopsy just to be reassured of the benign nature of the findings. The RCI may assist the clinician in this situation with a systematic determination of what is probably normal versus what is abnormal. This is accomplished by the grading of the acetic acid signs, margins, color, and vessels.

> Using a systematic determination of what is probably normal versus what is abnormal through the grading of acetic acid signs, margins, color, and vessels, the colposcopist can best select the most severe area to biopsy.

It is recognized that most high-grade lesions have absent vessels; thickened, dull-white epithelium; and distinct, definable margins. In contrast, normal physiologic metaplasia usually display absent vessels. However, the color of the lesion is white but semitransparent, and the margins are often indistinct and confluent with the surrounding mature squamous epithelium (Figs. 9–79 and 9–80). Additionally, normal metaplastic epithelium usually contains gland openings, and the acetowhite change of normal metaplastic epithelium often occupies most of the circumference of the transformation zone and is always contiguous with the NSCJ.

CONCLUSION

Target biopsy followed by ablation or excision is the mainstay of management of cervical lesions that can be adequately visualized. For the colposcopist who does not progress beyond whimsical estimates of lesion prominence (which cannot differentiate minor from high-grade lesions), the colposcope will never be more than a simple aid to the collection of directed biopsy specimens. Unfortunately, in situations in which the colposcopist's only option is passive response to the histopathology report, optimal management of the patient's disease will not occur.

Because the most prominent areas of colposcopic change do not necessarily coincide with the areas of greatest histologic abnormality, less experienced colposcopists may not be able to select the most abnormal sites for directed biopsy. Peripheral areas of prominent acetowhite change tend to be overinterpreted, and the subtle acetowhite change of high-grade CIN near the external os tends to be easily overlooked. Using colposcopic criteria that are based on critical analysis, rather than "pattern recognition," is the best solution.

It is easy to derive the four proven colposcopic criteria, and they can be quickly compiled into an index that helps the clinician recognize lesion severity while colposcopy is performed. Of course, using the colposcopic index to infer approximate histologic findings does not eliminate the importance of biopsy. Skilled physicians will conscientiously follow the triage rules, including the need to collect carefully selected target biopsy specimens.

For the practicing clinician, the value of these individual colposcopic signs is maximized by combining them into a weighted scoring system. The overall predictive accuracy of the combined colposcopic index is greater than 95%.[1-3]

Hence, the formal calculation of this colposcopic index produces a meaningful clinical assessment of lesion severity, against which the clinician can reconcile the cytologic and histologic findings.

colposcopic impression may not accurately reflect the histologic severity.

- Because prominent areas of colposcopic change do not necessarily coincide with areas of greatest histologic severity, large areas of minor-grade lesions or squamous metaplasia are often overinterpreted, and subtle areas of high-grade lesions are easily overlooked.

- Although the final diagnosis is ultimately determined by the histologic interpretation, the colposcopic impression is a necessary safeguard against inaccurate or confusing histologic diagnoses.

- Margins are scored based on whether they are feathered, straight, or peeling.

- Color is determined by the degree of acetowhite change obtained following the application of copious amounts of 3% to 5% acetic acid. In practice, most lesions are scored in the intermediate category based on color (score 1).

- Vessels are scored based on how prominent (coarse) they are, but it is recognized that most high-grade lesions lack visible vessels.

- Iodine staining is graded by the uptake of diluted Lugol's solution into the epithelium and may range from partial uptake to total rejection of iodine. Normal columnar epithelium, as well as epithelial altering conditions such as vaginitis or atrophy, is not scored in this category.

- Each of the four categories is assigned a score. The calculation of the scoring is cumulative; therefore, the numerator fluctuates, and the denominator is fixed at eight.

- A lesion that scores five or higher is typically high grade, whereas a score of two or lower usually indicates low-grade disease.

SUMMARY OF KEY POINTS

- The RCI uses four colposcopic criteria (acetowhite reaction, color, margins, and vessels) to formulate an accurate colposcopic impression and to aid in the selection of the most appropriate sites for colposcopically directed biopsy.

- If only acetowhite change and abnormal vessels are accepted as descriptors of preinvasive lesions, the

References

1. Reid R, Stanttope CR, Herschman BR, et al: Genital warts and cervical cancer. IV. A colposcopic index for differentiating subclinical papillomaviral infection from cervical intraepithelial neoplasia. Am J Obstet Gynecol 1984;149:815.
2. Reid R, Herschman BR, Crum CP, et al: Genital warts and cervical cancer. V. The tissue basis of colposcopic change. Am J Obstet Gynecol 1984;149:293.
3. Reid R, Scaizi P: Genital warts and cervical cancer. VI. An improved colposcopic index for differentiating benign papillomaviral infections from high-grade cervical intraepithelial neoplasia. Am J Obstet Gynecol 1985;153:611.

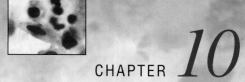

• Alan G. Waxman

CHAPTER *10*

Low-Grade Squamous Intraepithelial Lesion

The Bethesda System combines cervical intraepithelial neoplasia grade 1 and human papillomavirus changes into the descriptive category of *low-grade squamous intraepithelial lesion*.

The Bethesda System of nomenclature for cervical cytology combines the histologic diagnoses of cervical intraepithelial neoplasia (CIN) grade 1 and human papillomavirus (HPV) changes into the descriptive diagnostic category of *low-grade squamous intraepithelial lesion* (LSIL).[1] In this chapter, the virology, cytology, and histology as well as the colposcopic findings that characterize low-grade lesions will be discussed. The features that distinguish true dysplastic changes from benign findings resulting from the process of squamous metaplasia or posttreatment repair will be delineated. Finally, the special situations encountered by the colposcopist evaluating women with LSIL who are at various stages of life (adolescence, pregnancy, postmenopausal state) will be addressed.

VIROLOGY OF LOW-GRADE LESIONS

Unlike high-grade squamous intraepithelial lesion, LSIL contains both low-risk and high-risk HPV types.

Low-grade lesions of the cervix reflect the pathologic effects of infection with HPV. Although more than 80 HPV viral types have been identified, only 30 are known to infect the anogenital tract. HPV has been divided into low-risk and high-risk types based on their association with high-grade squamous intraepithelial lesions (HSIL) and invasive cervical cancer.[2] Although several of the low-risk HPV types (most commonly types 6 and 11) are frequently found in LSIL, it is important to note that high-risk HPV types, including types 16, 18, 45, 56, 31, 33, and 35, are also found in LSIL.[3, 4] Investigators in the atypical squamous cells of undetermined significance (ASCUS)/LSIL Triage Study (ALTS) found high-risk HPV types in as many as 86.1% of women with cervical

LSIL. HPV type 16 was the most common type and was found in 24.8% of cervices. This large, multicenter trial was designed, in part, to determine whether the presence of high-risk types of HPV could predict which low-grade lesions had malignant potential. However, the LSIL arm of the study needed to be discontinued when the high frequency of high-risk HPV types in LSIL was discovered. In contrast to HSIL, in which infection with a single HPV type is the rule, it has been observed that multiple HPV types are commonly found in LSIL.[3, 5] In the ALTS, multiple HPV types were found in 58.9% of women with LSIL.[5]

The cytopathic effects of HPV include the appearance of the characteristic koilocyte with an enlarged, irregular nucleus and a perinuclear "halo" in the cytoplasm.

The mechanisms of infection with HPV have been well studied. The virus is thought to enter the epithelium through microlacerations that occur most commonly during sexual intercourse. The relatively thin metaplastic epithelium is more accessible to the virus than is the thicker, more mature squamous epithelium. The virus infects the basal epithelial cells, sheds its capsid, and exists in the host nucleus in an episomal state, separate from the host genome.

When as yet poorly identified cofactors are present, and in the absence of successful suppression by the cell-mediated immune system of the host, HPV viral replication and cell proliferation may be stimulated. As the epithelial cells mature and move away from the basement membrane toward the surface epithelium, HPV may reacquire its capsid and begin replication and proliferation within the intermediate and superficial cells. In this form, LSIL is a productive viral infection. The intermediate and superficial epithelial cells will have many virions in each cell. Morphologically, the cells will show the cytopathic effects of HPV, including the appearance of the characteristic koilocyte with an enlarged, irregular nucleus and a perinuclear "halo" in the cytoplasm. Colposcopically, LSIL may have the appearance of a flat acetowhite lesion or an exophytic condyloma.[3, 6, 7] For most low-grade lesions, this is the ultimate expression of the HPV infection. The cytopathic effects of the viral infection will be manifested, but the lesions will never become truly preinvasive.

> **Integration of HPV DNA has been found in the majority of squamous cell carcinomas of the cervix but has been found much less frequently in preinvasive cervical lesions where HPV remains as an episomal particle.**

An alternative developmental pathway has been proposed for those low-grade lesions destined to become high-grade lesions. The HPV DNA is thought to leave its episomal state and become integrated into the DNA of the host cells in the basal layer of the epithelium. As these cells mature, they move progressively toward the surface of the epithelium, retaining their dysplastic characteristics, including an enlarged, irregular nucleus and a relatively reduced cytoplasmic volume. Integration of the viral HPV DNA has been found in the majority of squamous cell cervical cancers but has been found much less frequently in preinvasive lesions where HPV remains as an episomal particle.[3]

The question has been raised as to whether lesions destined to progress to high grade may in some cases arise not from LSIL but from a separate population of cells.[4] In a small series of cases in which the two grades of CIN coexisted, Park et al found different HPV types in adjacent CIN 1 and CIN 3 lesions.[8]

FACTORS AFFECTING THE DEVELOPMENT OF LSIL

> **Factors associated with the development of LSIL include young age, presence of high-risk HPV types, and duration of HPV infection.**

Only a minority of women who are HPV positive will develop LSIL. Factors associated with the development of LSIL include young age, presence of high-risk HPV types, and duration of HPV infection. Both the incidence of HPV infection and the development of LSIL appear to peak in young women in late adolescence and the early twenties and decline thereafter. The acquisition of HPV is felt to reflect the onset of sexual activity in women with an immature transformation zone, whereas the clearance of HPV correlates with cell-mediated immunologic response and a decline in the number of new sexual partners.[4]

> **The acquisition of HPV reflects the onset of sexual activity in women with an immature transformation zone.**

Moscicki and colleagues proposed that the rate at which the cervix undergoes squamous metaplasia over time is a key factor in the development of LSIL. They monitored young college women with periodic colpophotographs and documented changes in the area of immature squamous metaplasia before development of LSIL. They were able to demonstrate that the development of LSIL correlated with the rate of recent squamous metaplasia but not with the area of cervical ectopy per se.[6]

Several studies have shown that the incidence of cervical infection with HPV is associated with young age.[4, 5, 7, 10] Manos and associates found that although the incidence of low-grade lesions declined with age, this trend was negated when controlling for HPV status.[11]

> **Factors related to the development of squamous intraepithelial lesion include infection with high-risk HPV types and persistence of HPV infection.**

The transient nature of HPV infection in young women, even with high-risk viral types, has been well documented.[9, 10, 12] Ho and coworkers followed a cohort of college women over 3 years and found that 43% of those who were HPV negative on entering the study acquired HPV infection during the study period. The median duration of these incident infections was 8 months. Seventy percent of those who became HPV positive during the study reverted to negative status after 12 months, and 91% tested negative after 24 months. Only 5.1% of women who were HPV positive during the 3-year study period developed squamous intraepithelial lesion. Of these, 93% had low-grade lesions. This included women who were HPV positive at the start of the study as well as those who developed the infection during the study period. Factors related to the development of squamous intraepithelial lesion included infection with a high-risk HPV type and persistence of HPV infection for at least 6 months.[9] Moscicki et al confirmed the transient nature of HPV infection in college-aged women by requiring multiple consecutive negative assessments to document clearance of HPV. During the study, the development of LSIL was associated with persistent lesions, and the association of persistent HPV positivity was a strong factor for the development of HSIL.[10]

> **Cytologically and histologically, LSIL is characterized by enlargement of the cell nucleus to at least three times the size of the normal nucleus of an intermediate cell.**

HISTOLOGIC AND CYTOLOGIC CHARACTERISTICS OF LSIL

Histologically and cytologically, LSIL is characterized by enlargement of the cell nucleus to at least three times the size of a normal intermediate cell nucleus. The epithelial cells also exhibit moderate variation in nuclear size and shape, hyperchromatic chromatin, and frequent binucleation[1] (Fig. 10–1). The cytoplasm is frequently pushed to the periphery of the cell, thus creating the koilocyte with its characteristic perinuclear halo or cytoplasmic clearing (Fig. 10–2). At the cellular level, findings of LSIL may be present without development of koilocytosis. Histologically, there is loss of normal progressive cellular differentiation in the lower third of the epithelium but progres-

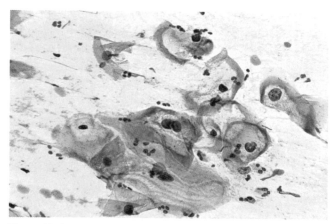

Figure 10-1. Pap smear classified as epithelial cell abnormality, low-grade squamous intraepithelial lesion. In this smear, koilocytes can be seen, characterized by somewhat enlarged nuclei with chromatin abnormalities, irregularities in nuclear contour, and distinctive perinuclear haloes. In addition, two binucleated cells are identified; binucleation is another characteristic feature of human papillomavirus effect.

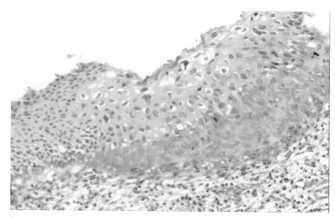

Figure 10-3. Cervical intraepithelial neoplasia grade 1, cervical biopsy. The epithelium lacks maturation in the lower third of the epithelial thickness and shows disorderly basal cells with some crowding of cells within the parabasal area. Multinucleated cells are seen near the surface, and koilocytosis is present. There is mild, superficial, chronic inflammation in the stroma.

sive normal cell maturation in the upper two thirds of the epithelial layers (Fig. 10–3). By contrast, CIN 2 or CIN 3 reflects the loss of progressive cellular maturation extending to encompass the upper two thirds of the epithelium.[1]

For LSIL to be accurately diagnosed, both nuclear enlargement and nuclear atypia must be present.

Rigorous attention to these nuclear abnormalities is essential to prevent cytologic misclassification of minor cellular changes into the category of LSIL. It has been suggested that nuclear enlargement with atypia is neces-

sary to make the diagnosis of LSIL. A frequent source of a false-positive LSIL result is the diagnosis of koilocytosis based on the presence of the perinuclear halo with nuclear irregularity and hyperchromasia but without the requisite nuclear enlargement. More than two thirds of such patients are HPV negative.[1, 13]

It has been found that histologic CIN is confirmed more often in younger women with LSIL than in older women with the same cytologic abnormality.

Age plays a role in the histologic confirmation of LSIL detected on cytology. Wright and colleagues found that histologic CIN was confirmed more often in women younger than 29 years with cytologic LSIL than in those older than 29 years, which was the median age of the study population. On the other hand, histologic confirmation of CIN was equal among younger and older women who had a cytologic diagnosis of HSIL.[14]

NATURAL HISTORY OF LSIL

Seventy to eighty percent of low-grade lesions remain unchanged over time or resolve spontaneously without treatment, especially in younger women. In a significant proportion, however, a higher-grade lesion develops. Nasiell et al followed 555 women with cytologic evidence of CIN 1. Only those who progressed to CIN 3 were treated. During the study, 62% of the women returned to normal, while 16% progressed to CIN 3 and were subsequently treated. Two patients who dropped out of the study were found 2 and 6 years later to have invasive cervical cancer.[15] Melnikow and associates performed a meta-analysis of studies that followed women who did not receive treatment after abnormal cytologic diagnosis. They reported that whereas 47.4% of women with LSIL returned to normal cytology within 2 years, 20.8% progressed to CIN

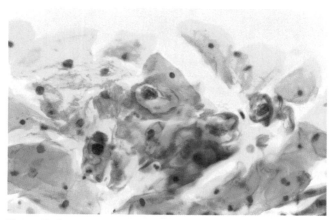

Figure 10-2. Epithelial cell abnormality, low-grade squamous intraepithelial lesion with changes of human papillomavirus. In the near center of this smear, a cell with a similarly enlarged, irregular nucleus with a distinctive perinuclear halo and clearing of the cytoplasm can be seen. Adjacent to it are several additional cells with similar findings admixed with superficial and intermediate squamous cells.

2 or CIN 3, and 0.15% progressed to cancer.[16] These studies demonstrate that although a proportion of women with LSIL may develop high-grade lesions or invasive cancer, a large number, if not most, will exhibit spontaneous lesion regression.

A significant percentage of low-grade lesions resolve spontaneously without treatment or merely persist over time.

The actual proportions of low-grade lesions that regress and progress and the rates of change over time have not been fully elucidated. This is due in part to methodologic difficulties inherent in performing natural history studies. Unless all study patients with normal and abnormal cytology undergo colposcopy and directed biopsies, it is impossible to accurately classify which cervix is truly normal and which harbors some degree of dysplasia. The effect of biopsy further confounds the ideal study design, because it is known that performance of a biopsy can accelerate regression, thus altering the natural history of the lesion. Moreover, the false-negative rate of the Papanicolaou (Pap) test has been reported to be as high as 51%,[17] ensuring some degree of misclassification in studies of natural history based on cytology alone. Positive but underinterpreted LSIL cytology is also a concern. Kinney et al, reporting on colposcopically directed biopsies of 46,009 women, found that 15.2% of women with a cytologic diagnosis of LSIL had histologically confirmed CIN 2, CIN 3, or invasive cervical cancer.[18]

Combining HPV-associated koilocytosis with CIN 1 to create the Bethesda System category of LSIL remains controversial. Lonky et al compared colposcopically directed biopsy results of a well-screened population of women whose diagnosis of LSIL was based on HPV cytopathic effect with results of those whose LSIL diagnosis was based on CIN 1 alone without evidence of koilocytosis. Women with a diagnosis of LSIL and HPV cytopathic effect were more than twice as likely to be negative for CIN on colposcopy or biopsy. Additionally, women with Pap smears showing LSIL without HPV cytopathic effect were significantly more likely to harbor high-grade histologic lesions.[19] Kurman and associates justified combining cytologic findings of CIN 1 and HPV effect into LSIL by pointing to the behavior and virology of the two component lesions. They pointed to studies showing a 16% rate of progression to CIN 3 among women with CIN 1 and without HPV effect, compared with a 14% progression rate among those with HPV cytopathic changes. Furthermore, they noted that both CIN 1 and HPV changes are associated with a heterogeneous complement of high-risk and low-risk HPV types.[20]

COLPOSCOPIC FINDINGS OF LSIL

The degree of acetowhite change seen colposcopically in LSIL is variable. The acetic acid–mediated whiteness may appear as a pale, translucent, pink-white color (Fig. 10–4) or a dense, snow-white color (Fig. 10–5), depending on whether overt condylomatous changes are present

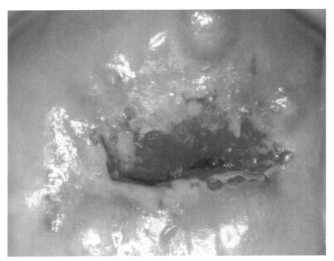

Figure 10–4. A low-grade lesion surrounding the os with translucent, mild, acetowhite changes and a nabothian cyst at 12 o'clock.

or not. The acetowhite appearance of dysplastic cervical lesions results when light directed from the colposcope is reflected off the different layers of cervical epithelium and the underlying network of basal capillaries at the stromal-epithelial junction. In cases of increased nuclear density of the epithelium (i.e., an increased nuclear-to-cytoplasmic [N/C] ratio), less light penetrates to the stroma and more is reflected back from the epithelium. Dysplastic epithelium is characterized by an increased N/C ratio. In cases of LSIL, this results from the relative enlargement of the cell nucleus to as much as three times that of a normal intermediate cell nucleus. The N/C ratio is less pronounced in LSIL than in HSIL, where the cytoplasm is contracted while the nucleus is enlarged.

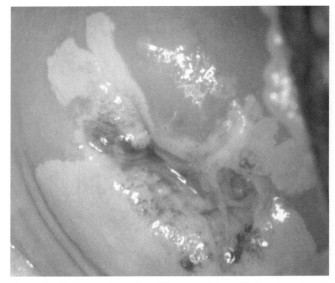

Figure 10–5. Low-grade lesion with snow-white epithelium, geographic borders, and fine punctuation and mosaic pattern noted near os.

The application of 3% to 5% acetic acid reveals the increased nuclear density of the dysplastic cervical epithelium. Although the mechanism by which diluted acetic acid causes dysplastic epithelium to appear white is not completely understood, it is felt that a major role is played by osmotic changes occurring in the cells. The hyperosmolar acetic acid partially dehydrates the cell, which has the effect of contracting the cytoplasmic volume and thus further increasing the N/C ratio. This transient increase in relative nuclear density creates an increase in the amount of white light reflected back to the eyepiece of the colposcope. Over time, the acetic acid effect fades as water returns to the intracellular compartment. In low-grade lesions without overt condylomatous changes, the epithelium appears as a pale, relatively translucent, pink-white color. The acetowhite reaction of LSIL is more gradual in onset and more transient in duration than are the acetowhite changes observed in higher-grade dysplasia.

The acetowhite reaction of LSIL is more gradual in onset and more transient in duration than what occurs when higher-grade dysplasia is present.

Condylomatous changes resulting from certain types of HPV, most notably types 6 and 11, may present on the cervix as exophytic condylomata acuminata (Fig. 10–6) or as flat to slightly raised "satellite lesions" (Fig. 10–7). These lesions may or may not be contiguous with the transformation zone and frequently appear as multiple, small, well-circumscribed acetowhite lesions on the portio vaginalis of the cervix (Fig. 10–8). They may extend onto the vagina as well (Fig. 10–9). Histologically, condylomatous lesions are often characterized by surface keratinization resulting from hyperkeratosis or parakeratosis (Fig. 10–10). Colposcopically, most of the light projected

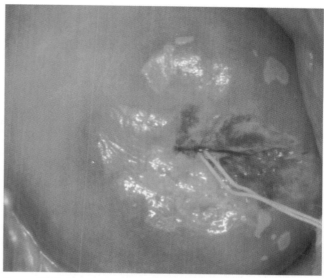

Figure 10–7. Peripheral patchy areas of faint acetowhite epithelium, as well as faint white epithelium on the posterior lip of the cervix. An intrauterine device string is visible at the os.

from the colposcope will reflect off the surface keratin with very little reaching the subepithelial capillaries, thus producing the dense, snow-white appearance after application of 3% to 5% acetic acid. Often, the surface keratin will appear white even without the application of acetic

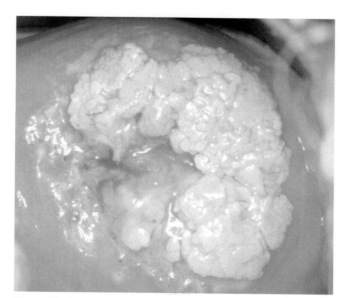

Figure 10–6. Exophytic cervical condyloma with a raised, irregular acetowhite surface.

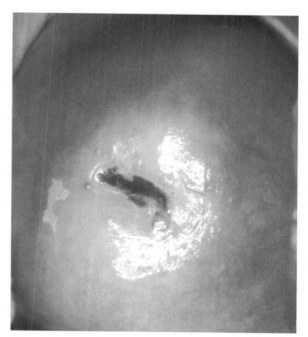

Figure 10–8. Satellite area of acetowhite epithelium on the portio of the cervix, not adjacent to the squamocolumnar junction.

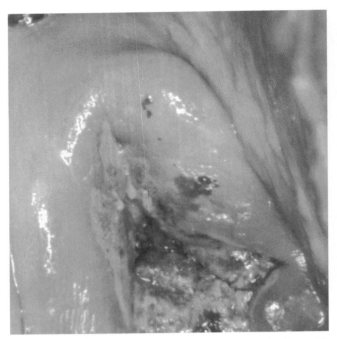

Figure 10–9. Example of low-grade lesion at 9 o'clock along with patchy low-grade changes of the left wall of the proximal vagina.

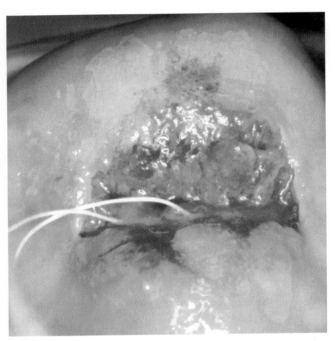

Figure 10–11. A low-grade lesion with geographic borders and fine punctation at 12 o'clock.

acid, as in leukoplakia. It will take up Lugol's solution poorly and appear as white to pale yellow iodine staining.[21]

> **Condylomatous lesions may vary in surface contour, from flat lesions with fine punctation, to slightly raised areas with asperities, to florid, exophytic condylomata acuminata.**

Condylomatous lesions may vary in surface contour from flat, acetowhite lesions with fine punctation (Fig. 10–11), to slightly raised areas with regular fine projec-

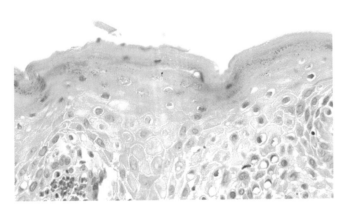

Figure 10–10. Cervical biopsy with slight hypergranulosis and mild hyperkeratosis. No definite evidence of human papillomavirus change is identified in this view.

tions called asperities, to florid, exophytic condylomata acuminata (Figs. 10–12 and 10–13). Flat, acetowhite satellite lesions are sometimes referred to as flat condylomata.[21]

> **Unlike the exophytic lesions of invasive cancer, condylomata do not exhibit atypical vessels or areas of necrosis.**

Each papilla in an exophytic condylomata acuminata has a central ascending and descending capillary loop that may be more easily seen after the diluted acetic acid has begun to fade (Fig. 10–14). Condylomata may be difficult to distinguish from high-grade lesions if they have only a minimally raised surface with shallow projections. The central capillary loops may appear as punctation.[21] The distinction between condylomata acuminata and invasive cancer may also be confusing. Contact bleeding may be present, especially in the presence of an accompanying vaginal or cervical infection. However, unlike the exophytic lesions of invasive cancer, condylomata do not exhibit atypical vessels or areas of necrosis (Fig. 10–15).

> **Terms used to describe the margins of noncondylomatous low-grade lesions include *feathered, flocculated*, and *geographic*.**

In noncondylomatous, low-grade intraepithelial lesions, the surface contours are usually flat. The margins may be indistinct, with the acetowhite changes noted at the squamocolumnar junction fading into the background color of the mature squamous epithelium (Fig. 10–16).

The margins may also appear irregular (Fig. 10–17), as opposed to the sharp, straight margins of high-grade lesions. Numerous terms are used to describe the margins of low-grade lesions, including *feathered* as on the tail of a turkey, *flocculated* like gathered cloth, or *geographic*

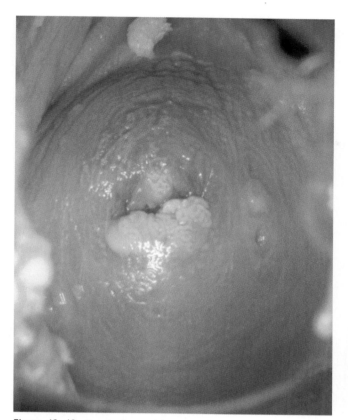

Figure 10–12. Exophytic condyloma at the os as well as near the cervicovaginal reflection.

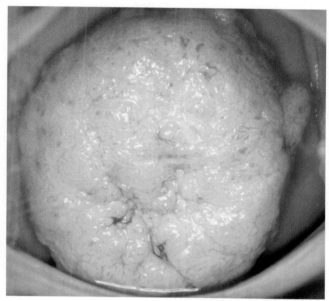

Figure 10–14. Large exophytic condyloma encompassing the entire cervix. The lesion is bright acetowhite, and as the acetic acid reaction fades slightly, looped vessels can be seen.

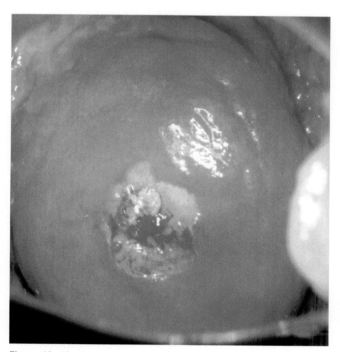

Figure 10–13. Low-grade lesion of the anterior lip of the cervix with an exophytic condyloma present at 12 o'clock.

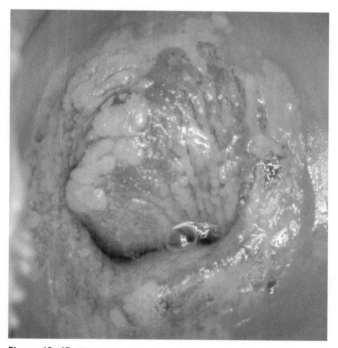

Figure 10–15. Ectropion with rim of faint acetowhite epithelium. In addition, there is raised, bright acetowhite epithelium at 12 o'clock with punctation consistent with condyloma.

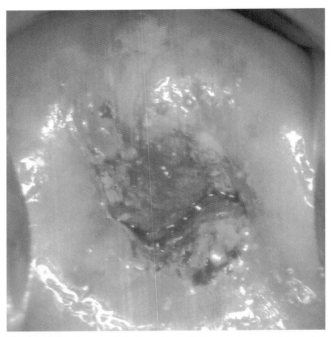

Figure 10-16. Low-grade lesion with indistinct borders and faint acetowhite epithelium.

with the maplike appearance of bays and peninsulas. LSIL may exhibit punctation and mosaic patterns (Fig. 10-18). Unlike high-grade lesions, however, the vessel patterns of low-grade lesions tend to be fine, of small caliber, regular in their distribution, and of normal intercapillary distance (50 to 250 μm). Atypical vessels are usually absent in low-grade lesions.

The colposcopic findings of low-grade lesions are variable. Hellberg and Nilsson reported the colposcopic appearance of 165 women with histologically confirmed CIN 1. The study patients demonstrated the following colposcopic findings: acetowhite epithelium in 52.1%, punctation in 22.4%, mosaic pattern in 18.2%, and atypical vessels in 2.4%.[22] Other, smaller series have reported these findings in the same order of frequency but with higher rates of the punctation and mosaic patterns, and acetowhite epithelium was reported as almost universally present.[23]

> **The colposcopic impression of low-grade disease is less precise and less reproducible than is the colposcopic impression of higher-grade lesions.**

Identifying the colposcopic findings and formulating a colposcopic impression of low-grade lesions can be more challenging in many ways than diagnosing high-grade lesions. The colposcopic impression of low-grade disease is less precise and less reproducible than the colposcopic impression of high-grade lesions.[23-25] Hopman et al reviewed eight studies that reported colposcopic impressions and histologic correlates in patients with satisfactory colposcopic examinations. They found that a colposcopic impression of CIN 1 accurately predicted the histologic

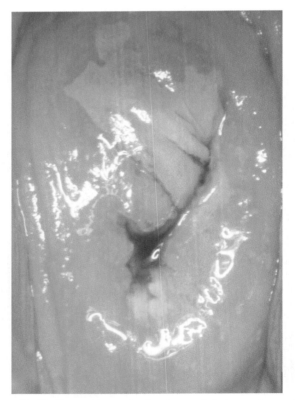

Figure 10-17. Geographic margins in a low-grade lesion on the anterior lip of the cervix. Squamocolumnar junction is not entirely visualized.

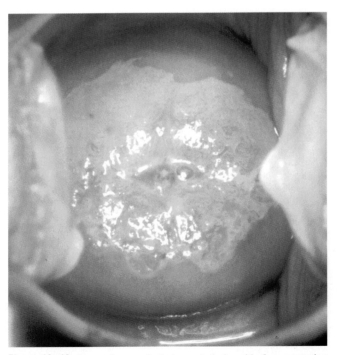

Figure 10-18. Large, low-grade lesion anteriorly with fine punctation and a faint mosaic pattern.

diagnosis only 42.8% of the time (range, 20% to 60%). This correlated with rates of 61.6%, 59% and 78.3% for no CIN, CIN 2, and CIN 3, respectively.[23] The study also found an intraobserver agreement of 66.7% when 23 expert colposcopists reviewed slide colpophotographs of varying degrees of dysplasia during two study sessions 2 to 3 months apart. The interobserver agreement for the two readings was only 52.4% and 51%, respectively. They found both interobserver and intraobserver concordance to be worse with CIN 1 and CIN 2 than with the categories of no CIN and CIN 3.[25]

COLPOSCOPIC MIMICS OF LOW-GRADE LESIONS

With the exception of characteristic findings of condylomata acuminata, the colposcopic findings of LSIL differ only by degree from those seen in immature squamous metaplasia. In immature squamous metaplasia, multiple layers of nuclear-dense reserve cells underlie the immature nonglycogenated metaplastic cells and the last remnants of the columnar layer. After application of diluted acetic acid, the nuclear-dense metaplastic epithelium frequently appears a pale acetowhite color (Fig. 10–19) that is less dense and more translucent than that observed in low-grade lesions (Fig. 10–20). Like LSIL, the margins are irregular and may be faint or indistinct. Fine mosaic and punctation patterns may also be seen. These acetowhite changes are especially prominent around gland openings and the new squamocolumnar junction.

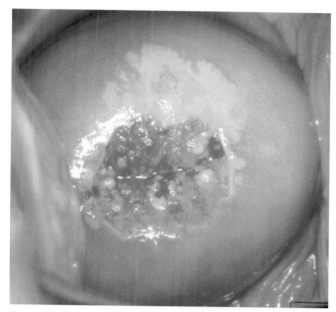

Figure 10–20. Low-grade lesion with geographic margins and a denser acetowhite appearance compared with the metaplasia seen in Figure 10–19.

Colposcopic findings of repair, which may be seen after treatment of CIN, are similar to those of squamous metaplasia. Pale acetowhite changes and even fine mosaic or punctation (Fig. 10–21) may be visible for the first 4 to 6 months after treatment with cryotherapy or loop excision.

The colposcopic examination is less sensitive in older women, especially if they are postmenopausal.

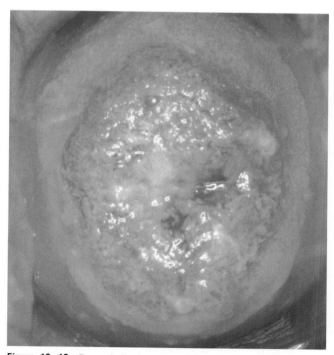

Figure 10–19. Congenitally large transformation zone with a band of metaplasia represented by mild acetowhite epithelium. The acetowhite changes of metaplasia can be confused with low-grade lesions.

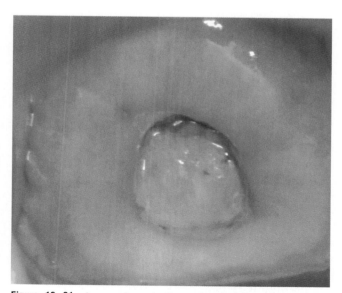

Figure 10–21. A normal cervix 2 months after loop electrosurgical excision. There is a mild protrusion of endocervical tissue out of the os that is undergoing metaplasia, giving a mild acetowhite appearance.

Caution must be exercised in making the colposcopic diagnosis of low-grade lesions in older women. This is especially true in postmenopausal women when squamous atrophy limits the epithelial strata to basal and parabasal layers. Zahm et al found that the acetowhite reaction, irregular surface contours, and distinct margins of high-grade lesions were more likely to be blunted in women age 35 years or older (Fig. 10–22). They observed that, even in older premenopausal women, the colposcopic examination was less sensitive than in younger women and that trivial findings had a higher frequency of harboring significant CIN.[26]

In pregnancy, low-grade lesions may be underdiagnosed colposcopically because of the normal physiologic changes that occur on the cervix.

To the colposcopist, the blunting of the acetowhite reaction in pregnancy may be problematic, because the cervix becomes increasingly edematous and congested. Economos et al[27] reported substantial underdiagnosis of the colposcopic impression in pregnant women. Fourteen percent of patients with a colposcopic impression of low-grade lesions actually had CIN 3 on directed biopsy. On the other hand, the estrogen-mediated eversion of the endocervix common in pregnancy may cause normal physiologic changes to be overdiagnosed colposcopically as low-grade dysplasia. Eversion permits the extension of squamous metaplasia centrally and creates the appearance of low-grade acetowhite change. The new proliferation of the endocervical papillae may also exhibit an acetowhite response on the tips. In pregnancy, the interpretation of low-grade lesions challenges even the most experienced colposcopist. See Chapter 20 for examples of lesions in pregnancy.

SUMMARY

The diagnosis of histologic and colposcopic LSIL requires rigorous attention not only to the characteristics of the lesion at the cellular and epithelial levels, but also to the patient's age and pregnancy status. Although the virology of CIN is becoming better understood, it is still not possible to reliably predict which low-grade lesions will regress spontaneously and in which women the finding of LSIL presages a progression to HSIL and, ultimately, invasive cervical cancer.

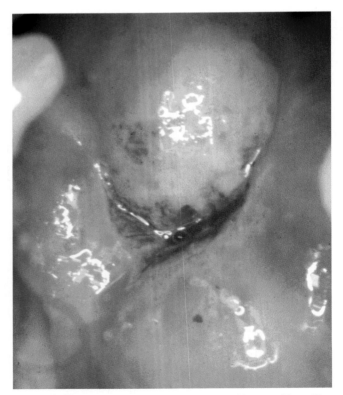

Figure 10–22. Cervix of a 50-year-old woman with acetowhite epithelium and ill-defined borders. The initial impression was a low-grade lesion, but biopsy revealed cervical intraepithelial neoplasia, grade 3.

SUMMARY OF KEY POINTS

- LSIL is associated with high-risk HPV types in up to 86% of cases.

- Unlike HSIL that reflects infection with a single HPV type, LSIL is associated with multiple HPV types in more than half of cases.

- Most low-grade lesions reflect the expression of an HPV infection rather than a true premalignant condition.

- Cytologic changes should not be characterized as "koilocytosis" or "HPV effect" based on a perinuclear halo alone. The nucleus must exhibit atypia, including enlargement to at least three times its normal size.

- The cytologic diagnosis of LSIL is more likely to be false positive in older women than in young women.

- A total of 70% to 80% of LSIL remains unchanged or resolves spontaneously over time. Less than 1% of LSIL progresses to invasive cervical cancer.

- Most women who are HPV positive do not develop LSIL.

- Persistence of HPV infection and infection with a high-risk HPV type are predictors of the development of squamous intraepithelial lesions.

- Cervical HPV infection is transient in most young women.

- Colposcopic findings of low-grade lesions are variable, and accurate colposcopic diagnosis of LSIL is less precise and less reproducible than in high-grade disease.

- Low-grade lesions may differ from squamous metaplasia only by degree.

- The acetowhite reaction of CIN may be blunted in older women and in pregnant women.

References

1. Kurman RJ, Solomon D: The Bethesda System for Reporting Cervical/Vaginal Cytologic Diagnoses: Definitions, Criteria, and Explanatory Notes for Terminology and Specimen Adequacy. New York, Springer-Verlag, 1994
2. Lorincz AT, Reid R, Jenson AB, et al: Human papillomavirus infection of the cervix: Relative risk associations of 15 common anogenital types. Obstet Gynecol 1992;79:328.
3. Park T, Fujiwara H, Wright TC: Molecular biology of cervical cancer and its precursors. Cancer 1995;76:1902.
4. Schiffman MH, Brinton LA: The epidemiology of cervical carcinogenesis. Cancer 1995;76:1888.
5. Atypical Squamous Cells of Undetermined Significance/Low-Grade Squamous Intraepithelial Lesions Triage Study (ALTS) Group: Human papillomavirus testing for triage of women with cytologic evidence of low-grade squamous intraepithelial lesions: Baseline data from a randomized trial. J Natl Cancer Inst 2000;92:397.
6. Moscicki AB, Burt VG, Kanowitz S, et al: The significance of squamous metaplasia in the development of low grade squamous intraepithelial lesions in young women. Cancer 1999;85:1139.
7. Reid R, Campion MJ: HPV-associated lesions of the cervix: Biology and colposcopic features. Clin Obstet Gynecol 1989;32:157.
8. Park J, Sun D, Genest DR, et al: Coexistence of low and high grade squamous intraepithelial lesions of the cervix: Morphologic progression or multiple papillomaviruses? Gynecologic 1998;70:368.
9. Ho GYF, Bierman R, Beardsley L, et al: Natural history of cervicovaginal papillomavirus infection in young women. N Engl J Med 1998;338:423.
10. Moscicki AB, Shiboski S, Broering J, et al: The natural history of human papillomavirus infection as measured by repeated DNA testing in adolescent and young women. J Pediatr 1998;132:277.
11. Manos MM, Sherman ME, Scott DR, et al: Human papillomavirus and cervical intraepithelial neoplasia. J Natl Cancer Inst 1993;85:1868.
12. Burk RD, Kelly P, Feldman F, et al: Declining prevalence of cervicovaginal human papillomavirus infection with age is independent of other risk factors. Sex Transm Dis 1996;23:333.
13. Cox JT, Massad LS, Lonky N, et al: ASCCP practice guidelines: Management guidelines for the follow-up of cytology read as low grade squamous intraepithelial lesion. J Lower Genital Tract Dis 2000;4:83.
14. Wright TC, Xiao WS, Koulos J: Comparison of management algorithms for the evaluation of women with low-grade cytologic abnormalities. Obstet Gynecol 1995;85:202.
15. Nasiell K, Roger V, Nasiell M: Behavior of mild cervical dysplasia during long-term follow-up. Obstet Gynecol 1986;67:665.
16. Melnikow J, Nuovo J, Willan AR, et al: Natural history of cervical squamous intraepithelial lesions: A meta-analysis. Obstet Gynecol 1998;92:727.
17. McCrory DC, Mather DB, Bastian L, et al: Evaluation of Cervical Cytology. Evidence Report/Technology Assessment No. 5. AHCPR Publication No. 99-E010. Rockville MD, Agency for Health Care Policy and Research, February 1999.
18. Kinney WK, Manos MM, Hurley LB, et al: Where's the high-grade cervical neoplasia? The importance of minimally abnormal Papanicolaou diagnoses. Obstet Gynecol 1998;91:973.
19. Lonky NM, Navarre GL, Saunders S, et al: Low-grade Papanicolaou smears and the Bethesda System: A prospective cytohistopathologic analysis. Obstet Gynecol 1995;85:716.
20. Kurman RJ, Malkasian GD, Sedlis A, et al: From Papanicolaou to Bethesda: The rationale for a new cervical cytology classification. Obstet Gynecol 1991;77:779.
21. Meisells A, Fortin R, Roy M: Condylomatous lesions of the cervix II. Cytologic, colposcopic, and histopathologic study. Acta Cytol 1977;21:379.
22. Hellberg D, Nilsson S: 20-year experience of follow-up of the abnormal smear with colposcopy and histology and treatment by conization or cryosurgery. Gynecol Oncol 1990;8:166.
23. Hopman EH, Kenemans P, Helmerhorst TJM: Positive predictive rate of colposcopic examination of the cervix uteri: An overview of literature. Obstet Gynecol Surv 1998;53:97.
24. Ismail SM, Colclough AB, Dinnen JS, et al: Observer variation in histopathological diagnosis and grading of cervical intraepithelial neoplasia. Br Med J 1989;298:707.
25. Hopman EH, Voorhorst FJ, Kenemans P, et al: Observer agreement on interpreting colposcopic images of CIN. Gynecol Oncol 1995;48:206.
26. Zahm DM, Ninkl I, Greinke C, et al: Colposcopic appearance of cervical intraepithelial neoplasia is age dependent. Am J Obstet Gynecol 1998;179:1298.
27. Economos K, Veridiano NP, Delke I, et al: Abnormal cervical cytology in pregnancy: A 17-year experience. Obstet Gynecol 1993;81:915.

History

A 19-year-old gravida 0, para 0 is referred to you with an abnormal Pap smear. She has been sexually active since age 16 years with four partners. She is a smoker.

Figure 10-23

This is her Pap smear

- What is the cytologic diagnosis?

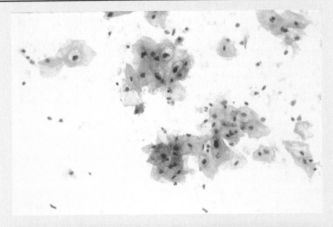

Figure 10-23.

Figure 10-24

This is a colpophotograph of her cervix after the application of 5% acetic acid.

- Is the transformation zone fully visualized?
- Describe what you see.

What is the next step in this patient's evaluation?

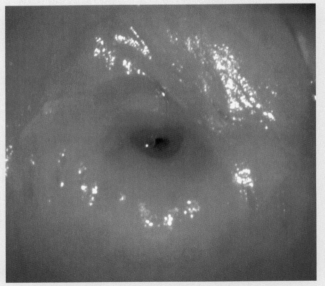

Figure 10-24.

Figure 10-25

This is a colpophotograph of the right vaginal fornix.

- What do you see?

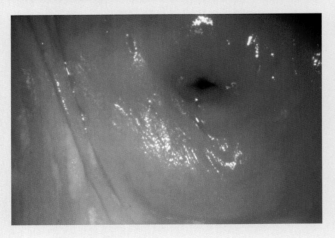

Figure 10-25.

236

Case Study 1 Answers

Figure 10-23
Several cells are seen with enlarged hyperchromatic nuclei, irregular nuclear borders, and sharply punched out perinuclear halos. These are koilocytes indicative of HPV infection.

Figure 10-24
The transformation zone is not fully visualized. Only normal squamous epithelium is seen.
There is no indication for an ectocervical biopsy. The ectocervical epithelium is normal. Because the transformation zone is in the endocervical canal and was not fully visualized, endocervical curettage is indicated. It is also necessary to evaluate the vagina for possible disease.

Figure 10-25
There are islands of acetowhite epithelium consistent with HPV change in the vagina. Biopsy confirmed the colposcopic impression.

Key Points of Case 1

Vaginal and vulvar disease may cause abnormalities on Pap smear. The vagina and vulva should be carefully evaluated, especially when evaluation of the cervix does not explain the cytologic abnormality.

Case Study 2 Questions

History
A 28-year-old gravida I, para I is sent to you for evaluation of a Pap smear suggestive of LSIL.

Figures 10–26 and 10–27
These are colpophotographs after the application of 5% acetic acid.

- Is the transformation zone fully visualized?
- Describe any colposcopic findings.

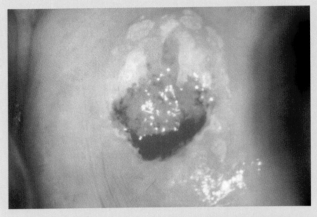

Figure 10–26.

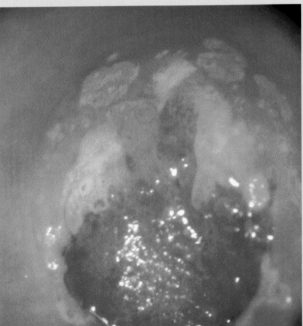

Figure 10–27.

Figure 10–28
The histology of the most severe colposcopic lesion is shown.

- What is your pathologic diagnosis?
- What are the management options in this patient?

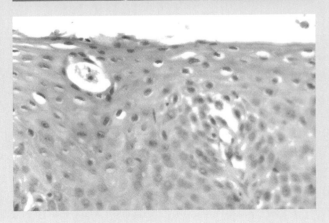

Figure 10–28.

Case Study 2 Answers

Figures 10–26 and 10–27

The squamocolumnar junction is seen along the posterior lip of the cervix, but in Figure 10–26, bleeding in the endocervical canal obscures the squamocolumnar junction anteriorly. In Figure 10–27, it is not possible to see the squamocolumnar junction despite removal of the blood, but by careful manipulation it was visible (not seen in these views).

There is bright acetowhite epithelium with a sharp geographic border seen adjacent to the squamocolumnar junction on the posterior lip of the cervix, with some other islands of grayer acetowhite epithelium distally.

Figure 10–28

Biopsy at the 6-o'clock position showed bland, well-spaced nuclei without hyperchromasia and only a few scattered perinuclear halos and "raisinoid" nuclei. This is metaplastic epithelium suggestive of some HPV changes.

There is little reason to treat this patient. Her cervical cytology, colposcopy, and biopsy did not show any evidence of high-grade disease, and even low-grade disease could not be confirmed by biopsy. She is best followed with colposcopy and repeat cytology in 6 months.

Key Points of Case 2

Women with low-grade cytology not confirmed on biopsy need not be treated. They may be followed with serial colposcopy and repeat cytology.

Case Study 3 Questions

History

A 43-year-old gravida III, para III is seen in your office. She is a smoker (one pack of cigarettes a day) with a history of genital warts 15 years ago. Her Pap smear is depicted in Figure 10–29.

Figure 10–29

- What do you see?
- What is your diagnosis?

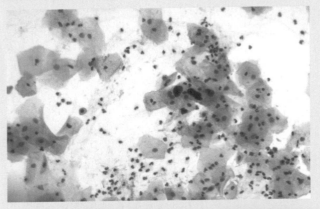

Figure 10–29.

Figure 10–30

This is a photograph of her cervix after the application of 5% acetic acid.

- Is the transformation zone fully visualized?
- Describe your findings.
- What is your colposcopic impression of the grade of the lesion?

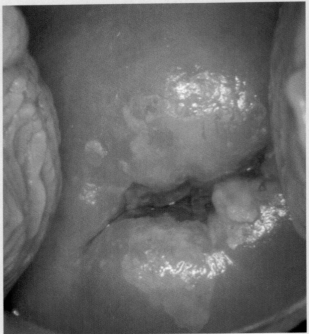

Figure 10–30.

Figure 10–31

A representative colposcopically directed biopsy was taken.

- What is your diagnosis?
- What should be the next step in this patient's management?

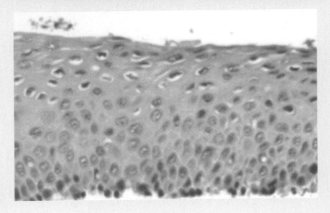

Figure 10–31.

Case Study 3 Answers

Figure 10–29

Several cells are seen with large, hyperchromatic nuclei but with abundant cytoplasm. This is consistent with a low-grade lesion.

Figure 10–30

The transformation zone is not fully visualized. Although the squamocolumnar junction is seen from 6 o'clock to 10 o'clock, there is acetowhite epithelium extending into the endocervical canal along the rest of the cervix. However, with some manipulation, the squamocolumnar junction was seen in its entirety (not shown). There is a gray-white lesion on both the anterior and the posterior lips of the cervix, although some of the lesion is a bit more translucent. The border is geographic. There are no vascular changes.

This appears to be a low-grade lesion.

Figure 10–31

There is nuclear crowding about one third to one half of the way to the epithelium with irregular, hyperchromatic nuclei and perinuclear halos seen on the surface. This is consistent with a CIN 1 to CIN 2 lesion with HPV changes.

It is acceptable to follow up a patient with a low-grade lesion with serial cytology and colposcopy. In a younger patient, this may even be the preferred approach. However, in this patient, several factors suggest that she should be treated. The lesion is a large three- to four-quadrant lesion. The patient is multiparous and beyond her reproductive age, and she is a smoker, placing her at greater risk for progression. The preferred management would be to treat her with cryotherapy, laser vaporization, or loop electrosurgical excision.

Key Point of Case 3

Treatment for minor-grade lesions must be individualized to the patient's age, her fertility desires, the extent of disease, and other associated risk factors.

Cytology, Colposcopy, and Histology of Low-Grade CIN

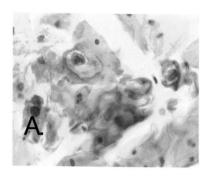

Features suggestive of a low-grade cervical lesion:
- Geographic borders
- Shiny acetowhite epithelium
- Absence of atypical vessels
- Satellite lesions
- Fine mosaic or punctation

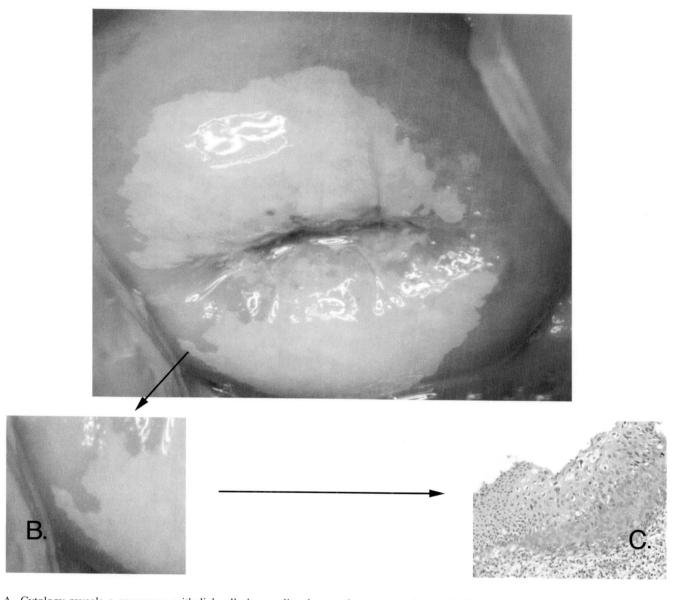

A. Cytology reveals a squamous epithelial cell abnormality: low-grade squamous intraepithelial lesion (LSIL) with changes of HPV. In the center is a cell with an enlarged, irregular nucleus; a distinctive perinuclear halo; and clearing of the cytoplasm. Adjacent are several cells with similar findings admixed with superficial and intermediate squamous cells. The background is clean.

B. Area of biopsy. Acetowhite epithelium with a geographic border and absent vessels.

C. Histology reveals CIN 1. The epithelium lacks maturation in the lower one third of the epithelium, and the disorderly basal cells exhibit some crowding within the parabasal area. Multinucleated cells are seen near the surface, and koilocytosis is present. There is mild, superficial, chronic inflammation in the stroma.

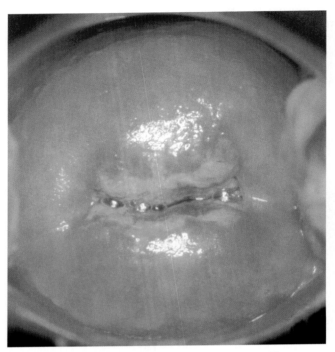

Plate 10–1. Acetowhite epithelium around the cervical os. The squamocolumnar junction cannot be seen. Biopsy confirmed cervical intraepithelial neoplasia, grade 1.

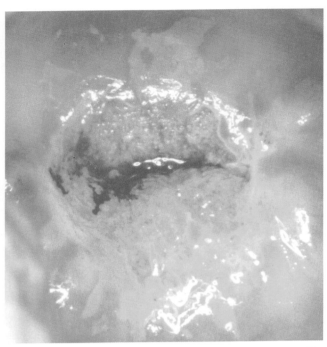

Plate 10–2. Faint acetowhite epithelium and geographic borders. The squamocolumnar junction is completely seen.

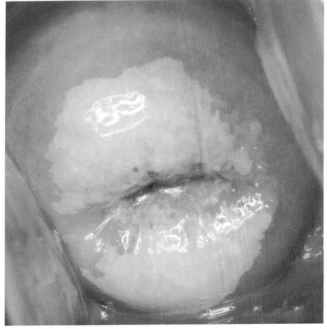

Plate 10–3. Large, low-grade lesion with snow-white epithelium and geographic border.

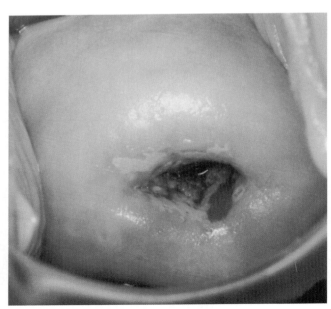

Plate 10–4. Low-grade lesion with geographic border.

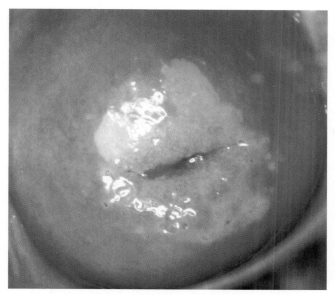

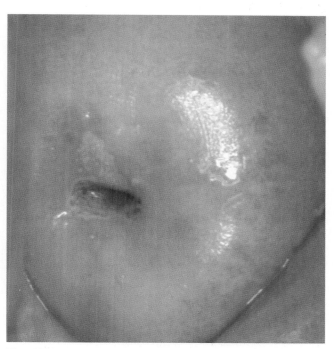

Plate 10-5. Faint area of acetowhite epithelium as well as a brighter area of acetowhite epithelium at 10 o'clock. Biopsies from 10 o'clock and 12 o'clock both revealed cervical intraepithelial neoplasia, grade 1. Satellite lesions are present.

Plate 10-6. Small, faint area of acetowhite epithelium and fine mosaic in a low-grade lesion.

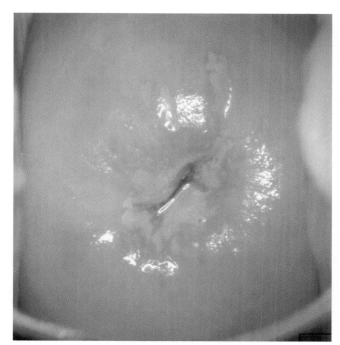

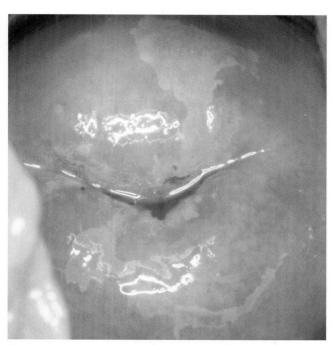

Plate 10-7. Central and satellite areas of acetowhite epithelium in a woman with a low-grade lesion.

Plate 10-8. Excellent example of geographic borders and faint acetowhite epithelium in a low-grade lesion.

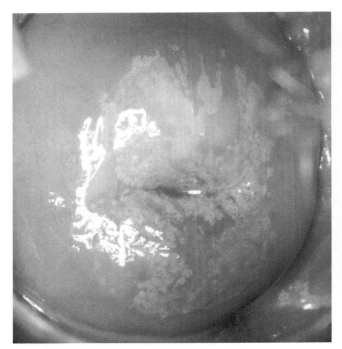

Plate 10-9. Low-grade lesion on the anterior lip of the cervix. Columnar epithelium is noted on the posterior lip.

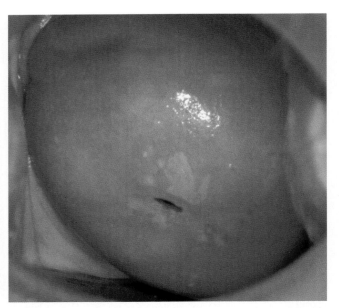

Plate 10-10. Satellite lesions exhibiting faint acetowhite epithelium that is not contiguous with the squamocolumnar junction. Biopsy confirmed cervical intraepithelial neoplasia, grade 1.

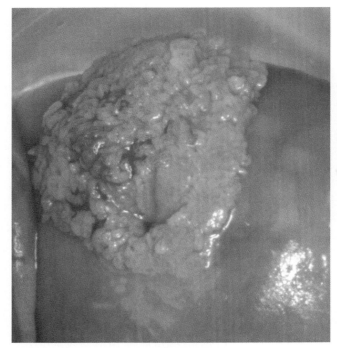

Plate 10-11. Large, exophytic condyloma of the cervix.

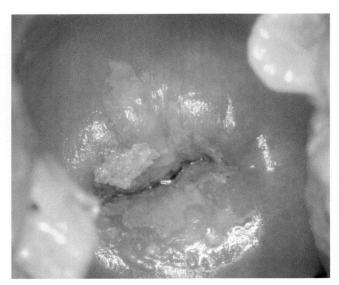

Plate 10-12. Low-grade lesions (flat condylomata) and an exophytic condyloma of the cervix at 11 o'clock.

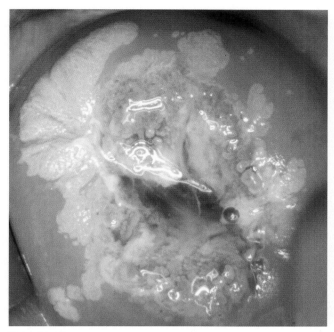

Plate 10-13. Large condyloma of the cervix with a hyperkeratotic, granular surface contour.

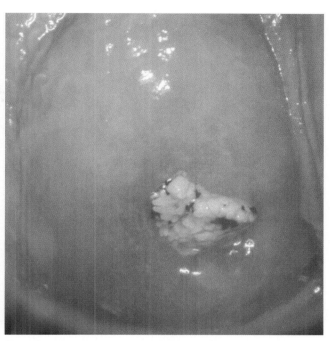

Plate 10-14. Exophytic condyloma at the cervical os.

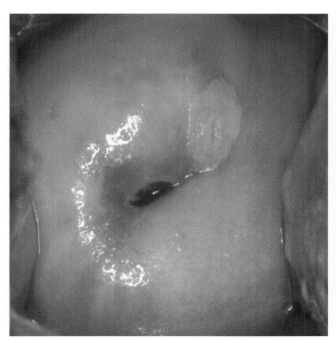

Plate 10-15. Inverted condyloma of the cervix.

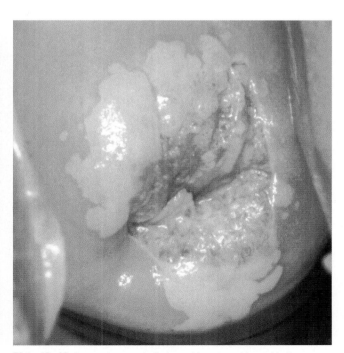

Plate 10-16. Large, low-grade lesion with snow-white epithelium, geographic borders, and absent vessels.

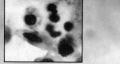

CHAPTER *11*

• Barbara S. Apgar
• Gregory L. Brotzman

High-Grade Squamous Intraepithelial Lesion

Unless their clinical setting is a referral practice, most colposcopists will evaluate primarily women with low-grade cervical lesions. Compared with low-grade squamous intraepithelial lesion (LSIL), high-grade squamous intraepithelial lesion (HSIL) may seem spectacular and impressive. However, if colposcopists concentrate only on features of preinvasive disease, subtle signs of invasive disease may be missed. The reduction in incidence of invasive cervical carcinoma is primarily due to the accurate diagnosis and treatment of high-grade cervical lesions and microinvasive disease.[1]

A substantial body of evidence has confirmed that the human papillomavirus (HPV) is the etiologic agent in cervical carcinogenesis. The worldwide prevalence of HPV in cervical cancer is about 99.7%.[2] The presence of HPV in virtually all cervical cancers implies that HPV has a stronger association with cervical cancer than does any other specific cause of human cancer. The cervical carcinogenesis model involves the following three steps: HPV infection, progression to a high-grade preinvasive lesion, and then invasion.[3] The central goal of colposcopy is to rule out invasive disease. It is important to remember that the majority of women who develop high-grade cervical disease or invasion have persistent HPV infection.[4] Inherent in this knowledge is the opportunity to identify the majority of women who are at risk for significant HPV-associated disease if they present for cytologic screening. Developing resources for targeting unscreened populations should be a top priority. It has been demonstrated that in the United States almost half of all cases of cervical cancer occurring annually are associated with inadequate Papanicolaou (Pap) smear screening or no screening at all.[5]

The best opportunity for prevention of invasive cervical carcinoma lies in screening women age 20 to 39 years when the incidence of cervical intraepithelial neoplasia (CIN), grade 3, is highest in the screened population.[6] In a targeted population of screened Icelandic women who were prospectively followed from 1966 to 1995, the rate of histologically verified CIN 2 or CIN 3 began to accumulate at 24 to 36 months after a normal cytologic

smear.[7] Among appropriately screened women, histologically verified CIN 2 or CIN 3 or invasive cancer is extremely uncommon after age 60 years.

RATES OF PROGRESSION

The approximate rate of progression from LSIL to HSIL ranges from 10% to 20%.

Although the natural history and progression from LSIL to HSIL are variable and uncommon, about 10% to 20% of women may progress to CIN 2 or CIN 3 after a cytologic diagnosis of LSIL.[8] In another study with a follow-up period of 18 months, 14% of low-grade CIN lesions progressed.[9] In this study, the regression rate was inversely related and the progression rate directly related to the grade of CIN. A more recent longitudinal study demonstrated that 18.6% of 342 women with LSIL progressed to CIN 2 or CIN 3.[10] From these data, it was determined that the approximate rate of progression from LSIL to HSIL ranges from 10% to 20%.

The rates of regression, persistence, and progression for CIN 2 were 54%, 16%, and 30%, respectively.

Unlike LSIL, HSIL has significant potential to progress to invasive cervical disease if left untreated.[11] Long-term studies, however, have demonstrated variable progression, persistence, and regression rates for HSIL. Failure to use a standard set of selection criteria and follow-up procedures contributes to the variations in study outcomes. Nasiell and colleagues conducted a natural history study of 894 women with CIN 2 over 50 to 78 months. The rates of regression, persistence, and progression for CIN 2 were 54%, 16%, and 30%, respectively.[12]

The progression rate in women with untreated carcinoma in situ is between 12% and 70%.

Very little is known about the actual progression rate of HSIL to cervical carcinoma. What little data are available come from a small series of women with carcinoma in situ (CIS) who inadvertently were not treated.[11] Review of published data suggests that the progression rate in women with untreated CIS is between 12% and 70%.[8, 13] The significant potential of HSIL to progress to microinvasive or invasive disease has led to the recommendation that these lesions be definitively treated rather than observed. There is a strong argument for the necessity of careful follow-up and the importance of active surveillance of abnormal findings after treatment of HSIL to ensure that any treatment failures are detected promptly.

CLASSIFICATION OF HSIL

It has been estimated that approximately 10% of the 50 million Pap smears performed annually in the United States will show some type of abnormality and that 5% of the abnormal smears will demonstrate findings of LSIL or worse.[14] In more recent studies, LSIL and atypical squamous cells of undetermined significance (ASCUS) are by far the most prevalent abnormal cytologic diagnoses.[15] In a study of 46,009 women who underwent routine cytologic screening, 3.5% had ASCUS, 0.9% LSIL, 0.5% atypical glandular cells of undetermined significance (AGUS), and 0.3% HSIL.

HSIL, as defined by the Bethesda System, encompasses the categories of moderate dysplasia (CIN 2) and severe dysplasia–carcinoma in situ (CIN 3). HSIL is characterized by more nuclear abnormalities, a less productive infection, a more restrictive set of HPV types, and a greater tendency to progress to invasive disease than when compared with LSIL.[16]

The decision to combine moderate and severe dysplasia and carcinoma in situ under the category of HSIL is based on the following findings:

1. They contain the same cell-to-cell morphology.
2. They share the same HPV associations with invasive cancer.
3. They have similar neoplastic potential.
4. They have similar ploidy abnormalities.

One commonly held belief is that most CIN 3 lesions evolve over time from preexisting CIN 1 lesions.

However, there is a debate as to whether CIN 2 and CIN 3 are the same biologic entities and whether they should be grouped under a single category (HSIL). Some believe that CIN incorporates two distinctly different categories of risk. One (CIN 1, koilocytosis) is reflective of the HPV infection, and the other (CIN 2 or CIN 3) is the true cancer precursor.[17] One commonly held belief is that most CIN 3 lesions evolve over time from preexisting CIN 1 lesions.[11] Adding more credibility to this hypothesis of a continuum is the observation that many women with cervical cancer have a previous history of a low-grade lesion.[18] About half of LSIL lesions behave as non-neoplastic, productive viral infections that exhibit a high

regression rate. However, the other half behaves as a preneoplastic lesion that either persists or progresses to a more advanced abnormality. Studies have suggested that the transit time from HSIL to cervical carcinoma is faster than that from LSIL to invasion.[19]

The National Breast and Cervical Cancer Early Detection Program data were analyzed for the years 1991 to 1995 (second screening) and included 312,858 low-income women age 18 years and older who received one or more Pap smears at screening sites across the United States with follow-up as necessary.[20] The age-adjusted rate of biopsy-confirmed CIN 2 or worse among women undergoing their first cytologic screening was 7.4 per 1000 Pap smears. Fifty-six percent of Pap smears reported as HSIL from the first screening cycle were found to have histologically confirmed CIN 2 or CIN 3. This large study demonstrated that rates of CIN 3 were higher than rates of CIN 2 among women 30 years and older in the first screening cycle and among women in the 30- to 39-year and the 50- 64-year age groups in subsequent screening cycles. These age-specific data are consistent with other reports that the rates of low-grade CIN are higher among reproductive-age women and that the rates of high-grade CIN and invasive disease are higher among older women; the data also bolster the argument that CIN 2 or CIN 3 progresses from lower grades of dysplasia.

Some have suggested that CIN 3 arises de novo. Others argue that CIN 2 should be grouped with CIN 1 rather than with CIN 3.

Kiviatt and others have questioned the continuum theory of CIN, and some have suggested that CIN 3 arises de novo.[11] Evidence in support of this theory is the fact that some women with CIN 2 or CIN 3 never had evidence of a preceding CIN 1.[21] This fact is substantiated by data that show that cytologically normal women who test positive for oncogenic HPV types may develop CIN 2 or CIN 3 without a previous history of CIN 1.[22] Others argue that CIN 2 and CIN 3 differ in their malignant potential and so should not be combined under one heading (HSIL). They argue that CIN 2 should be grouped with CIN 1 rather than with CIN 3.

LSIL consists of two different types of lesions that are biologically distinct.

Just as invasive cancer is monoclonal, so is HSIL. Park and associates, who found all their cases of HSIL to be monoclonal, confirmed this in a study.[23] In contrast, 32% of LSIL was polyclonal. In this particular study, which compared clonal status with HPV types, a strong association was observed between HPV type and clonal status. LSIL consists of two different types of lesions that are biologically distinct. One entity is monoclonal and is associated with the same HPV types present in HSIL. The second type of LSIL is polyclonal, is associated with other HPV types not usually associated with HSIL, and is usually recognized as low risk.

Ploidy can be correlated with the histologic grade of CIN.[24] Ploidy data strongly segregate HSIL from LSIL (78% aneuploidy versus 21% aneuploidy, respectively;

$P < .0001$). There is a significant association between aneuploidy and severity of the lesion. Ninety-four percent of CIN 3 lesions are aneuploid, compared with 55% of CIN 2 lesions and 14% of CIN 1 lesions. Aneuploidy appears to be strongly associated with the presence of oncogenic HPV types that are detected in 95% of HSIL.[25]

PREDICTING HSIL FROM CYTOLOGY, CERVICOGRAPHY, AND HPV TESTING

Most high-grade CIN and cancer occur in women with minor cytologic abnormalities, visible lower genital tract lesions, or both.

It has been shown that cytologic grading alone does not always reliably predict which women have histologic high-grade cervical cancer precursors or invasive disease. In a study by Lonky et al, the diagnosis of high-grade cervical disease occurred in 132 of 265 (50%) women with HSIL cytology, 329 of 1784 (18%) women with LSIL, and 278 of 3118 (9%) women with ASCUS.[26] Only 132 of 771 cases of high-grade cervical lesions (17%) and 5 of 13 cases of invasive cancer followed a cytologic diagnosis suggesting HSIL or invasion. Seventy-seven percent of histologic high-grade lesions were diagnosed after a minimally abnormal cytologic diagnosis. The authors suggested that most high-grade CIN and cancer may occur in women with minor cytologic abnormalities, visible lower genital tract lesions, or both. An earlier analysis of the Bethesda System demonstrated that approximately 22% of patients with LSIL have histologic-proved CIN 2 or CIN 3.[27] In studies correlating the cytologic diagnosis with the histologic diagnosis before the introduction of the Bethesda System, approximately 26% of women with mild dysplasia on cytology were shown to have moderate to severe dysplasia (CIN 2 or CIN 3) on histology.[28] Kinney and colleagues found that 39% of the total number of cases of histologic HSIL in a routine screening population were detected in the follow-up to ASCUS and that a total of 69% were detected in follow-up of cytologic diagnoses, including ASCUS, LSIL, and AGUS.[29]

The specificity of cervicography was 95% with a positive predictive value of 13.8%.

The efficacy of cervicography screening for detection of high-grade and invasive cervical disease was evaluated in a high-risk, population-based study of cervical neoplasia among 8460 Costa Rican women.[30] An abnormal result on cervigram led to the referral of 5.7% of women for colposcopy, resulting in detection of all invasive cancers and 49.3% of high-grade and invasive lesions combined. The specificity of cervicography was 95% with a positive predictive value of 13.8%. On the other hand, with cytologic screening, 6.9% of the women were found to have ASCUS or worse and were referred for colposcopy. Cytologic screening correctly identified 77.2% of women with HSIL or invasion and 94.2% of those who did not have disease. More than three times as many cases of HSIL and cancer were detected by cytology alone than were detected by cervicography. However, cervicography identified one cancer that cytology missed. Conventional cytologic screening resulted in higher sensitivity than that with cervicography (except for invasive disease), and there was only a small difference in specificity between the two methods. The lower sensitivity rate of cervicography is reflected in the fact that it is not of benefit in women with an incompletely visualized transformation zone (postmenopausal women). If the sensitivity of cervicography for detecting high-grade cervical lesions could be increased without the need for colposcopic referral, cervicography would be an excellent test because of its ease of use and low rate of technically defective cervigrams. Although cytology performed better than cervicography for detection of HSIL, cervicography appears particularly useful for detecting invasive lesions and for screening for HSIL in regions that lack effective cervical cytology screening programs.

In another study, 5550 women with preinvasive cervical lesions were randomized initially to either cytology alone or cytology plus cervicography; they were rescreened 1 year later with the same procedures.[31] Colposcopy was performed on all women with either abnormal cytology or abnormal cervigrams. Compared with cytology screening alone, screening with cytology and cervicography produced a 30% reduction in all grades of CIN lesions and a 43% reduction in CIN 2 and CIN 3. Most of the lesions detected by one method were not detected by the other, and it is possible that cervicography could detect lesions that do not express the cellular abnormalities necessary for cytologic detection.

Cervicography has performed favorably in smaller studies. The efficacy of combined repeat cytology and cervicography for the identification of HSIL among patients with an ASCUS or LSIL diagnosis was determined in a high-risk population.[32] A total of 24 of 187 patients with ASCUS were found to have histologic CIN 2 or CIN 3. A repeat Pap smear would have resulted in detection of 11 of 24 lesions (sensitivity, 46%), whereas a cervigram would have resulted in detection of 22 of 24 lesions (sensitivity, 92%). For LSIL, repeat Pap smear would have detected 29 of 37 lesions (sensitivity, 78%), whereas a cervigram would have detected 33 of 37 lesions (sensitivity, 89%).

HPV testing has been proposed as an adjunctive test to identify high-grade cervical disease in women with ASCUS cytology. In a study by Manos et al, HPV-based triage of women with ASCUS (reflex testing, performed out of the liquid media retained after performance of liquid-based cytologic testing) was more sensitive in detecting HSIL or worse, while referring fewer women to colposcopy and avoiding the need for follow-up visits to repeat cytologic testing.[15] Although this approach is more cost-effective if the patient does not have to return for separate HPV testing, other, smaller studies have not shown the same cost reduction.[33]

Overall, HPV testing is more sensitive than conventional cytology testing (88.4% versus 77.7%) for detection of high-grade lesions and cancer but is less specific (89% versus 94.2%).

HPV DNA testing by the Hybrid Capture (HC) II assay was strongly associated with detection of high-grade cervical lesions and cancers in a high-risk study population in Costa Rica.[3] HC II assay targets 13 oncogenic HPV types. Sensitivity for detection of high-grade lesions and cancer was 74.8%, and specificity was 93.4%. The authors stated that the sensitivity of HC II testing for the detection of high-grade lesions and cancer is likely to be high for all populations worldwide because the assay covers all known oncogenic HPV types. The study demonstrated that oncogenic HPV types could be present in women with minimally abnormal or normal Pap smears. The authors concluded that the percentage of patients referred to colposcopy, based on HPV testing and the specificity for detection of high-grade lesions or invasion, depends on the prevalence of HPV in the population. Overall, HPV testing is more sensitive than conventional cytology testing (88.4% versus 77.7%) for detection of high-grade lesions and cancer but is less specific (89% versus 94.2%).

FORMATION OF HSIL AND PROGRESSION TO INVASION

HSIL probably arises as a small focus within a lower-grade lesion that gradually expands and eventually replaces the original HPV-infected tissue.

Cervical cancers arise from precursor lesions that are graded according to severity of the degree of disruption of epithelial differentiation.[34] HSIL probably arises as a small focus within a lower-grade lesion that gradually expands and eventually replaces the original HPV-infected tissue. Some lesions may progress more rapidly than others. It is debatable whether high-grade CIN develops directly from a low-grade lesion or whether the presence of an oncogenic HPV type could lead directly to a high-grade lesion.[35] Several prospective studies have added validity to the progression theory.

The observation that the prevalence of HSIL peaks in women 25 to 34 years old and the hypothesis of a disease continuum with progression from HPV infection to HSIL to cancer was supported in data from the population-based study in rural Costa Rica.[16] In this study, the HSILs could be roughly divided into the equivalent of CIN 2 and CIN 3 with corresponding median ages of 33 years and 37 years, respectively. This division would roughly equate with the hypothetical transition time of more than 5 years from LSIL to HSIL. The mean age of women with cancer was 39 years, approximately 5 years older than the median age for HSIL. The authors suggested that HSILs progress to subclinical cancer in 9 to 10 years and that symptomatic cancer arises 4 to 5 years later.

No progression was seen in the absence of HPV positivity with high-risk HPV types.

Three hundred and forty-two patients with abnormal cytologic smears were monitored every 3 to 4 months by cytology, colposcopy, and HPV testing for a mean of 16.5 months.[36] Women with progressive CIN were defined as those developing lesions after a colposcopic impression of CIN 3 over more than two quadrants or those developing a cytologic smear with HSIL. Nineteen women developed progressive CIN disease, and, of these, all demonstrated continuous HPV positivity; in all cases, colposcopic biopsy revealed CIN 3. No progression was seen in the absence of HPV positivity with high-risk HPV types. The cumulative rate of progressive, histologically verified CIN was 17% after 36 months. In this study, continuous HPV positivity with oncogenic HPV types was a strong marker for progression to CIN 3. Another study demonstrated that HPV positivity (type 16) and the grade of histologic sample were independent predictive risk factors for progression to high-grade disease.[37]

The diagnosis of both LSIL and HSIL in the same cervical specimen may reflect lesions bordering between high and low grade, progression of disease, or even different HPV infections. In a study by Park and colleagues, 98 cervical specimens with a histologic diagnosis of LSIL or HSIL were reviewed by an independent panel of experts.[38] Of these specimens, 59% did not exhibit significant variation in grade (classification discrepancy), but 41% showed a one- or two-grade shift. Both low- and high-grade foci exhibited HPV positivity in 65% of the specimens. All the foci with a one-grade shift were the same HPV type. In contrast, a significantly higher proportion of lesions with a two-grade shift (CIN 1 to CIN 3) contained two different HPV types. The authors concluded that lesions containing LSIL and HSIL that span two grades (CIN 1 and CIN 2) most likely represent morphologic progression in a single infection. However, lesions containing histologic CIN 1 and CIN 3 may be attributed to either lesion progression or two coincident infections, both of which may be present in the same histologic sample. The latter finding has implications for both the diagnosis of CIN and the interpretation of the theory of morphologic progression from low-grade to high-grade lesion in the same case.

Follow-up examinations on HPV-positive women demonstrated that the rate of progression increases and the transit time decreases as the CIN becomes more severe. The probability that an untreated LSIL will progress to a higher grade is partially dependent on the grade of the lesion. As CIN progresses, the cells progressively evolve to a less differentiated cellular state. Increased vessel density (angiogenesis) is related to increased tumor growth.[39] Although little is known about the process of angiogenesis in preinvasive lesions, it has been determined that vessel density increases significantly with grade of CIN.[40] There is also a significant increase in vessel density during progression for CIN 3 to microinvasion.[41] From this study, it appears that the onset of angiogenesis occurs during the progression of neoplastic lesions. CIN can be considered a prevascular phase of neoplasm with no metastatic potential. However, once the neoplastic cells have crossed the basement membrane, the tumor possesses the potential to control its own growth. Angiogenesis then becomes a tumor initiator with significant prognostic potential.

RISK FACTORS ASSOCIATED WITH HSIL

> **Cigarette smoking is related not only to the size of the lesion but also to the degree of dysplasia. Smoking more than 20 cigarettes per day appears to increase the risk of CIN 2 or CIN 3 in women who have minor cytologic abnormalities.**

Risk factors for low-grade and high-grade preinvasive cervical lesions appear to differ substantially. The variables of high-risk HPV types, multiple pregnancies, and smoking appear to be independent risk factors for CIN 2 or CIN 3.[42] In one study, the most prominent variable differentiating women with CIN 3 from women without CIN was detection of high-risk HPV types, followed by smoking and multiple pregnancies. Cigarette smoking is related not only to the size of the lesion but also to the degree of dysplasia. Smoking more than 20 cigarettes per day appears to increase the risk of CIN 2 and CIN 3 in women who have minor cytologic abnormalities.[43] In another study, the significant risk factors for high-grade CIN were current cigarette smoking, long-term contraceptive use, and presence of HPV type 16.[44] The presence of HPV 16 was associated with an 8.7-fold elevation in estimated relative risk (RR) for high-grade lesions. The estimated RR of high-grade CIN in current cigarette smokers was 2.4 compared with that of never-smokers, and it increased with the number of pack-years of exposure. Long-term users of oral contraceptive pills had an estimated RR for high-grade CIN of 1.9 compared with that of never-users. In contrast, the presence of HPV 16, oral contraceptive use, and cigarette smoking had little or no relationship to low-grade CIN.

> **Among smokers, the risk of high-grade CIN increased in parallel with the time of exposure and the number of years of smoking.**

In another study of the progression of low-grade to high-grade cervical lesions, women with CIN 2 or CIN 3 were compared with women with CIN 1 to determine risk factors associated with the most severe lesions.[45] After controlling for age, education, ethnicity, and frequency of Pap smear sampling, infection with HPV type 16 was associated with high-grade lesions but not with viral load or infection with multiple HPV types. The risk of CIN 3 increased with number of cigarettes smoked per day and decreased with frequency of condom use, but no such effect was seen for CIN 2. The authors suggested that although infection with HPV type 16 was associated with high-grade lesions, additional cofactor association such as cigarette smoking might be required for neoplastic progression. In another study of young Brazilian women, current cigarette smoking was strongly associated with CIN 2 or CIN 3. Among smokers, the risk of high-grade CIN increased parallel to the time of exposure and the number of years of smoking.[46] In these same women, the risk of being HPV positive for oncogenic types was significantly higher in those with CIN 2 or CIN 3 compared with those with lower-grade lesions. The authors suggested that high-risk HPV types and current cigarette

smoking could be synergistic for the development of cervical carcinogenesis.

Results of a study of 291 women suggested that among women whose median age was 33 years with a single cytologic smear showing LSIL, the prevalence of high-grade lesions (CIN 2 or CIN 3) increased in less educated women reporting one or more full-term pregnancies and in never-smokers.[47] The risk of CIN 2 or CIN 3 tended to increase with the number of sexual partners. Compared with women reporting one sexual partner, the multivariate odds ratios of CIN 2 and CIN 3 were 1.4 and 2.3, respectively, for women reporting two to three, or four or more, sexual partners ($P < .05$). The risk was also increased in current smokers and never-smokers. This study agrees with others[48] in that the risk of CIN is higher among smokers and women of low socioeconomic standing, especially if they have multiple sexual partners.

It has been suggested that minority women experience a high number of HPV-associated lesions.[49] It was shown that in 971 Hispanic women, 13.2% were positive for high-risk HPV types. Older age and oral contraceptive use were inversely associated with the high-risk HPV types. Single status and lifetime number of sexual partners were positively associated with an increased risk for HSIL. It was suggested that sexual behavior of the male partner may influence the rate of HPV infection in this population.

The role of immunosuppression in HSIL is discussed in Chapter 21.

HPV TYPES IN HSIL

A distinction has been made among HPV types of low, intermediate, and high oncogenic potential. Clinically, HPV types have been divided into low-risk types (types 6, 11, 42, 43, 44) and high-risk types (types 16, 18, 31, 33, 35, 52, 58). Comparisons of the strength of association between specific HPV type and disease severity have indicated that HPV types can be classified into specific categories based on risk.[50] RR for HPV types 31, 33, 35, 51, and 52 (RR, 23 to 168.6) peak in the HSIL category. The under-representation of these types in invasive cancers is the basis for designating them as intermediate-risk types. Overall, the presence of an intermediate-risk type confers an approximate RR of 71.9 for occurrence of HSIL and 31.1 for occurrence of invasive cancer.

> **HPV type 16 is the most important viral subtype; it is detected in 47.1% of invasive cancers, 47.1% of HSILs, and 16.2% of LSILs.**

HPV types 16, 18, 45 and 56 are associated with invasive cancer. RR estimates for HPV type 16 rise significantly between LSIL (RR, 36.9) and HSIL (RR, 235.7) and flatten out between HSIL and invasive cancer (RR, 260). Type 16 is almost equally common in both HSIL and invasive cancer and is the most important viral subtype, being detected in 47.1% of invasive cancers, 47.1% of HSILs, and 16.2% of LSILs.[50] In the Costa Rica study, the majority of HSILs and cancers were associated with previously identified oncogenic HPV types, particularly HPV 16, which was detected in almost 50% of both HSIL and cancer.[16] HPV 58 was the second most common HPV type in HSILs and the third most common type in cancer. This finding is in contrast with other studies that found that HPV 58 was not common in women with cancer from Central America or South America.[51]

> **The RRs of LSIL and HSIL in women infected with HPV types 18, 45, and 56 are roughly comparable for LSILs (RR, 32.7) and HSILs (RR, 65.1) but rise dramatically in women with invasive cancers (RR, 296.1).**

> **HPV type 18 is detected 2.6 times more commonly with invasive cancer that occurred within 1 year of a normal cytologic smear.**

> **HPV type 18 is consistently associated with cervical adenocarcinomas and less frequently associated with invasive squamous cell carcinomas of the cervix.**

The RRs of LSIL and HSIL in women infected with HPV types 18, 45, and 56 are roughly comparable for LSILs (RR, 32.7) and HSILs (RR, 65.1) but rise dramatically in women with invasive cancers (RR, 296.1).[50] HPV type 18 was the second most common HPV type among women with cancer in the Costa Rica study but not among those with HSIL.[16] This indicates that these viral types are highly represented in invasive cancer but are underrepresented in preinvasive lesions, including HSIL. HPV type 18 is detected 2.6 times more commonly with invasive cancer that occurred within 1 year of a normal cytologic smear. This may explain the rapid transit time to invasion in women infected with HPV 18 and could explain why the survival of patients with cervical cancer appears worse if they harbor HPV 18.[52] HPV 18 is consistently associated with cervical adenocarcinomas and less frequently associated with invasive squamous cell carcinomas of the cervix, which implies that it is more efficient in inducing malignant changes in glandular cells than in squamous cells.[53]

Up to 14% of cytologically normal women harbor oncogenic HPV types.

It has been demonstrated that up to 14% of cytologically normal women harbor oncogenic HPV types.[20, 54] In a study of 17,654 cytologically normal women, a total of 380 incident cases and 1037 matched controls were followed prospectively.[55] Compared with HPV-negative women, women who tested positive for HPV DNA at study enrollment were 3.8 times (95% confidence interval [CI], 2.6 to 5.5) more likely to have LSIL subsequently diagnosed for the first time during follow-up, and they

were 12.7 times (95% CI, 6.2 to 25.9) more likely to develop HSIL. The LSILs harboring oncogenic HPV types are probably the most likely to persist and progress.[23]

There is a significant association of the severity of histologic grade with oncogenic HPV types.[24] Nearly all women with HSIL harbor oncogenic HPV types if accurate testing of HPV is employed. Although lower risk HPV types can be found in HSIL, HSIL is characterized by the presence of oncogenic HPV types that are the same as those found in invasive cancer. Harboring a high-risk HPV type is associated with a twofold to threefold increased risk of CIN 3.[56] HPV DNA can be detected in more than 95% of HSIL. Only a small percentage of HSIL contains more than one HPV type. For HPV types 16, 18, and 33, 20% are detected in LSIL, and 78% are detected in HSIL. One study demonstrated that 84% of histologic CIN 3 contained high levels of at least one of the following HPV types: 16, 18, 31, 33, and 35.[57]

Epidemiologic study has demonstrated that HPV type 16 is the most common type of HPV in cytologically normal women and that this type carries the highest risk of progression to CIN 2 or CIN 3 and invasion. The differences in biologic characteristics among intratypic HPV 16 variants have been elucidated and include prototype-like variants and non–prototype-like variants.[58] Whether women in this study attended a university or sexually transmitted disease clinic, a greater risk of histologically confirmed CIN 2 or CIN 3 was associated with HPV 16 non–prototype-like variants. Among university students, those with HPV 16 non–prototype-like variants were 6.5 (95% CI, 1.6 to 27.2) times more likely to develop CIN 2 or CIN 3 than were those with prototype-like variants. Women presenting to a sexually transmitted disease clinic were similarly affected (RR, 4.5; 95% CI, 0.9 to 23.8). The authors suggested that the increased risk of CIN 2 and CIN 3 associated with these non–prototype-like variants may represent a difference in the biologic behavior of HPV types. Interestingly, results indicating increased risk for CIN 2 and CIN 3 in nonprototype variants were not explained by risk factors implicated in studies mentioned previously, including number of sexual partners, persistent HPV 16 positivity, nonwhite ethnicity, and infection with other HPV types. Other important points made by the authors include the suggestion that some types of cells may be more permissive for viral replication and may result in an overgrowth of a particular HPV variant. The authors stated that it is likely that the histologic classification of CIN 2 and CIN 3 may not accurately reflect biologic potential for progression. Genomic differences underlying the increased risk of progression to CIN 2 and CIN 3 remain to be elucidated.

High-grade CIN develops quickly in women with persistent HPV 16 infection.

It has been demonstrated that the persistence of HPV infection is higher among women infected with high-risk HPV types than among women with other HPV types.[59]

In a study that prospectively evaluated women who were positive for HPV 16 but had normal cytology, significantly more women in the persistently positive group subsequently developed histologic CIN.[60] Lesions in women with persistent HPV type 16 were more severe than those in women infected for a short time. Based on this 2-year study, the probability of CIN developing in women with persistent HPV 16 infection and normal cytology was 44%. Koutsky and coworkers reported a cumulative incidence of 28% of developing CIN in cytologically normal women in a 2-year period.[20] Both studies demonstrated that high-grade CIN develops quickly in women with persistent HPV 16 infection.

Oncogenic HPV types were detected less frequently and in lower concentration in cytologic smears from incident CIN 2 and CIN 3 than in smears from prevalent CIN 2 and CIN 3.[54] In this study, HPV status in women with a history of normal cytology and histologic CIN 2 or CIN 3 (incident CIN 2 or CIN 3) was compared with the CIN 2 or CIN 3 diagnosed in 40 patients with a history of abnormal cytology (prevalent CIN 2 or CIN 3). Smears of incident CIN 2 or CIN 3 were HPV positive in 50% of cases compared with 80% in prevalent CIN 2 or CIN 3. Oncogenic HPV types were significantly less common in smears from incident CIN 2 or CIN 3 compared with prevalent CIN 2 or CIN 3 (36.1% versus 72.5%, respectively). Viral load in HPV-positive smears of prevalent CIN 2 or CIN 3 was significantly higher than that of incident CIN 2 or CIN 3 ($P = .0005$).

It has been demonstrated that the prevalence of HPV 16 increases from 24.5% to 50.2% based on increasing degree of severity of CIN and age of patient.[42] The prevalence of oncogenic HPV among women with CIN 1 (57.8%) as well as CIN 2 or CIN 3 (59.4%) was significantly higher than that among women who were cytologically normal or who had HPV-associated changes only in the biopsy specimens. In this study, women with histologic CIN 2 or CIN 3 had the highest rate of oncogenic HPV in the youngest age group (77.8%), and this prevalence gradually decreased with increasing age (40% in women older than 40 years). Overall, the high prevalence of oncogenic HPV associated with abnormal histology was found largely among women younger than 30 years. The frequency of detection of high-risk HPV among women with all grades of CIN was age dependent. However, the prevalence of histologic CIN 2 or CIN 3 significantly increased with increasing age.

Acquisition of HPV infection is predominantly influenced by sexual behavior.

Although most young women exhibit low-grade cervical lesions, some harbor oncogenic types that could potentially induce progression of the lesion. It was shown that more than 60% of 661 sexually active female adolescents harbored at least one of the following oncogenic HPV types: 16, 18, 31, 33, or 35.[61] On the basis of this study, it can be noted that oncogenic-related HPV types are common in adolescents, and the strong association with number of sexual partners suggests that acquisition of HPV infection is predominantly influenced by sexual behavior.

Young women who were HPV positive appeared to eliminate HPV over a relatively short period and also appeared to be at low or no risk of developing significant disease. Those who remain HPV positive for approximately 2 years have significant risk of developing HSIL.

Continued HPV positivity and presence of squamous intraepithelial lesion occur synchronously and, coupled with a high viral load, make the probability of regression unlikely.

Young women who were HPV positive were followed for more than 2 years; they appeared to eliminate HPV over a relatively short period and also appeared to be at low or no risk of developing significant disease.[62] However, during follow-up examinations, 40% of the young women in this study were identified as having different subtypes of HPV, suggesting that the appearance of HPV DNA is related to sexual behavior and acquisition of new sexual partners. In women undergoing spontaneous regression of HPV, a high degree of persistent HPV negativity was found as the study interval increased. However, a substantial number of young women remained intermittently HPV positive. This suggests that HPV remains latent in some women, with the potential to undergo reactivation at some point. It has been suggested that women who remain HPV positive for approximately 2 years have significant risk of developing HSIL.[63] Continued HPV positivity and presence of a squamous intraepithelial lesion occur synchronously and, coupled with a high viral load, make the probability of regression unlikely.[4] This is especially significant when the squamous intraepithelial lesion demonstrates HPV type specificity. Women with a low level of type-specific persistent infection or non–type-specific persistent infection do not seem to demonstrate the same high progression rates.

Older women who are HPV positive are more likely to have their HPV persist for more than 6 months.

The 5-year clearance rate of HPV is 92%.

Older women may have fewer sexual partners and may be exposed to fewer HPV types. From past exposure, older women may also have acquired immunity to HPV. Older women who are HPV positive are more likely to have their HPV persist for more than 6 months. Women with HSIL tend to be older than those with LSIL. Studies have demonstrated that the peak incidence of cervical cancer in women older than 40 years may be related to a combination of older age and persistence of high-risk HPV types.[64] Untreated women with cervical epithelial abnormalities exhibit a significantly increased risk of subsequent disease progression if they harbor HPV 16 or HPV 18.[65] In a population-based study, it was demonstrated that the 5-year clearance rate of HPV was 92% and that the only HPV infection that persisted was related to HPV type 16.[66] It has also been shown in younger women that HPV type 16 has a slower clearance rate than does HPV type 18 or the low-risk HPV types.[67] This implies that if a woman harbors many years of persistent oncogenic HPV types, she is more likely to eventually show signs of more serious disease.

CYTOLOGY OF HSIL

Although the nuclei of an HSIL are about the same size as those seen in an LSIL, the nuclei appear larger because of the decrease in the cytoplasmic area.

The cells of high-grade cervical lesions are characterized by progressive dedifferentiation, smaller cell size, marked nuclear atypia, and decreased amounts of cytoplasm.[68] The cell size becomes smaller as the grade of squamous intraepithelial lesion becomes more severe. In HSIL, the overall cell size is as small or smaller than the basal or parabasal cells in normal tissue. In contrast, the cells of a low-grade lesion are approximate in size to a normal intermediate cell. The cells also become more elongated as they become more dysplastic. Although the nuclei of an HSIL lesion are about the same size as those seen in an LSIL lesion, the nuclei appear larger because of the decrease in the cytoplasmic area (Fig. 11–1).[69]

Overall, compared with lower-grade lesions, there is a marked increase in the nuclear-cytoplasmic ratio in HSIL. Usually, only a small rim of cytoplasm remains around the nucleus of a highly dysplastic cell. When the nuclei of HSIL are surrounded by very little cytoplasm ("naked nuclei"), the nuclei appear more prominent. The nuclear outlines become more irregular as the dysplastic process evolves. Hyperchromasia is usually prominent, and the

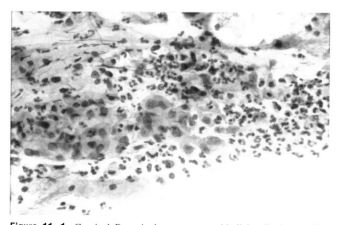

Figure 11–1. Cervical Papanicolaou smear: epithelial cell abnormality, high-grade squamous intraepithelial lesion. Dysplastic epithelial cells are seen mixed with acute inflammatory cells. The epithelial cells show moderate nuclear pleomorphism with coarse nuclear chromatin and irregular nuclear outlines. The background is otherwise clean.

chromatin may be finely or coarsely granular and may exhibit clumping of chromatinic material.[68] Nucleoli are usually absent. The cells may occur singly, in poorly defined sheets, or in syncytial aggregates with poorly defined cytoplasmic borders.

Most HSILs do not contain abundant evidence of the cytopathic effect of HPV.

Most HSILs do not contain abundant evidence of the cytopathic effect of HPV.[70] Koilocytosis, a cellular feature of LSIL, is usually absent in HSIL, reflecting the absence of a productive HPV infection. Abnormal mitotic figures frequently observed in histologic sections of HSIL are not commonly seen in cytologic smears.

Some HSILs are composed of cells with more abundant but abnormally keratinized cytoplasm. These cells may be shed singly or in dense clusters and have enlarged hyperchromatic nuclei often displaying smudged chromatin. The nuclear size and cellular shape are variable. At times, these keratinized lesions may be indistinguishable from invasive lesions.

Table 11–1 summarizes the cytologic abnormalities of HSIL.

It is recognized that some cytologic smears previously diagnosed as normal in women with current HSIL are found to contain abnormal cells on retrospective review.[71] HSIL may be misinterpreted as abnormal mature squamous cells or immature metaplastic cells. The differential diagnosis can be challenging for the pathologist. The small, single cells of HSIL are the abnormal cells most difficult to detect in routine screening and are one cause for false-negative reports.[68] The atypical immature squamous metaplastic type cells (AISMTs) account for the most commonly missed or misinterpreted cells.[72] AISMTs are most commonly missed because of screening errors in women with HSIL. AISMTs are small cells with hyperchromatic nuclei, increased nuclear-cytoplasmic ratio, and nuclear irregularities, and they can be confused with the cells of HSIL. However, none of the nuclear features of AISMTs specifically fit the marked nuclear atypia of HSIL. The most difficult feature to accurately assign is increased nuclear-cytoplasmic ratio. Wright et al believe that the most helpful feature in distinguishing HSIL from immature metaplasia is the absence of nuclear pleomorphism in the metaplastic cells. It should also be stressed that the term AISMT[73] is not accepted by all pathologists.

The small, single cells of HSIL can be missed if the background of the smear contains profuse inflammatory cells. The true nuclear enlargement and increased nuclear cytoplasmic ratio of HSIL can also be difficult to assess if extensive cytolysis has occurred.

HISTOLOGY OF HSIL

Progressing CIN is marked by a proliferation of atypical basaloid cells with an increased nuclear-cytoplasmic ratio and variability in nuclear size.

As the grade of CIN becomes more severe, the cells become more dedifferentiated or immature. Preinvasive

▼ Table 11–1

Cytologic Abnormalities of High-Grade Squamous Intraepithelial Lesions
Small size of cells
Increasing dedifferentiation of cells
Abnormal chromatin distribution or clumping
Nuclear membrane irregularity
Increased nuclear-cytoplasmic ratio
Elongated cells
Variability of nuclear size
Irregular nuclear membranes
Absence of prominent nuclei
Single cells or syncytial sheets of cells

cervical lesions are subdivided histologically based on the degree of proliferation of abnormal, dedifferentiated, "basaloid" cells. Normally, the basal layer of the epithelium is at least two cell layers thick. Progressing CIN is marked by a proliferation of atypical basaloid cells with an increased nuclear-cytoplasmic ratio and variability in nuclear size. In all grades of CIN, the basement membrane remains intact, and there is no extrusion of basaloid cells into the underlying stroma.

As the dysplastic process advances, the desmosomes no longer effectively attach the epithelium to the basement membrane. Clinically, this process is reflected in the peeling edges of high-grade lesions.

As the dysplastic process advances, the basaloid cells exhibit less glycogen and lose the ability to adhere to one another. On an ultrastructural level, the cells begin to lose the surface microridges and develop the presence of abundant microvilli. The desmosomes and junctional units are lost. The desmosomes no longer effectively attach the epithelium to the basement membrane. Clinically, this process is reflected in the peeling edges of high-grade lesions.

As the CIN progresses, advancing layers exhibit less cytoplasmic maturation, and the cytoplasmic borders become less distinct. In a full-thickness intraepithelial neoplasia, it may not be possible to distinguish the characteristic basal, intermediate, and superficial cell layers. The higher grades of CIN tend to be characterized by more mitotic activity in the upper layers. As the mitotic activity increases, basaloid cells replace normal cells in the superficial layers.

Normal cells are diploid, and condyloma acuminatum is often polyploid, but HSILs and invasive cancers are generally aneuploid.

Normal cells are diploid, and condyloma acuminatum is often polyploid, but HSILs and invasive cancers are generally aneuploid. As aneuploidy develops, cellular mitotic activity commences throughout all layers of the epithelium. This evidence of a derangement in DNA replication may result in multiple mutations in the genetic structure, and some of these mutations may activate oncogenes and result in the progression of the neoplastic process.[74]

Aneuploid lesions have more marked nuclear atypia, more cellular disorganization, and the presence of abnormal mitotic figures.

A number of studies have compared histologic features with ploidy levels and found that cervical lesions with diploid or polyploid DNA contents generally retain polarity of the basal cell layer and lack abnormal mitotic figures.[74] On the other hand, aneuploid lesions have more marked nuclear atypia, more cellular disorganization, and the presence of abnormal mitotic figures. The best histologic correlate of aneuploidy is abnormal mitotic figures, usually present in the superficial layers of the epithelium.[74] Although an epithelial lesion exhibiting abnormal mitotic figures should be classified as HSIL, HSIL lacking abnormal mitotic figures should still be classified as CIN 2 or CIN 3 if other well-known features of HSIL are present. Although koilocytosis is a characteristic of low-grade lesions, some high-grade cervical epithelial lesions will exhibit koilocytosis in the superficial layers but should still be classified as high-grade CIN if they meet the remaining high-grade criteria.

The following histologic features should be used to differentiate LSIL from HSIL:

1. Distribution of dedifferentiated basal cells
2. Extent of dedifferentiation
3. Degree of nuclear atypia

Higher grades of CIN tend to involve more superficial layers of the epithelium. When one third to two thirds of the epithelium is involved, the lesion is classified as CIN 2. When more than two thirds of the epithelium is involved, it is classified as CIN 3. In the lower grades of CIN, only the basal layer is dedifferentiated, and the upper layers retain their cytoplasmic differentiation despite the presence of some cellular disorganization (Fig. 11–2).

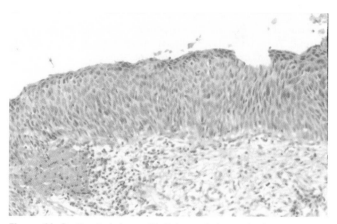

Figure 11–2. Cervical intraepithelial neoplasia grade 3 biopsy. The epithelium has complete loss of maturation of keratinocytes with marked crowding and vertical orientation of the nuclei. There is virtually no maturation of the squamous epithelial cells from the basal to the superficial layer. Within the submucosa there is mild, superficial, chronic inflammation.

COLPOSCOPY OF HSIL

It is easier to determine that a cervix is either normal or very abnormal than it is to distinguish between minor degrees of change.

The high sensitivity and low specificity of colposcopy are most likely due to "overcalling" of low-grade lesions.

It is easier to distinguish high-grade lesions of the cervix from low-grade lesions than it is to distinguish low-grade lesions from normal findings or from an inflammatory process.[75] In a meta-analysis evaluating the performance of colposcopy, Mitchell et al selected articles from 1960 to 1996 that studied a population of patients with abnormal cytology who were subsequently evaluated with colposcopy. The analysis demonstrated that the high sensitivity and low specificity of colposcopy are most likely due to "overcalling" of low-grade lesions. The specificity of colposcopy improved when the threshold was set to distinguish high-grade lesions and cancer from less severe abnormalities. The likelihood ratios showed much higher shifts between low-grade and high-grade lesions than between normal cervix and low-grade lesions. The authors attributed this finding to the fact that vascular atypia is the hallmark of higher-grade lesions. In a study by Hopman and colleagues, intraobserver and interobserver agreement in interpreting colposcopic images of CIN 3 were 70% and 76.9%, respectively.[76] These authors, too, found it easier to determine that a cervix was either normal or very abnormal than to distinguish between minor degrees of change. For the colposcopist attempting to carefully identify high-grade disease, these findings are reassuring. Ismail and associates found a similar agreement among histopathologists in the diagnosis of CIN 3.[77]

High-grade cervical lesions may be found anywhere in the transformation zone, but most are seen close to the squamocolumnar junction.

If the colposcopist fails to note the less obvious but more severe central lesion, as demonstrated by a lesion with an internal margin, the colposcopic biopsy may be misdirected and the patient may subsequently be undertreated.

Treatment is based on the highest grade of CIN present, regardless of the other grades of CIN that may be present. High-grade cervical lesions may be found anywhere in the transformation zone, but most are seen close to the squamocolumnar junction. It has been suggested that CIN 2 or CIN 3 begins as a small focus of highly dysplastic epithelium near the squamocolumnar junction, probably in an area of immature squamous metaplasia, and eventually expands peripherally.[78] Areas of high-grade CIN can also form at the proximal edge of the field of a preexisting low-grade lesion. The detection of an internal line of demarcation (internal margin) that separates a central area of significant colposcopic atypia from a much larger field of lower-grade acetowhite epi-

thelium is a reliable sign of high-grade cervical disease (Fig. 11–3).[79] This observation highlights the centripetal structure of CIN, with the less-differentiated, higher-grade component being more centrally located and the better-differentiated portion residing at the periphery.[80] In general, the most abnormal area of a lesion will be contiguous with the squamocolumnar junction. This is an important point, because a large lesion may have rather spectacular (but low-grade) geographic change at its peripheral margin but centrally harbor a more ominous high-grade lesion. If the colposcopist fails to note the less obvious but more severe central lesion, as demonstrated by a lesion with an internal margin, the colposcopic biopsy may be misdirected, and the patient may subsequently be undertreated.

Colposcopically, a flat or raised surface contour, a symmetrical shape, a straight peripheral margin, and a dull, oyster-white color distinguish high-grade lesions.

The application of 3% to 5% acetic acid assists in the delineation of the colposcopic features of CIN 2 and CIN 3. The specific findings of high-grade disease include characteristic margins, color, vessel pattern, and iodine staining. Colposcopically, a flat or raised surface contour, a symmetrical shape, a straight peripheral margin, and a dull, oyster-white color distinguish high-grade lesions.[79]

The size of the transformation zone and of the lesion, the intensity of the color, the distinctiveness of the margins, the pattern of the vessels, and the presence of micropapillae as independent findings were highly correlated with the histologic grade. Variation in the acetowhite color was the most important finding, with an odds ratio of 16; coarse vessels versus no vessels had an odds ratio of 10,

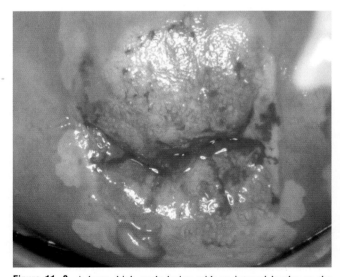

Figure 11–3. A large, high-grade lesion with an internal border on the anterior lip of the cervix. Note how the geographic peripheral color changes abruptly toward the os, taking on a denser, whitish color. A coarse mosaic is also present. Disease is present on the posterior lip of the cervix as well. Multiple punch biopsies revealed cervical intraepithelial neoplasia, grade 3.

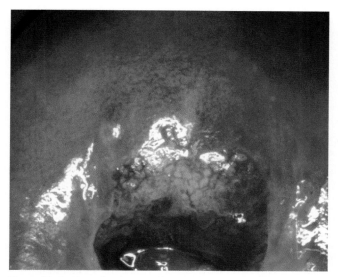

Figure 11-4. Example of green filter examination showing accentuation of mosaic.

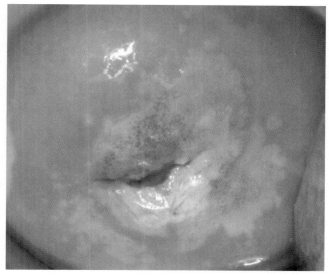

Figure 11-5. Peripheral low-grade squamous intraepithelial lesion, with irregular margins and central high-grade squamous intraepithelial lesion with coarse punctation anteriorly, and with dense acetowhite epithelium and internal margin at 3 o'clock to 5 o'clock. Biopsy revealed cervical intraepithelial neoplasia, grade 2.

fine vessels versus no vessels had an odds ratio of 1.6, and large and medium-sized lesions showed odds ratios of 3.6 and 2, respectively.

Because colposcopic findings represent a wide spectrum of morphologic change, it is difficult to predict the histologic grade unless specific grading criteria are used. The relationship between specific colposcopic diagnostic findings and histologic grade of the lesion was examined in 896 women.[81] Results indicated that the size of the transformation zone and of the lesion, the intensity of the color, the distinctiveness of the margins, the pattern of the vessels and the presence of micropapillae as independent findings were highly correlated with the histologic grade ($P < 0.0001$). The likelihood of finding a higher histologic grade was estimated as an odds ratio (OR). Variation in the acetowhite color was the most important finding with an OR of 16 (95% CI, 10 to 26). Coarse vessels versus no vessels had an OR of 10 (95% CI, 3.2 to 34). Fine vessels versus no vessels had an OR of 1.6 (CI, 1.1 to 2.5). Large and medium-sized lesions showed ORs of 3.6 and 2, respectively. Results of this study demonstrated that the approximate colposcopic correlation within one histologic grade was found in 88.3% of the women (see Chapter 9 on colposcopic grading systems).

Not all high-grade lesions exhibit abnormal vessel patterns, so the absence of vessels does not imply that the lesion lacks significance.

When viewed with a red-free (green) filter before the application of 3% to 5% acetic acid, high-grade lesions may exhibit abnormal vessel patterns such as mosaic and punctation (Fig. 11-4). These patterns may disappear after the application of 3% to 5% acetic acid owing to the constriction of narrow vessels by the intense swelling of the dysplastic epithelium.[79] Not all high-grade lesions exhibit abnormal vessel patterns, so the absence of vessels does not imply that the lesion lacks significance. In fact,

punctation and mosaic patterns are seen more often in low-grade CIN.

The presence or absence of a vascular pattern is not diagnostic of either a high-grade lesion or a low-grade lesion.

As the metabolic rate increases within HSIL, vascular dilation resists the constrictive effects of epithelial swelling, thus resulting in persistence of the mosaic and punc-

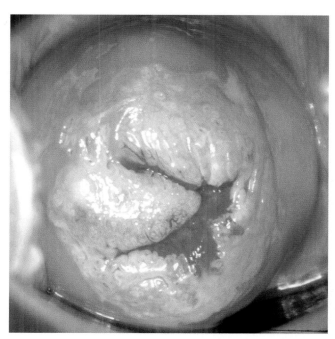

Figure 11-6. Large, high-grade squamous intraepithelial lesion with coarse mosaic at 10 o'clock to 11 o'clock.

tation patterns after the application of acetic acid. But the presence or absence of a vascular pattern is not diagnostic of either a high-grade lesion or a low-grade lesion. As the intercapillary distance of the vessels increases, the vessel patterns appear coarser, and the vessels can achieve significant dilation (Figs. 11–5 and 11–6). As lesion severity progresses, the abnormal vessels may transition to atypical vessels as the vessels begin to run horizontally across the epithelium.

It has been demonstrated that 20% of patients younger than 35 years with documented CIN 2 or CIN 3 present with trivial colposcopic findings of doubtful significance. This compares with 88% of patients older than 35 years with CIN 2 or CIN 3 who present with trivial findings. As many as 38% to 55% of cases of documented CIN 2 or CIN 3 could be missed in older women.

It has been demonstrated that 20% of patients younger than 35 years with documented CIN 2 or CIN 3 present with trivial colposcopic findings of doubtful significance. This compares with 88% of patients older than 35 years with CIN 2 or CIN 3 who present with trivial findings.[82] This study suggests that the sensitivity of colposcopy is decreased and that cervical lesions are undergraded in older women. As many as 38% to 55% of cases of documented CIN 2 or CIN 3 could be missed in this age group.

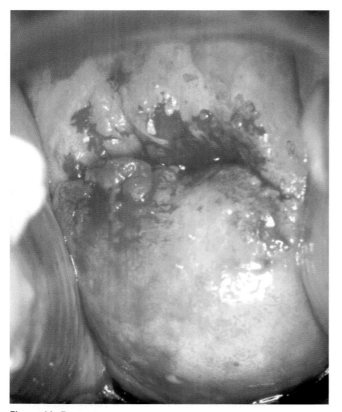

Figure 11–7. High-grade squamous intraepithelial lesion: dense aceto-white epithelium on the anterior lip that is peeling off after being touched with a cotton-tipped applicator.

▼ Table 11–2

Colposcopic Findings of High-Grade Cervical Intraepithelial Neoplasia

Margin
Sharp and distinct
Internal margin possibly present within lower-grade lesion
Rolled or peeling edges

Color
Denser white than low-grade lesions
Dull, not shiny
Acetowhite reaction tending to remain for a longer time

Vascular Pattern
Coarse punctation and/or mosaic
Wide intercapillary distance of vessels
Mosaic with central punctation (umbilication)

Iodine Staining
Rejects iodine

Care must be taken when examining a high-grade lesion to avoid detaching the surface epithelium by abrasion. As cervical lesions become more abnormal, the desmosomal anchors loosen, allowing the overlying diseased epithelium to more easily detach from the basement membrane. Colposcopically, this epithelial detachment is exhibited as a rolled or peeling margin (Fig. 11–7). Care must be taken when examining a high-grade lesion to avoid detaching the surface epithelium by abrasion. Sometimes, manipulation with a cotton-tipped applicator alone for the purposes of better visualization of the cervix is enough to detach the epithelium. If the cervical biopsy specimen is submitted to pathology unattached to the basement membrane and underlying stroma, it is impossible to determine the grade of the lesion or if the lesion is invasive, often yielding the unsatisfying report of "dysplasia—unable to grade."

Table 11–2 summarizes the colposcopic findings of HSIL.

An adequate number of biopsies should be taken if there is any suspicion of microinvasive or invasive cancer.

An adequate number of biopsies should be taken if there is any suspicion of microinvasive or invasive cancer. If the colposcopist takes only one biopsy, it is more likely that a small focus of microinvasive disease could be missed. Multiple punch biopsies are recommended in the assessment of large, complex, high-grade lesions.

SUMMARY OF KEY POINTS

- Among appropriately screened women, histologically verified CIN 2, CIN 3, or invasive cancer is extremely uncommon after age 60 years.

- The progression rate of CIN 1 is about 10% to 20%, of CIN 2 about 30%, and of CIN 3 up to 70%.

- It is uncertain whether CIN 3 lesions evolve over time from preexisting CIN 1 lesions or arise de novo as CIN 3 lesions.

- The histopathologic entity termed LSIL consists of two different types of lesions that are biologically distinct. One entity is monoclonal and is associated with the same HPV types present in HSIL. The other is polyclonal, is associated with other HPV types not usually associated with HSIL, and is usually recognized as low risk.

- Cytologic grading alone does not always reliably predict which women have histologic high-grade cervical cancer precursors or invasive disease.

- Most high-grade CIN and cancer may occur in women with either minor cytologic abnormalities, visible lower genital tract lesions, or both.

- Overall, HPV testing is more sensitive than conventional Pap smear testing for detection of high-grade lesions and cancer, but it is less specific.

- HSIL probably arises as a small focus within a lower-grade lesion that gradually expands and replaces the original HPV-infected tissue.

- CIN does not progress in the absence of HPV positivity with high-risk HPV types.

- High-risk HPV types and current cigarette smoking could be synergistic for the development of cervical carcinogenesis. The risk of high-grade CIN increases in parallel with the time of exposure and the number of years of smoking. Smoking more than 20 cigarettes per day appears to increase the risk of CIN 2 and CIN 3 in women who have minor cytologic abnormalities.

- HPV type 18 is consistently associated with cervical adenocarcinomas and less frequently associated with invasive squamous cell carcinomas of the cervix.

- Up to 14% of cytologically normal women harbor oncogenic HPV types. Compared with HPV-negative women, women who tested positive for HPV DNA were 3.8 times more likely to develop LSIL and 12.7 times more likely to develop HSIL.

- Nearly all women with HSIL harbor oncogenic HPV types if accurate testing of HPV is employed.

- High-grade CIN develops quickly in women with persistent HPV type 16 infection.

- Young women who are HPV positive and who eliminate HPV over a relatively short period are at low risk for developing significant disease. Women who remain HPV positive for approximately 2 years have significant risk of developing HSIL.

- The 5-year clearance rate of HPV is 92%.

- Older women who are HPV positive are more likely to have their HPV persist for more than 6 months.

- Although the nuclei of an HSIL are about the same size as those seen in an LSIL, the nuclei appear larger because of the decrease in the cytoplasmic area.

- Koilocytosis, a cellular feature of LSIL, is usually absent in HSIL, reflecting the absence of a productive HPV infection.

- As the dysplastic process advances, the desmosomes no longer effectively attach the epithelium to the basement membrane. Clinically, this process is reflected in the peeling edges of high-grade lesions.

- It is easier to determine that a cervix is either normal or very abnormal than it is to distinguish between minor degrees of change. The high sensitivity and low specificity of colposcopy are most likely due to "overcalling" of low-grade lesions.

- High-grade cervical lesions may be found anywhere in the transformation zone, but most are seen close to the squamocolumnar junction.

- The size of the transformation zone and of the lesion, the intensity of the color, the distinctiveness of the margins, the pattern of the vessels, and the presence of micropapillae are independent findings that correlate highly with the histologic grade. Variation in the acetowhite color was the most important finding correlating with HSIL, followed by coarse vessels versus no vessels, fine vessels versus no vessels, and large and medium-sized lesions.

- The presence or absence of a vascular pattern is not diagnostic of either a high-grade lesion or a low-grade lesion.

- It has been demonstrated that 20% of patients younger than 35 years with documented CIN 2 or CIN 3 present with trivial colposcopic findings of doubtful significance, compared with 88% of patients older than 35 years with CIN 2 or 3 who present with trivial findings.

References

1. Schiffman M, Herrero R, Bergstrom R, et al: Detection of preinvasive cancer of the cervix and the subsequent reduction in invasive cancer. J Natl Cancer Inst 1993;85:1050.
2. Walboomers JM, Jacobs MV, Manos MM, et al: Human papillomavirus is a necessary cause of invasive cervical cancer worldwide. J Path 1999;189:12.
3. Schiffman M, Herrero R, Hildesheim A, et al: HPV DNA testing in cervical cancer screening. Results from women in a high-risk province of Costa Rica. JAMA 2000;283:87.
4. Ho GY, Burk RD, Klein, S et al: Persistent genital human papillomavirus infection as a risk factor for persistent cervical dysplasia. J Natl Cancer Inst 1995;87:1365.

5. Schwartz PE, Hadjimicharl O, Lowell DM, et al: Rapidly progressive cervical cancer: The Connecticut experience. Am J Obstet Gynecol 1996;175:1105.
6. Smith HA: Cervical intraepithelial neoplasia grade III (CIN III) and invasive cervical carcinoma: The yawning gap revisited and the treatment of risk. Cytopathol 1999;10:161.
7. Sigurdsson K: Trends in cervical intra-epithelial neoplasia in Iceland through 1995: Evaluation of targeted aged groups and screening intervals. Acta Obstet Gynaecol Scand 1999;78:486.
8. Ostor AG: Natural history of cervical intraepithelial neoplasia: A critical review. Int J Gynecol Path 1993;12:.
9. Syrjanen K, Vayrynen M, Saarikoski S, et al: Natural history of cervical human papillomavirus (HPV) infections based on prospective follow-up. Br J Obstet Gynaecol 1985;92:1086.
10. Duggan MA, McGregor SE, Stuart GC, et al: The natural history of CIN I lesions. Eur J Gynaecol Oncol 1998;19:338.
11. Kiviat N: Natural history of cervical neoplasia: Overview and update. Am J Obstet Gynecol 1996;175:1099.
12. Nasiell K, Roger V, Nasiell M: Behavior of mild cervical dysplasia during long-term follow-up. Obstet Gynecol 1986;67:665.
13. Paavonen J, Stevens CE, Wolner-Hanssen P, et al: Colposcopic manifestations of cervical and vaginal infections. Obstet Gynecol Surv 1988;43:716.
14. Kurmun RJ, Henson DE, Herbst AL, et al: Interim guidelines for management of abnormal cervical cytology. JAMA 1994;271:1866.
15. Manos MM, Kinney WK, Hurley LB, et al: Identifying women with cervical neoplasia. Using human papillomavirus DNA testing for equivocal results. JAMA 1999;281:1605.
16. Herrero R, Hildesheim A, Bratti C, et al: Population-based study of human papillomavirus infection and cervical neoplasia in rural Costa Rica. J Natl Cancer Inst 2000;92:464.
17. Wright TC, Kurman RT: A critical review of the morphologic classification system or preinvasive lesions of the cervix: The scientific basis for shifting the paradigm. Papillomavirus Rep 1994;5:175.
18. Burghardt E, Ostor AG: Site and origin of squamous cervical cancer: A histomorphologic study. Obstet Gynecol 1983;62:117.
19. Richart RM, Townsend DE, Crisp W, et al: An analysis of "long-term" follow-up results in patients with cervical intraepithelial neoplasia treated by cryotherapy. Am J Obstet Gynecol 1980;137:823.
20. Lawson HW, Lee MC, Thames SF, et al: Cervical cancer screening among low-income women: Results of a national screening program, 1991–1995. Obstet Gynecol 1998;92:745.
21. Koutsky LA, Holmes KK, Critchlow CW, et al: A cohort study of the risk of cervical intraepithelial neoplasia grade 2 or 3 in relation to papillomavirus infection. N Engl J Med 1992;327:1272.
22. Cuzick J, Szarewski A, Terry G, et al: Human papillomavirus testing in primary cervical screening. Lancet 1995;345:1533.
23. Park TW, Richart RM, Sun XW, Wright TC: Association between human papillomavirus type and clonal status of cervical squamous intraepithelial lesions. J Nat Cancer Inst 1996;88:317.
24. Monsonego J, Valensi P, Zerat L, et al: Simultaneous effects of aneuploidy and oncogenic human papillomavirus on histological grade of cervical intraepithelial neoplasia. Br J Obstet Gynaecol 1997;104:723.
25. Rihet S, Lorenzato M, Clavel C: Oncogenic human papillomaviruses and ploidy in cervical lesions. J Clin Path 1996;49:892.
26. Lonky NM, Sadeghi M, Tsadik GW, Petitti D: The clinical significance of the poor correlation of cervical dysplasia and cervical malignancy with referral cytologic results. Am J Obstet Gynecol 1999;181:560.
27. Lonky NM, Navarre GL, Saunders S, et al: Low-grade Papanicolaou smears and the Bethesda System: A prospective cytohistopathologic analysis. Obstet Gynecol 1995;85:716.
28. Campion MJ, McCance DJ, Cuzick J, Singer A: Progressive potential of mild cervical atypia: Prospective cytological, colposcopic, and virological study. Lancet 1986;2:237.
29. Kinney WK, Manos MM, Hurley LB, et al: Where's the high-grade cervical neoplasia? The importance of the minimally abnormal Papanicolaou diagnoses. Obstet Gynecol 1998;91:973.
30. Schneider DL, Herrero R, Bratti C, et al: Cervicography screening for cervical cancer among 8460 women in a high-risk population. Am J Obstet Gynecol 1999;180:290.
31. Autier P, Coibion M, De Sutter P, Wayemberg M: Cytology alone versus cytology and cervicography for cervical cancer screening: A randomized study. Obstet Gynecol 1999;93:353.
32. Eskridge C, Begneaud WP, Landwehr C: Cervicography combined with repeat Papanicolaou test as triage for low-grade cytologic abnormalities. Obstet Gynecol 1998;92:351.
33. Wright TC, Sun XW, Koulos J: Comparison of management algorithms for the evaluation of women with low-grade cytologic abnormalities. Obstet Gynecol 1995;85:202.
34. Schoell WM, Janicek MF, Mirhashemi R: Epidemiology and biology of cervical cancer. Semin Surg Onc 1999;16:203-.
35. Downey GP, Bavin PJ, Deery AR, et al: Relation between human papillomavirus type 16 and potential for progression of minor-grade cervical disease. Lancet 1994;344:432.
36. Remmink AJ, Walboomers JM, Helmerhorst TJ, et al: The presence of persistent high-risk HPV genotypes in dysplastic cervical lesions is associated with progressive disease: Natural history up to 36 months. Int J Cancer 1995;61:3061.
37. Konno R, Paez C, Sato S, et al: HPV, histologic grade and age. Risk factors for the progression of cervical intraepithelial neoplasia. J Reprod Med 1998;43:561.
38. Park J, Sun D, Genest DR, et al: Coexistence of low and high grade squamous intraepithelial lesions of the cervix: Morphologic progression or multiple papillomaviruses? Gynecol Oncol 1998;70:386.
39. Stafl A, Mattingly RF: Angiogenesis of cervical neoplasia. Am J Obstet Gynecol 1975;121:845.
40. Smith-McCune KK, Weidner N: Demonstration and characterization of the angiogenic properties of cervical dysplasia. Cancer Res 1994;54:800.
41. Tjalma W, Sonnemans H, Weyler J, et al: Angiogenesis in cervical intraepithelial neoplasia and the risk of recurrence. Am J Obstet Gynecol 1999;181:554.
42. Adam E, Berkova Z, Daxnerova Z, et al: Papillomavirus detection: Demographic and behavioral characteristics influencing the identification of cervical disease. Am J Obstet Gynecol 2000;182:257.)
43. Daly SF, Doyle M, English J, et al: Can the number of cigarettes smoked predict high-grade cervical intraepithelial neoplasia among women with mildly abnormal cervical smears? Am J Obstet Gynecol 1998;179:399.
44. Brisson J, Morin K, Fortier M, et al: Risk factors for cervical intraepithelial neoplasia: Differences between low and high-grade lesions. Am J Epidemiol 1994;140:700.
45. Ho, GY, Kadish AS, Burk RD, et al: HOV 16 and cigarette smoking as risk factors for high-grade cervical intra-epithelial neoplasia. Int J Cancer 1998;78:281.
46. Roteli-Martins CM, Panetta K, Alves VA, et al: Cigarette smoking and high-risk HPV DNA as predisposing factors for high-grade cervical intraepithelial neoplasia (CIN) in young Brazilian women. Acta Obstet Gynecol Scand 1998;77:678.
47. Parazzini F, Sideri M, Restelli S, et al: Determinants of high-grade dysplasia among women with mild dyskaryosis on cervical smear. Obstet Gynecol 1995;86:754.
48. Luesley D, Blomfield P, Dunn J, et al: Cigarette smoking and histological outcome in women with mildly dyskaryotic cervical smears. Br J Obstet Gynaecol 1994;101:49.
49. Giuliano AR, Papenfuss M, Schneider A, et al: Risk factors for high-risk type papillomavirus infection among Mexican-American women. Cancer Epidemiol Biomarkers Prev 1999;8:615.
50. Lorincz AT, Reid R, Jenson B, et al: Human papillomavirus infection of the cervix: Relative risk associations of 15 common anogenital types. Obstet Gynecol 1992;79:328.
51. Bosch FX, Manos MM, Munoz N, et al: Prevalence of human papillomavirus in cervical cancer: A worldwide perspective. J Natl Cancer Inst 1995;87:796.
52. Burges RA, Monk BJ, Kurosaki T, et al: Human papillomavirus type 18: Association with poor prognosis in early stage cervical cancer. J Natl Cancer Inst 1996;88:1361.
53. Stoler MH: A brief synopsis of the role of human papillomaviruses in cervical carcinogenesis. Am J Obstet Gynecol 1996;175:1091.
54. Schneider A, Zahm DM, Greinke C, et al: Different detectability of high-risk HPV in smears from incident and prevalent high-grade squamous intraepithelial lesions of the cervix. Gynecol Oncol 1997;65:399.
55. Kjellberg L, Wang Z, Wiklund F, et al: Sexual behavior and papillomavirus exposure in cervical intraepithelial neoplasia: A population-based case-control study. J Gen Virology 1999;80(pt 2):391.

56. Cuzick K, Terry G, Ho L, et al: Type-specific human papillomavirus DNA in abnormal smears as a predictor of high-grade cervical intraepithelial neoplasia. Br J Cancer 1994;69:167.

57. Xi LF, Koutsky LA, Galloway DA, et al: Genomic variation of human papillomavirus type 16 and risk for high grade cervical intraepithelial neoplasia. J Natl Cancer Inst 1997;89:796.

58. Hildesheim A, Shiffman MH, Gravitt PE, et al: Persistence of type specific human papillomavirus infection among cytologically normal women. J Infect Dis 1994;169:235.

59. Harmsel BT, Smedts F, Kuijpers J, et al: Relationship between human papillomavirus type 16 in the cervix and intraepithelial neoplasia. Obstet Gynecol 1999;93:46.

60. Moscicki AB, Palefsky J, Gonzales J, Schoolnik GK: Human papillomavirus in sexually active adolescent females: Prevalence and risk factors. Pediatr Res 1990;28:507.

61. Moscicki AB, Palefsky J, Smith G, et al: Variability of human papillomavirus DNA testing in a longitudinal cohort of young women. Obstet Gynecol 1993;82:578.

62. Koutsky LA: Role of epidemiology in defining events that influence transmission and natural history of anogenital papillomavirus infections. J Natl Cancer Inst 1991;83:978.

63. Romney SL, Ho GYF, Palan PR, et al: Effects of B-carotene and other factors on outcome of cervical dysplasia and human papillomavirus infection. Gynecol Oncol 1997;65:483.

64. Woodman CB, Rollason T, Ellis J, et al: Human papillomavirus infection and risk of progression of epithelial abnormalities of the cervix. Br J Cancer 1996;73:553.

65. Elfgren K, Kalantari M, Bogerger B, et al: A population-based five-year follow-up study of cervical human papillomavirus infection. Am J Obstet Gynecol 2000;183:561.

66. Moscicki AB, Shiboski S, Broering J, et al: The natural history of human papillomavirus infection as measures by repeated DNA testing in adolescent and young women. J Pediatr 1998;132:277.

67. Bonfiglio TA: The cytopathology of squamous epithelial lesions of the cervix and vagina. In Bonfiglio TA, Erozan YS (eds): Gynecologic Cytopathology. Philadelphia, Lippincott-Raven, 1997, pp 7–10.

68. Kurman RJ, Solomon D: The Bethesda System for Reporting Cervical/Vaginal Cytologic Diagnoses. New York, Springer-Verlag, 1994, pp 48–59.

69. Sato S, Maruta J, Ito K, et al: Prognostic features of cervical dysplasia associated with specific types of HPV DNA and cytologic feature characteristic of HPV infections in dysplasia. Acta Cytol 1998;42:1377–1381.

70. Montes MA, Cibas ES, DiNisco SA, Lee KR: Cytologic characteristics of abnormal cells in prior "normal" cervical/vaginal Papanicolaou smears from women with a high- grade squamous intraepithelial lesion. Cancer 1999;87:45.

71. Hatem F, Wilbur DC: High grade squamous cervical lesions following negative Papanicolaou smears: False-negative cervical cytology or rapid progression. Diag Cytopath 1995;12:135.

72. Crum CP, Egawa K, Fu YS et al: Atypical immature metaplasia (AIM): A subset of human papillomavirus infection of the cervix. Cancer 1983:51:2214.

73. Wright TC, Kurman RJ, Ferenczy A: Precancerous lesions of the cervix. In Kurman RJ (ed): Blaustein's Pathology of the Female Genital Tract. New York, Springer-Verlag, 1994, pp 229–277.

74. Mitchell MF, Schottenfeld D, Tortolero-Luna G, et al: Colposcopy for the diagnosis of squamous intraepithelial lesions: A meta-analysis. Obstet Gynecol 1998;91:626.

75. Hopman EH, Voorhorst FJ, Kenemans P, et al: Observer agreement on interpreting colposcopic images of CIN. Gynecol Oncol 1995;58:206.

76. Ismail SM, Colclough AB, Dinnen JS, et al: Observer variation in histopathological diagnosis and grading of cervical intraepithelial neoplasia. Br Med J 1989:298:707.

77. Tidbury P, Singer A, Henkins D: CIN 3: The role of lesion size in invasion. Br J Obstet Gynaecol 1992;99:583.

78. Campion MJ, Greenberg MD, Kazamel TI: Clinical manifestations and natural history of genital human papillomavirus infections. Obstet Gynecol Clinics North Am 1996;23:783.

79. Boonstra H, Aalders JG, Koudstaal, J et al: Minimal extension and appropriate topographic position of tissue destruction for treatment of cervical intraepithelial neoplasia. Obstet Gynecol 1990;75:227.

80. Kierkegaard O, Byrjalsen C, Hansen KC, et al: Association between colposcopic findings and histology in cervical lesions: The significance of the size of the lesion. Gynecol Oncol 1995;57:66.

81. Zahm DM, Nindl I, Greinke C, et al: Colposcopic appearance of cervical intraepithelial neoplasia is age dependent. Am J Obstet Gynecol 1998;179:1298.

Case Study 1 Questions

History

A 29-year-old gravida II, para II had an LSIL Pap smear 2 years ago but is just now presenting to the colposcopy clinic for evaluation. She is a smoker and has a history of chlamydia.

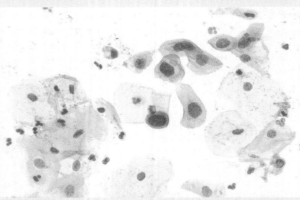

Figure 11–8

This is her Pap smear. What do you see?

Figure 11–8.

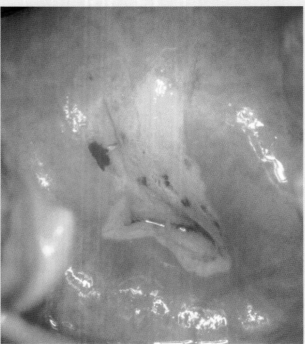

Figure 11–9

This is a colpophotograph of her cervix after the application of 5% acetic acid.

- Is this an adequate examination?
- Are the findings normal or abnormal?
- Describe what you see.

Figure 11–9.

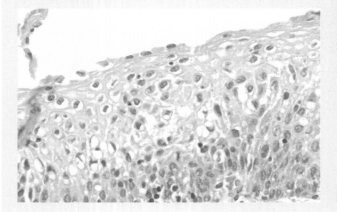

Figure 11–10

A biopsy is taken from the 6-o'clock position and is represented in Figure 11–10.

- What is your pathologic diagnosis?
- Based on your diagnosis, what treatment options would be appropriate for this patient?

Figure 11–10.

Case Study 1 Answers

Figure 11-8

This slide represents an HSIL Pap smear. There are cells in the center of the field that are consistent with HSIL with moderate nuclear pleomorphism and nuclear chromatin hyperchromasia.

Figure 11-9

There is an area of acetowhite epithelium near the os that extends into the canal. If the squamocolumnar junction cannot be seen, this would be an unsatisfactory examination. With an endocervical speculum, the squamocolumnar junction could be seen extending 1 cm into the os.

Figure 11-10

The biopsy demonstrates CIN 2 with koilocytosis. In the parabasal area, nuclear crowding is present, and the cells within the epithelium lack some degree of maturation, although maturation is present in the upper half of the epithelium. Some of the cells near the surface show distinct perinucelar halos with binucleation and features of koilocytosis. Appropriate treatment consists of loop excision or a cone biopsy. Laser ablation or cryotherapy is not appropriate because the disease extends greater than 5 mm into the os.

Key Point of Case 1

If an adequate or satisfactory colposcopic examination cannot be obtained in the face of HSIL cytology and a lesion extending into the endocervical canal, excision of the transformation zone (cone biopsy) is needed.

History

This 25-year-old gravida I, para I presents with a Pap test showing an HSIL. Last year, she was treated with electrosurgical loop excision for a CIN 3 lesion. The margins of the specimen were positive at that time. She is sexually active and uses condoms for birth control. She smokes one pack of cigarettes a day.

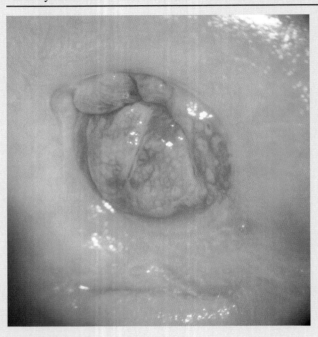

Figure 11-11.

Figure 11-11
This is a colpophotograph of her cervix after the application of 5% acetic acid.

- Is the transformation zone fully visualized?
- Describe what you see.
- What is the differential diagnosis for this lesion?

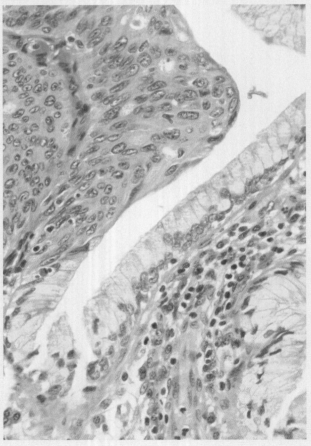

Figure 11-12.

Figure 11-12
This is a biopsy of the most severe colposcopic lesion.

- What is your histologic diagnosis?
- What is the next step in this patient's evaluation?

Case Study 2 Answers

Figure 11–11

The transformation zone is not fully visualized. The ectocervical squamous epithelium ends in an abrupt circular rim characteristic of a previously treated cervix. There is acetowhite epithelium with a mosaic pattern seen medial to this ectocervical rim. The mosaic tiles are irregular in shape and size, and some have a central punctuation. This is highly suggestive of a high-grade lesion, but the possibility must be considered that this is just immature squamous metaplasia.

Figure 11–12

An endocervical crypt is seen. At the lower portion of the photomicrograph, normal columnar epithelium is seen with basally placed nuclei and cells in a "picket-fence" arrangement. But at the upper portion of the crypt, the columnar cells have been replaced by a dysplastic squamous epithelium whose nuclei are disordered and reach to the top of the epithelium. This is a high-grade intraepithelial lesion.

The patient has an unsatisfactory colposcopy and a recurrent high-grade lesion. She needs a cone biopsy for treatment and to exclude the possibility of more advanced disease in the endocervical canal.

Key Point of Case 2

It is difficult to distinguish between immature metaplasia and recurrent dysplasia following treatment for CIN. When in doubt, a biopsy is always indicated.

Case Study 3 Questions

History

This 30-year-old gravida 0, para 0 presents with a Pap smear showing an LSIL. She is sexually active and uses condoms for birth control. She has had five previous sexual partners. She smokes two packs of cigarettes a day.

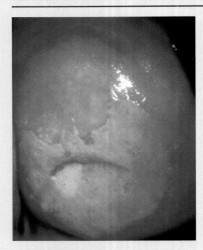

Figure 11–13.

Figures 11–13 and 11–14

Figure 11–13 is a colpophotograph of her cervix after the application of 5% acetic acid. Figure 11–14 is a colpophotograph of her cervix after the application of Lugol's iodine.

- Is the transformation zone fully visualized?
- Describe what you see.
- What is the most appropriate site for a directed biopsy?

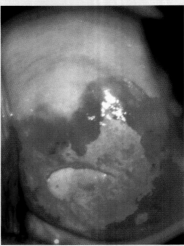

Figure 11–14.

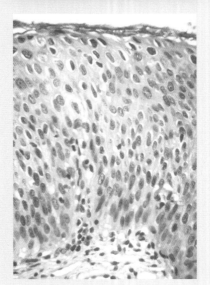

Figure 11–15.

Figure 11–15

- This is a biopsy of the most severe colposcopic lesion.
- What is your histologic diagnosis?

Case Study 3 Answers

Figures 11–13 and 11–14

The transformation zone is not fully visualized. A large area of low-grade acetowhite epithelium with an irregular geographic border replaces most of the transformation zone. In Figure 11–14, this can be seen as a variegated area of patchy iodine uptake. This is consistent with low-grade CIN. However, at the 7-o'clock position, there is a patch of higher-grade acetowhite epithelium (Figure 11–13) that is more starkly non-staining with Lugol's iodine (Figure 11–14). This appearance of a "lesion within a lesion" is called an internal margin and is very highly suggestive of a high-grade lesion. The biopsy should come from this area. Biopsies of the outer lesion are not necessary and may be misleading.

Figure 11–15

The biopsy shows full-thickness change with disordered, hyperchromatic, dysplastic nuclei. This is a CIN 3 lesion.

Key Point of Case 3

A lesion within a lesion (internal margin) is very highly suggestive of a high-grade lesion. The biopsy should be from the inner lesion.

Cytology, Colposcopy, and Histology of High-Grade CIN

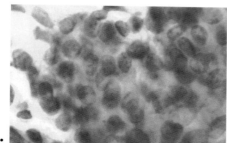

A.

Features suggestive of a high-grade lesion:
- Dense acetowhite epithelium
- Internal border
- Coarse mosaic
- Coarse punctation

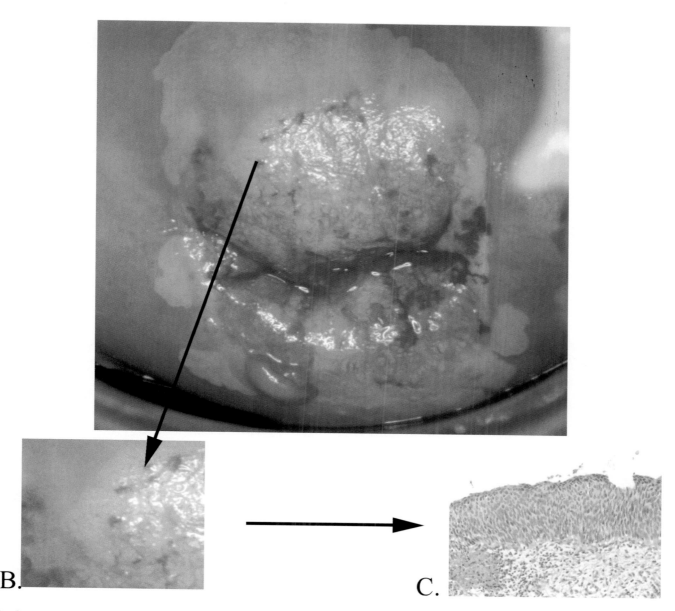

B.

C.

A. Cytology reveals a squamous epithelial cell abnormality: high-grade intraepithelial lesion (HSIL). This group of dysplastic epithelial cells demonstrates marked crowding and overlapping with moderate nuclear pleomorphism. There is nuclear chromatin hyperchromasia and an apparent abnormal mitotic figure in one cell.

B. Area of biopsy. Acetowhite epithelium with punctation and an internal border.

C. Histology reveals CIN 3. The epithelium has complete loss of maturation of keratinocytes with marked crowding and vertical orientation of the nuclei. There is virtually no maturation of the squamous epithelial cells from the basal to the superficial layer. Within the submucosa, there is mild, chronic inflammation.

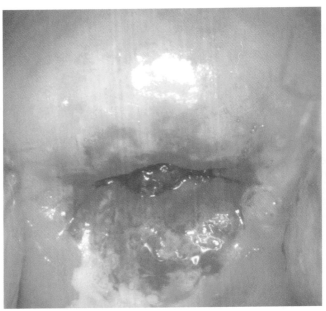

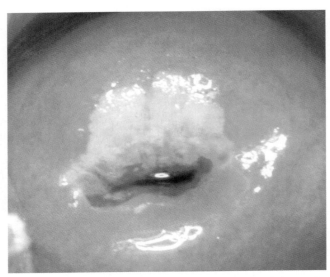

Plate 11-2. Acetowhite epithelium of the anterior lip of the cervix. Cervical intraepithelial neoplasia, grade 2 found on biopsy.

Plate 11-1. Focal area of dense acetowhite epithelium on the posterior lip of the cervix. Cervical intraepithelial neoplasia grade 2 found on biopsy.

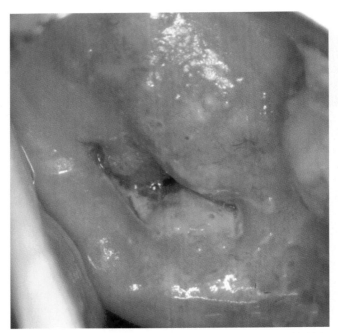

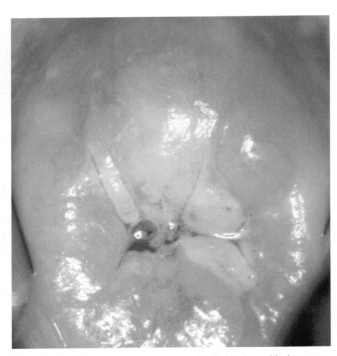

Plate 11-3. Dense acetowhite epithelium at the os consistent with high-grade squamous intraepithelial lesion. The squamocolumnar junction cannot be seen at 4 o'clock, so this is an unsatisfactory examination. Although there is no disease on the anterior lip, the transformation zone is extensive, as evidenced by the presence of several nabothian cysts.

Plate 11-4. High-grade squamous intraepithelial lesion with dense acetowhite epithelium, slight punctation at 12 o'clock, and sharp margins. The squamocolumnar junction is not seen in this image.

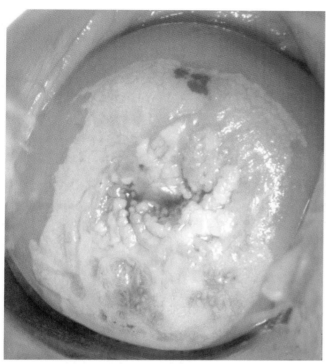

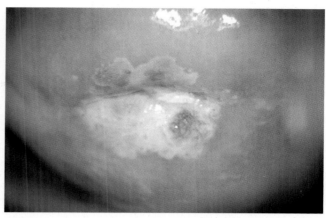

Plate 11-6. Low-grade lesion with fine mosaic on the anterior lip and high-grade lesion with coarse mosaic on the posterior lip. Biopsy at 12 o'clock revealed cervical intraepithelial neoplasia, grade 1 and cervical intraepithelial neoplasia, grade 3 at 5 o'clock.

Plate 11-5. This cervix has a large transformation zone with peripheral immature metaplasia and faint mosaic pattern, along with an area of dense acetowhite epithelium centrally. A biopsy at 9 o'clock revealed metaplasia, whereas a biopsy at 4 o'clock revealed cervical intraepithelial neoplasia, grade 3.

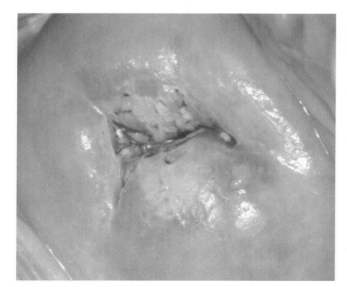

Plate 11-7. Well-defined focal area of acetowhite epithelium at 6 o'clock and, less prominently, at 12 o'clock. Biopsy revealed cervical intraepithelial neoplasia, grade 2.

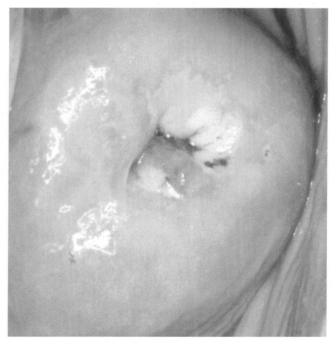

Plate 11-8. Dense acetowhite epithelium surrounding the os, and mucus is also present. The squamocolumnar junction cannot be seen. Biopsy revealed cervical intraepithelial neoplasia, grade 3.

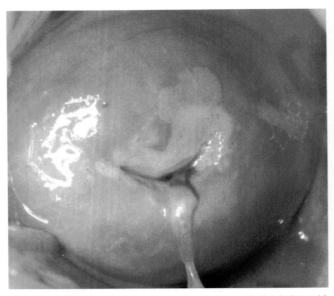

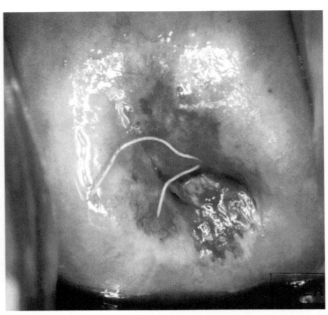

Plate 11–9. Peripheral low-grade squamous intraepithelial lesion with geographic margins and mild, acetowhite epithelium with a central, dense acetowhite lesion. The squamocolumnar junction is not seen. Peripheral biopsy revealed cervical intraepithelial neoplasia, grade 1, and central biopsy revealed cervical intraepithelial neoplasia, grade 2.

Plate 11–10. Dense acetowhite epithelium is noted near the internal os posteriorly, along with a coarse mosaic pattern. Biopsy revealed cervical intraepithelial neoplasia, grade 3.

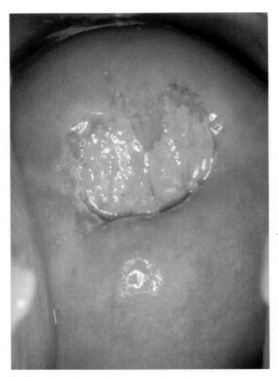

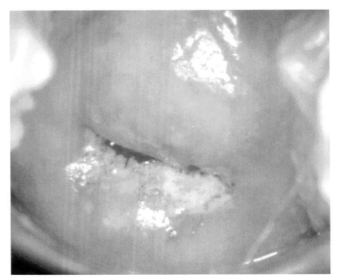

Plate 11–11. High-grade squamous intraepithelial lesion with dense acetowhite epithelium and coarse punctation on the left posterior cervix. The squamocolumnar junction is not seen.

Plate 11–12. Acetowhite epithelium that extends into the canal, becoming a denser acetowhite near the os. Visualization of the upper border of the lesion is important because the most abnormal region of the lesion is usually at the squamocolumnar junction. The biopsies showed cervical intraepithelial neoplasia, grade 2.

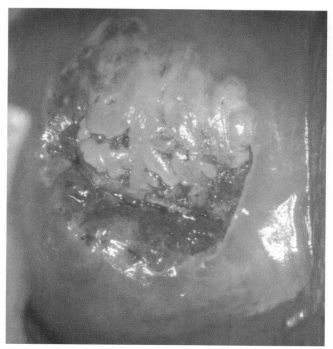

Plate 11-13. Cervical intraepithelial neoplasia grade 2 lesion of the anterior lip of the cervix.

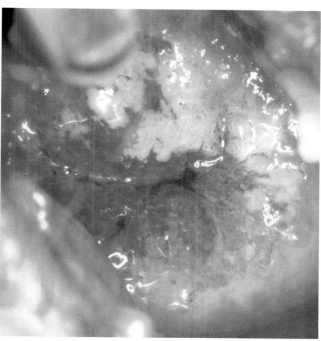

Plate 11-14. High-grade squamous intraepithelial lesion with dense acetowhite epithelium and coarse punctation noted at 2 o'clock.

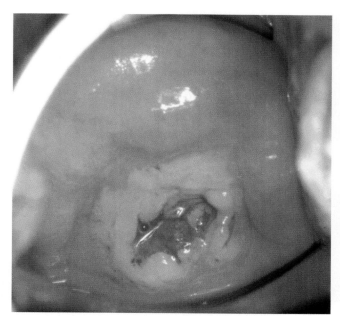

Plate 11-15. Acetowhite epithelium near the os in a patient who is post laser treatment, 1 year earlier. A biopsy at 6 o'clock revealed cervical intraepithelial neoplasia, grade 2.

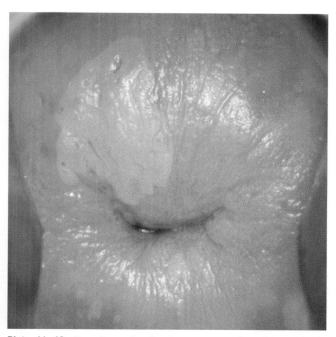

Plate 11-16. Hyperkeratosis after laser surgery gives this cervix its granular appearance. There is a large, well-circumscribed area of acetowhite epithelium at the 9-o'clock to 12-o'clock position that represents residual posttreatment cervical intraepithelial neoplasia.

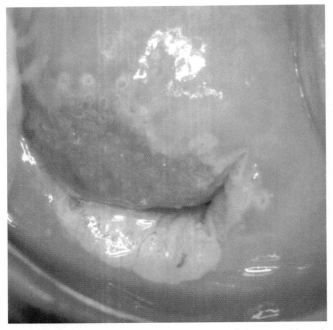

Plate 11–17. Well-demarcated peripheral border of the acetowhite epithelium on the posterior lip of the cervix. Cervical intraepithelial neoplasia, grade 3, was found on biopsy.

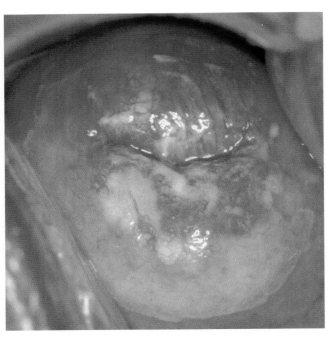

Plate 11–18. Large transformation zone with mild acetowhite epithelium peripherally and dense acetowhite epithelium with coarse mosaic pattern mainly at 7 o'clock and 11 o'clock. Biopsy revealed cervical intraepithelial neoplasia, grade 3.

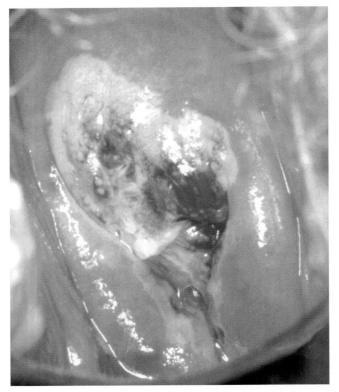

Plate 11–19. High-grade lesion with dense acetowhite epithelium and coarse mosaic that extends into the canal. The upper limits of the lesions could not be seen, and the patient underwent a cone biopsy. The pathology was cervical intraepithelial neoplasia, grade 3.

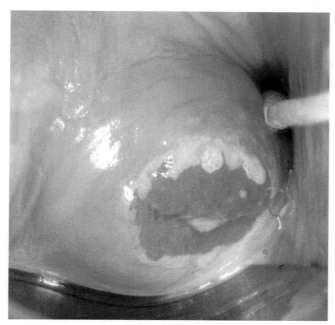

Plate 11–20. Adequate examination with mild acetowhite epithelium anteriorly and a central, 12-o'clock, denser acetowhite area with coarse punctation. A biopsy of the area of punctation revealed cervical intraepithelial neoplasia, grade 2.

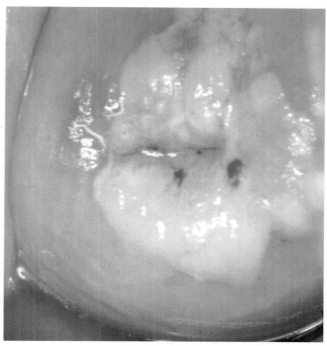

Plate 11–21. Large, high-grade lesion with dense acetowhite epithelium, no vessels, and an inadequate examination.

- R. Kevin Reynolds
- Kelly J. Manahan

CHAPTER *12*

Squamous Cervical Cancer: Invasion and Microinvasion

INCIDENCE

Since the early 1960s, the incidence of cervical cancer in the United States has declined by 87%.

In much of the world, cervical cancer remains the most common cancer diagnosis in women. Only in nations with health care systems that provide screening and treatment of preinvasive lesions is the incidence of cervical cancer substantially lower. Since the early 1960s, cervical cancer incidence has declined by 87% in the United States.[1] Although the reasons for this decline in mortality are complex, the trend has clearly followed the widespread acceptance of Papanicolaou (Pap) smear screening to identify patients with treatable preinvasive disease. A total of 13,700 new diagnoses of cervical cancer and 4900 cervical cancer deaths occurred in the United States in 1998.[2]

COLPOSCOPIC ASSESSMENT OF INVASIVE AND MICROINVASIVE LESIONS

When a visible lesion is identified on the cervix, or when a squamous intraepithelial lesion is diagnosed on Pap smear, visual and colposcopic inspection of the cervix and vagina with directed biopsy, endocervical assessment with either curettage or brushing for cytology, and bimanual pelvic examination are warranted. Many authors have attempted to distinguish the colposcopic appearance of preinvasive cervical neoplasia from microinvasive or invasive cervical carcinoma.[4, 5]

A lack of abnormal colposcopic findings does not always indicate an absence of cervical pathology.

The premise on which colposcopy is based is that dysplastic lesions and cancers have visually distinct morphology that can be recognized by the skilled colposcopist. Abnormal colposcopic findings indicative of microinvasive and invasive cervical carcinomas are similar to those described in previous chapters for preinvasive cervical neoplasia. Although microinvasive and invasive cervical carcinomas are often assumed to demonstrate progressively more abnormal findings on a continuum beginning with preinvasive disease, published evidence does not support this assumption. The most severe lesions do not always demonstrate the most abnormal colposcopic findings. Likewise, a lack of abnormal colposcopic findings does not always indicate an absence of cervical pathology.

Colposcopic detection of microinvasive and invasive disease can be difficult. Although many authors report that colposcopy is of value in detecting early invasive disease, these same authors report a significant problem with inaccuracy of colposcopic diagnosis.[6, 7] In a retrospective review of 180 patients with microinvasive and occult invasive squamous cell carcinoma of the cervix, Benedet defined the accuracy rate of colposcopy as the percentage of patients with a satisfactory colposcopic examination who were correctly diagnosed on the basis of this examination.[7] In this series, patients were correctly identified as having microinvasive carcinoma only 73% of the time. Patients with occult invasive squamous cell carcinoma of the cervix were detected with an accuracy rate of 87%. In a similar population-based study of 61 patients with microinvasive disease, Paraskevaidis and associates reported a colposcopic sensitivity of only 50%.[8] Hopman and coworkers, in a review of the relevant literature, found that nearly 50% of cases of microinvasive disease were missed by colposcopic assessment.[9] In one report, underdiagnosis of microinvasive carcinoma was 100% with colposcopic examination.[10] Hopman and colleagues also found interobserver agreement of colposcopic impression about half the time among 23 experienced colposcopists.[11] These studies highlight the limitations of colposcopic assessment in the detection of microinvasive and invasive lesions.

Nearly 50% of cases of microinvasive carcinoma may be missed by colposcopic examination.

A number of abnormal colposcopic findings are reported to be associated with microinvasive and invasive cervical cancer. These include atypical vessels, necrosis, ulceration, and exophytic mass (Figs. 12–1, 12–2, 12–3, and 12–4). Many abnormal colposcopic findings are also associated with intraepithelial neoplasia, as reported in previous chapters. These include acetowhite epithelium, punctation, mosaic, atypical vessels, and keratosis. Some colposcopic findings, such as unusual friability, necrosis, ulceration, and exophytic mass, may also be associated with benign conditions such as infections and trauma. Atypical vessels are surface capillaries that have unusual patterns such as hairpin loops, abnormal branching, commas, starbursts, and corkscrews. Nabothian cysts may have surface vascularity, but these can be distinguished from atypical vascular patterns because of the normal pattern of vessel arborization and the characteristic hemispheric contour of the cyst (Figs. 12–5 and 12–6). Necrosis of neoplastic tissue may be noted by a color change resulting in a yellow-to-tan appearance, often associated with friability (Fig. 12–7). Invasive lesions may demonstrate endophytic growth, leading to ulceration, or exophytic growth, resulting in an irregularly shaped mass protruding from the cervical surface.

Many authors report a constellation of these findings that may be more indicative of microinvasive or invasive disease. Sugimori and coworkers, in a review of 46 patients with microinvasive and invasive carcinoma, reported thick, white, elevated lesions with sharply demarcated margins in 85% of patients with microinvasive disease, whereas this condition was noted in only 41% of patients with carcinoma in situ.[6] Sugimori and associates demonstrated that when mosaic, punctation, and acetowhite epithelium were noted, microinvasive carcinoma was more likely when the lesion encompassed the circumference of the external os and when the lesion was

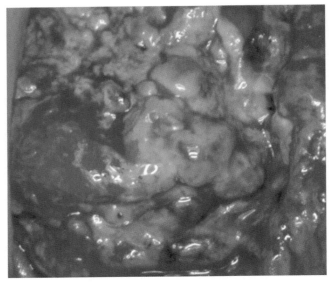

Figure 12–2. Example of necrosis and yellow appearance of the cervical epithelium.

sharply demarcated. Other studies have not confirmed these observations.[12, 13] Liu and coworkers reported that 40% of patients with a microinvasive cancer demonstrated mosaic, punctation, and acetowhite epithelium; 37% were found to have only two of these abnormalities; 18% had only one; and 5% had no abnormal colposcopic findings at all.[5] In a retrospective review of 228 patients, Noda evaluated the ability of colposcopy to discriminate among dysplasia, carcinoma in situ, and microinvasive carcinoma.[4] Twenty-five percent of patients with microinvasive disease had lesions that demonstrated a mosaic pattern, 14% harbored punctation, 25% had acetowhite

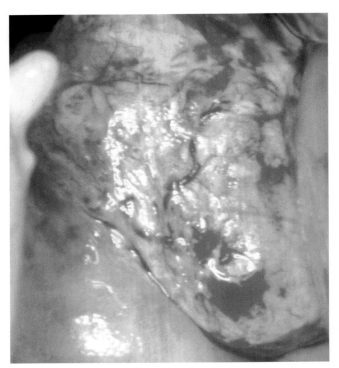

Figure 12–1. Cancer with cervical mass and large atypical vessels present.

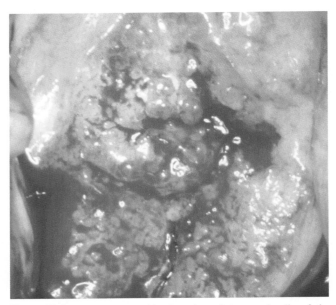

Figure 12–3. Large cancer with ulceration of the anterior lip of the cervix; overall yellow, necrotic appearance, and friability.

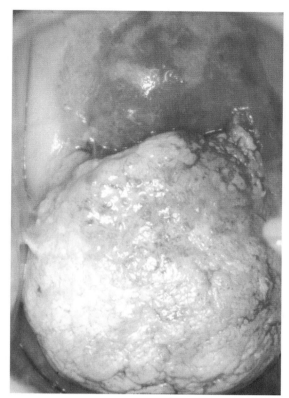

Figure 12–4. Large, fungating mass on the posterior lip of the cervix with dense acetowhite epithelium and atypical vessels. Image provided by Dr. Vesna Kesic.

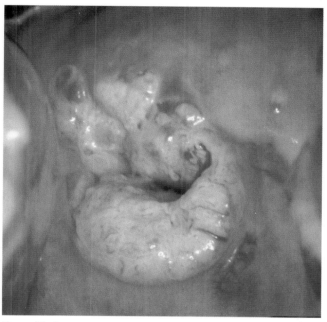

Figure 12–6. Nonbranching atypical vessels on the surface of a raised, acetowhite mass on the posterior lip of the cervix. There are also two nabothian cysts at 2 o'clock.

epithelium, and 50% showed keratosis. The triad of mosaic, punctation, and acetowhite epithelium appeared in approximately 20% of patients with microinvasive carcinoma. Paraskevaidis and colleagues reported that 34% of patients with microinvasive disease had no abnormal colposcopic findings.[8]

The frequency of the finding of atypical vessels increases as the depth of invasion increases.

It has long been believed that the pathognomonic colposcopic finding indicative of microinvasive or invasive

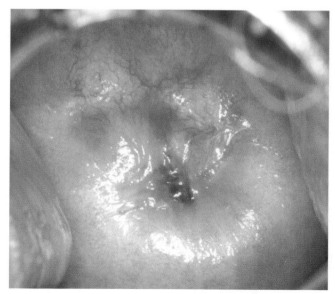

Figure 12–5. Normal, arborizing vessels and nabothian cysts.

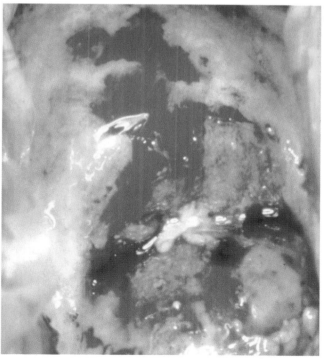

Figure 12–7. Cancer with necrosis, friability, and a diffuse yellow appearance.

disease is the presence of atypical vessels.[9] Koller first described atypical vessels as vessels that are 2 to 10 times wider than normal capillaries and are irregular in width, shape, and course.[14] Authors have reported the presence of atypical vessels in microinvasive cancer in anywhere from 0% to approximately 80% of patients. Several reported that the frequency of atypical vessels increased with increasing depth of invasion.[4, 5, 9] Liu and associates reported that 32% of patients with invasion of less than 3 mm in depth had atypical vessels, whereas 100% of patients with invasion of 3 to 5 mm had atypical vessels.[5] Van Meir and colleagues reported that atypical vessels were not found in any patients with less than 3 mm of invasion but were found in all patients with 3 to 5 mm of invasion.[13] A proposed explanation for the lack of atypical vessels with microinvasive disease is that neovascularization may not be necessary for the development of small lesions.[5] Folkman indicated that tumors up to 2 to 3 mm in diameter can survive by diffusion alone without requiring angiogenesis.[15]

ADDITIONAL DIAGNOSTIC BIOPSY PROCEDURES

If colposcopic-directed biopsy reveals a lesion invading more than 5 mm below the basement membrane, no further histologic data are required for staging.

Following colposcopic assessment with directed biopsies, additional biopsy material may be required to accurately stage the cervical lesion. If the colposcopically directed biopsy reveals a lesion invading more than 5 mm below the basement membrane, no further histologic data are required to stage the lesion. If invasion less than or equal to 5 mm below the basement membrane is detected, complete assessment of the cervical portio is required to rule out the presence of deeper invasion. Treatment by conization should be reserved for special cases that are discussed in detail later in this chapter. Ablative therapy, such as cryocautery or CO_2 laser photoablation, is always contraindicated once invasion is documented.

HISTOPATHOLOGY

The American Joint Commission on Cancer (AJCC), in cooperation with the American College of Surgeons and the American Cancer Society, has proposed universal adoption of the World Health Organization (WHO) system titled the International Histological Classification of Tumors.[17] The AJCC classification of cervical cancer types is divided into three major categories: squamous carcinoma, adenocarcinoma, and other types (Table 12–1). The squamous types are divided into preinvasive and invasive groups, and the invasive category can be further subdivided into keratinizing, nonkeratinizing, and verrucous types. Squamous cancer accounts for at least 75% of cervical cancers; it is discussed later in this chapter.[1] Adenocarcinoma will be addressed in Chapter 13.

Invasive squamous cervical cancer is usually composed of compact nests of neoplastic squamous cells invading the subepithelial stroma. The size, shape, and degree of keratinization vary widely. At least two systems for grading of squamous carcinoma are currently used. The AJCC system defines the grades as well differentiated (G1), moderately differentiated (G2), poorly differentiated (G3), or undifferentiated (G4).[17] For practical reasons, the older morphologic grading system proposed by Reagan and Ng is more widely used. Using the Reagan and Ng nomenclature, well-differentiated carcinoma is called large-cell keratinizing type, whereas moderately differentiated carcinoma is defined as large-cell nonkeratinizing type, and poorly differentiated tumors are termed small-cell nonkeratinizing type.[18] Small-cell nonkeratinizing tumors are of squamous origin and are distinct from small-cell neuroendocrine tumors. When small cells predominate in a tumor, immunohistochemical analysis aids in determining the correct cell type.

In well-differentiated squamous carcinoma of the cervix, the most prominent feature is the presence of keratin, often deposited in keratin pearls.

In well-differentiated squamous carcinoma of the cervix, the most prominent feature is the presence of keratin, often deposited in keratin pearls. Keratin pearls are eosinophilic, concentric whorls surrounded by epithelial nests (Fig. 12–8). Well-differentiated squamous carcinoma cells are usually oval or polygonal in shape and have distinct intercellular bridges. Nuclei are usually large, hyperchromatic, and irregularly shaped.[1, 19]

The cells and nuclei of moderately differentiated tumors are more pleomorphic, and mitotic figures are more frequent. Cellular borders and intercellular bridges are less distinct. Dyskeratosis and abnormal intracellular keratin formation are often present, but keratin pearl formation is rare (Fig. 12–9).

▼ Table 12–1

AJCC Classification of Cervical Cancer Histopathology

Cervical intraepithelial neoplasia, grade 3
Squamous cell carcinoma in situ
Squamous cell carcinoma
    Invasive
    Keratinizing
    Nonkeratinizing
    Verrucous
Adenocarcinoma in situ
Adenocarcinoma
    Invasive carcinoma
    Endocervical carcinoma
    Endometrioid carcinoma
    Clear cell carcinoma
    Adenosquamous carcinoma
    Adenoid cystic carcinoma
Small-cell carcinoma (neuroendocrine)
Undifferentiated carcinoma

AJCC, American Joint Committee on Cancer.
Data from Fleming ID, Cooper JS, Henson DE, et al (eds): AJCC Cancer Staging Handbook. Philadelphia, Lippincott-Raven, 1998.

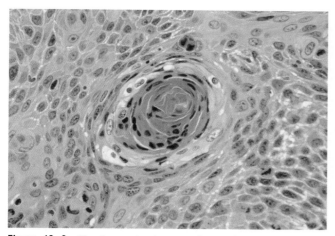

Figure 12–8. Keratin pearls demonstrating eosinophilic, concentric whorls surrounded by epithelial nests.

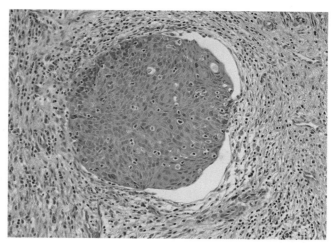

Figure 12–10. Histology demonstrating lymphovascular space invasion.

Poorly differentiated carcinomas are characterized by large, irregular nuclei; frequent mitotic figures; minimal cytoplasm; and areas of necrosis. Cells may be oval or fusiform in shape. Keratin formation is rare or absent. The differential diagnosis for cells with these characteristics includes small-cell neuroendocrine and sarcoma tumor types. Immunohistochemical analysis may be required to reach the correct diagnosis.[1, 19]

The presence of lymphovascular space invasion (LVSI) has significant impact on treatment planning and prognosis, which are discussed later in this chapter. LVSI is diagnosed when malignant cells are detected in a lumen that is lined with endothelial cells (Fig. 12–10). The differential diagnosis includes tissue-processing artifact, where retraction of tissue during fixation causes an apparent lumen.[1] Unlike with true LVSI, a lining of endothelial cells will not be seen at the border of the lumen.

Discriminating between dysplastic and microinvasive lesions can be difficult, particularly if the biopsy specimen has been cut tangentially. When squamous carcinoma first breeches the basement membrane, the invading squamous cells appear better differentiated than adjacent dysplastic epithelial cells appear. Features include larger cells with abundant eosinophilic cytoplasm and occasional keratin pearl formation. The leading edge of the invasive focus appears ragged, with neoplastic cells appearing to drop off the epithelium and into the stroma.[1, 20] A marked, local, acute inflammatory response is often noted at the site of invasion. By convention, the depth of stromal invasion is measured perpendicularly from the nearest basement membrane to the base of the lesion (Fig. 12–11). If the origination site of the tumor is not obvious, depth is measured from the basement membrane of the nearest surface epithelium. If the invasive focus arises from the base of a gland, depth is measured from the site of origin of the invasive focus to the deepest portion of the invasive lesion.

An unusual variant of squamous cervical carcinoma is verrucous carcinoma. This tumor is usually associated with human papillomavirus (HPV) type 6, and its papillary appearance is often mistaken clinically for a giant

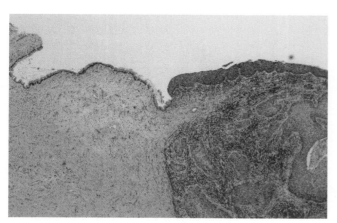

Figure 12–9. Large-cell, nonkeratinizing carcinoma.

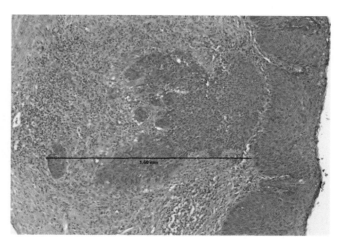

Figure 12–11. Microinvasion.

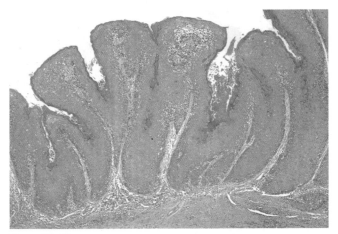

Figure 12–12. Verrucous carcinoma.

condyloma.[21, 22] The tumor is exophytic in nature. Microscopic features include bland-appearing cells with a low mitotic index and an undulating surface (Fig. 12–12). Fibrovascular cores are absent in the papillary structure of the tumor, which offers a useful distinction in comparison with the prominent fibrovascular cores noted in condyloma. The stromal-epithelial interface is often described as having a pushing border with a broad, smooth appearance. These tumors tend to recur locally, and metastasis is uncommon.[21–23]

STAGING OF CERVICAL CANCER

Staging using the International Federation of Gynecology and Obstetrics system includes selective use of colposcopy and directed biopsy, intravenous pyelogram, chest x-ray, cystoscopy, and sigmoidoscopy.

Patients must be staged to determine appropriate treatment and to offer accurate counsel regarding prognosis. Figure 12–13 demonstrates a pictorial description of clinical staging for cervical cancer. There are two staging systems in widespread use today. The more commonly used international standard for staging is defined by the International Federation of Gynecology and Obstetrics (FIGO) in conjunction with the WHO.[17] The FIGO cervical cancer staging criteria were revised in 1995 (Table 12–2). By convention, when there is disagreement regarding staging, the less advanced stage is chosen for statistical consistency. Stage is based primarily on clinical examination that includes bimanual pelvic and rectovaginal examination. When determining stage using the FIGO system, tests that may officially be used include biopsy, colposcopy, intravenous pyelogram (IVP), chest x-ray, cystoscopy, and sigmoidoscopy. Tests that may not be used to officially stage include computed tomography (CT), magnetic resonance imaging (MRI), lymphangiogram, and surgical findings from laparoscopy and laparotomy. Tests should be used selectively based on the

physical examination. For example, cystoscopy or sigmoidoscopy is recommended when the clinical examination suggests a stage III or stage IV lesion, but it is not cost-effective for stage I and stage II lesions because of low yield.[24] CT scans, although not allowable for staging purposes, may be useful for treatment planning in some cases. CT scanning of the abdomen and pelvis is unlikely to detect lymphadenopathy for stage 1B1 lesions owing to the low expected incidence of lymphatic metastases, but it would be much more likely to identify lymph node metastases in larger stage IB2, stage II, and stage III lesions where para-aortic node metastases occur in 18% to 33% of patients.[25] Lymphangiography and MRI scans are considered optional and are not routinely ordered. By convention, once a patient has been staged, the stage is not changed even if subsequent testing or surgery indicates that the tumor is more or less advanced than was originally believed.

The AJCC, using the tumor, nodes, and metastasis (TNM) staging system, has defined a parallel staging system.[17] The American College of Surgeons requires use of the AJCC system for accreditation of tumor registries. The AJCC definition of the tumor categories corresponds to the FIGO staging system. When surgery is the primary treatment, the histologic findings permit the case to be assigned a pathologic stage that is designated postsurgical TNM (pTNM). A comparison of the FIGO and AJCC staging systems is presented in Tables 12–2 and 12–3.

Both the FIGO and AJCC staging systems are applicable to all histologic types, including glandular neoplasms.

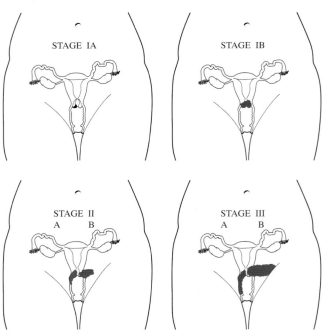

Figure 12–13. Pictorial description of clinical staging for cervical cancer. This figure illustrates findings the examiner may appreciate on bimanual and rectovaginal examination. The dotted line in the stage IA diagram illustrates the line of resection for a cold-knife cone biopsy. The A and B substages for stages II and III disease are represented on the patient's right and left sides, respectively.

▼ Table 12–2

Cervical Cancer Staging: FIGO and AJCC Systems

FIGO Stage	Primary Tumor	AJCC TNM
—	Primary tumor cannot be assessed	TX
0	Carcinoma in situ	Tis
I	Carcinoma confined to the cervix (disregard extension to corpus)	T1
IA1	Measurable invasion ≤3 mm in depth and 7 mm in diameter	T1a1
IA2	Measurable invasion >3 and ≤5 mm in depth as well as ≤7 mm in diameter	T1a2
IB1	Lesion of >5 mm depth and/or >7 mm diameter, but ≤4 cm in diameter	T1b1
IB2	Lesion of >4 cm diameter	T1b2
II	Tumor extends beyond the cervix but not to the pelvic wall; tumor may involve vagina, but not the lower third	T2
IIA	No parametrial involvement	T2a
IIB	Parametrial involvement	T2b
III	Tumor extends to the pelvic wall or may involve the lower third of the vagina	T3
IIIA	No extension to pelvic wall	T3a
IIIB	Extension to pelvic wall; includes all cases with hydronephrosis or nonfunctioning kidney	T3b
IV	Spread beyond true pelvis or involvement of bladder or rectal mucosa	T4
IVA	Tumor invades bladder or rectal mucosa and/or extends beyond true pelvis; bullous edema is not sufficient to classify invasion	T4a
IVB	Distant metastases	T4b

FIGO Stage	Regional Lymph Nodes	AJCC TNM
—	Regional lymph nodes cannot be assessed	NX
—	No regional lymph node metastasis	N0
—	Regional lymph node metastasis	N1

FIGO Stage	Distant Metastasis	AJCC TNM
—	Distant metastasis cannot be assessed	MX
—	No distant metastasis	M0
—	Distant metastasis, including para-aortic node metastases	M1

AJCC, American Joint Committee on Cancer; FIGO, International Federation of Gynecology and Obstetrics; TNM, tumor, nodes, and metastasis.
Data from Fleming ID, Cooper JS, Henson DE, et al (eds): AJCC Cancer Staging Handbook. Philadelphia, Lippincott-Raven, 1998.

However, the microinvasive cancer entity has not been defined for adenocarcinoma, primarily because of controversy regarding the lack of a reproducible reference point for measurement of lesion depth. This contrasts with squamous lesions, where depth is measured perpendicular to the nearest basement membrane to determine depth of invasion.

Surgical staging to obtain pelvic and para-aortic nodes

before treatment has been evaluated in several clinical trials. An extrafascial surgical approach has been shown to cause less radiation-associated morbidity.[26] Surgical staging has not been shown to improve survival.[27] With the exception of clinical trials, surgical staging is not routinely performed.

Treatment of Cervical Cancer

Disease confined to the cervix is defined as stage I. The substage (i.e., IA1, IA2, IB1, IB2) is based on depth and diameter of invasion within the cervix. This correlates well with likelihood of metastases as well as survival.

Microinvasive Carcinoma, Stage IA1 and IA2

Patients with 3 mm or less of invasion may be offered conservative surgery, including fertility-sparing cold-knife conization or loop electrosurgical excision.

Stage IA lesions are referred to as microinvasive. The clinical significance of microinvasive cancer is that it is an empirically defined subset of stage I disease, in which lymph node metastasis and recurrence are rare. Because many women who develop cervical cancer are in their

▼ Table 12–3

Cervical Cancer Stage Grouping, AJCC System

Stage	T	N	M
Stage 0	Tis	N0	M0
Stage IA1	T1a1	N0	M0
Stage IA2	T1a2	N0	M0
Stage IB1	T1b1	N0	M0
Stage IB2	T1b2	N0	M0
Stage IIA	T2a	N0	M0
Stage IIB	T2b	N0	M0
Stage IIIA	T3a	N0	M0
Stage IIIB	T1	N1	M0
	T2	N1	M0
	T3a	N1	M0
	T3b	Any N	M0
Stage IVA	T4	Any N	M0
Stage IVB	Any T	Any N	M1

AJCC, American Joint Committee on Cancer.
Data from Fleming ID, Cooper JS, Henson DE, et al (eds): AJCC Cancer Staging Handbook. Philadelphia, Lippincott-Raven, 1998.

early reproductive years, it is helpful to define a group of patients with little risk of recurrence so that fertility-sparing treatment may be considered. The definition of microinvasive cervical carcinoma has been a point of controversy and confusion for many years. Three widely accepted definitions of microinvasive disease are those of the FIGO and the Society of Gynecologic Oncologists (SGO) and a Japanese definition.[28] The FIGO definition specifies tumor depth and width, whereas the SGO definition specifies tumor depth but excludes multifocal lesions and LVSI. The Japanese definition specifies tumor depth, confluence, and cell type and excludes LVSI. The one variable that is specified in each of the three definitions is depth of invasion, although the actual depth varies for each definition. Many studies have analyzed the risk of metastasis to lymph nodes based on depth of invasion within the cervical lesion. Collectively, the data indicate that the risk of nodal metastasis with invasion beyond the basement membrane of less than or equal to 3 mm is 0.5% and that the risk of nodal spread with depth of invasion over 3 mm is 8.2%.[29] Only 1 of 397 patients with cervical stromal invasion less than or equal to 3 mm was found to have lymph node metastasis.[30] These data support the practice of offering conservative surgery, including fertility-sparing cervical conization, to patients with less than or equal to 3 mm of invasion. Simple hysterectomy would be recommended for patients not wishing to remain fertile.

The presence of lymphovascular space invasion and stromal invasion greater than 3 mm carries a significant risk of recurrence.

Another predictor of metastatic disease and recurrence in patients with microinvasive cervical carcinoma is the presence of LVSI. In 1994, the Gynecologic Oncology Group analyzed the risk of nodal metastases in the presence of LVSI.[31] In patients with 3 to 5 mm of invasion and with LVSI, 15.6% had pelvic node metastasis, whereas only 0.9% of patients had evidence of pelvic node metastases in the absence of LVSI. Van Nagell and coworkers reported no nodal metastases and no recurrences in 17 patients with invasion of less than 3 mm and LVSI. However, 25% of patients with stromal invasion from 3.1 to 5 mm and LVSI developed recurrent disease.[30] Creasman and colleagues reviewed 114 patients with microinvasive cervical carcinoma and reported that 2 of 25 patients with less than 1 mm of invasion had lymphovascular involvement and that neither patient developed recurrent disease.[31] Although each of these studies has a small number of patients, the data suggest that the presence of LVSI and stromal invasion greater than 3 mm carries a significant risk of recurrence. The recurrence risk appears to be low with invasion of less than 3 mm, despite the presence of LVSI.

Stage IA1

Accepted surgical treatments for microinvasive disease include simple hysterectomy, using either the abdominal or the vaginal approach, or cervical cone biopsy, using cold-knife conization or the loop electrocautery excision procedure. Tseng and associates reported that 12 patients with microinvasive cervical carcinoma of less than 3 mm of invasion managed by cold-knife conization alone developed no recurrences after a mean follow-up of 6.7 years.[32] In a prospective study of the management of 29 patients with microinvasive cervical carcinoma managed by LEEP, all patients had a depth of invasion of less than 3 mm, and no patient was noted to have LVSI. After 25 months of follow-up, none of these patients developed recurrence.[33] However, a case of widespread lymph node metastasis in a patient with microinvasive cervical carcinoma measuring 0.8 mm has been reported.[34] In another report, a patient with 0.2 mm of invasion and positive LVSI demonstrated bulky pelvic lymph node metastases at the time of laparotomy.[30] Patients must be informed of the slight but ever-present risk of recurrent disease despite appropriate conservative management.

Stage IA2

Appropriate treatment for stage IA2 includes radical hysterectomy with pelvic lymphadenectomy, modified radical hysterectomy with pelvic lymphadenectomy, or radiation therapy.

Stage IA2 disease is defined as invasion of greater than 3 mm but less than 5 mm in depth and tumor diameter no greater than 7 mm in width. Appropriate treatment for this stage includes radical hysterectomy with pelvic lymphadenectomy, modified radical hysterectomy with pelvic lymphadenectomy, or radiation therapy. Although radical hysterectomy (described in Table 12–4) results in excellent long-term survival for patients with stage IA2 disease, a modified radical hysterectomy may likewise prove to be curative, with fewer potential complications and less morbidity.[35] The modified radical hysterectomy has been reported to have less overall morbidity, especially with regard to urinary tract dysfunction.[36] Several studies suggest that tumor volume less than or equal to 1 cm can be successfully treated with a modified radical approach with comparable survival rates. In a retrospective review, Magrina and coworkers reported that 47 patients with tumor volume less than or equal to 2 cm treated with a modified radical hysterectomy had a 5-year survival of 100% with no recurrences.[37] These studies suggest that a modified radical hysterectomy provides adequate disease resection. However, no consensus definition of acceptable tumor size or volume has been accepted to define the patient population best suited for this approach, which limits the acceptability of modified radical hysterectomy for many oncologists.

Other suggested indications for modified radical hysterectomy include microinvasion with lymphovascular invasion, adjuvant hysterectomy following radiation therapy with small-volume residual carcinoma, or medial parametrial thickening or a positive endocervical curettage.[28] Although this approach has been reported to be a reasonable option, it must be understood that no advantage in performing a modified radical hysterectomy has been shown for patients with these indications.

Stage IA2 lesions may also be treated with intracavitary radiation therapy alone.[19, 38, 39] Although some authors report that external pelvic radiotherapy is not re-

▼ Table 12-4

Comparison of Hysterectomy Types

Anatomic Structure	Extrafascial	Modified Radical	Radical
Uterus	Removed	Removed	Removed
Ovaries	Optional removal	Optional removal	Optional removal
Cervix	Removed	Removed	Removed
Vaginal margin	None	1-2 cm margin	>2-3 cm margin
Ureters	Not mobilized	Dissected through broad ligament	Dissected through broad ligament
Cardinal ligaments	Divided at uterine border	Divided where ureter transits the broad ligament	Divided at pelvic sidewall
Uterosacral ligaments	Divided at cervical border	Partially resected	Divided near sacral origin
Bladder	Mobilized to base of cervix	Mobilized to upper vagina	Mobilized to middle vagina
Rectum	Not mobilized	Mobilized below cervix	Mobilized below middle vagina

quired for these tumors, patients with 3 to 5 mm of invasion and LVSI will have an 8.2% risk of pelvic nodal metastasis. Consideration should be given to treating these patients with both external radiation therapy and intracavitary implants.

Stages IB and IIA

Stage IB or IIA cervical cancer is effectively treated with either radical pelvic surgery or radiation therapy, with nearly equal likelihood of survival regardless of treatment modality.

Stage IB or IIA cervical cancer is effectively treated with either radical pelvic surgery or radiation therapy, with nearly equal likelihood of survival.[40-42] The surgical approach is preferred in younger patients because of the ability to preserve ovarian hormone production and vaginal pliability for sexual function.[43-45] The choice of surgical or radiation therapy depends on tumor characteristics, medical condition of the patient, and preferences of the oncologist and the patient. Preferences are often based on the difference in treatment-related complications rather than on the difference in likelihood of long-term survival.[19] Acute surgery-related complications include intraoperative bleeding and postoperative infection. Delayed postsurgical complications include vesicovaginal and ureterovaginal fistulae that occur in less than 2% of cases.[46-48] Loss of ovarian function occurs in up to 40% of surgically treated cervical cancer patients with ovarian preservation.[49, 50] In comparison, radiation-associated complications include diarrhea in both the acute and the chronic setting, as well as stricture or fistula formation that is prone to occur 2 or more years after treatment. The incidence of chronic diarrhea may range between 3% and 40% depending on the volume of small bowel radiated and the total radiation dose. The likelihood of stricture or fistula formation varies with the radiation dose administered and the medical condition of the patient. Strictures, perforation, and formation of fistulae occur in about 5% of patients who undergo pelvic radiation.[51]

The surgical procedure of choice for treatment of stage IB or stage IIA cervical cancer is radical hysterectomy with pelvic lymphadenectomy.

The surgical procedure of choice for treatment of stage IB or stage IIA cervical cancer is radical hysterectomy with pelvic lymphadenectomy. A radical hysterectomy differs from a simple, or extrafascial, hysterectomy by including resection of the cardinal and uterosacral ligaments of the uterus and removal of the upper portion of the vagina.[28, 52, 53] Several hysterectomy techniques are compared in Table 12-4. Extrafascial hysterectomy has no place in the treatment of invasive cervical cancer, with the exception of combined radiation and surgery protocols for unusual tumor distributions such as the so-called barrel-shaped cervix.[54-56]

Radiation therapy for stage IB and stage IIA cervical cancer treatment usually includes external beam treatment and intracavitary implants. External beam radiotherapy (teletherapy) is administered in daily fractions for approximately 5 weeks. In addition, intracavitary implants, using either the low dose rate afterloading technique or the more recently developed high dose rate afterloading technique, are recommended.[19] Specific doses and treatment schedules vary, although clinical outcomes for the various regimens are generally similar.

Stages IIB and III

There seems to be little justification for empirically treating the para-aortic nodes in patients with stage IIB or stage III lesions unless metastasis has been clearly documented.

Patients with stage IIB and stage III tumors used to be treated with radiation therapy alone. Standard radiation therapy treatment includes external radiation therapy to the pelvis using a daily four-field box technique, typically administering 4500 to 5000 cGy. An additional boost to areas with bulky tumor is often necessary. In addition to external radiation therapy, an intracavitary implant is required to attain a tumoricidal dose of radiation. Intracavitary therapy using a tandem and ovoids application for small tumors or an interstitial template for large tumors allows optimization of the final radiation dose to the tumor while minimizing the dose to the bladder and rectum.

In 1999, the National Cancer Institute issued a Clinical Announcement citing five clinical trials, all of which demonstrated significant improvement of survival rates for patients treated with radiation and concurrent chemotherapy. The five trials did not use the same chemotherapy drugs, schedules, or dosages, although cisplatin was included in all five protocols.[57-59] A combination of radiation and chemotherapy has become the standard approach for treatment of patients with locally advanced cervical cancer. However, optimization of the chemotherapy drug regimens, dosages, and schedules requires further study.

Patients with pelvic lymph node metastasis or with bulky cervical primary lesions have a significant risk of metastasis to the para-aortic nodes. Patients with stage 2B lesions have involved para-aortic nodes in 12.8% of cases.[19] Para-aortic nodes are not included in the standard pelvic port for radiation therapy, potentially resulting in undertreatment of these patients. The Radiation Therapy Oncology Group reported on a clinical trial in which patients who were randomized to receive para-aortic node radiation in addition to standard pelvic radiotherapy were likely to survive for 5 years 67% of the time, versus 55% in the control group.[60] Severe or life-threatening toxicities were four times more likely in the group receiving para-aortic radiation. A similar randomized trial reported by the European Organization for Research on Treatment of Cancer did not show survival benefit for patients receiving para-aortic radiation.[61] Until further studies can resolve this conflict, there seems to be little justification for empirically treating the para-aortic nodes in patients with stage IIB or stage III lesions unless metastasis has been clearly documented.

Stage IV and Recurrent Cervical Cancer

> **When disease extends beyond the cervix, 5-year survival falls to 65% for patients with stage II lesions, to 45% for patients with stage III lesions, and to less than 10% for patients with stage IV lesions.**

Treatment of stage IVA disease involving the bladder or the rectal mucosa may include either combined chemotherapy and radiation or pelvic exenteration, an ultraradical surgical procedure that removes uterus, tubes, ovaries, vagina, bladder, and rectum.[62, 63] Exenteration is usually reserved for patients with vesicovaginal or rectovaginal fistula before treatment. Treatment of widely metastatic disease (stage IVB) consists of individualized therapy, including combinations of radiation and chemotherapy, depending on location and extent of metastases. The most active chemotherapy drugs include cisplatin, fluorouracil, ifosfamide, and bleomycin.[19] Long-term survival is unlikely. Surgery is indicated only for palliation in patients with distant metastases. Recurrent cervical cancer that is confined to the pelvis is treated based on the type of treatment originally administered. Patients with recurrence who were initially treated with surgery may be treated with radiation therapy to the pelvis or to other sites of metastasis. Central pelvic recurrence in patients previously treated with radiation may be amenable to pelvic exenteration.[63] Reconstructive surgical techniques allow

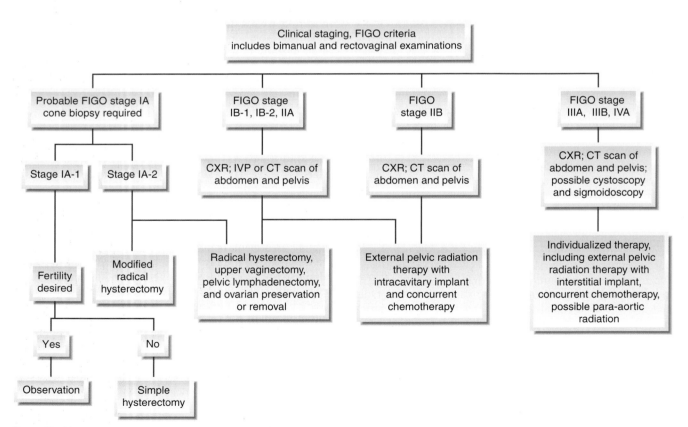

Figure 12–14. Management of invasive cervical cancer.

restoration of bladder, rectal, and vaginal function via continent urinary conduit formation, low rectal reanastomosis, and vaginoplasty, respectively. Figure 12–14 presents a summary diagram for the management of cervical cancer.

Survival

Five-year survival of patients with microinvasive squamous carcinoma of the cervix (stage IA1) is 99%, even when conservative surgical therapy is used to preserve fertility.[19] Patients with larger lesions still confined to the cervix (stages IA2, IB1, and IB2) have an approximately 90% likelihood of 5-year survival, whether they are treated with surgery or with radiation.[40, 41] In the subset of patients who are treated surgically and who have no evidence of lymph node metastases, 96% survive 5 years. However, when disease extends beyond the cervix, 5-year survival falls to 65% for patients with stage II lesions, to 45% for patients with stage III lesions, and to less than 10% for patients with stage IV lesions. Recurrent disease in the pelvis that is treated with radiation results in long-term survival of up to 45% of patients. Pelvic exenteration for central pelvic recurrence can potentially salvage up to 60% of patients.[63] Ten percent to 15% of patients with metastatic recurrent cervical cancer treated with chemotherapy have objective responses. Progression-free intervals are typically no longer than a year.[19]

SUMMARY OF KEY POINTS

- Colposcopic findings specific to microinvasive and invasive cervical carcinoma may be absent or may overlap with findings of intraepithelial lesions.

- If histology reveals a lesion invading more than 5 mm below the basement membrane, no further histologic data are required for staging. If invasion is less than 5 mm below the basement membrane, complete assessment of the cervical portio is required to rule out the presence of deeper invasion.

- Cone biopsy has been the accepted diagnostic tool for evaluation of the portio if colposcopy is unsatisfactory, endocervical curettage is positive, or invasion is less than 5 mm. LEEP may be a reasonable alternative in some circumstances.

- Staging of cervical cancer is primarily based on clinical examination and appropriate testing. Tests that may not be used to officially stage disease include CT, MRI, lymphangiogram, laparoscopy, and laparotomy.

- Microinvasive cancer is a subset of stage I disease and implies that risk of recurrence is rare and that fertility-sparing treatment may be considered.

- Although radical hysterectomy for patients with stage IA2 disease results in excellent long-term survival, modified radical hysterectomy may likewise be curative with less potential for complica-

tions and morbidity. Treatment with external radiation therapy and intracavitary implants may also be considered.

- Stage IB or IIA cervical cancer can be effectively treated with either radical pelvic surgery or radiation therapy, but the surgical approach is preferred in younger patients.

- Patients with stages IIB and III cervical cancer demonstrate significantly improved survival rates if they are treated with radiation and concurrent chemotherapy.

- Treatment of widely metastatic disease (stage IVB) consists of combinations of radiation and chemotherapy, including cisplatin, fluorouracil, ifosfamide, and bleomycin.

- Five-year survival rates of patients with cervical cancer are as follows: stage IA1—99%; stages IA2, IB1, and IB2—90%; stage II—65%; stage III—45%; and stage IV—less than 10%.

References

1. Ferenczy A, Winkler B: Carcinoma and metastatic tumors of the cervix. In Kurman RJ (ed): Blaustein's Pathology of the Female Genital Tract, 3rd ed. New York, Springer Verlag, 1987.
2. Landis SH, Murray T, Bolden S, et al: Cancer statistics, 1998. CA Cancer J Clin 1998;48:6.
3. Hinselmann H: Verbesserung der inspektionsmoglichkeiten von vulva, vagina und portio. Munch Med Wschr 1925;1733.
4. Noda S: Colposcopic differential diagnosis of dysplasia, carcinoma in situ and microinvasive carcinoma of the cervix. Aust N Z J Obstet Gynaecol 1981;21:37.
5. Liu WM, Chao KC, Wang KI, et al: Colposcopic assessment in microinvasive carcinoma of the cervix. Chin Med J 1989;43:171.
6. Sugimori H, Matsuyama T, Kashimura M, et al: Colposcopic findings in microinvasive carcinoma of the uterine cervix. Obstet Gynecol Survey 1979;34:804.
7. Benedet JL, Anderson GH, Boyes DA: Colposcopic accuracy in the diagnosis of microinvasive and occult invasive carcinoma of the cervix. Obstet Gynecol 1985;65:557.
8. Paraskevaidis E, Kitchener HC, Miller ID, et al: A population-based study of microinvasive disease of the cervix—a colposcopic and cytologic analysis. Gynecol Oncol 1992;45:9.
9. Hopman EH, Kenemans P, Helmerhorst TJM: Positive predictive rate of colposcopic examination of the cervix uteri: An overview of literature. Obstet Gynecol Survey 1998;53:97.
10. Edebiri AA: The relative significance of colposcopic descriptive appearances in the diagnosis of cervical intraepithelial neoplasia. Int J Gynecol Obstet 1990;33:23.
11. Hopman EH, Voorhorst FJ, Kenemans P, et al: Observer agreement on interpreting colposcopic images of CIN. Gynecol Oncol 1995;58:206.
12. Choo YC, Chan OLY, Hsu C, et al: Colposcopy in microinvasive carcinoma of the cervix: An enigma of diagnosis. Br J Obstet Gynaecol 1994;91:1156.
13. Van Meir JM, Wielenga G, Drogendijk A: Colposcopic analysis of 20 patients with microinvasive carcinoma of the uterine cervix. Obstet Gynecol Survey 1979;21:37.
14. Koller O: The Vascular Patterns of the Uterine Cervix. Philadelphia, FA Davis, 1963.
15. Folkman J: Tumor angiogenesis: Therapeutic implications. New Engl J Med 1971;285:1182.
16. Mitchell MF: Preinvasive diseases of the female lower genital tract. In Gershenson DM, DeCherney AH, Curry SL (eds): Operative Gynecology. Philadelphia, WB Saunders, 1993.

17. Cervix uteri. In Fleming ID, Cooper JS, Henson DE, et al (eds): AJCC Cancer Staging Handbook. Philadelphia, Lippincott-Raven, 1998.

18. Reagan JW, Ng ABP: The cellular manifestations of uterine carcinogenesis. In Norris NJ, Hertig AT, Abell MR (eds): The Uterus. Baltimore, Williams & Wilkins, 1973.

19. Stehman FB, Perez CA, Kurman RJ, et al: Uterine cervix. In Hoskins WJ, Perez CA, Young RC (eds): Principles and Practice of Gynecologic Oncology. Philadelphia, Lippincott-Raven, 1997.

20. Cherry CP, Glucksmann A: Lymphatic embolism and lymph node metastasis in cancers of the vulva and uterine cervix. Cancer 1955; 8:564.

21. Okagaki T, Clark BA, Zachow KR: Presence of human papillomavirus in verrucous carcinoma of the vagina: Immunohistochemical, ultrastructural, and DNA hybridization studies. Arch Pathol Lab Med 1984;108:567.

22. Rando RF, Sedlacek TV, Hunt J, et al: Verrucous carcinoma of the vulva associated with an unusual type 6 human papillomavirus. Obstet Gynecol 1986;67:70.

23. Kashimura M, Tsukamoto N, Matsukama K, et al: Verrucous carcinoma of the uterine cervix: Report of a case with follow-up of 6½ years. Gynecol Oncol 1984;19:204.

24. Shingleton HM, Fowler WC, Koch GG: Pretreatment evaluation in cervical cancer. Am J Obstet Gynecol 1971;110:385.

25. Lagasse LD, Creasman WT, Shingleton HM, et al: Results and complications of operative staging in cervical cancer: Experience of the Gynecologic Oncology Group. Gynecol Oncol 1980;9:90.

26. Berman ML, Lagasse LD, Watring WG, et al: The operative evaluation of patients with cervical carcinoma by an extraperitoneal approach. Obstet Gynecol 1977;50:658.

27. Nelson JH, Macasaet MA, Lu T, et al: The incidence and significance of para-aortic lymph node metastases in invasive carcinoma of the cervix. Am J Obstet Gynecol 1974;118:749.

28. Morrow CP, Curtin JP: Surgery for cervical neoplasia. In Gynecologic Cancer Surgery. New York, Churchill Livingstone, 1996, p 472.

29. Cavanagh D, Ruffalo EH, Marsden DE: Gynecologic Cancer: A Clinico-Pathologic Approach. East Norwalk, CT, Appleton-Lange, 1985, p 79.

30. Van Nagell JR, Greenwell N, Powell DF, et al: Microinvasive carcinoma of the cervix. Am J Obstet Gynecol 1983;145:981.

31. Creasman WT, Fetter BF, Clarke-Pearson, et al: Management of stage IA carcinoma of the cervix. Am J Obstet Gynecol 1985;153:164.

32. Tseng CJ, Horng SG, Soong YK, et al: Conservative conization for microinvasive carcinoma of the cervix. Am J Obstet Gynecol 1997;176:1009.

33. Paraskevaidis E, Kitchener HC, Kalantaridou SN, et al: Large loop conization for early invasive cervical cancer. Int J Gynecol Cancer 1997;7:95.

34. Collins HS, Burke TW, Woodward JE, et al: Widespread lymph node metastases in a patient with microinvasive cervical carcinoma. Gynecol Oncol 1989;34:219.

35. Photopulos GJ, Vander Zwagg R: Class II radical hysterectomy shows less morbidity and good treatment efficacy compared to class III. Gynecol Oncol 1991;40:21.

36. Magrina JF, Goodrich MA, Weaver AL, et al: Modified radical hysterectomy: Morbidity and mortality. Gynecol Oncol 1995;59:277.

37. Magrina JF, Goodrich MA, Lidner TK, et al: Modified radical hysterectomy in the treatment of early squamous cervical cancer. Gynecol Oncol 1999;72:183.

38. Nelson JH, Averette HE, Richart RM: Detection, diagnostic evaluation and treatment of dysplasia and early carcinoma of the cervix. CA Cancer J Clin 1975;25:134.

39. Seski JC, Abell MR, Morley GW: Microinvasive squamous carcinoma of the cervix: Definition, histologic analysis, late results of treatment. Obstet Gynecol 1977;50:410.

40. Newton M: Radical hysterectomy or radiotherapy for stage I cervical cancer. Am J Obstet Gynecol 1975;123:535.

41. Morley GW, Seski JC: Radical pelvic surgery versus radiation therapy for stage I carcinoma of the cervix (exclusive of microinvasion). Am J Obstet Gynecol 1976;126:785.

42. Roddick JW, Greenlaw: Treatment of cervical cancer. Am J Obstet Gynecol 1971;119:754.

43. Webb GA: The role of ovarian conservation in the treatment of carcinoma of the cervix with radical surgery. Am J Obstet Gynecol 1975;122:476.

44. Abitbol NM, Davenport JH: Sexual dysfunction after therapy for cervical carcinoma. Am J Obstet Gynecol 1974;119:181.

45. Siebel M, Freeman MG, Graves WL: Carcinoma of the cervix and sexual function. Obstet Gynecol 1979;55:484.

46. Allen HH, Collins JA: Surgical management of carcinoma of the cervix. Am J Obstet Gynecol 1977;127:741.

47. Artman LE, Hoskins WJ, Bibro MC, et al: Radical hysterectomy and pelvic lymphadenectomy for stage IB carcinoma of the cervix: Twenty one years experience. Gynecol Oncol 1987;28:8.

48. Hoskins WJ, Ford JH Jr, Lutz MH, et al: Radical hysterectomy and pelvic lymphadenectomy for the management of early invasive cancer of the cervix. Gynecol Oncol 1976;4:278.

49. Anderson B, LaPolla J, Turner D, et al: Ovarian transposition in cervical cancer. Gynecol Oncol 1993;4:206.

50. Feeney DD, Moore DH, Look KY, et al: The fate of the ovaries after radical hysterectomy and ovarian transposition. Gynecol Oncol 1995;56:3.

51. Letschert JG: The prevention of radiation induced small bowel complications. Eur J Cancer 31A:1361,1995.

52. Extraperitoneal pelvic lymph node dissection with modified radical hysterectomy. In Gallup DG, Talledo OE: Surgical Atlas of Gynecologic Oncology. Philadelphia, WB Saunders, 1994.

53. Radical hysterectomy with pelvic lymph node dissection. In Gallup DG, Talledo OE: Surgical Atlas of Gynecologic Oncology. Philadelphia, WB Saunders, 1994.

54. Hopkins MP, Peters WA, Anderson W, et al: Invasive cervical cancer treated initially by standard hysterectomy. Gynecol Oncol 1990;36:7.

55. Nelson AJ, Fletcher GH, Wharton JT: Indications for adjunctive conservative extrafascial hysterectomy in selected cases of carcinoma of the uterine cervix. AJR Am J Roentgenol 1975;123:91.

56. Gallion HH, Van Nagell JR, Donaldson GS, et al: Combined radiation therapy and extrafascial hysterectomy in the treatment of stage IB barrel-shaped cervical cancer. Cancer 1985;56:262.

57. Whitney CW, Sause W, Bundy BN, et al: A randomized comparison of fluorouracil plus cisplatin versus hydroxyurea as an adjunct to radiation therapy in stages IIB-IVA carcinoma of the cervix with negative para-aortic nodes. A gynecologic oncology group and southwest oncology group study. J Clin Oncol 1999;17:1339.

58. Morris M, Eifel PJ, Lu J, et al: Pelvic radiation with concurrent chemotherapy versus pelvic and para-aortic radiation for high risk cervical cancer: A randomized Radiation Therapy Oncology Group clinical trial. New Engl J Med 1999;340:1137.

59. Rose PG, Bundy BN, Watkins EB, et al: Concurrent cisplatin-based chemoradiation improves progression-free and overall survival in advanced cervical cancer: Results of a randomized Gynecologic Oncology Group study. New Engl J Med 1999;340:1144.

60. Rotman M, Choi K, Guze C, et al: Prophylactic irradiation of the para-aortic node chain in stage IIB and bulky stage IB carcinoma of the cervix: Initial results of RTOG 7920. Int J Radiat Oncol Biol Phys 1990;19:513.

61. Haie C, Pejovic MH, Gerbaulet A, et al: Is prophylactic para-aortic irradiation worthwhile in the treatment of advanced cervical carcinoma? Results of controlled clinical trial of the EORTC radiotherapy group. Radiother Oncol 1988;11:101.

62. Million RR, Rutledge F, Fletcher GH: Stage IV carcinoma of the cervix with bladder invasion. Am J Obstet Gynecol 1972;113:239.

63. Morley GW, Hopkins MP, Lindenauer SM, et al: Pelvic exenteration, University of Michigan: 100 patients at 5 years. Obstet Gynecol 1989:74:934.

Case Study 1 Questions

History

A 63-year-old gravida II, primipara II whose last Pap smear and gynecologic examination were 30 years ago during her last pregnancy, is referred to you.

Figure 12-15
This is her Pap smear.

- Describe what you see.

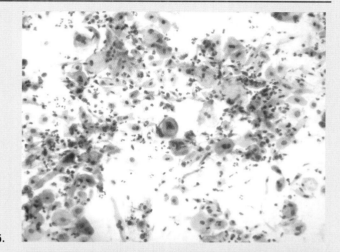

Figure 12-15.

Figure 12-16
This is a photograph of her colposcopic findings.

- What do you see?

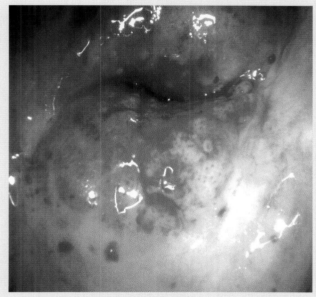

Figure 12-16.

Figure 12-17
This is a biopsy of the cervix at the 6-o'clock position.

- What is your diagnosis?
- What is the appropriate next step in this patient's management?

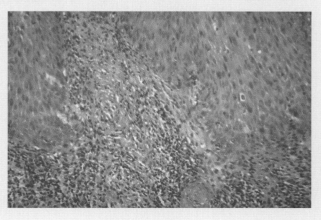

Figure 12-17.

Case Study 1 Answers

Figure 12–15

There are several keratinized cells with larger hyperchromatic nuclei and pink cytoplasm. The shape of the cells is elongated and bizarre, suggestive of malignancy.

Figure 12–16

The cervix is atrophic, which makes the colposcopic changes less prominent. Acetowhite epithelium is seen with coarse punctation. Some of the punctation tends to be slightly linear or comma shaped. The borders of the lesions are not well seen. This is a high-grade lesion.

Figure 12–17

Although the surface of the lesion is not seen in this view, there are spindle-shaped, crowded, hyperchromatic nuclei extending toward the surface of the epithelium, suggestive of a high-grade lesion. However, at the bottom, a small tongue of neoplastic epithelium can be seen below the basement membrane. This is a microinvasive lesion.

The next step in the patient's management is a cone biopsy. When microinvasive cancer is seen on a punch biopsy, one can never be certain that there is not frankly invasive cancer elsewhere in the cervix. In the postmenopausal patient, treatment with an extrafascial hysterectomy following the cone biopsy is appropriate. Bypassing the cone biopsy and treating the patient with potentially occult or frankly invasive cancer with an extrafascial hysterectomy would compromise her care and would eliminate the ability to treat her with a radical hysterectomy.

Key Point of Case 1

The diagnosis of microinvasive cervical cancer can be made only by excision of the entire transformation zone (cone biopsy).

Case Study 2 Questions

History

A 30-year-old gravida 0, primipara 0 is referred to you for evaluation of a Pap smear showing atypical squamous cells of undetermined significance.

Figures 12–18 and 12–19

- Describe what you see.

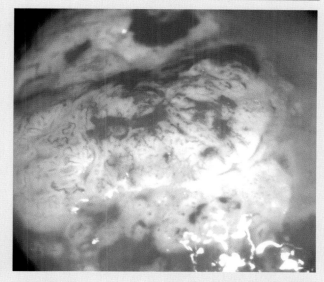

Figure 12–18.

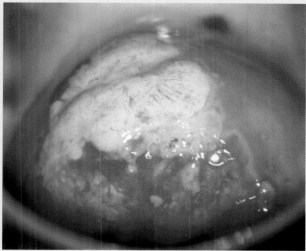

Figure 12–19.

Figure 12–20

- What is the diagnosis?
- What is the proper management of this case?

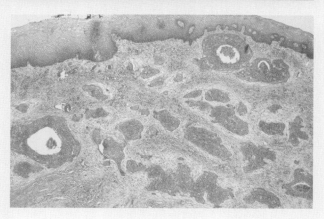

Figure 12–20.

Case Study 2 Answers

Figures 12–18 and 12–19

On the anterior lip of the cervix, there is a dense, raised, acetowhite lesion with atypical vessels, including comma shapes and curlicues. This is consistent with an invasive cancer.

Figure 12–20

This is a frankly invasive cancer, with infiltrating cancer seen throughout under the basement membrane.

This woman needs to be treated with a radical hysterectomy. For a FIGO stage I lesion, radical radiation is inappropriate because it will irradiate her ovaries and cause premature menopause. Less aggressive therapy (cone biopsy or simple hysterectomy) would not be curative.

Key Point of Case 2

Recognize the appearance of an invasive cancer.

Cytology, Colposcopy, and Histology of Invasive Squamous Cell Cancer

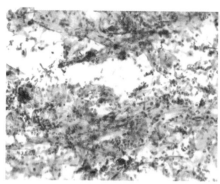

A.

Features suggestive of cancer:
- **Raised surface contour**
- **Atypical vessels**
- **Dense acetowhite epithelium**
- **Friability**
- **Ulceration**
- **Yellow color**

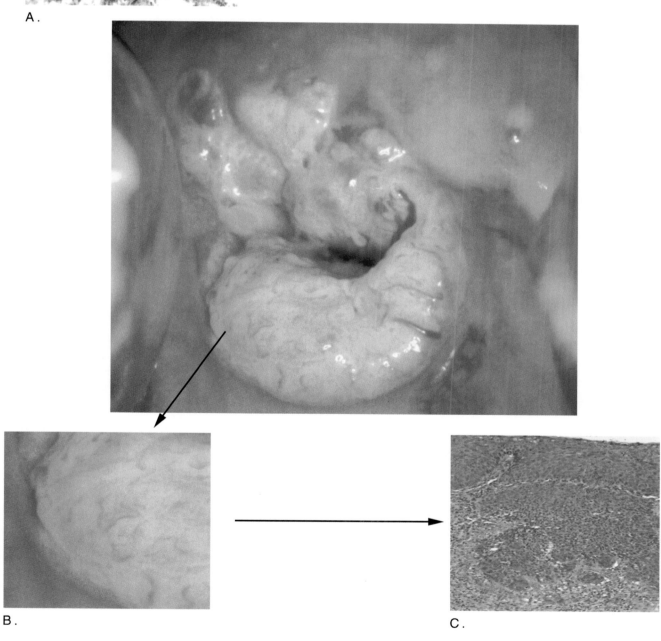

B.

C.

A. Cytology reveals only inflammatory changes because of superficial necrosis produced by the cancer.

B. Area of biopsy. Dense acetowhite epithelium with atypical blood vessels.

C. Histology reveals squamous cell cancer. The basement membrane of the epithelium is breeched, and the abnormal cells extend into the stroma.

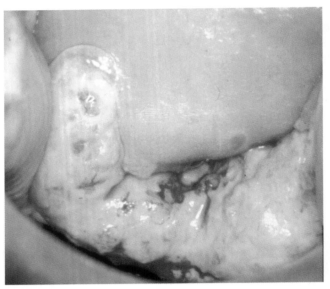

Plate 12-1. Large, raised cancer, yellow in appearance, on the posterior lip of the cervix. There is an ulcer at 6 o'clock and atypical vessels throughout the mass.

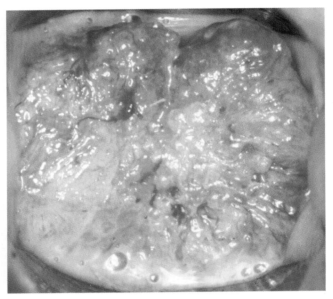

Plate 12-2. Fungating cancer with obliteration of the os and multiple atypical vessels.

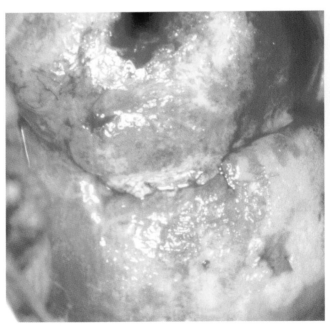

Plate 12-3. Mass on the anterior lip of cervix with atypical vessels and yellow appearance. There is also leukoplakia of the posterior lip of the cervix.

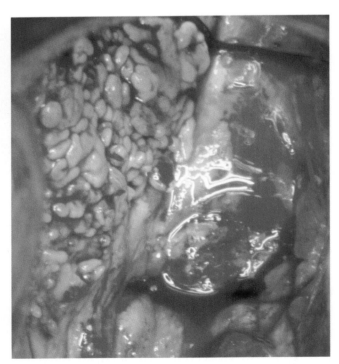

Plate 12-4. Papillary tumor of the cervix.

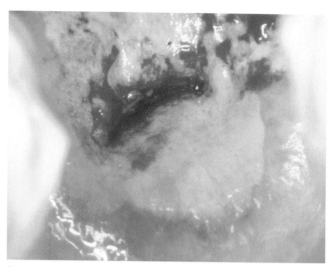

Plate 12–5. Example of microinvasive cancer. There is dense aceto-white epithelium and coarse punctation with a rolled edge at 10 o'clock. Contact bleeding is present on the upper right cervix.

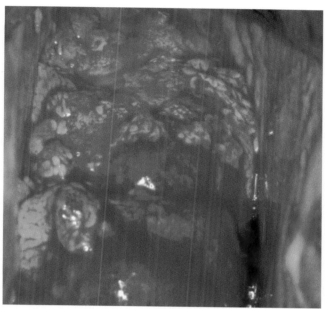

Plate 12–6. Large, fungating, nodular cancer that completely distorts the normal cervical anatomy, accompanied by bleeding.

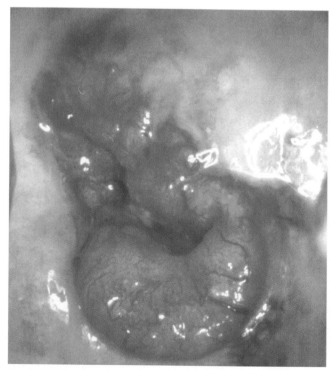

Plate 12–7. Raised fleshy mass almost circumferentially involving the central cervix. Note the multiple atypical vessels. This is Figure 12–6 before the application of 5% acetic acid.

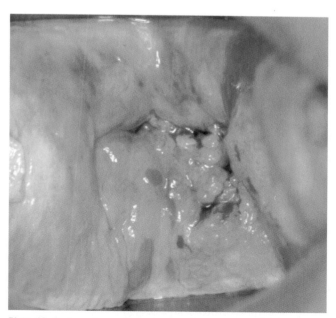

Plate 12–8. Irregular surface contour of a cancer involving primarily the central, posterior portion of the cervix. Image provided by Dr. Vesna Kesic.

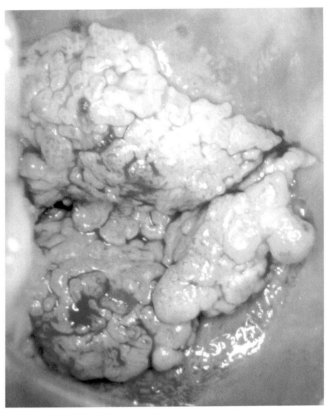

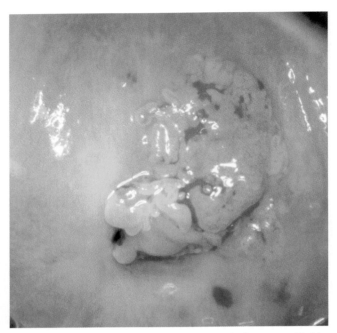

Plate 12-10. Papillary cancer with atypical vessels. Image provided by Dr. Vesna Kesic.

Plate 12-9. Cervical cancer with an encephaloid appearance and scattered atypical vessels. This could be confused with a condyloma.

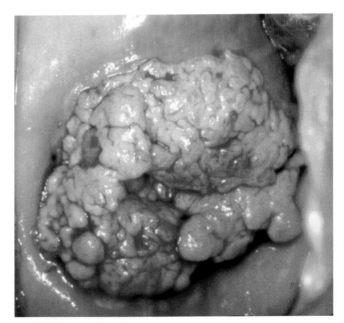

Plate 12-11. Cancer with encephaloid appearance and scattered atypical vessels.

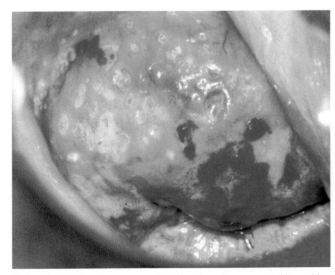

Plate 12-12. Invasive cancer with bleeding, dense acetowhite epithelium, and superficial spread on the anterior aspect of the cervix.

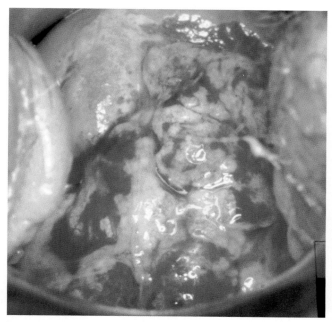

Plate 12-13. Cancer with an irregular, papillary surface; dense aceto-white epithelium, and atypical vessels.

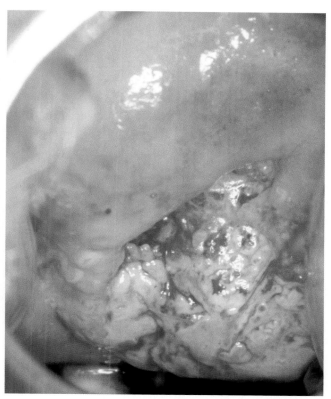

Plate 12-14. Cancer with irregular, yellow papillary surface.

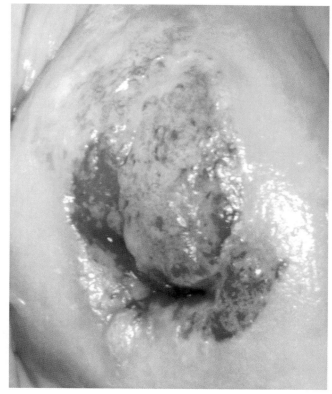

Plate 12-15. Bizarre vessels over all the cervix and a nodule at 7 o'clock.

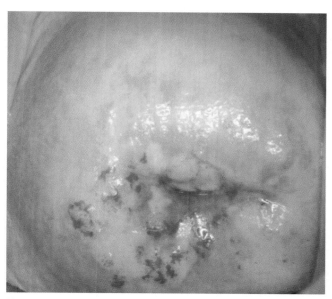

Plate 12-16. Multiple atypical vessels in a patient with microinvasive carcinoma.

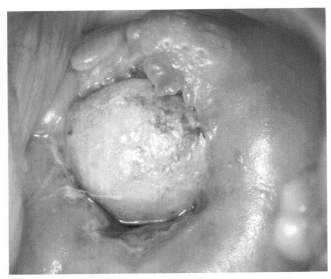

Plate 12–17. Large endocervical mass with acetowhite epithelium, mosaic, and papillary necrosis. Biopsy showed invasive cancer.

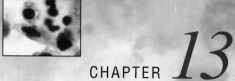

Colposcopic Features of Cervical Adenocarcinoma in Situ and Adenocarcinoma and Management of Preinvasive Disease

Adenocarcinoma in situ (ACIS) of the uterine cervix, first described in 1953 by Friedell and McKay,[1] is part of a morphologic spectrum of intraepithelial disease (like squamous disease) ranging from mild changes to severe abnormalities. The entire spectrum is referred to as *cervical intraepithelial glandular neoplasia* (CIGN).[2, 3] It has been divided into two grades: low-grade and high-grade CIGN. Low-grade CIGN includes glandular atypia (nonneoplastic changes associated with inflammation and radiotherapy) and glandular dysplasia (atypical hyperplasia of less severe changes than those of ACIS). High-grade CIGN consists solely of ACIS.[4–6]

Two percent of intraepithelial lesions are ACIS, whereas adenocarcinoma composes 6% to 18% of invasive cervical cancers, indicating either that intraepithelial transit time to invasion is brief or that intraepithelial disease is underdiagnosed.

ACIS arises in a synchronous fashion involving the surface and superficial endocervical crypts. The exact nature of this metamorphosis is poorly understood, but the conversion from normal glandular cells to ACIS is not believed to be related to the atypical metaplastic process that produces squamous disease. Two percent of intraepithelial lesions are ACIS, whereas adenocarcinoma composes 6% to 18% of invasive cervical cancers. This is perplexing and indicates either that intraepithelial transit time to invasion is brief or that intraepithelial disease is underdiagnosed.[7–10] Regardless of whether adenocarcinoma is found in the in situ or the invasive form, 46% to 72% of cases have concurrent squamous lesions (i.e., are of mixed disease).[11–13]

ACIS appears to be increasing in incidence. It is now found more commonly in younger women ranging in age from 29 to 46 years, with an average age of 35.8 years.

ACIS appears to be increasing in incidence. It is now found more commonly in younger women ranging in age from 29 to 46 years, with an average age of 35.8 years.[2, 14–16] The early diagnosis of glandular disease still represents a real challenge for clinicians, who are likely to miss the lesions because of the absence of clinical indicators, normal cytology, or cytology suggestive of squamous disease and because of unfamiliarity with the disease's newly delineated colposcopic presentations.[16–22] It is hoped that this text and atlas will enable more colposcopists to become familiar with the features of this disease.

COLPOSCOPY IN GLANDULAR DISEASE

ACIS only slightly changes the surface contour of the cervix. Often, the neoplastic "glands" are buried beneath the surface.

Historically, authors have complained that colposcopy has not been helpful in identifying ACIS. This is because the disease only slightly changes the surface contour and because often the neoplastic "glands" are buried beneath the surface.[15, 23] Because ACIS is still relatively rare, very few colposcopists have the opportunity to collect a sizable series and gain experience with colposcopic identification. Colposcopists are trained to recognize patterns in the transformation zone associated with normal squamous epithelium, squamous metaplasia, squamous cervical intraepithelial neoplasia, and squamous cell cancer. They have not been taught to identify the subtle alterations of the columnar epithelium that signal a developing or established glandular abnormality. But this is changing. These lesions exhibit certain features that can lead the enlightened colposcopist to suspect a glandular lesion is present and to search for it.[21–22]

Most glandular lesions lie within or close to the transformation zone.

Diagnostic excisional biopsy must always be performed when ACIS is found on punch biopsy or when ACIS is suspected cytologically or colposcopically but not proven histologically.

Most glandular lesions lie within or close to the transformation zone. Squamous disease, especially in younger women, is usually colposcopically visible, whereas ACIS (by itself or in mixed disease) can lie proximally, involving the cervical canal, or can lie beneath metaplastic epithelium or an abnormal transformation zone and thus be out of colposcopic view.[12, 21–22] Because of the location of the ACIS, the exfoliative cytology of mixed disease may indicate only a squamous abnormality, thus influencing the colposcopist to look exclusively for a squamous lesion and to be satisfied upon finding it. Furthermore, the colposcopic biopsy may confirm the squamous lesion, with ACIS being detected only on a subsequent excision or within a hysterectomy specimen. Diagnostic excisional biopsy must always be performed when ACIS is found on punch biopsy or when ACIS is suspected cytologically or colposcopically but not proven histologically.

THREE PRESENTATIONS OF ACIS AND ADENOCARCINOMA

The most common colposcopic appearance of glandular disease is a papillary expression resembling an immature transformation zone. The second most common form is a flat, variegated red and white area resembling an immature transformation zone. The least common presentation is one or more isolated, elevated, individual, densely acetowhite lesions overlying columnar epithelium.

Three colposcopic appearances of glandular disease have been described.[21, 22] The most common form is a papillary expression resembling an immature transformation zone. After acetic acid is applied, discrete patches of somewhat acetowhite, fused villi, varying in size, can be identified. They look like the fused villous processes of early, normal metaplasia (Fig. 13–1), and this is why lesions are dismissed without sampling.[21–23] The second most common form is a flat, variegated red and white area resembling an immature transformation zone (Fig. 13–2).[21, 22] The least common presentation is one or more isolated, elevated, individual, densely acetowhite lesions overlying columnar epithelium (Fig. 13–3).[21, 22] The degree of acetowhiteness exhibited by glandular disease reflects the degree of villous fusion (the more fusion, the whiter the lesion) and the histologic pseudostratification of columnar cells with their enlarged hyperchromatic nuclei.[21, 22]

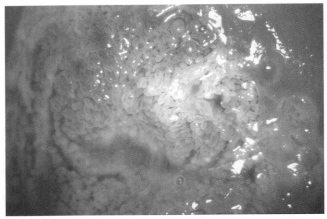

Figure 13–1. Cervical adenocarcinoma in situ involves centrally the left upper quadrant from the 12-o'clock to the 3-o'clock position. Faint acetowhite, papillary-like fusion overlies columnar epithelium, mimicking the fusing villi that occur in the metaplastic process that converts normal columnar to normal squamous metaplasia. The fact that fusion and acetowhiteness are focal rather than diffuse is an indication this is more than metaplasia. (From Wright VC, Shier RM: Colposcopy of Adenocarcinoma in Situ and Adenocarcinoma of the Cervix. Houston, Biomedical Communications, 2000.)

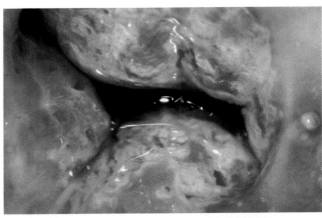

Figure 13–2. An adenocarcinoma-in-situ lesion displaying large "gland" or crypt openings. The lesion occupies the endocervical canal, and what is visible exhibits a patchy red and white color after acetic acid. It exhibits an irregular surface and looks somewhat like an immature transformation zone. (From Wright VC, Shier RM: Colposcopy of Adenocarcinoma in Situ and Adenocarcinoma of the Cervix. Houston, Biomedical Communications, 2000.)

When glandular and squamous diseases coexist, the squamous component is more likely to be noted because it is more likely to be visible.

When glandular and squamous diseases coexist, the squamous component is more likely to be noted because it is more likely to be visible. Glandular lesions can abut the squamous lesion, be sandwiched between two squamous lesions, or lie above the squamous lesion (Fig. 13–4).[21, 22, 24, 25] Squamous cancer is present in approximately 4% to 5% of mixed disease cases.

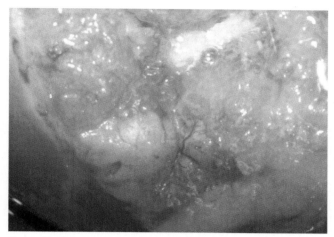

Figure 13–3. A well-defined, elevated, and densely acetowhite adeno-carcinoma in situ overlies columnar epithelium at the 6- to 8-o'clock position. It is not in contact with the squamous border. A large, branching, taproot-like blood vessel courses its surface. (From Wright VC, Shier RM: Colposcopy of Adenocarcinoma in Situ and Adenocarcinoma of the Cervix. Houston, Biomedical Communications, 2000.)

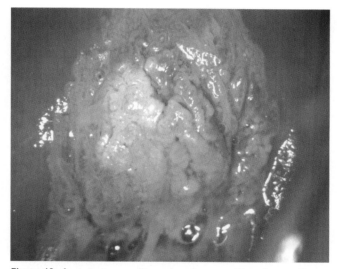

Figure 13–4. A fusing, papillary, densely acetowhite adenocarcinoma-in-situ lesion lies in the upper quadrant. Peripherally, encircling it from the 9-o'clock to the 3-o'clock position, is an associated low-grade squamous intraepithelial lesion. (From Wright VC, Shier RM: Colposcopy of Adenocarcinoma in Situ and Adenocarcinoma of the Cervix. Houston, Biomedical Communications, 2000.)

NEW CRITERIA FOR DIFFERENTIATING CERVICAL DISEASES

The standard colposcopic criteria of Kolstad and Stafl and Reid's colposcopic grading index apply to squamous and not glandular lesions.

Because there is no single colposcopic appearance that characterizes glandular dysplasia, ACIS, and adenocarcinoma and because colposcopic appearances of these enti-

ties often mimic other conditions, their colposcopic diagnosis has been less than satisfactory. Furthermore, the five standard colposcopic criteria of Kolstad and Stafl[26] (vascular patterns, intercapillary distance, surface contour, color tone, and clarity of demarcation) apply to squamous and not glandular lesions. The same is true of Reid's colposcopic grading index.[27] More recently, however, a new set of colposcopic criteria has been recommended for differentiating among metaplasia, condylomata, squamous intraepithelial neoplasia, squamous cell carcinoma, metaplasia, and glandular disease.[21, 22, 28] The criteria are

- lesion location over columnar epithelium, not contiguous with the squamocolumnar junction;
- large "gland" or crypt openings;
- papillary structure;
- budding;
- patchy red and white coloration;
- waste-thread, tendril, root, and character-writing blood vessels; and
- single or multiple dots produced at the tips of papillary projections by looped vessels.

Punctation, mosaic patterns, and corkscrew vessels, although common in squamous disease, do not appear in glandular disease.

Some features can be used to eliminate a lesion from consideration, such as punctation and true mosaic pattern (which are present only in squamous intraepithelial lesions) and corkscrew vessels (which are associated only with invasive squamous disease). Although many colposcopically recognized features are common to a variety of diseases, paying attention to surface contour and vascular configurations can greatly help the colposcopist discover glandular disease (Table 13–1)[21, 22, 28] when it is present and differentiate it from other conditions.

WHEN TO SUSPECT GLANDULAR LESIONS

Glandular lesions can lie lateral to a squamous lesion; between two squamous lesions; or, more commonly, above the squamous component within the endocervical canal.

The existence of two or more squamous lesions separated by glandular-appearing epithelium is highly suggestive of a glandular lesion. Primary (i.e., not post treatment) squamous lesions do not "skip"; they are always contiguous.

The following colposcopic features alert the colposcopist that a glandular lesion might be present:

- Elevated lesions, especially those exhibiting irregular surfaces, that overlie the columnar epithelium. The differential diagnosis includes metaplasia, condylo-

Surface Topography and Blood Vessel Patterns in Different Cervical Diseases*

	Metaplasia	Condylomata	CIN	ACIS	Adeno-carcinoma	Invasive Squamous Disease	Micro-glandular Hyperplasia
Surface Patterns							
Lesions overlying columnar epithelium not contiguous with the squamocolumnar junction	•	•		•	•		•
Lesions with very large gland openings				•	•		
Papillary lesions	•	•		•	•	•	•
Epithelial budding	•	•					
Patchy red and white lesions (transformation zone–like)	•						
Blood Vessel Patterns							
Punctation			•				
Mosaicism			•				
Corkscrew						•	
Waste thread		•		•		•	
Tendril				•	•		
Root	•			•	•		
Character writing	•	•		•	•		
Single and multiple dots	•	•		•	•		•

* Bullets indicate conditions in which they can be found.
ACIS, adenocarcinoma in situ; CIN, cervical intraepithelial neoplasia.
Adapted from Wright VC, Shier RM: Colposcopy of Adenocarcinoma in Situ and Adenocarcinoma of the Cervix. Houston, Biomedical Communcations, 2000.

mata, ACIS, adenocarcinoma, and microglandular hyperplasia (Figs. 13–5, 13–6, 13–7, and 13–8).

- Lesions with large "gland" or crypt openings in association with other abnormal colposcopic features. Many ACIS lesions occupy the endocervical canal entirely or in part. They are patchy red and white (not uniformly dense white like high-grade squamous intraepithelial neoplasia) (see Fig. 13–2). Frequently, the openings produce excessive mucus.
- Papillary lesions. Papillary excrescences must be differentiated from the normal papillary glandular mu-

cosa (the grapelike villous structures of columnar epithelium), metaplasia, condylomata, ACIS, adenocarcinoma, squamous cell carcinoma, and microglandular hyperplasia (Figs. 13–9, 13–10, and 13–11; see also Figs. 13–1, 13–4, 13–7, and 13–8).

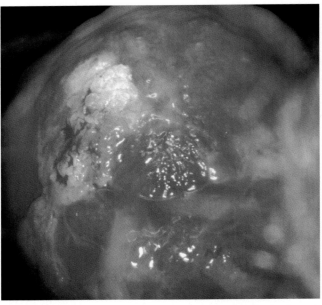

Figure 13–6. This cervical adenocarcinoma is well-defined, elevated, and densely acetowhite and has a papillary surface. It lies over columnar epithelium. Notably, it is not in contact with the squamous border. (From Wright VC, Shier RM: Colposcopy of Adenocarcinoma in Situ and Adenocarcinoma of the Cervix. Houston, Biomedical Communications, 2000.)

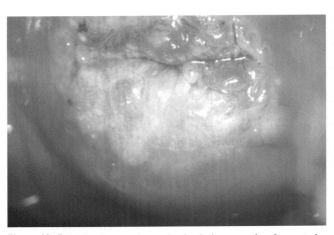

Figure 13–5. This adenocarcinoma-in-situ lesion occupies the posterior cervix. It is elevated and fairly well demarcated, has an irregular surface, and is patchy red and acetowhite.

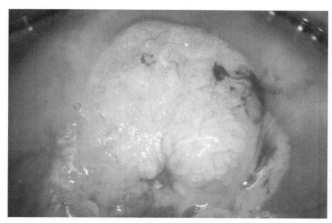

Figure 13–7. This adenocarcinoma is well defined and densely aceto-white. It exhibits a papillary surface. Dots (tips of the afferent and efferent vessels) can be seen in the tips of some papillary excrescences. It resembles a condylomatous lesion. (From Wright VC, Shier RM: Colposcopy of Adenocarcinoma in Situ and Adenocarcinoma of the Cervix. Houston, Biomedical Communications, 2000.)

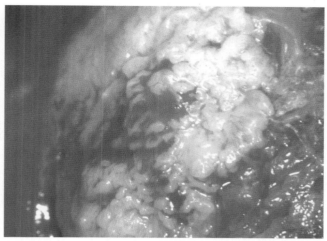

Figure 13–9. Large, densely acetowhite, fused papillary excrescences of a cervical adenocarcinoma. It is obviously friable and somewhat gray-ish. (From Wright VC, Shier RM: Colposcopy of Adenocarcinoma in Situ and Adenocarcinoma of the Cervix. Houston, Biomedical Communications, 2000.)

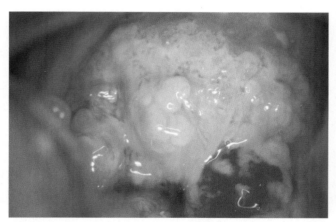

Figure 13–8. Large, fused, densely acetowhite, polypoid masses of microglandular hyperplasia. Colposcopically, the lesion mimics a cervi-cal adenocarcinoma (see Figs. 13–7 and 13–9). (From Wright VC, Shier RM: Colposcopy of Adenocarcinoma in Situ and Adenocarcinoma of the Cervix. Houston, Biomedical Communications, 2000.)

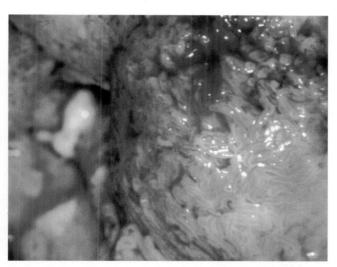

Figure 13–10. The villous structures of a papillary adenocarcinoma. Some scattered single dots are seen in the tips of excrescences, and looped vessels are noted within projections seen from the side. (From Wright VC, Shier RM: Colposcopy of Adenocarcinoma in Situ and Adenocarcinoma of the Cervix. Houston, Biomedical Communications, 2000.)

Figure 13–11. An adenocarcinoma that resembles an atypically devel-oping transformation zone. It is patchy red and acetowhite and exhibits fusion of the papillary projections. Scattered dots appear in the tips of some excrescences seen head-on. (From Wright VC, Shier RM: Colpos-copy of Adenocarcinoma in Situ and Adenocarcinoma of the Cervix. Houston, Biomedical Communications, 2000.)

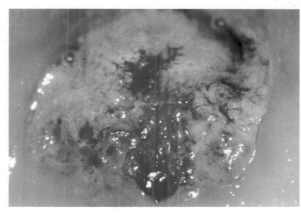

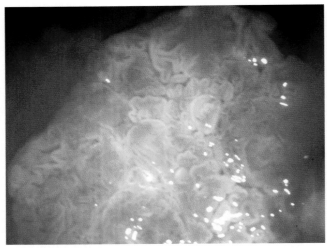

Figure 13-12. Cervical adenocarcinoma in situ containing papillary processes with scalloped edges and budding. Blood vessels creating character writing–like patterns are noted in several locations peripherally between the 11-o'clock and 1-o'clock positions. (From Wright VC, Shier RM: Colposcopy of Adenocarcinoma in Situ and Adenocarcinoma of the Cervix. Houston, Biomedical Communications, 2000.)

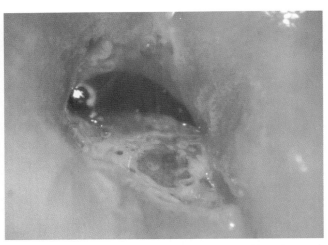

Figure 13-14. A variegated, patchy red and acetowhite adenocarcinoma-in-situ lesion involving the endocervical canal. The large gland opening at the 11-o'clock position is surrounded by an elevated, papillary excrescence. (From Wright VC, Shier RM: Colposcopy of Adenocarcinoma in Situ and Adenocarcinoma of the Cervix. Houston, Biomedical Communications, 2000.)

- Epithelial budding. ACIS can proliferate like "cactus budding." When it is observed colposcopically, a differentiation should be made among immature metaplastic epithelium, immature condylomata, and ACIS (Figs. 13–12 and 13–13).
- Lesions with a patchy red and white surface. When such a surface coloration is seen, the colposcopist should differentiate between a developing normal transformation zone, ACIS, and invasive adenocarcinoma (Figs. 13–14, 13–15, and 13–16; see also Fig. 13–2).
- Atypical blood vessel formations. Adenocarcinoma in situ can demonstrate a variety of blood vessel patterns. The common ones are waste thread (Fig. 13–17), tendril (Fig. 13–18), and single and multi-

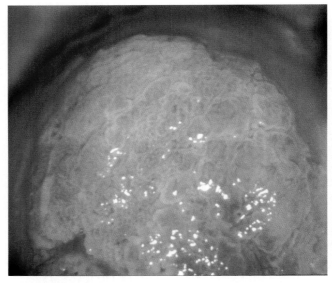

Figure 13-13. Normal metaplastic epithelium displaying epithelial budding and several reverse pseudomosaic areas of white halos surrounding central vascular points. Colposcopically, it appears similar to the adenocarcinoma-in-situ lesion shown in Figure 13–12. (From Wright VC, Shier RM: Colposcopy of Adenocarcinoma in Situ and Adenocarcinoma of the Cervix. Houston, Biomedical Communications, 2000.)

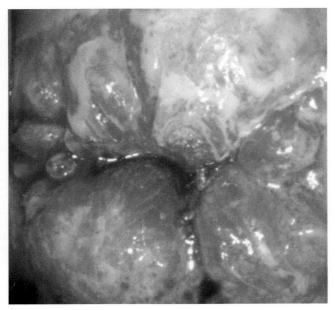

Figure 13-15. A large, four-quadrant, cervical adenocarcinoma in pregnancy (37 weeks' gestation). It is patchy red and acetowhite and resembles a developing transformation zone.

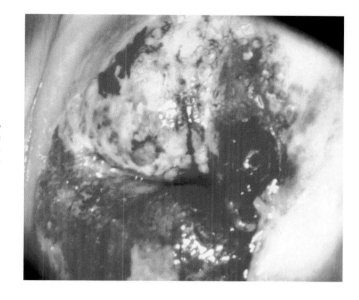

Figure 13-16. An adenocarcinoma-in-situ lesion from the 9-o'clock to the 12-o'clock position. It is variegated red and acetowhite. The surface is slightly irregular. (From Wright VC, Shier RM: Colposcopy of Adenocarcinoma in Situ and Adenocarcinoma of the Cervix. Houston, Biomedical Communications, 2000.)

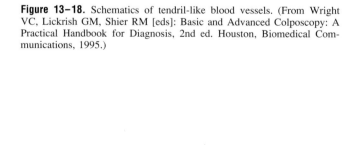

Figure 13-17. Schematics of waste thread–like blood vessels drawn from actual colpophotographs. (From Wright VC, Lickrish GM, Shier RM [eds]: Basic and Advanced Colposcopy: A Practical Handbook for Diagnosis, 2nd ed. Houston, Biomedical Communications, 1995.)

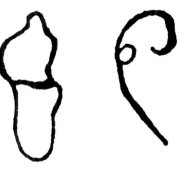

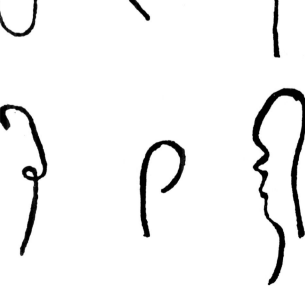

Figure 13-18. Schematics of tendril-like blood vessels. (From Wright VC, Lickrish GM, Shier RM [eds]: Basic and Advanced Colposcopy: A Practical Handbook for Diagnosis, 2nd ed. Houston, Biomedical Communications, 1995.)

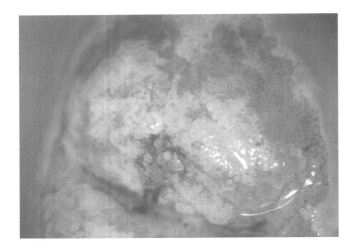

Figure 13–19. An adenocarcinoma-in-situ lesion displaying acetowhite, fused villous structures. The lesion appears variegated red and acetowhite. The angioarchitecture pattern includes single and multiple dots in the tips of projections. The lesion lies on columnar epithelium not in contact with the squamocolumnar junction. (From Wright VC, Shier RM: Colposcopy of Adenocarcinoma in Situ and Adenocarcinoma of the Cervix. Houston, Biomedical Communications, 2000.)

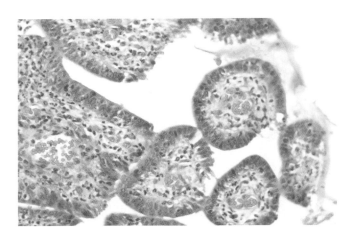

Figure 13–20. Histology of Figure 13–19. The centrally placed blood vessels in the projection sections are responsible for the single and multiple dots seen colposcopically. (From Wright VC, Shier RM: Colposcopy of Adenocarcinoma in Situ and Adenocarcinoma of the Cervix. Houston, Biomedical Communications, 2000.)

ple dots (Figs. 13–19 and 13–20), in association with some very bizarre formations such as taproot, tuberous root, and character writing (Figs. 13–21, 13–22, 13–23, 13–24, 13–25, 13–26, and 13–27). Although atypical blood vessel formations can be seen in both ACIS and adenocarcinoma, they are more common in the latter. Punctation, mosaic patterns, and corkscrew vessels, although common in squamous disease, do not appear in glandular disease.

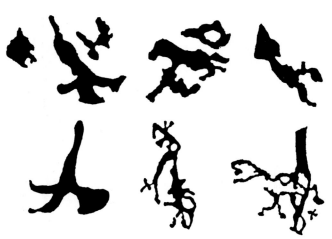

Figure 13–21. Schematics of rootlike blood vessels. (From Wright VC, Shier RM: Colposcopy of Adenocarcinoma in Situ and Adenocarcinoma of the Cervix. Houston, Biomedical Communications, 2000.)

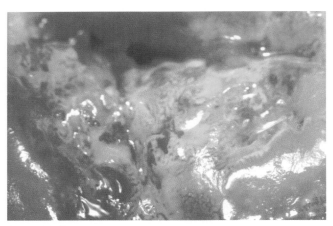

Figure 13–22. Irregular, dilated, tuberous, rootlike blood vessels in a cervical adenocarcinoma. Character-writing vascular forms are interspersed. (From Wright VC, Lickrish GM, Shier RM [eds]: Basic and Advanced Colposcopy: A Practical Handbook for Diagnosis, 2nd ed. Houston, Biomedical Communications, 1995.)

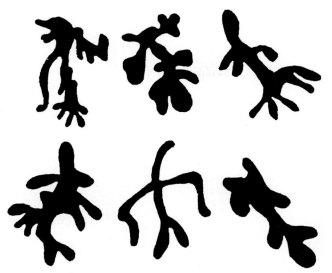

Figure 13–23. Schematics of character writing–like blood vessels. (From Wright VC, Shier RM: Colposcopy of Adenocarcinoma in Situ and Adenocarcinoma of the Cervix. Houston, Biomedical Communications, 2000.)

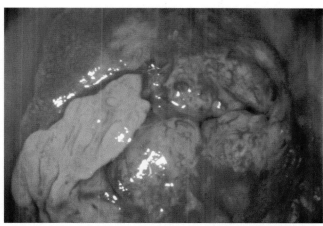

Figure 13–25. A case of mixed disease. The high-grade squamous intraepithelial lesion/cervical intraepithelial neoplasia grade 3 lies between the 6-o'clock and 10-o'clock positions. The adenocarcinoma-in-situ lesion is located between the 12-o'clock and 6-o'clock positions. Numerous rootlike and character writing–like vessels are evident in the glandular lesion. (From Wright VC, Shier RM: Colposcopy of Adenocarcinoma in Situ and Adenocarcinoma of the Cervix. Houston, Biomedical Communications, 2000.)

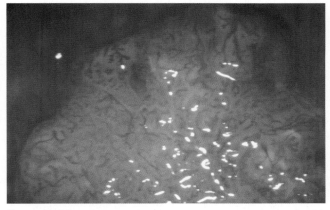

Figure 13–24. A variety of blood vessel patterns are seen in this adenocarcinoma-in-situ lesion. These include character writing–like, taproot-like, waste thread–like, and tendril-like patterns. (From Wright VC, Lickrish GM, Shier RM [eds]: Basic and Advanced Colposcopy: A Practical Handbook for Diagnosis, 2nd ed. Houston, Biomedical Communications, 1995.)

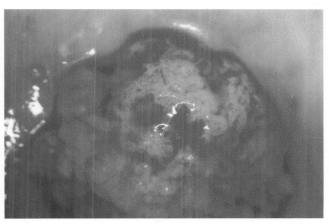

Figure 13–26. This friable, papillary cervical adenocarcinoma contains waste thread–like and tendril-like vessels. It is patchy red and acetowhite. (From Wright VC, Shier RM: Colposcopy of Adenocarcinoma in Situ and Adenocarcinoma of the Cervix. Houston, Biomedical Communications, 2000.)

Figure 13–27. Character writing–like blood vessels in a cervical adenocarcinoma. (From Wright VC, Shier RM: Colposcopy of Adenocarcinoma in Situ and Adenocarcinoma of the Cervix. Houston, Biomedical Communications, 2000.)

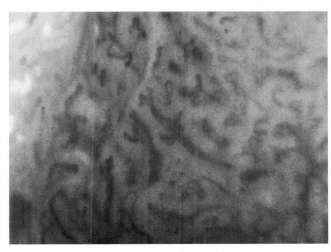

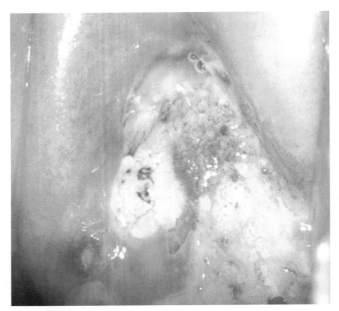

Figure 13–28. Centrally and to the left is an elevated, dense, aceto-white ACIS lesion (proven on excision). It is separated by normal-appearing columnar epithelium from a much larger, densely aceto-white microinvasive squamous cell cancer (seen on the right). (From Wright VC, Shier RM: Colposcopy of Adenocarcinoma in Situ and Adenocarcinoma of the Cervix. Houston, Biomedical Communications, 2000.)

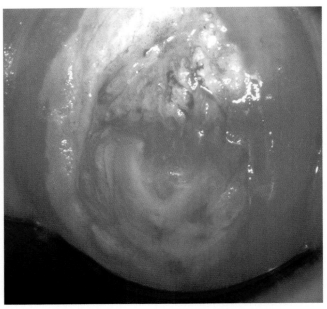

Figure 13–30. Central is the papillary, patchy, and variegated red-and-white (immature transformation zone–like) ACIS lesion (proven on excision). Peripherally from 6 to 12 o'clock is a dense acetowhite area with punctation that was proven to be an HSIL (CIN 3) lesion. (From Wright VC, Shier RM: Colposcopy of Adenocarcinoma in Situ and Adenocarcinoma of the Cervix. Houston, Biomedical Communications, 2000.)

- High-grade squamous lesions. Glandular lesions can lie lateral to a squamous lesion; between two squamous lesions; or, more commonly, above the squamous component (within the endocervical canal) (Figs. 13–28, 13–29, and 13–30; see also Figs. 13–4 and 13–25). The cytology frequently reflects only the squamous component (usually high grade). Thus, the colposcopist is programmed mentally for

squamous disease and most likely gives no thought to the possibility of a coexisting glandular component. When the cytology is high-grade squamous, colposcopists should automatically be aware that a glandular component might be present and should look for it. The existence of two or more squamous lesions separated by glandular-appearing epithelium is highly suggestive of a glandular lesion (see Fig. 13–29). Primary (i.e., not post treatment) squamous lesions do not "skip"; they are always contiguous.

DIFFERENTIAL DIAGNOSES IN GLANDULAR DISEASE

The differential diagnosis for ACIS in a histologic specimen includes microglandular hyperplasia, mesonephric duct hyperplasia, tubal or serous metaplasia (ciliated cell metaplasia), cervical endometriosis, cervical adenocarcinoma, adenomatoid proliferation ("tunnel clusters"), glandular dysplasia, and glandular atypia (inflammatory related). Making this determination is the pathologist's responsibility.[29]

FACTORS THAT INFLUENCE MANAGEMENT

The following nine factors influence management:

- Patient age
- Lesion location (ectocervical, endocervical, or both)
- Three-dimensional lesion geometry (linear length of disease and underlying crypt depth)

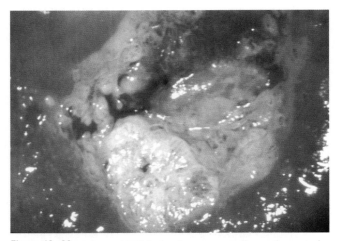

Figure 13–29. A large ACIS lesion is seen centrally on the posterior cervical lip. It is dividing an HSIL lesion located between 10 and 11 o'clock and between 3 and 5 o'clock. (From Wright VC, Shier RM: Colposcopy of Adenocarcinoma in Situ and Adenocarcinoma of the Cervix. Houston, Biomedical Communications, 2000.)

- Potential for ACIS to be buried under metaplastic or dysplastic epithelium
- Presence of a squamous component
- Possible multifocal lesions (skip lesions)
- Specimen margin status post excision
- Patient's desire for fertility
- Patient compliance[28]

Younger women are more likely to have ectocervical expression, shorter linear length of the lesion, and lesser depth of crypt involvement. Rarely do lesions extend across the entire glandular epithelium.

The majority of women with ACIS are of reproductive age, and many wish to maintain fertility. In addition, age is closely related to location of lesion, lesion extent, and depth of subsurface (i.e., crypt) involvement. Younger women are more likely to have ectocervical expression, shorter linear length of the lesion, and lesser depth of crypt involvement. Rarely do lesions extend across the entire glandular epithelium.[12, 16, 17, 30] Linear length of disease (distance over the tissue surface between caudal and cephalad edges) does not usually exceed 15 mm.[11, 16, 30] However, Östör reported a linear length of 30 mm in a 45-year-old patient.[16] Nicklin et al found that women younger than 36 years had a mean lesion length of 5.6 mm, whereas women 36 years and older had a mean lesion length of 10.8 mm.[30] This difference was found to be statistically significant at the 0.05 probability level in 37 patients. Only 1 of 14 younger women, in a subseries of 31, had a linear length of more than 10 mm. But 9 of 17 women—more than half—in the older group had lesion lengths of more than 10 mm, with a maximum of 25 mm.

Younger women had lesser depth of disease than did older women.

Crypt involvement is usually superficial (average, 2.5 mm) and usually does not exceed 4 mm below the surface.[12, 16, 17, 29] The Nicklin group found that younger women had lesser depth of disease than did older women; only 2 of 14 younger women had depth more than 2 mm, but 9 of 17—again more than half—older women had depth of more than 2 mm, up to 6 mm.[30] Invariably, normal crypts are seen beneath involved ones. The involved crypts can be focal, or, more rarely, may intermingle with normal ones. The transition between normal and neoplastic epithelium, whether on the surface or in the lining of the crypt, is abrupt.

At least half of all ACIS cases have an associated squamous component. With mixed disease, it is very unusual to find both squamous and glandular neoplasia in the same crypt.

At least half of all ACIS cases have an associated squamous component (cervical intraepithelial neoplasia or squamous cell cancer). With mixed disease, it is very unusual to find both squamous and glandular neoplasia in

the same crypt. In about half of ACIS cases, the disease has been identified beneath the transformation zone (whether normal metaplastic or dysplastic) (Fig. 13–31).[12] ACIS is categorized as multifocal (so-called skip lesions) if an uninvolved, complete, radial cervical section separated two sections involved with ACIS. Multifocal lesions are rare and are probably not found in more than 15% of cases.[12, 16, 30]

ACIS has many architectural and histologic patterns. The architectural patterns include cribriform, epithelial budding, and papillary formations. The histologic patterns are the endometrioid, the endocervical, and the intestinal.[16] These are probably responsible for the varying colposcopic appearances, although they play no role in patient management.[28]

Smaller, more ectocervical lesions in younger women are more easily managed conservatively with smaller, cylindrical excisions. In older women, excision may be required at or above the internal os.

Smaller, more ectocervical lesions in younger women are more easily managed conservatively with smaller, cylindrical excisions. These specimens can probably be designed to encompass all diseased tissue, taking age, potential for buried disease, lesion location, and geometry into consideration. In older women, excision may be required at or above the internal os, which may affect

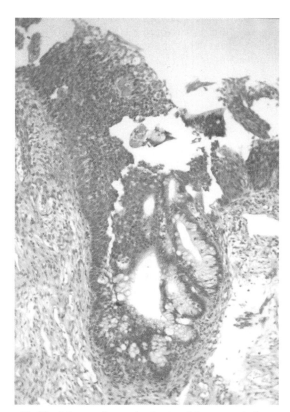

Figure 13–31. Adenocarcinoma in situ involving a cervical crypt and opening through dysplastic squamous epithelium. The adenocarcinoma-in-situ lesion is buried beneath the squamous lesion.

cervical competence, but it is likely that women with disease entirely in the canal, requiring a large specimen to produce negative margins, will be generally past reproductive age.

WHEN ACIS IS A SURPRISE FINDING

If ACIS is a surprise finding at histology, the colposcopist should repeat the colposcopic examination and try to locate the lesion and the squamocolumnar junction in relation to the external os. This information will be used to plan the radius and height of the cylindrical specimen to be excised.[28]

WHY NOT TO PROCEED TO HYSTERECTOMY

All patients with biopsy-proven ACIS, regardless of their age, fertility status, or lesion location, require an excisional biopsy. It is never appropriate to proceed directly to simple, class I hysterectomy (removal of all cervical tissue in an extirpated specimen).

All patients with biopsy-proven ACIS, regardless of their age, fertility status, or lesion location, require an excisional biopsy. It is never appropriate to proceed directly to simple, class I hysterectomy (removal of all cervical tissue in an extirpated specimen). Should the patient actually harbor adenocarcinoma, she needs a more radical procedure, not a simple one. It is on the basis of the excised specimen's margins that the step after excision is determined.[15, 28, 29]

MANAGEMENT OF ADENOCARCINOMA IN SITU

Excision

The height of the cylinder to be excised depends on the location of the squamocolumnar junction and the theoretical linear limit of in situ disease measured along the cervical surface.

The wider the location of the squamocolumnar junction on the surface of the ectocervix, the less likely that in situ disease will be extremely high within the endocervical canal.

The height of the cylinder to be excised depends on the location of the squamocolumnar junction and the theoretical linear limit of in situ disease measured along the cervical surface (see Figs. 13–1 to 13–4, 13–12, 13–14, 13–16, 13–24, and 13–25). One must estimate the upper limit of diseased tissue going toward, into, or up the endocervical canal from the squamocolumnar junction. The wider the location of the squamocolumnar junc-

tion on the surface of the ectocervix, the less likely that in situ disease will be extremely high within the endocervical canal.

A circle 5 to 7 mm outside the junction is where the circumferential excision line of the cylindrical specimen should be located.

Some have advocated excising a specimen with a height of 20 to 25 mm, measured from the most external curvature of the cervix, to incorporate most (estimated to be 95%[31]) ACIS, but this excision does not take into consideration the location of the disease, the location of the squamocolumnar junction, or the patient's age. A more individualized approach should be considered to account for the distribution of disease (Fig. 13–32). A circle 5 to 7 mm outside the junction is where the circumferential excision line of the cylindrical specimen should be located. The extra 5 to 7 mm should take care of any buried glandular disease under squamous tissue, should it exist, as well as any endocervical (lateral) crypt involvement. This procedure may be further modified in the presence of peripheral squamous disease (see Figs. 13–25 and 13–28 to 13–30). When the lesion can be identified, it may be possible to determine the height of the cylinder, taking into consideration the patient's age. The ideal excisional outcome is for all the margins to be negative, including the ectocervical, the deep, and the upper margins.

Methods of Excision

Excision is better done with the scalpel or the Ultrapulse carbon dioxide laser along the deep margin, with scalpel excision or tonsil snare cut at the apex. Electrosurgical loop excision can cause considerable distortion of specimen histology and can make interpretation of the margins difficult.

Excision is better done with the scalpel or the Ultrapulse CO_2 laser along the deep margin, with scalpel excision or tonsil snare cut at the apex. These two approaches create the proper cylindrical excision and produce an upper cut with margins that can be interpreted. Although monopolar electrosurgical loop excision has been advocated, it can cause considerable distortion of specimen histology that can make interpretation of the margins difficult or even impossible. This is because electric current always follows the path of least resistance, and the mucus in glandular mucosa provides less resistance (Figs. 13–33 and 13–34). In this circumstance, it may not be possible to differentiate between ACIS and adenocarcinoma, particularly if a positive margin exists. The distortion within the specimen will likely be equal in the remaining uterine cervix, thus hindering further cervical assessment (see Figs. 13–33 and 13–34).

When the Excised Specimen Has Negative Margins

Most studies indicate that when the specimen margins are negative, patients desiring future childbearing can be conservatively managed.

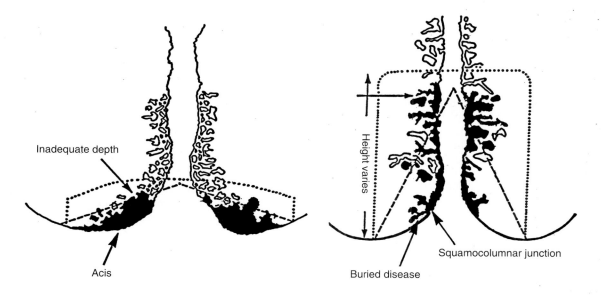

Inadequate depth

Acis

Height varies

Squamocolumnar junction

Buried disease

- - - - Cone shaped profile (inadequate)

• • • • Large cylinder ideal

Figure 13–32. Schematics of conical and cylindrical excision lines for two lesion locations. A cylindrical shape better accounts for the distribution of disease in both circumstances. The cylinders' widths and heights depend on the location of the adenocarcinoma in situ, the location of the squamocolumnar junction, and any presence of squamous disease.

Negative margins are associated with persistent ACIS and occasionally with adenocarcinoma in 12.5% of cases that proceed to hysterectomy, so patients with negative margins must be counseled about the importance of compliance and the risks of conservative management.

Most studies indicate that when the specimen margins are negative, patients desiring future childbearing can be conservatively managed.[2, 11, 15, 31–33] Negative margins are associated with persistent ACIS (found in an extirpated uterus) in 12.5% of cases that proceed to hysterectomy.[15, 17, 31, 34] On occasion, adenocarcinoma has been reported as well, even after negative margins. Therefore, patients with negative margins who choose to be followed this way must be counseled about the importance of compliance and the risks of undetected persistent and recur-

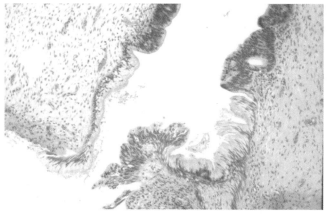

Figure 13–33. ACIS occupies the upper part of the cervical crypt. Beneath is pseudostratified glandular epithelium induced by electric current. The distorted area mimics the adenocarcinoma in situ. (From Wright VC, Shier RM: Colposcopy of Adenocarcinoma in Situ and Adenocarcinoma of the Cervix. Houston, Biomedical Communications, 2000.)

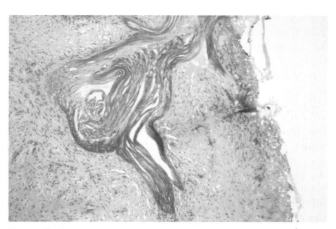

Figure 13–34. Complete destruction of glandular epithelium because of electric current. Histologic interpretation is impossible.

rent disease, because follow-up screening may be unreliable.[19, 20, 35] Although hysterectomy has been heretofore advocated for all ACIS patients, some colposcopists, including the author, have been carefully and conscientiously following up women who continue to have children. The colposcopists use colposcopy, cytology, and endocervical curettage, with biopsy when indicated, every 4 months for 1 year and every 6 months thereafter.[28, 32] Once reproduction is complete, some patients are still recommended for hysterectomy, but it is not clear whether this is mandatory in the compliant patient.[7, 28, 34]

When Excision Margins Are Reported As Positive

> **Surgical excision margins have been reported as positive in 25% to 57.5% of ACIS cases.**

Surgical excision margins have been reported as positive in 25% to 57.5% of ACIS cases.[15, 32, 36, 38, 40] The ectocervical margin was involved in 2.2% to 17.5% of cases, and the endocervical or deep margin was positive in 27.5% to 40%[15, 36, 38, 40] of cone-shaped specimens. With better colposcopic recognition of this disease, cylindrical specimens, and more individualized surgical approaches, fewer positive margins can be expected.[21, 22]

> **Because of the high risk of residual ACIS or adenocarcinoma, cylindrical excision producing negative margins is required.**

Positive margins are of great clinical significance because of the high risk of residual ACIS (46% of cases) or adenocarcinoma (16.7% of cases)[2, 15–16, 36, 37]; therefore, repeat cylindrical excision (probably higher and wider) producing negative margins is required, even in patients who do not want future children. It is not appropriate to proceed to simple, class I hysterectomy because invasive cancer may be present, in which case the patient needs a more radical procedure.

SUMMARY

ACIS and adenocarcinoma exhibit many different colposcopic patterns. Many intraepithelial lesions resemble a normally developing transformation zone, and this similarity explains why the lesions are missed at colposcopy. However, colposcopists can learn to differentiate the lesions from a normal transformation zone and from their colposcopic mimics using newer criteria expressed in Table 13–1. Critical attributes are surface topography and blood vessel configuration. Biopsy is always required, and, when biopsy shows ACIS, excision is necessary to determine the true histology. Before hysterectomy, an excisional procedure that produces a specimen with negative margins is necessary. Repeat excision is required until margins are clear. When this is not possible, a more radical procedure is required. Some clinicians, after appropriate counseling, have chosen to follow up compliant patients without hysterectomy, even those who desire no

future childbearing. Many patients still proceed to hysterectomy after any childbearing is complete.

SUMMARY OF KEY POINTS

- Two percent of intraepithelial lesions are ACIS, whereas adenocarcinoma composes 6% to 18% of invasive cervical cancers, indicating either that intraepithelial transit time to invasion or that intraepithelial disease is underdiagnosed.

- ACIS appears to be increasing in incidence. It is now found more commonly in younger women.

- ACIS alters the cervical surface contour very little. Often, the neoplastic glands are buried beneath the surface.

- Most glandular lesions lie within or close to the transformation zone.

- Diagnostic excisional biopsy must always be performed when ACIS is found on punch biopsy or suspected cytologically or colposcopically but not proven histologically.

- The most common colposcopic appearances of glandular disease are a papillary expression resembling an immature transformation zone; a flat, variegated red and white area resembling an immature transformation zone; and more isolated, elevated, individual, densely acetowhite lesions overlying columnar epithelium.

- At least half of all ACIS cases have an associated squamous component.

- When glandular and squamous diseases coexist, the squamous component is more likely to be noted because it is more likely to be visible.

- Squamous cell carcinoma is present in approximately 4% to 5% of mixed disease cases.

- The standard colposcopic criteria of Kolstad and Stafl and Reid's colposcopic grading index apply to squamous but not glandular lesions.

- Colposcopic criteria for identifying glandular disease are lesion location over columnar epithelium; large gland or crypt openings; papillary structure; budding; patchy red and white coloration; waste thread–like, tendril-like, rootlike, or character writing–like blood vessel patterns; and single or multiple dots produced at the tips of papillary projections by looped vessels.

- Punctation and mosaic vessel patterns and atypical corkscrew vessels are common in squamous disease but do not appear in glandular disease.

- Glandular lesions can lie lateral to a squamous lesion, between two squamous lesions or, more commonly, above the squamous component within the endocervical canal.

- The appearance of two or more squamous lesions separated by glandular-appearing epithelium is highly suggestive of a glandular lesion.

- Younger women are more likely to have ectocervical expression, shorter linear length of the lesion, and lesser depth of crypt involvement.

- Smaller, more ectocervical lesions in younger women are more easily managed conservatively with smaller cylindrical excisions. In older women, excision may be required at or above the internal os.

- All patients with biopsy-proven ACIS, regardless of their age, fertility status, or lesion location, require an excisional biopsy to exclude adenocarcinoma.

- The height of the cylinder to be excised depends on the location of the squamocolumnar junction and the theoretical linear limit of in situ disease measured along the cervical surface.

- Most studies indicate that when the specimen margins are negative, patients desiring future childbearing can be conservatively managed.

- Negative margins are associated with persistent ACIS and occasional adenocarcinoma, so patients with negative margins must be counseled about the importance of compliance and the risks of conservative management.

- Surgical excision margins are reported positive in 25% to 57.5% of ACIS cases.

References

1. Friedell GH, McKay DG: Adenocarcinoma in situ of the endocervix. Cancer 1953;6:887.
2. Cullimore JE, Luesley DM, Rollason TP, et al: A prospective study of conization of the cervix in the management of cervical intraepithelial glandular neoplasia (CIGN): A preliminary report. Br J Obstetr Gynecol 1992;99:314.
3. Gloor E, Hurlimann J: Cervical intraepithelial neoplasia (adenocarcinoma in situ and glandular dysplasia). Cancer 1986;58:1272.
4. Anderson MC: Glandular lesions of the cervix: Diagnostic and therapeutic dilemmas. Baillières Clin Obstet Gynecol 1995;9:105.
5. Kurman RJ, Norris HJ, Wilkinson EJ: Tumours of the cervix, vagina and vulva. In Rosai J, Sobin LH (eds): Atlas of Tumour Pathology, Third Series, Fascicle 4. Washington, DC, Armed Forces Institute of Pathology, 1992, pp 77–83.
6. Scully RE, Bonfiglio TA, Kurman RJ, et al: Histological typing of female genital tract tumours. In Scully RE, Poulsen HE, Sobin LH (eds): WHO International Histological Classification of Tumours, 2nd ed. Geneva, World Health Organization, 1994, pp 43–44.
7. Christopherson WM, Nealson N, Gray LA: Noninvasive precursor lesions of adenocarcinoma and mixed adenosquamous carcinoma of the cervix uteri. Cancer 1979;44:975.
8. Boon ME, Baak JPA, Kurver PJH: Adenocarcinoma in situ of the cervix. Cancer 1981;48:768.
9. Ng ABP: Microinvasive adenocarcinoma and precursors of adenocarcinoma of the uterine cervix. In Wied GL, Koss LG, Regan JW (eds): Compendium on Diagnostic Cytology. Chicago, Tutorials of Cytology USA, 1983, pp 148–154.
10. Reagan JW, Ng APB: The cells of uterine adenocarcinoma, 2nd ed. Basel, Karger S, 1973, pp 96–112.
11. Andersen ES, Arffmann E: Adenocarcinoma in situ of the uterine cervix: A clinicopathologic study of 36 cases. Gynecol Oncol 1989;35:1.
12. Colgan TJ, Lickrish GM: The topography and invasive potential of cervical adenocarcinoma in situ, with and without associated squamous dysplasia. Gynecol Oncol 1990;36:246.
13. Weisbrot IM, Stabinsky C, Davis AM: Adenocarcinoma in situ of the uterine cervix. Cancer 1972;29:1179.
14. Schwartz SM, Weiss NS: Increased incidence of adenocarcinoma of the cervix in young women in the United States. Am J Epidemiol 1986;124:1045.
15. Muntz HG, Bell DA, Lage JM. et al: Adenocarcinoma in situ of the uterine cervix. Obstet Gynecol 1992;80:935.
16. Östör AG, Pagano R, Davoren RAM, et al: Adenocarcinoma in situ of the cervix. Int J Gynecol Pathol 1984;3:179.
17. Andersen ES, Arffmann E: Adenocarcinoma in situ of the uterine cervix: A clinicopathologic study of 36 cases. Gynecol Oncol 1989;35:1.
18. Laverty CR, Farnsworth A, Thurlse J, Bowditch R: The reliability of a cytological prediction of a cervical adenocarcinoma in situ. Aust N Z J Obstet Gynecol 1988;28:307.
19. Nguyen GK, Jeannot AB: Exfoliative cytology of in situ and microinvasive adenocarcinoma of the uterine cervix. Acta Cytol 1984;28:461.
20. Mitchell H, Medley G, Gordon I, Giles G: Cervical cytology reported as negative and risk of adenocarcinoma of the cervix: No strong evidence of benefit. Br J Cancer 1995;71:894.
21. Wright VC, Shier RM: Why adenocarcinoma in situ and adenocarcinoma are often missed by colposcopists. In Wright VC, Shier RM: Colposcopy of Adenocarcinoma in Situ and Adenocarcinoma of the Cervix. Houston, Biomedical Communications, 2000, pp 1–4.
22. Wright VC: Colposcopy of adenocarcinoma in situ and adenocarcinoma of the uterine cervix: Differentiation from other cervical lesions. J Low Gen Tr Dis 1999;3:83.
23. Coppleson M, Atkinson KH, Dalrymple JC: Cervical squamous and glandular neoplasia: Clinical features and review of management. In Coppleson M (ed): Gynecologic Oncology. Edinburgh, Churchill Livingstone, 1992, pp 571–607.
24. Lickrish GM, Colgan TJ, Wright VC: Colposcopy of adenocarcinoma in situ and adenocarcinoma of the cervix. Obstet Gynecol Clin North Am 1993;20:111.
25. Wright VC, Lickrish GM: Colposcopy of adenocarcinoma in situ and invasive adenocarcinoma of the cervix. In Wright VC, Lickrish GM, Shier RM (eds): Basic and Advanced Colposcopy - A Practical Handbook for Diagnosis, 2nd ed. Houston, Biomedical Communications, 1995, pp 12-1–12-13.
26. Kolstad P, Stafl A: Terminology and definitions. In Atlas of Colposcopy. Oslo, Universitetsforlaget, 1972, pp 21–25.
27. Reid R, Scalzi P: Genital warts and cervical cancer—VII. An improved colposcopic index for differentiating benign papillomaviral infections from high-grade cervical intraepithelial neoplasia. Am J Obstet Gynecol 1985;153:611.
28. Wright VC: Society of Obstetricians and Gynaecologists of Canada Clinical Practice Guidelines on Adenocarcinoma In Situ of the Cervix: Clinical features and review of management. JSOGC 1999;77:699.
29. Lickrish GM, Colgan T: Management of adenocarcinoma in situ of the uterine cervix. In Wright VC, Liskrish GM, Shier RM (eds): Basic and Advanced Colposcopy: A Practical Handbook for Treatment. Houston, Biomedical Communications, 1995, pp 30-5–30-7.
30. Nicklin JL, Wright RG, Bell JR, et al: A clinicopathological study of adenocarcinoma in situ of the cervix. The influence of cervical HPV infection and other factors, and the role of conservative surgery. Aust N Z J Obstet Gynaecol 1991;31:179.
31. Bertrand M, Lickrish GM, Colgan TJ: The anatomic distribution of cervical adenocarcinoma in situ: Implications for treatment. Obstet Gynecol 1987;157:21.
32. Wolf J, Levenback C, Malpica A, et al: Adenocarcinoma in situ of the cervix: Significance of cone biopsy margins. Obstet Gynecol 1996;88:82.
33. Im DI, Duska LR, Recension NB: Adequacy of conization margins of adenocarcinoma in situ of the cervix as a predictor of residual disease. Gynecol Oncol 1995;59:179.
34. Weisbrot IM, Stabinsky C, Davis AM: Adenocarcinoma in situ of the uterine cervix. Cancer 1972;29:1179.
35. Laverty CR, Farnsworth A, Thurlse J, et al: The reliability of a

cytological prediction of a cervical adenocarcinoma in situ. Aust N Z J Obstet Gynaecol 1988;29:307.

36. Poynor EA, Barakat RR, Hoskins WJ: Management and follow-up of patients with adenocarcinoma in situ of the uterine cervix. Gynecol Oncol 1995;57:158.

37. Hopkins M, Roberts JA, Schmidt RW: Cervical adenocarcinoma in situ. Obstet Gynecol 1988;71:842.

38. Wildrich T, Kennedy AW, Myers TM, et al: Adenocarcinoma in situ of the uterine cervix: Management and outcome. Gynecol Oncol 1996;61:304.

39. Denechy TR, Gregori CA, Brun JJ: Endocervical curettage, cone margins, and residual adenocarcinoma in situ of the cervix. Obstet Gynecol 1997;90:1.

40. Azodi M, Setsuko KC, Rutherford TZ, et al: Adenocarcinoma in situ of the cervix: Management and outcome. Gynecol Oncol 1999; 73:348.

41. Wright VC, Davies E, Riopelle MA: Laser cylindrical excision to replace conization. Am J Obstet Gynecol 1984;150:704.

Case Study 1 Questions

History

A 33-year-old woman who has no children but is desirous of a family is referred to your colposcopy clinic for investigation because of a Papanicolaou (Pap) test reported as atypical glandular cells of undetermined significance (AGUS). One of the following colposcopic images is her lesion, and it corresponds to the histology that represents the lesion. The other two are mimics. All colpophotographs were taken after application of 5% acetic acid. Using Table 13–1,

- Describe what you see for each colpophotograph.
- Identify the adenocarcinoma in situ (ACIS)/adenocarcinoma.

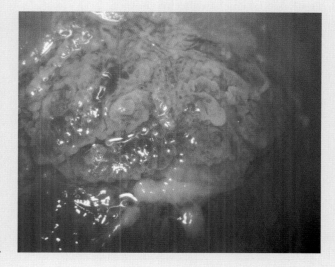

Figure 13–35.

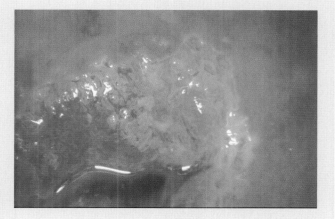

Figure 13–36.

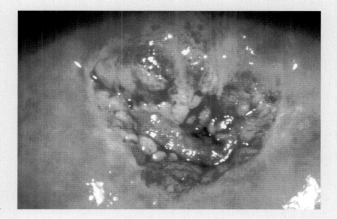

Figure 13–37.

Case Study 1 Answers

Figure 13–35

This is immature metaplasia of the anterior cervical lip. It is characterized by early fusion of the villous structures of the ectopy, resulting in a variegated red-and-white appearance. The overall formation appears papillary, and the process is occurring over columnar epithelium. In the tips of some of the excrescences, single dotlike angioarchitecture is seen.

Figure 13–36

This is the ACIS/adenocarcinoma lesion involving the anterior cervical lip. It appears variegated red and white, and the changes overlie the columnar epithelium. Numerous fused-like papillary excrescences are seen. In the tips of some of the excrescences is single dotlike angioarchitecture.

Figure 13–37

This is microglandular hyperplasia involving the external os and lower endocervical canal. Large, globular, fused masses of tissue overlie the columnar epithelium. They have a pronounced yellow color resembling the color of chicken fat. (From Wright VC, Shier RM: Colposcopy of Adenocarcinoma in Situ and Adenocarcinoma of the Cervix. Houston, Biomedical Communications, 2000.)

Figure 13–38

This is the histology of the cylindrically excised specimen from the lesion seen in Figure 13–36. The margins were negative. It was also representative of the colposcopically directed biopsy that was taken. It shows an ACIS lesion with both endocervical and intestinal cell types (the latter at the papillary surface). Interspersed between the abnormal ACIS excrescences are two papillary projections of normal columnar epithelium (tall columnar cells with basally situated nuclei. The linear length of the ACIS lesion measured 5.8 mm histologically, and the maximal depth of crypt involvement measured 1.61 mm.

Key Points of Case 1

Colposcopy cannot differentiate between ACIS and adenocarcinoma. Hence, if the biopsy demonstrates ACIS, a cylindrical excision producing negative margins must follow to exclude adenocarcinoma.

Cervical glandular disease has many mimics, the most common being an immature transformation zone (compare Figs. 13–35 and 13–36).

The histologic finding of normal epithelium between ACIS in the same histologic section (see Fig. 13–36) does not constitute multifocality (skipped lesions). In this case, the finding is seen in the same histologic section. ACIS is categorized as a multifocal only if an unequivocal, complete cervical section separates two sections involved with ACIS.

Because the margins of the excised specimen were negative, this woman can be managed conservatively with patient counseling because she wants to have children.

Microglandular hyperplasia is a benign progesterone-induced lesion. The lesion can shed cells that may be interpreted as AGUS. Frequently, it has a yellow hue and can mimic both ACIS and adenocarcinoma (see also Fig. 13–8).

Case Study 2 Questions

History

This 30-year-old woman had a Pap test reported as high-grade squamous intraepithelial lesion (HSIL).

Figure 13–39

This is the colpophotograph of her cervix after 5% acetic acid application.

- Describe what you see.
- Make your differential diagnosis.
- Decide where you would biopsy.

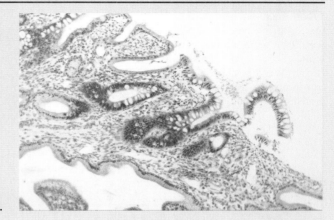

Figure 13–38.

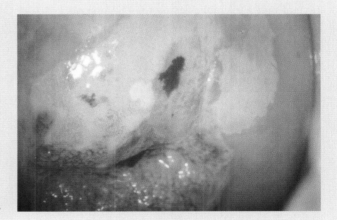

Figure 13–39.

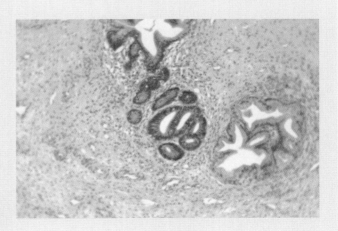

Figure 13–40.

Case Study 2 Answers

Figure 13–39

An HSIL (acetowhite with punctation) is being separated by a variegated red-and-white lesion centrally. When such an observation is made, the area causing the split is suspect for glandular disease. Biopsies would be recommended from at least one of the acetowhite areas and the variegated red-and-white area. (From Wright VC, Shier RM: Colposcopy of Adenocarcinoma in Situ and Adenocarcinoma of the Cervix. Houston, Biomedical Communications, 2000.)

Figure 13–40

This histology is representative of the variegated red-and-white ACIS lesion located between the two parts of the acetowhite HSIL. The neoplastic epithelium is characterized by increased cellularity and disorganization in comparison with the normal glandular epithelium, which shows tall columnar cells with basally situated nuclei. The linear length of the ACIS lesion measured 4.97 mm, and the maximal depth of crypt involvement was 2.3 mm. Buried ACIS disease extended 0.69 mm beneath the high-grade squamous lesion.

Key Points of Case 2

In cases of mixed disease (ACIS and squamous), the majority of the abnormal Pap smears reflect squamous disease with no clue that a glandular lesion is present. Thus, the colposcopist is mentally programmed to find the squamous lesion with no thought that a glandular lesion may be present.

The splitting of a squamous lesion is suspect of a glandular lesion, and a biopsy must be taken from this area. In general, in the absence of previous treatment, high-grade squamous lesions are dense white from border to border.

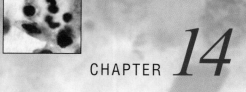

CHAPTER *14*

• Burton A. Krumholz

Vagina: Normal, Premalignant, and Malignant

The vulvovaginal boundary (Hart's line) demonstrates clear histologic differences between the vaginal and the vulvar epithelia.

In the resting position, the vagina forms a fibromuscular tube that is flattened from anterior to posterior.[1] It connects the uterine cervix with the vestibule of the vagina. The vulvovaginal boundary (Hart's line)[2] can be clearly demarcated by the application of diluted iodine solution (half-strength Lugol's solution or Schiller's solution). This boundary demonstrates clear histologic differences between the vaginal and the vulvar epithelia. The vagina is characterized by a large degree of elasticity that reaches its maximum during childbirth. The entire length of the vagina is located between the rectum posteriorly and the urinary bladder and urethra anteriorly. The posterior wall measures about 11 cm in length, whereas the anterior wall measures only 8 cm. The posterior vaginal fornix is adjacent to the pouch of Douglas, which is lined by peritoneum and allows for communication to the lowest point of the peritoneal cavity.

The vaginal wall consists of three layers: the epithelial layer, the muscular coat, and the vaginal fascia.

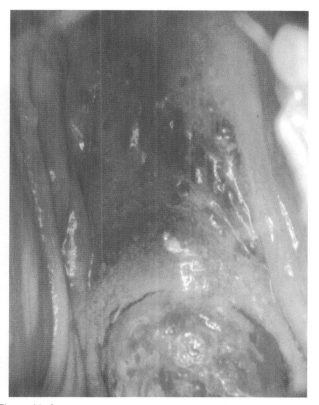

Figure 14–1. Cervical deformity and vaginal transformation zone in a 24-year-old patient with no history of diethylstilbestrol exposure. Vaginal acetowhitening represents an area of adenosis found in 3% to 4% of women.

Figure 14–2. Cervical deformity (ridge and pseudopolypoid configuration) with extensive vaginal transformation zone in a diethylstilbestrol-exposed woman.

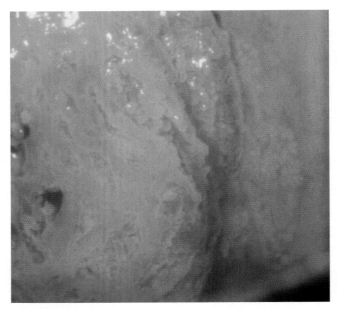

Figure 14–3. Extensive cervicovaginal transformation zone demonstrating crypts, folds, gland openings, and grapelike villi.

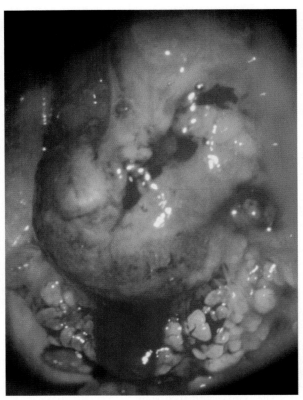

Figure 14–5. Normal cervical transformation zone and exaggerated grapelike villi in the posterior fornix of a diethylstilbestrol-exposed patient.

Histologically, the vaginal wall consists of three layers: the epithelial layer, the muscular coat, and the vaginal fascia. The epithelial layer consists of a stratified squamous epithelium and a lamina propria that is subject to age and hormonal influences. The lamina propria contains a dense network of elastic fibers that continue to proliferate until about the age of 40 years. In elderly women, the

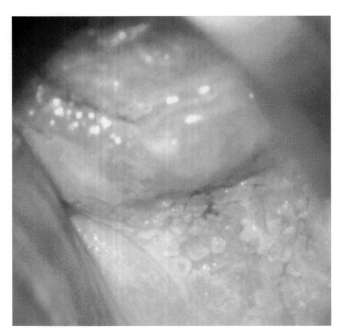

Figure 14–4. Grapelike villi in the posterior vaginal fornix of a diethylstilbestrol-exposed patient.

fibers swell and often exist only in fragments. The vaginal epithelium forms transverse folds called rugae. Traditionally, it has been stated that the vaginal epithelium has few, if any, glands. More recent descriptions of the vaginal epithelium reveal the presence of glandular elements or their metaplastic counterpart in 3% to 4% of women. These areas have been described as adenosis, although they represent normal vaginal variants or remnants from embryologic development (Figs. 14–1, 14–2, 14–3, 14–4, and 14–5). These areas may also be described as a vaginal transformation zone.[3]

Although the cyclic hormonal changes in the vaginal epithelium are less pronounced than those in the endometrium, they are apparent on cytologic examination. Glycogen content is highest during ovulation and is significantly decreased in estrogen deficiency states.

PREMALIGNANT AND MALIGNANT VAGINAL DISEASE

Cruveilhier first described vaginal cancer in 1826.[4] Vaginal intraepithelial neoplasia (VAIN) was subsequently described more than 100 years later at the Mayo Clinic in 1933 and was reported by Hummer et al in 1970.[5]

In 1981, Woodruff noted that fewer than 300 cases of

VAIN had been reported in the literature, suggesting that VAIN was a rare condition.[6]

Vaginal neoplasms account for 1% to 4% of all gynecologic malignancies.

Epidemiology

Women with VAIN 1 and VAIN 2 tend to be younger than those with VAIN 3.

Vaginal neoplasms account for 1% to 4% of all gynecologic malignancies.[7] With the increase in cytologic screening and colposcopy, the frequency of detection has increased. Additionally, there appears to be a real increase in the number of women with human papillomavirus (HPV)-related disease that could also account for an increase in the number of cases of VAIN detected. As with other squamous lesions of the lower female genital tract, HPV appears to be the primary initiator of these vaginal lesions.[8]

The true incidence of VAIN is difficult, if not impossible, to assess.[9] Because women with VAIN are usually asymptomatic, and because the majority of cases are found after an abnormal Papanicolaou (Pap) smear, the frequency can be related to the prevalence of cytologic screening in a population. Reported incidences vary by as much as 0.2[10] to 2 per 100,000.[11] The true incidence is probably somewhere in the middle of this 1000-fold range. With increased cytologic screening, the condition may be more readily diagnosed and found to be more prevalent.[12]

VAIN can occur at any age, but the highest incidence rates are observed in women older than 60 years.

Although VAIN can occur at any age, the highest incidence rates are observed in women older than 60 years, with the mean age of diagnosis of VAIN 3 at about 53 years.[5] As with cervical intraepithelial neoplasia (CIN) and vulva intraepithelial neoplasia (VIN), which may be present at the same time or follow at a later time, VAIN is identified more frequently in younger women. Patients with VAIN 1 and VAIN 2 tend to be younger than those with VAIN 3. In young women with VAIN, an association with HPV is common.

It is postulated that VAIN 1 and VAIN 2 are representative of more benign viral proliferation, whereas VAIN 3 is considered a true cancer precursor.

In 1% to 3% of patients with cervical neoplasia, vaginal neoplasia will either coexist or occur at a later date.[13] In an early study, the time interval from an earlier diagnosis of CIN 3 to a current diagnosis of VAIN 3 varied from less than 2 years to as much as 17 years.[5] The age range of patients was from 24 to 75 years, with a mean age of 52 years.[6] Several more recent reports[14-17] indicate a wider range, somewhere between 19 and 86 years. There appears to be about a 15-year average difference, possibly reflecting different etiologies or different disease processes. It has been postulated that VAIN 1 and VAIN 2 are representative of more benign viral proliferation, whereas VAIN 3 is a true cancer precursor.

Compared with CIN development, the development of VAIN following HPV infection may require a greater period of time and may occur less frequently because of the different type of epithelium from which VAIN arises.

Predisposing Causes

The etiology of VAIN has not been conclusively determined, but it appears that exposure to a sexually transmitted carcinogenic agent (i.e., HPV) is the most likely predisposing factor. The precise relationship between HPV and VAIN is unknown, but it may involve a multistep process associated with cofactors such as sexual activity, other infectious agents (herpes simplex virus and Epstein-Barr virus), smoking, immune status, and genetic predisposition.

Compared with CIN development, the development of VAIN following HPV infection may require a greater period of time and may occur less frequently because of the different type of epithelium from which VAIN arises. Coppleson et al[3] stated that most cases of VAIN arise within a transformation zone (Fig. 14–6). They believed

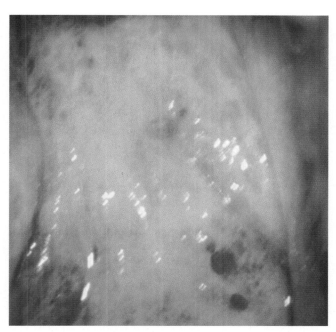

Figure 14–6. Atypical adenosis in the vaginal vault characterized by acetowhitening and atypical vessels. Patient is a 30-year-old woman who had a radical hysterectomy at age 15 years for clear-cell adenocarcinoma of the cervix.

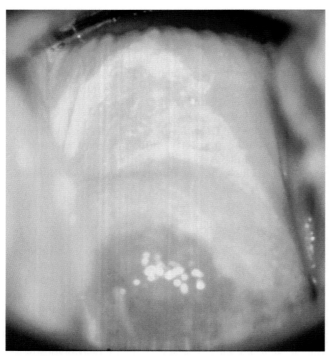

Figure 14–7. Grade 2 acetowhitening of cervix and anterior vaginal fornix reveals a sharp border, a slightly raised surface, and an irregular mosaic. Biopsies reported as concurrent cervical intraepithelial neoplasia grade 3 and vaginal intraepithelial neoplasia grade 3.

that the occurrence of metaplasia on the vaginal wall carries the same biologic significance as it does on the cervix. Although VAIN is less common and arises from a more obscure natural history, the authors believed that VAIN could occur in the original squamous epithelium of the vagina.

In 1987, Schneider et al[18] reported on the presence of HPV in the vagina of posthysterectomy patients and noted an increase in associated VAIN. In this study, 5% of HPV-positive patients (all had HPV 16) had VAIN. In the same year, Bornstein et al[19] identified HPV in five diethylstilbestrol (DES)-exposed women with VAIN. Confirming that CIN and VAIN share a common etiology would explain reports that describe 36% to 48% of patients with VAIN as having concurrent CIN.[14, 16] Fifty-one to sixty-two percent of women with VAIN have been treated for CIN, and as many as 25% have undergone hysterectomies for CIN as well. Almost 75% of women with VAIN have preceding or coexisting squamous carcinomas of the cervix or vulva.[15, 20–22] Gemmell[23] stated that despite these figures, VAIN occurs in less than 1% of women who have undergone hysterectomy for CIN in a 10-year follow-up period.

VAIN has also been reported to occur after hysterectomy for benign conditions. In 1986, Lenehan et al[15] reported that 40% of women with VAIN had undergone hysterectomies for non-neoplastic disorders, indicating that hysterectomy itself may be a risk factor for subsequent VAIN. It was postulated that development of VAIN was related to trauma to the vaginal tissue at the time of surgery.

It has been suggested that radiation therapy is a predisposing factor for VAIN occurring 10 to 15 years after therapy.[24–26] The radiation may sensitize the epithelium to subsequent development of neoplasia. It is unknown if these radiation-induced lesions are associated with HPV.

VAIN, along with other lower genital tract neoplasias, occurs more frequently in immunocompromised women. In these patients, VAIN is more often multifocal, persistent, and aggressive.[20, 27]

Reports by Robboy et al[28] in 1984 and Bornstein et al[8] in 1987 have also shown an increased incidence of VAIN in DES-exposed women. This may be due to the fact that 35% to 40% of these women have a transformation zone that extends into the vagina (Fig. 14–7).

Pathology

Microscopically, the features of VAIN are similar to those of CIN, and both conditions have problems of subjectivity in diagnosis and grading of disease severity.

VAIN is defined as "the spectrum of intraepithelial changes beginning with a generally well-differentiated neoplasm, traditionally classified as mild dysplasia, and ending with invasive carcinoma."[29] The intraepithelial changes include nuclear pleomorphism, loss of polarity, abnormal mitosis, and loss of differentiation as cells progress from the basement membrane to the surface epithelium and are confined to the squamous epithelium above the basement membrane.[29]

Microscopically, the features of VAIN are similar to those of CIN, and similar problems of subjectivity in diagnosis and grading of disease severity exist. Despite this, the traditional grading of CIN has been applied to VAIN. Full-thickness epithelial involvement is termed VAIN 3, whereas VAIN 1 and VAIN 2 denote the presence of cytologic atypia in the lower one third or two thirds of the epithelium. Lopes et al[9] suggested that it may be more useful with regard to treatment and potential for malignant transformation to simply divide VAIN into low-grade (VAIN 1 and VAIN 2) and high-grade (VAIN 3) lesions. Using the traditional grading system, VAIN occurs 52% of the time as VAIN 1, 19% of the time as VAIN 2, and 29% of the time as VAIN 3.

Sherman and Paull[30] demonstrated that the cytologic and histologic grading of VAIN is moderately reproducible but also noted that the cytologic diagnosis of VAIN 2 is employed infrequently and rarely matches the diagnosis in the corresponding histology. For this reason, they suggested that differentiating VAIN 2 from VAIN 3 is unnecessary.

Careful evaluation of the progressive potential of the various cervical, vaginal, and vulvar lesions has led Jenkins to suggest that despite the similarities among CIN, VIN, and VAIN, there is no guarantee that there are parallel similarities in etiology or biologic behavior.[31]

Although the natural history of VAIN has not been clearly defined, most low-grade VAIN lesions probably regress spontaneously without treatment, and because most of the lesions are asymptomatic, they may not be clinically identified.

Natural History

> **The progression of VAIN to vaginal carcinoma appears to be far less frequent than the progression of CIN to cervical carcinoma.**

If screening methods for detection of vaginal cancer are to be effective, vaginal neoplasia must pass through a preclinical phase in which it is detectable. Whether VAIN represents that preclinical state is unknown. The natural history of VAIN has not been clearly defined. Most low-grade VAIN lesions are asymptomatic and probably regress spontaneously without treatment. Therefore, they may not be clinically identified. The risk of progression from VAIN to an invasive vaginal carcinoma appears to be far lower than the risk for CIN progressing to cervical carcinoma. VAIN 3 lesions are thought to have a greater potential for malignant transformation than VAIN 1 lesions have. Studies by Aho and colleagues[14] and Petrilli and associates[32] indicated that although VAIN seems to regress in some patients (Aho—18 of 23 [78%]; Petrilli—6 of 12 [50%]), it may persist in others (Aho—3 of 23 [13%]; Petrilli—6 of 12 [50%]) or may eventually progress to invasive cancer (Aho—2 of 23 [9%]; Petrilli—0 of 12 [0%]). VAIN 1 lesions are more likely to regress. Lesions not associated with CIN or VIN showed a higher rate of regression (91%) than did those associated with CIN or VIN (67%). Four of the five women with VAIN 3 in Aho et al's study demonstrated regression of the lesion, and one woman progressed to invasion.

Clinical Features

> **The most common clinical presentation of VAIN is in a patient who has undergone a hysterectomy for CIN 3 or cervical carcinoma.**

VAIN is usually asymptomatic, and patients become aware of the disease only after an abnormal Pap smear is reported (Figs. 14–8 and 14–9). VAIN most commonly presents in women who have undergone hysterectomy for CIN (carcinoma in situ) (Figs. 14–10, 14–11, and

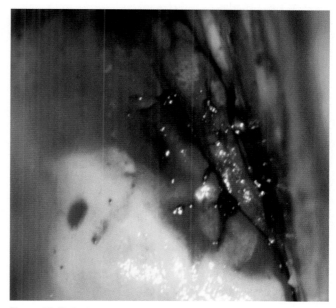

Figure 14–9. Iodine staining with half-strength Lugol's solution defines the nonstaining areas that coincide with the previously noted poorly defined white lesions. Biopsy reported as vaginal intraepithelial neoplasia grade 2.

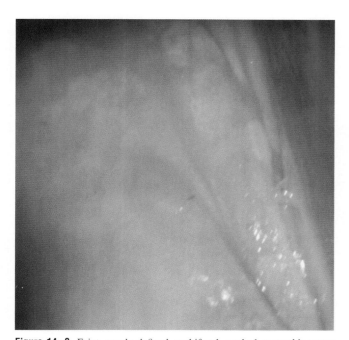

Figure 14–8. Faint, poorly defined, multifocal, grade 1 acetowhite areas in the left anterior vaginal fornix in a patient with persistent high-grade squamous intraepithelial lesion on cervical cytology who had no identifiable cervical lesion (see also Fig. 14–9).

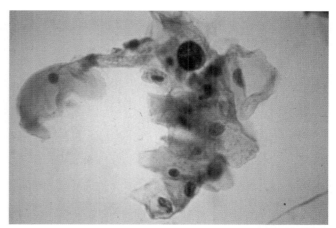

Figure 14–10. Vaginal cytology of a 46-year-old woman taken 4 years posthysterectomy for cervical intraepithelial neoplasia grade 3. The presence of nuclear enlargement and hyperchromasia is consistent with high-grade squamous intraepithelial lesion of the vagina.

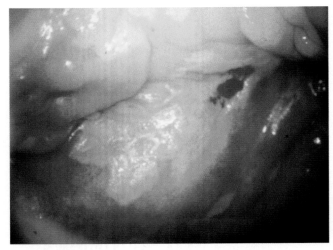

Figure 14–11. Wide area of acetowhite change with well-defined borders at the vaginal vault. There is a small ulcer at the vaginal apex. A few isolated satellite lesions can be seen.

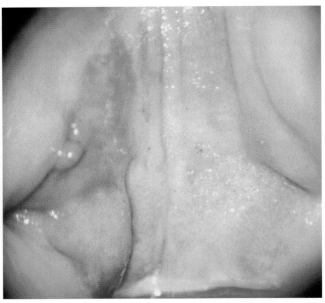

Figure 14–13. The vaginal apex of a woman 10 years after hysterectomy before the application of acetic acid. There is a large erythematous area with foci of vascular prominence (see also Fig. 14–14).

14–12).[33] Women occasionally complain of postcoital bleeding or an unusual vaginal discharge, although these symptoms are uncommon. Occasionally, a color change in the vaginal epithelium may alert the clinician to an area of abnormal epithelium (Figs. 14–13 and 14–14).

VAIN affects the upper third of the vagina in 85% to 92.4% of cases.[15, 17] About half of these cases are multifocal.[14–16] Only rarely, as in an immunosuppressed woman, will the entire vagina be involved. Because the presenting lesions are often located on the anterior or posterior vaginal wall, they may be hidden by the speculum (Fig. 14–15). VAIN may occur with vaginal condylomata. VAIN lesions may be leukoplakic (Figs. 14–16, 14–17, and 14–18), erythematous, or ulcerated[34] (Figs. 14–19 and 14–20). Immunosuppressed patients with HPV-associated cervical disease are also at risk for vaginal involvement and should undergo a thorough vaginal examination.

> **VAIN lesions may be leukoplakic, erythematous, or ulcerated, and the lesions are multifocal in about half of cases.**

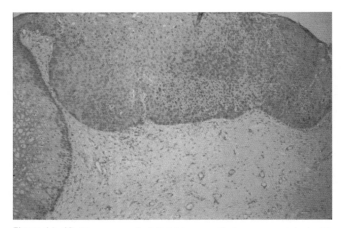

Figure 14–12. Biopsy reveals full-thickness cell changes consistent with a diagnosis of vaginal intraepithelial neoplasia grade 3.

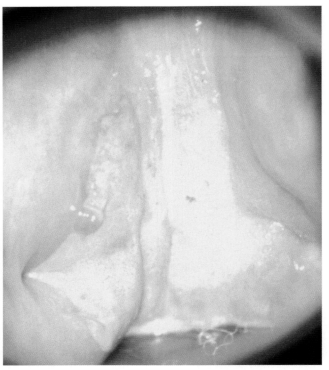

Figure 14–14. The same area after the application of acetic acid solution. The erythematous region has developed a well-demarcated acetowhiteness dipping into the "dog ear" at the right apex. Biopsy showed vaginal intraepithelial neoplasia grade 3.

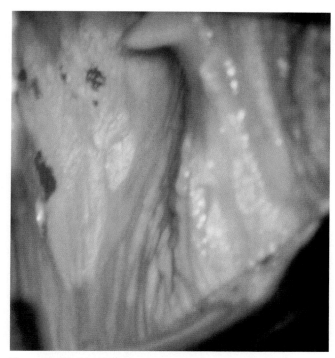

Figure 14–15. Multifocal acetowhite patches in left lateral vaginal fornix. (The cervix, not seen, is normal.) Biopsy showed vaginal intraepithelial neoplasia grade 2 to grade 3.

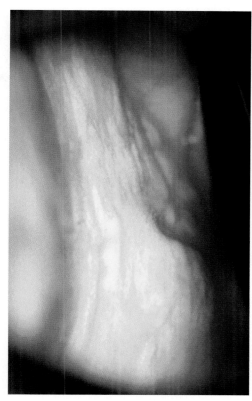

Figure 14–17. Diffuse, multifocal, slightly raised areas of acetowhiteness seen tangentially along the left upper vaginal sidewall (see also Fig. 14–18).

Detection

The primary method of detecting VAIN is by cytologic examination of asymptomatic women. However, VAIN lesions should be suspected in women with cervical or vulvar neoplasia, lower genital tract condylomata, or abnormal cytologic smears after hysterectomy; in women after pelvic irradiation; or in women with abnormal cytology in the absence of a recognizable cervical lesion.

The detection of VAIN in a woman with a cervix is usually associated with a concurrent or previous diagnosis of CIN. In these situations, careful colposcopic examination of the entire lower genital tract must be performed before proceeding to a cone biopsy. This is especially important in women in whom an abnormal smear persists

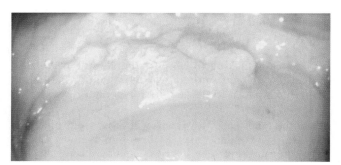

Figure 14–16. Raised white hyperkeratotic area along the anterior fornix. Biopsy reported as vaginal intraepithelial neoplasia grade 1 with warty changes.

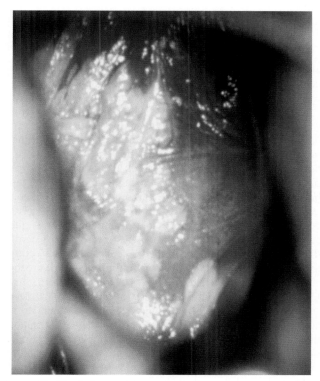

Figure 14–18. Iodine staining with half-strength Lugol's solution clearly defines the large area of atypical vaginal epithelium. Biopsy is reported as vaginal intraepithelial neoplasia grade 3.

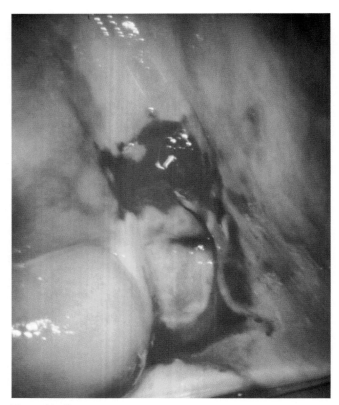

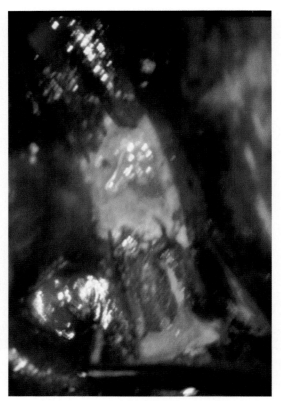

Figure 14–19. Patient previously treated with laser ablation for vaginal intraepithelial neoplasia grade 3 returned with a Papanicolaou smear of high-grade squamous intraepithelial lesion. Colposcopy revealed a focally denuded area mixed with poorly adherent acetowhite epithelium (see also Fig. 14–20).

Figure 14–20. Iodine staining with half-strength Lugol's solution reveals nonstaining in the denuded areas. Biopsy shows vaginal intraepithelial neoplasia grade 3.

after treatment of a cervical lesion. Nwabineli and Monaghan[35] found that 103 of 4147 women (2.5%) treated for CIN by laser had coexisting vaginal abnormalities.

Despite the fact that most VAIN is found in women who have undergone hysterectomy, the necessity for vaginal cytologic screening after hysterectomy has been questioned. This is particularly true when the hysterectomy is done for benign disease. Fetters et al[36] reviewed the recommendations of major organizations and major textbooks of gynecology and performed a MEDLINE computer search for the years from 1966 through 1995. They concluded that data do not support screening for vaginal cancer in women following total hysterectomy for benign disease. Women who have had a subtotal hysterectomy and still have a cervix should continue to be screened according to established guidelines. Women with maternal DES exposure or with a history of abnormal cytologic smears or gynecologic malignancy should continue to receive vaginal screening. Fetters and colleagues concluded that diligence is needed to distinguish between populations at increased risk for vaginal cytologic abnormalities and those with little or no risk. Their conclusions were supported by Pearce et al,[37] who found that the probability of an abnormal Pap smear was 1.1% and that the positive predictive value for detecting vaginal cancer was

0%. The prevalence of vaginal dysplasia after hysterectomy for benign disease was between 0.13% and 0.15%. On the basis of similar data, Piscitelli et al[38] recommended vaginal cytology every 5 years. Fox et al[39] studied women older than 50 years and concluded that these women had a 10-fold decreased risk of an abnormal Pap smear and that the majority of the abnormalities were false positives. Noller[40] believed that the use of the Pap smear after hysterectomy for benign disease should become an antiquated procedure. Furthermore, from an ethical perspective, Fetters et al[36] decried the use of deceit to gain compliance for health maintenance examinations. A patient should not be asked to return for a vaginal cytologic smear when the underlying motive is to perform a breast examination or to provide another preventive health service.

Evidence is lacking to support the routine performance of cytologic sampling of the vagina in women who have had a hysterectomy for benign disease.

On the other hand, a woman with a previous diagnosis of CIN 3 who undergoes a total hysterectomy should have screening cytology every 6 months during the first postoperative year, and then, if all cytology in the first year is normal, she can revert to usual screening intervals.[23]

The presence of benign glandular cells in vaginal smears of women following hysterectomy has been described and appears to pose no significant risk for subsequent development of vaginal cancer.[41-43]

EVALUATION AND DIAGNOSIS

Colposcopic Examination of the Vagina

Colposcopic examination of the vagina is indicated for the evaluation of abnormal cytology whenever cervical colposcopy is negative, after treatment of CIN, or after hysterectomy for CIN or invasive disease. Other indications for vaginal colposcopy include HPV-associated disease in immunocompromised women, history of maternal DES exposure, or inspection or palpation revealing the presence of gross vaginal lesions, suspected VAIN, or extensive HPV-associated lesions in the vagina.[2]

The goal of the colposcopic examination is to identify the presence of preinvasive or invasive disease, to determine the extent of disease, and to select appropriate therapy (Table 14-1). Colposcopic examination of the vagina is more tedious and difficult than colposcopy of the cervix, and it is frequently described as more technically challenging. The large surface area of the vagina, the presence of vaginal rugae, posthysterectomy "dog ears," and multifocal disease increase the technical difficulty of vaginal colposcopy for the clinician and make this examination lengthy, uncomfortable, and potentially stressful for the patient. The speculum blades obscure a 360-degree view of the vagina, and the colposcopic grading in the vagina is not as accurate as in the cervix.

> Colposcopy of the vagina is more tedious and difficult than colposcopy of the cervix and is frequently described as more technically challenging.

Vaginal colposcopy is performed in the modified dorsal lithotomy position. If possible, it is preferable to raise the buttocks 5 to 10 degrees. A thorough inspection of the vulvar vestibule is completed before the application of 3% to 5% acetic acid. An appropriately sized speculum should be chosen and carefully inserted into the vagina. The size of the speculum should be deep enough to view the distal vagina but also allow easy rotation so the entire vagina may be visualized. Although lubricants should not be used, the use of a diluted solution of 1% to 4%

lidocaine may ease the discomfort of the examination. A tampon soaked in the solution may be inserted for 3 to 5 minutes before insertion of the speculum, or direct mucosal application of the solution may be performed during colposcopic examination. In instances where a Pap smear may need to be performed, the latter approach is preferred.

The vagina is then thoroughly moistened with 5% acetic acid. Because this solution is stronger than the frequently used 3% acetic acid solution, it accentuates the more subtle vaginal lesions more rapidly and effectively. It may be necessary to continuously reapply acetic acid during a prolonged examination. The vaginal mucosal folds are inspected for acetowhite changes by rotating and withdrawing the speculum and observing the epithelium as it rolls over the speculum blades during withdrawal of the speculum. The application of half-strength Lugol's solution to the vaginal mucosa after examination for acetowhite changes is frequently helpful in identifying multifocal areas of epithelial change or areas that were previously undetected. Lugol's solution will dehydrate the vaginal epithelium. If the vaginal speculum needs to be withdrawn and reinserted, a thin coating of lubricating jelly on the speculum can ease the process. The use of an iris hook or similar appliance can help expose hidden areas by stretching the mucosa and flattening the rugae, thus enhancing the identification of acetowhite areas. In the patient who has had a hysterectomy, the iris hook can aid visualization of the epithelium at the vaginal angles or within the "dog ears."

> The use of an iris hook or similar appliance can help expose hidden areas by stretching the mucosa and flattening the rugae, thus enhancing the identification of acetowhite areas. In the patient who has had a previous hysterectomy, the iris hook can aid visualization of the epithelium at the vaginal angles or within the "dog ears."

Biopsy sites in the vagina should be selected at the time of colposcopic examination. The ancillary tools that may be helpful in vaginal colposcopy are listed in Table 14-2. The use of diluted iodine solution aids in selecting sites for biopsy, especially when the lesions are multifocal (Fig. 14-21). The vaginal epithelium should also be palpated to detect any indurated areas. Cervical punch biopsy instruments are normally used to obtain the sample. It is helpful to elevate the biopsy site with an iris hook (Fig. 14-22) or a single-toothed tenaculum to en-

▼ Table 14-1

Indications for Vaginal Colposcopy

Abnormal cytology in a woman
    With a normal cervix after colposcopy or therapy
    Without a cervix after hysterectomy
CIN in an immunocompromised patient
In utero DES exposure
Gross lesions by inspection or palpation
Suspected VAIN or vaginal carcinoma
Widespread lower genital tract HPV infection

DES, diethylstilbestrol; HPV, human papillomavirus; VAIN, vaginal intraepithelial neoplasia.

▼ Table 14-2

Ancillary Tools for Vaginal Colposcopy

Colposcope with variable magnification
Topical anesthesia
5% acetic acid
Skin or iris hook, mirror, and endocervical speculum
Half-strength Lugol's solution
Topical estrogen cream

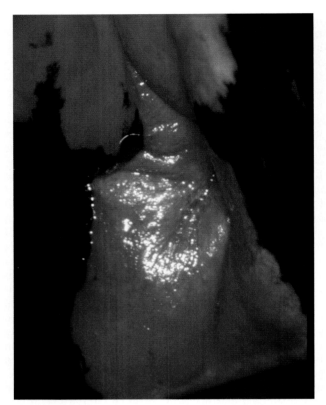

Figure 14–21. Half-strength Lugol's solution or Schiller's solution may be used to stain normal, well-differentiated squamous epithelium so that it can be differentiated from nonstaining areas that are not normal.

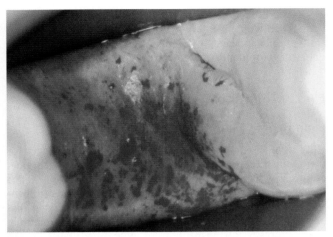

Figure 14–23. Atrophic vaginal epithelium frequently shows areas of ecchymosis and petechial hemorrhage (see also Fig. 14–24).

Atrophic changes of the vaginal mucosa of the postmenopausal patient may be cytologically mistaken for VAIN. The use of topical estrogen may result in maturation of the vaginal epithelium and reversal of this cytologic misdiagnosis. These atrophic changes may also mask the colposcopic appearance of VAIN. Topical estrogen cream may reverse these changes as well. The colposcopic examination should be repeated after daily application of topical estrogen in the vagina for 3 weeks (Figs. 14–23 and 14–24). Use of an oral estrogen preparation may not sufficiently reverse the vaginal atrophy.

Vascular patterns tend to be absent in VAIN 1 but present in VAIN 3. Any lesion exhibiting atypical vessels or mosaic or punctation should be biopsied.

sure that the stroma is included in the specimen so invasive cancer can be excluded. However, caution should be exercised during the biopsy, because the vaginal epithelium may be only 1 mm thick, and a deep biopsy may go through the full thickness of the vaginal wall, whereas an overly superficial biopsy will not exclude invasion. When a vaginal biopsy cannot be obtained in the office with use of local anesthesia, an evaluation under general anesthesia may become necessary. It is rarely necessary to suture the vagina after punch biopsy. Bleeding is generally controlled with the application of Monsel's solution (ferric subsulfate) and local pressure or with insertion of a tampon.

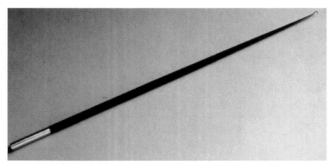

Figure 14–22. Small hook that can be used to evert the vaginal "dog ears." The hook is helpful in manipulating the vaginal tissues with little discomfort.

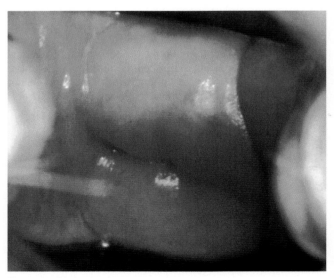

Figure 14–24. Three weeks after the use of topical estrogen creams, the vagina has a normal appearance.

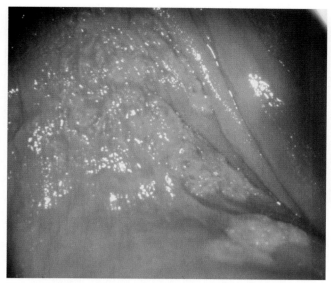

Figure 14-25. The anterior vaginal fornix shows a wide area of aceto-white change with a warty surface contour and an isolated warty lesion on the anterior portio of the cervix. Biopsies reported vaginal intraepithelial neoplasia grade 3 and cervical intraepithelial neoplasia grade 3.

Colposcopic Findings in the Vagina

Colposcopic patterns may reflect findings that are slightly more severe than the histologic diagnosis. Prediction of histology from atypical colposcopic appearances, especially the lower grades of VAIN (Fig. 14-25), is more difficult in the vagina than on the cervix. Vascular patterns tend to be absent in low-grade (VAIN 1) lesions but present in VAIN 3 lesions (Fig. 14-26). Iodine staining may show partial uptake or no staining in low-grade lesions but may be strongly nonstaining in VAIN 3 lesions. Lesions that are raised, exophytic, or nodular, along with those that exhibit atypical vessels, coarse punctation, or mosaic and ulceration must raise suspicion for invasion.

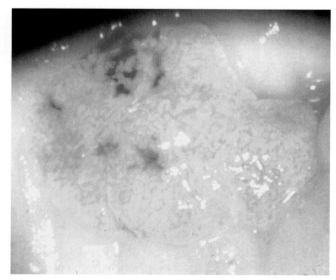

Figure 14-26. Raised papillary area of the vaginal vault 6 months after hysterectomy. The area shows mosaic and punctation as well. Biopsy reported as vaginal intraepithelial neoplasia grade 3.

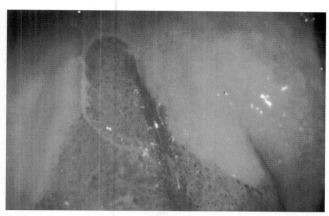

Figure 14-27. Colposcopy of the vagina of a 70-year-old woman. Hysterectomy was done 25 years earlier for uterine myomata. She has had no Papanicolaou smear in 15 years. Recent Papanicolaou smear shows high-grade squamous intraepithelial lesion. The view at high magnification shows a well-defined lesion with coarse punctation.

Because there is not a strong correlation between vaginal colposcopy and histology, biopsy of all suspicious lesions is critical.

If lesions are present, the surface pattern tends to be irregular, possibly owing to the looser configuration of the vaginal walls. Punctation may be noted in the aceto-white epithelium. Mosaic patterns and leukoplakia of the vagina are rare (Figs. 14-27 and 14-28). Lesions are

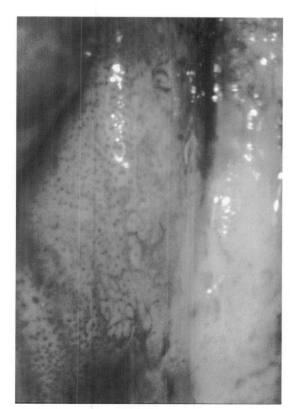

Figure 14-28. The same patient as in Figure 14-27 with a magnified view of the right posterior vaginal wall. There is a large area of acetowhiteness with coarse punctation and mosaic. The biopsy diagnosis is vaginal intraepithelial neoplasia grade 3.

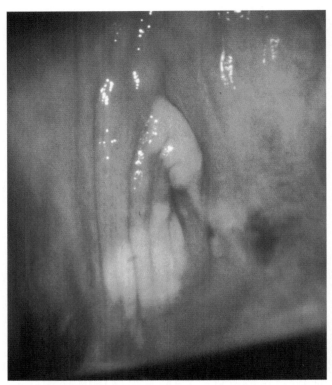

Figure 14–29. Focal grade 3 acetowhite change at the right upper corner of the vaginal vault near the posthysterectomy "dog ear." Biopsy reported as vaginal intraepithelial neoplasia grade 3.

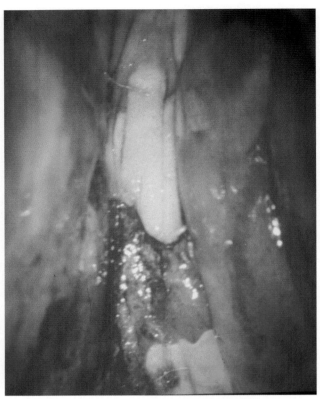

Figure 14–31. The upper vaginal cuff of a 72-year-old woman with a prior hysterectomy noted to have an abnormal Papanicolaou smear. Colposcopy revealed two large areas of grade 3 acetowhite change with peeling and curled edges. Biopsy showed vaginal intraepithelial neoplasia grade 3.

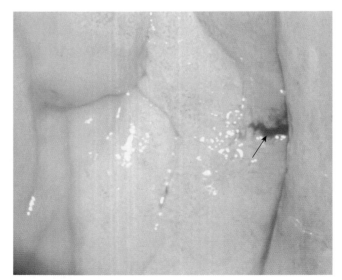

Figure 14–30. Vaginal vault reveals a large acetowhite region with a small focal ulcer (*arrow*). Biopsy shows vaginal intraepithelial neoplasia grade 3.

commonly seen following hysterectomy for CIN if the area of vaginal extension has not been completely excised. Another common finding is an acetowhite lesion that is either flat or slightly raised and has a sharp border. These lesions can be multifocal and may show a micropa-

pillary surface similar to subclinical condyloma (Figs. 14–29, 14–30, 14–31, 14–32, and 14–33).

The colposcopic appearances of clinical and subclinical HPV lesions are similar to those on the cervix. They may be grossly visible or seen only with the colposcope. They are frequently characterized by the presence of microspikes or exhibit a micropapillary appearance. They are generally keratinized and appear snow white after the application of 5% acetic acid. Flat condylomata may exist as multifocal lesions and be indistinguishable from VAIN, with which they may coexist. It may be difficult to distinguish VAIN and flat condylomata by cytology, colposcopy, and histology.

Colposcopically, vaginal cancer may present as an exophytic lesion with true erosions or ulcerations and atypical vessels.

Cancer of the vagina is most often an extension of a squamous cell cancer of the cervix, or it may arise from vulvar cancer or represent secondary invasion from another site. Rarely, vaginal cancer arises as a primary lesion. The colposcopic features of vaginal squamous cancer are similar to those of other lower genital tract squamous carcinomas. Exophytic tumor and true erosions or ulcerations may be present. Examination of the vascu-

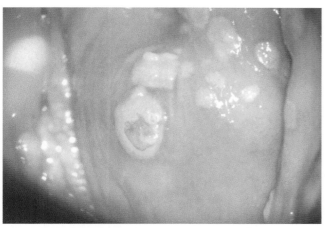

Figure 14−32. The upper vagina of a 29-year-old woman with no known immunocompromise had been treated repeatedly for several years for recurrent cervicovaginal condylomata and recurrent cervical intraepithelial neoplasia grade 3 and vaginal intraepithelial neoplasia grade 3. Several months after hysterectomy, colposcopy was performed and revealed irregular, patchy, grade 2 to grade 3 acetowhite changes that were multifocal. Biopsy was reported as vaginal intraepithelial neoplasia grade 3.

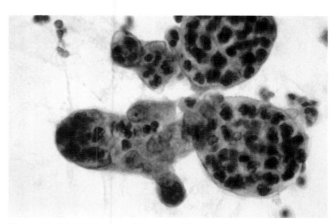

Figure 14−34. Vaginal cytology of a 68-year-old woman 2 years after hysterectomy for well-differentiated endometrial adenocarcinoma. The cells are consistent with endometrial adenocarcinoma (see also Fig. 14−35).

lature may reveal atypical corkscrew-like or spaghetti-like vessels similar to those that might be seen on the cervix.

Adenocarcinoma of the vagina is more likely to be metastatic in origin, although primary disease has been reported[44] (Figs. 14−34 and 14−35). Whether these primary, non−clear-cell adenocarcinomas arise in areas of adenosis is unknown.[45, 46] Clear-cell adenocarcinomas arise within areas of adenosis and are extremely rare. Melanoma of the vagina has been reported, and there were 120 cases in the English literature as of 1987. These highly malignant tumors compose about 2.5% of all primary vaginal malignancies.[47]

Other vaginal lesions that may mimic invasive cancer include traumatic ulcers and erosions such as tampon ulcers and pessary injuries, atrophic and postirradiation changes, endometriosis, posthysterectomy granulation tissue, prolapse of the tubal fimbria following hysterectomy,

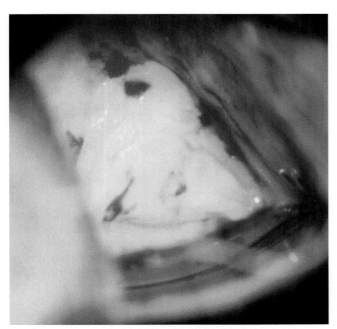

Figure 14−33. One year after hysterectomy, the upper vagina of an 80-year-old woman revealed thick acetowhite and hyperkeratotic areas at the vault of the vagina. Minor vascular atypia was noted. Biopsy was reported as vaginal intraepithelial neoplasia grade 3.

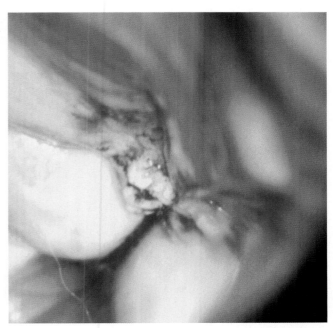

Figure 14−35. Upper left vaginal corner displays a small focal area of raised acetowhiteness with vascular atypia. Biopsy was reported as recurrent endometrial adenocarcinoma.

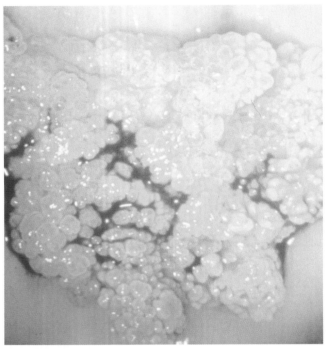

Figure 14–36. Raised papillary area of the vaginal vault 6 months after hysterectomy. Biopsy revealed condylomata acuminata.

post-traumatic vaginal adenosis, and a variety of inflammatory disorders (Figs. 14–36 to 14–43).

> **The therapeutic modalities available for VAIN include observation, surgical excision, ablation, radiation, and topical chemotherapy.**

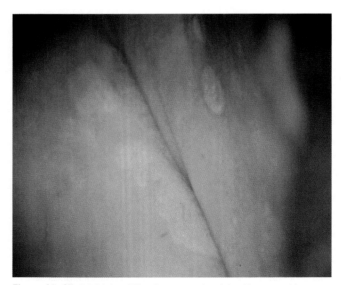

Figure 14–37. Multiple, diffusely arranged, minimally acetowhite areas in the left anterior vaginal fornix. Biopsy reported as flat condyloma.

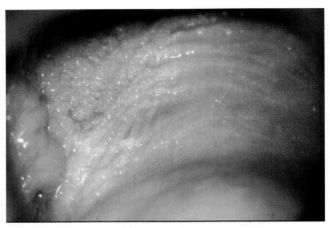

Figure 14–38. Diffuse, raised, irregular areas along the anterior vaginal fornix. The areas are micropapillary and confluent. Biopsy showed condylomata acuminata.

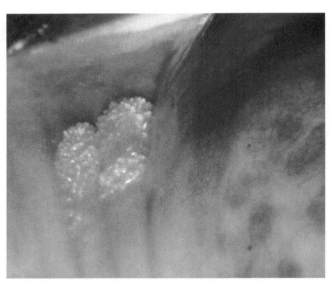

Figure 14–39. Isolated focus of a micropapillary lesion in the right anterior fornix. Biopsy showed condylomata acuminata.

THERAPY

The options available for managing VAIN include observation, surgical excision, ablation or destruction, radiation, and topical chemotherapy. Observation without treatment of VAIN may be justified in young patients and in those with minor-grade lesions. It may be better to delay aggressive interference and adopt watchful waiting if the possibility exists that the lesion will regress.

All methods of therapy for VAIN have a reasonably good success rate as long as there is consistent follow-up. The treatment options depend on the diagnostic and technical skills of the clinician, the clinician's personal experience, and the equipment available. The treatments are

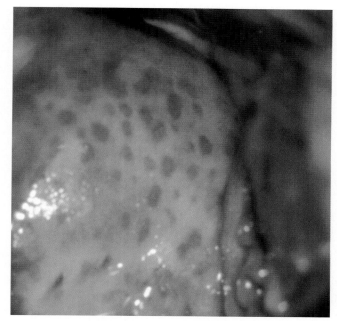

Figure 14–40. Upper vaginal vault, seen with green filter, shows diffuse pattern of "strawberry" epithelium as seen in trichomoniasis vaginalis and other severe vaginal inflammations.

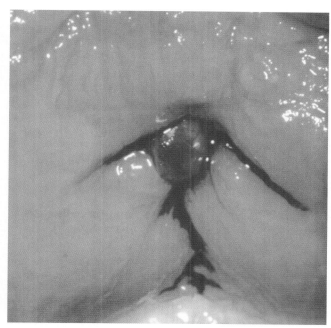

Figure 14–42. A focal, red, raised area in the upper vagina of a woman 3 months after hysterectomy in an area of granulation tissue.

modified and influenced by the size, location, and number of lesions; the age and health status of the patient; and her willingness to comply with follow-up appointments.

A significant factor in determining the optimal therapy for VAIN rests on whether or not the patient has had a prior hysterectomy for CIN. Soutter[48] suggested that post-hysterectomy VAIN might be prevented by carefully assessing the vagina with colposcopy or, at least, iodine staining before hysterectomy to assess for the presence of vaginal disease. Furthermore, Ireland and Monaghan[49] demonstrated that abnormal epithelium was likely to be buried behind sutures used to close the vaginal vault, thus

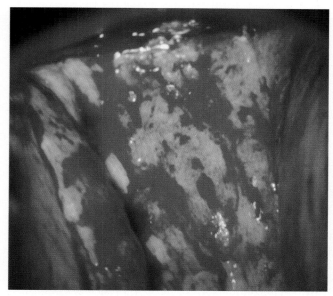

Figure 14–41. Vaginal vault with extensive areas of friable tissue and diffuse areas of atypical vessels. These are seen in a 76-year-old woman with vault prolapse and pessary use for several years. Biopsy revealed marked inflammation. Local therapy with topical estrogen cream and an antibiotic cream resulted in a return to normal.

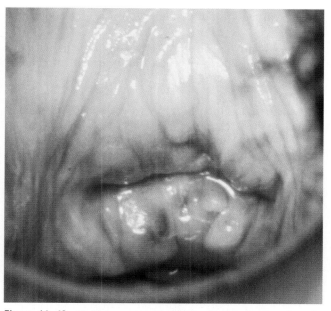

Figure 14–43. Multiple cysts with bluish discoloration noted at the vaginal vault 2 years after hysterectomy for endometriosis. Biopsy revealed endometriosis.

rendering the VAIN lesions invisible and inaccessible. This report showed that 28% of those treated surgically proved to have unexpected invasive disease. On the basis of these data, Soutter concluded that neither laser vaporization nor topical chemotherapy (fluorouracil) should be used as the sole treatment for women with posthysterectomy VAIN and that surgical excision should be strongly considered. Successful surgical excision or partial vaginectomy with laser, as reported by Julian et al,[50] is dependent on the experience and skills of the surgeon.

Surgical Treatment of VAIN

> **If the VAIN lesion is small and unifocal, office excisional biopsy may be sufficient therapy.**

If lesions are small and isolated, office biopsy excision may be sufficient as primary treatment, but care must be taken to ensure that the patient will return for follow-up visits because other lesions are frequently noted after the primary excision.[8] For lesions in young women that may be somewhat larger but still well demarcated, the lesions may be treated by excising strips of epithelium with a small electrosurgical loop electrode. It is essential to avoid deep tissue penetration (beyond 1 to 2 mm) with the loop to prevent injury to adjacent bowel or bladder.[51, 52]

Wharton et al[53] suggested that if there is any suspicion of invasion or if the patient is older than 40 to 45 years, the treatment of choice is partial vaginectomy. Clearly, excision is warranted when there is a need for extended sampling and when there is a significant discrepancy among cytology, colposcopy, and biopsy. The advantage of the procedure is that it provides a specimen for pathologic evaluation. Partial vaginectomy, however, will often result in shortening of the vagina, significant blood loss, and occasional need for a skin graft. Cure rates are reported to be as high as 90%. If invasion is found, the patient will require further therapy, usually radiation.

> **If there is any suspicion of invasion or if the patient is older than 40 to 45 years, the treatment of choice is partial vaginectomy.**

Partial vaginectomy for VAIN can also be accomplished by laser excision.[50] This approach has the advantage of allowing the surgeon to work in a smaller space and may result in less blood loss and less shortening of the vagina. This operative technique requires presurgical treatment of the vagina with topical estrogen in the postmenopausal patient. Before the procedure, the vagina is re-evaluated with colposcopy. Diluted iodine solution can be used to outline the most caudad extent of the VAIN. The laser is then used to outline the extent of the vaginal involvement. Saline solution containing a diluted concentration of a vasoconstrictive agent such as epinephrine or vasopressin is injected beneath the epithelium and serves as a "backstop" for the laser energy. Using cutting power, the incision is started at the lowest posterior margin. Under the continuous visual control of the operating microscope, the edge is elevated and the incision is continu-

ously undercut until the vaginal apex is reached. The procedure is repeated, advancing the incision under the anterior vaginal wall. The apex is finally undercut, and the specimen is removed. Any bleeding points are coagulated with the laser. Postoperatively, the patient may use daily topical estrogen cream in the vagina. No attempt is made to suture or otherwise close the vaginal defect. This approach allows for re-epithelialization of the vagina. The benefit of having a histology specimen is significant if there is concern that invasion may be present. This procedure is appropriate for use by an experienced colposcopist and laser surgeon when the diagnosis cannot be otherwise made by a simpler and less invasive technique.

> **If invasion is found after either biopsy or surgical excision of VAIN, radiation therapy may be indicated.**

If invasion is found after either biopsy or surgical excision of VAIN, radiation therapy may be indicated. DeBuben's[54] intracavitary brachytherapy has been used for treatment of both VAIN and early invasive vaginal carcinoma. The intravaginal application of both high dose rate and low dose rate has been used, with excellent therapeutic results.[55–61] The major concerns with this form of therapy are the possibility of radiation-induced cancer and the potential adverse effects on sexual function.[62, 63]

Laser Vaporization of VAIN

> **When all areas of abnormal epithelium have been fully visualized and sampled by adequate biopsies and there is no suspicion of invasion, laser vaporization of VAIN can be performed.**

When there is no suspicion of invasion, laser ablation by vaporization of the epithelium can be performed. This approach is acceptable only if the areas of abnormal epithelium have been fully visualized and sampled by adequate biopsy.[64–81] The optimal depth of destruction is 1.5 mm. Although this depth was chosen empirically by early investigators, Benedet and colleagues[77] carefully studied histology specimens and performed microscopic measurements with a calibrated micrometer to determine the range of epithelial thickness in both involved and uninvolved vaginal tissue. The significant range of involvement in dysplastic vaginal epithelium ranged from 0.1 to 1.4 mm. Therapeutic success rates for this form of therapy vary between 80% and 85%. Adverse effects of laser vaporization include high, unexplained fevers[78] and later development of vaginal adenosis in the treated areas.[79]

Topical Chemotherapy

> **Topical chemotherapy, such as fluorouracil, has been used as an intravaginal treatment of VAIN with reported cure rates of 80% to 85%.**

The use of the topical cytotoxic antimetabolite fluorouracil for the treatment of preinvasive disease of the vagina was first reported by Woodruff and associates,[80] who

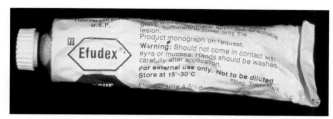

Figure 14–44. Use of fluorouracil cream has been a popular method to treat diffuse vaginal intraepithelial neoplasia.

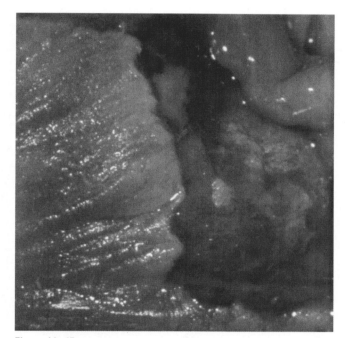

Figure 14–45. An area of denuded epithelium at the vaginal vault. This was noted after the use of intravaginal fluorouracil cream and represents a local "burn" of the vaginal mucosa.

noted successful results in eight of nine treated patients. In 1978, Piver[81] reported on the use of 20% fluorouracil, and, in 1981, Sillman and colleagues described the use of fluorouracil in "chemosurgery."[82] Subsequent reports from several authors[83-89] indicated cure rates that ranged from 80% to 85%. Most of the reported protocols used 5% fluorouracil cream (1.5 to 2 g per intravaginal application) (Fig. 14–44). Various regimens have been used, and all have had similar outcomes. The most commonly used regimen consists of an intravaginal application of 2 g of the 5% fluorouracil cream for 5 to 7 consecutive nights. A thick application of zinc oxide ointment or petroleum jelly is applied to the introitus and the vulvar skin before insertion of the fluorouracil cream to protect the area from irritation, ulceration, and sloughing. Use of a vaginal tampon does not appear to protect the vulva and may reduce the effectiveness of the fluorouracil. The patient is re-evaluated 12 weeks after initiation of therapy. If the patient still has disease, therapy with fluorouracil cream can be repeated once weekly for 10 weeks, or the patient

can be treated with laser therapy. Petrilli et al[32] and Krebs and Helmkamp[90] reported on successive treatments with carbon dioxide laser and topical fluorouracil after a failed first attempt at treatment with fluorouracil.

The side effects of fluorouracil therapy range from minimal to severe. In some cases, the treatments must be discontinued because the side effects are severe. The most common side effects are vaginal burning and dyspareunia.

In a study of long-term sequelae following fluorouracil therapy, Krebs and Helmkamp[90] found that 4 of 25 women developed chemical mucositis 2 to 4 weeks after therapy and 11.4% had acute ulcers. A total of 5.7% of the treated women developed chronic ulcers lasting longer than 6 months (Fig. 14–45), and these numbers increased if there was continued prophylactic use of the cream. Most of the patients who developed ulcers were symptomatic, with a serosanguineous or watery discharge and postcoital or irregular bleeding. Only 50% of these ulcers healed without treatment. The development of vaginal adenosis after treatment has also been reported. Because of the potential adverse events associated with fluorouracil therapy, its use should be confined to treating extensive, widespread, multifocal high-grade VAIN that cannot be treated with other, potentially less morbid modalities.

Other Treatments for VAIN

Cryosurgical therapy has not found a niche in the management of VAIN. The imprecise and unpredictable degree of tissue destruction associated with cryosurgery limits its value for a disease process that is frequently multifocal and is most commonly found in the upper vagina, where potential damage to adjacent organs is greater.[91-93]

Isolated descriptions of the use of other topical agents for treatment of VAIN have been reported. The agents described include interferon, 2,4-dinitrochlorobenzene, and retinoids; more recently, there have been anecdotal reports on the use of imiquimod, especially in immunocompromised patients.[94-96]

INVASIVE CANCER

The most common invasive cancers of the vagina are metastasized from the endometrium, the cervix, or the ovary. Primary squamous cell cancer of the vagina is rare.

The most common invasive cancers of the vagina are metastatic from the endometrium, the cervix, or the ovary. Choriocarcinoma and any intra-abdominal cancer can metastasize to the vagina. Primary squamous cell cancer of the vagina is rare. Peters et al[97] described six patients with superficial or microinvasive vaginal cancer arising in a field of carcinoma in situ, three of whom had no associated cervical lesion. Woodruff and Parmley[98] described a series of malignant tumors arising in the vagina that are not commonly seen in the lower genital tract. These included sarcoma botryoides, endodermal sinus tumor, malignant melanoma, and tumors of the para-

▼ Table 14–3

Classification of Carcinoma of the Vagina

Squamous Cell Carcinoma

Keratinizing
Nonkeratinizing
Verrucous
Warty (condylomatous)

Adenocarcinoma

Clear cell
Endometrioid
Mucinous
Endocervical
Intestinal
Mesonephric

Others

Adenosquamous
Adenoid cystic
Adenoid basal
Carcinoid
Small cell
Undifferentiated

Data from Scully RE, Bonfiglio TA, Kurman RJ: Vulva. In Scully RE (ed): Histological Typing of Female Genital Tract Tumors, 2nd ed. Berlin, Springer-Verlag, 1994, p 9.

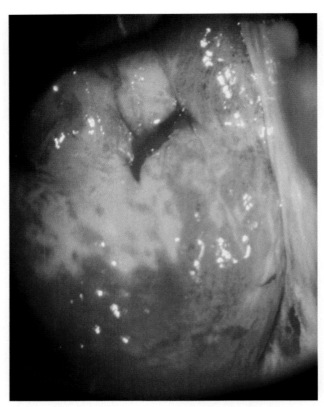

Figure 14–47. Diffuse acetowhitening, mild vascular atypia, and a central ulcer of the vaginal vault. Biopsy reported as early invasive squamous cell carcinoma of the vagina.

vestibular glands—various malignant variants of fibromas and myomas and lymphomas.

The World Health Organization has published a classification of carcinomas of the vagina[99] (Table 14–3). Squamous cell cancers include keratinizing, nonkeratinizing, verrucous, and warty (condylomatous) types (Figs. 14–46, 14–47, 14–48, 14–49, and 14–50). Adenocarcinomas include clear-cell, endometrioid, mucinous, and

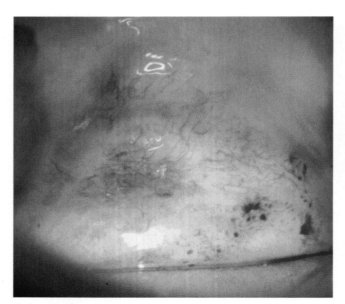

Figure 14–46. Marked vascular atypia and coarse punctation seen at colposcopy. Biopsy revealed early squamous cell carcinoma of the vagina.

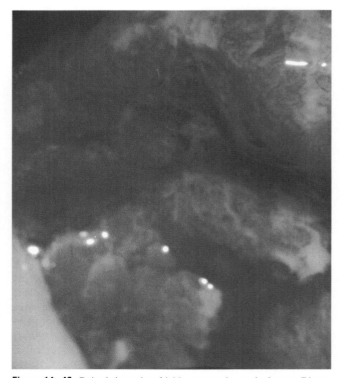

Figure 14–48. Raised, irregular, friable area at the vaginal apex. Biopsy revealed invasive squamous cell carcinoma of the vagina.

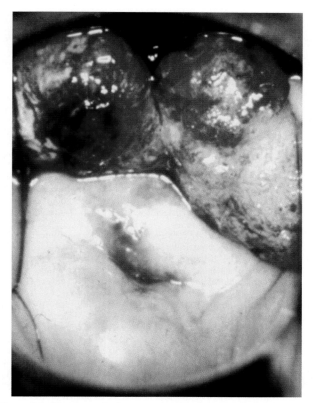

Figure 14–49. Large, bulky mass in the upper vagina with marked atypical vessels in an area of acetowhiteness in the left anterior vagina. Biopsy showed invasive squamous cell carcinoma.

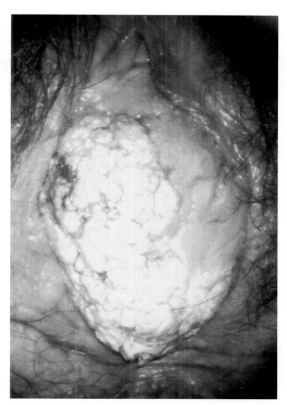

Figure 14–50. Vaginal vault prolapse in a 76-year-old woman after prior hysterectomy revealed a thick hyperkeratotic area over the right two thirds of the prolapsed vaginal epithelium. Biopsy revealed invasive squamous cell carcinoma.

mesonephric types. Other vaginal cancers include adenosquamous, adenoid cystic, and adenoid basal, as well as carcinoid, small-cell, and undifferentiated types.

Most vaginal cancers are initially asymptomatic but may be associated with vaginal discharge, postcoital staining, or malodor. A high index of suspicion is often required to make an early diagnosis. If colposcopic findings are present, atypical vessels are usually seen.

SUMMARY OF KEY POINTS

- Vaginal neoplasms account for 1% to 4% of all gynecologic malignancies.

- VAIN is being identified more frequently in younger women and is usually associated with HPV infection.

- VAIN 1 and VAIN 2 are representative of more benign viral proliferation, whereas VAIN 3 may be a true cancer precursor.

- Between 36% an 48% of women with VAIN have concurrent CIN.

- The natural history of VAIN has not been clearly defined. Most low-grade VAIN probably regresses spontaneously without treatment. The risk of progression of VAIN 3 to invasion appears to be far less than the risk of progression of CIN to cervical carcinoma.

- Patients with VAIN are usually asymptomatic and become aware of their condition only after an abnormal Pap smear is reported.

- The most common clinical presentation for VAIN is in a patient who has undergone hysterectomy for CIN 3. Presenting lesions are usually located on the anterior or posterior vaginal walls and may be hidden by the speculum.

- Evidence at this time does not indicate the need to continue routine Pap smears in women who have had hysterectomies for benign disease.

- Patients with a history of abnormal cytologic smears or gynecologic malignancy should continue to be screened.

- Colposcopic examination of the vagina is more technically difficult than is colposcopy of the cervix. The application of half-strength Lugol's solution to the vaginal mucosa after examination with 5% acetic acid may be helpful in identifying multifocal areas of epithelial change or areas that are difficult to detect by gross visual inspection.

Continued on following page

- Vascular patterns tend to be absent in VAIN 1 but present in VAIN 3. Lesions that are raised, exophytic, or nodular or exhibit abnormal or atypical vessels should raise suspicion for invasion.

- Treatment for VAIN should be carefully individualized. VAIN therapies may include observation of VAIN 1, surgical excision, ablation, radiation, and topical chemotherapy. The treatments are modified and influenced by the size, location, and number of the lesions; the age and health status of the patient; the need to preserve vaginal function; and the patient's compliance with follow-up appointments.

- If VAIN lesions are small, office biopsy excision may be sufficient. For larger but well-demarcated lesions, excision with the electrosurgical loop electrode may be sufficient. For more extensive and severe lesions, partial vaginectomy, possibly with laser, may be appropriate.

- If there is any suspicion of invasion, or if the patient is older than 40 to 50 years, partial vaginectomy is the treatment of choice, and cure rates approach 90%.

- If there is no suspicion of invasion, laser vaporization can be performed. Therapeutic success rates vary between 80% and 85%.

- Use of topical chemotherapy (i.e., fluorouracil) for treatment of VAIN results in reported cure rates of 80% to 85%. However, adverse effects are common and include irritation, ulceration, and sloughing. The use of fluorouracil should be confined to treating extensive, multifocal VAIN.

- A total of 5.7% of women treated with intravaginal fluorouracil develop chronic vaginal ulcers lasting longer than 6 months.

References

1. Platzer W, Poisel S, Hafez ESE: Functional anatomy of the human vagina. In Hafez ESE, Evans TN (eds): The Human Vagina. London, Elsevier, 1978, pp 41–53.
2. Davis GD: Colposcopic examination of the vagina. Obstet Gynecol Clin North Am 1993;20:217.
3. Coppleson M, Pixley E, Reid B: The vagina. In Coppleson MC, Pixley E (eds): Colposcopy, 3rd ed. New York, Charles C Thomas, 1985, pp 403–434.
4. Cruveilhier J: Varices des veines du ligament rond, simulant une hernie inguinale: Anomalie remarquable dans la disposition general du peritoine: Cancer ulcere la parol anterieure du vagin et bas-sond de la vessie. Bull Soc Anat Paris 1826;1:199.
5. Hummer WK, Mussey E, Decker DG, Dockerty MG: Carcinoma in situ of the vagina. Am J Obstet Gynecol 1970;108:1109.
6. Woodruff JD: Carcinoma in situ of the vagina. Clin Obstet Gynecol 1981;24:485.
7. DeSaia PJ, Morrow CP, Townsend DE (eds): Synopsis of Gynecologic Oncology. New York, John Wiley & Sons, 1975.
8. Townsend DE: Intraepithelial neoplasia of the vagina. In Coppleson M (ed): Gynecologic Oncology. Edinburgh, Churchill Livingstone, 1992, pp 493–499.
9. Lopes A, Monaghan JM, Roberston G: Vaginal intraepithelial neoplasia. In Luesley D, Jordan J, Richart RM (eds): Intraepithelial Neoplasia of the Lower Genital Tract. Edinburgh, Churchill Livingstone, 1995, pp 169–176.
10. Timonen S, von Numers C, Meyer B: Dysplasia of the vaginal epithelium. Gynecologica 1966;162:125.
11. Cramer DN, Cutler SJ: Incidence and histology of malignancies of the female genital organ in the U.S. Am J Obstet Gynecol 1974; 118:443.
12. Hollingworth A, Cuzick J: The epidemiology of precancerous lesions of the female lower genital tract. In Clinical Practice of Gynecology. London, Elsevier Science, 1990, pp 1–21.
13. Graham JB, Meigs JV: Recurrence of tumour after total hysterectomy for carcinoma in situ. Am J Obstet Gynecol 1952;64:1159.
14. Aho M, Vesterinen E, Meyer B, et al: Natural history of vaginal intraepithelial neoplasia. Cancer 1991;68:195.
15. Lenehan PM, Meffe F, Lickrish GM: Vaginal intraepithelial neoplasia: Biologic aspects and management. Obstet Gynecol 1986;68:189.
16. Mao CC, Chao KC, Lian YC, Ng HT: Vaginal intraepithelial neoplasia: Diagnosis and management. Chin Med J (Taipei) 1990; 46:35.
17. Audet-Lapointe P, Body G, Vauclair R, et al: Vaginal intraepithelial neoplasia. Gynec Oncol 1990;36:232.
18. Schneider A, de Villiers EM, Schneider V: Multifocal squamous neoplasia of the female genital tract: Significance of human papillomavirus infection of the vagina after hysterectomy. Obstet Gynecol 1987;70:294.
19. Bornstein J, Kaufman RH, Adam E, Adler-Storhz K: HPV associated with vaginal intraepithelial neoplasia in women exposed to DES in utero. Obstet Gynecol 1987;97:58.
20. Sillman FH, Sedlis A, Boyce JG: A review of lower genital intraepithelial neoplasia and the use of topical 5-fluorouracil. Obstet Gynecol Survey 1985;40:1990.
21. Benedet JL, Sanders BH: Carcinoma in situ of the vagina. Am J Obstet Gynecol 1984;148:695.
22. Kanbour AI, Klionsky B, Murphy AI: Carcinoma of the vagina following cervical cancer. Cancer 1974;34:1838.
23. Gemmell J, Holmes DM, Duncan ID: How frequently need vaginal smears be taken after hysterectomy for cervical intraepithelial neoplasia? Br J Obstet Gynecol 1990;97:635.
24. Novak ER, Woodruff JD: Postirradiation malignancies of the pelvic organs. Am J Obstet Gynecol 1959;77:617.
25. Rutledge F: Cancer of the vagina Am J Obstet Gynecol 1967;97: 635.
26. Taylor ES: Discussion: Cancer of the vagina. Am J Obstet Gynecol 1967;97:635.
27. Halpert R, Fruchter RG, Sedlis A, et al: Human papillomavirus and lower genital neoplasia in renal transplant patients. Obstet Gynecol 1986;68:251.
28. Robboy SJ, Noller KL, O'Brien P, et al: Increased incidence of cervical and vaginal dysplasia in 3,980 diethylstilbestrol (DES) exposed young women: Experience of the National Collaborative DES-Adenosis (DESAD) Project. JAMA 1984;252:2979.
29. Ferenczy A, Wright TC: Anatomy and histology of the cervix. In Kurman RJ (ed): Blaustein's Pathology of the Female Genital Tract, 4th ed. New York, Springer-Verlag, 1994, p 185.
30. Sherman ME, Paull G: Reproducibility of pathologic diagnosis and correlation of smears and biopsies. Acta Cytol 1993;37:699.
31. Jenkins D: The pathology of lower genital tract premalignancy. In Clinical Practice of Gynecology. Edinburgh, Elsevier Science, 1990, pp 51–85.
32. Petrilli ES, Townsend DE, Morrow CP, Nakao CY: Vaginal intraepithelial neoplasia: Biologic aspects and treatment with topical 5-fluorouracil and the carbon dioxide laser. Am J Obstet Gynecol 1980;138:321.
33. Wharton JT, Tortolero-Luna G, Linares AC, et al: Vaginal intraepithelial neoplasia and vaginal cancer. Obstet Gynecol Clin North Am 1996;23:325.
34. Rhodes-Morris HE: Treatment of vulvar intraepithelial neoplasia and vaginal intraepithelial neoplasia. Clin Consult Obstet Gynecol 1994;6:44.
35. Nwabineli NJ, Monaghan JM: Vaginal epithelial abnormalities in patients with CIN: Clinical and pathological features and management. Brit J Obstet Gynecol 1991;98:25.
36. Fetters MD, Fischer G, Reed BD: Effectiveness of vaginal Papanicolaou smear screening after total hysterectomy for benign disease. JAMA 1996;275:940.
37. Pearce KF, Haefner HK, Sarwar SF, Nolan TE: Cytopathological

findings on vaginal Papanicolaou smears after hysterectomy for benign gynecologic disease. N Engl J Med 1996;335:1559.

38. Piscitelli JT, Bastian LA, Wilkes A, Simel DL: Cytologic screening after hysterectomy for benign disease. Am J Obstet Gynecol 1995; 173:424.

39. Fox J, Remington P, Layde P, Klein G: The effect of hysterectomy on the risk of an abnormal screening Papanicolaou test result. Am J Obstet Gynecol 1999;180:1104.

40. Noller KL: Screening for vaginal cancer. N Engl J Med 1996;335: 1599.

41. Ponder TB, Easley KO, Davila RM: Glandular cells in vaginal smears from posthysterectomy patients. Acta Cytol 1997;41: 1701.

42. Bewtra C: Columnar cells in posthysterectomy vaginal smears. Diagn Cytopathol 1992;8:342.

43. Ramirez PE, Valente PT: Paradoxical glandular cells in vaginal cuff cytology: Metaplasia versus neoplasia. Acta Cytol 1995;980.

44. Clement PB: Adenocarcinoma in situ of the vagina: A case report. Cancer 1979;43:2479.

45. Stafl A, Mattingly RF: Vaginal adenosis: A precancerous lesion? Am J Obstet Gynecol 1974;120:666.

46. Scurry J, Planner R, Grant P: Unusual variants of vaginal adenosis: A challenge for diagnosis and treatment. Gynecol Oncol 1991;41: 172.

47. Liu LY, Hou YJ, Li JZ: Primary malignant melanoma of the vagina: A report of seven cases. Obstet Gynecol 1987;70:569.

48. Soutter WP: Commentary: The treatment of vaginal intraepithelial neoplasia after hysterectomy. Br J Obstet Gynecol 1988;95: 961.

49. Ireland D, Monaghan JM: The management of the patient with abnormal vaginal cytology following hysterectomy. Br J Obstet Gynecol 1988;95:973.

50. Julian TM, O'Connell BJ, Gosewehr JA: Indications, techniques, and advantages of partial laser vaginectomy. Obstet Gynecol 1992; 80:140.

51. Ferenczy A: Personal communication, September 1993.

52. Patsner B: Treatment of vaginal dysplasia with loop excision: Report of five cases. Am J Obstet Gynecol 1993;169:179.

53. Wharton JT, Tortolero-Luna G, Linares AC, et al: Vaginal intraepithelial neoplasia and vaginal cancer. Obstet Gynecol Clin North Am 1996;23:325.

54. DeBuben I: Radium in the treatment of cancer of the vagina. Surg Gynecol Obstet 1931;52:844.

55. Brown GR, Fletcher GH, Rutledge FN: Irradiation of "in-situ" and invasive squamous cell carcinomas of the vagina. Cancer 1971;28: 1278.

56. Usherwood MM: Management of vaginal carcinoma after hysterectomy. Am J Obstet Gynecol 1975;122:352.

57. Woodman CB, Mould JJ, Jordan JA: Radiotherapy in the management of vaginal intraepithelial neoplasia after hysterectomy. Br J Obstet Gynecol 1988;95:976.

58. Oliver JA: Severe dysplasia and carcinoma in situ of the vagina. Am J Obstet Gynecol 1979;134:133.

59. Stock RG, Mychalczàk B, Armstrong JG, et al: The importance of brachytherapy technique in the management of primary carcinoma of the vagina. J Radiat Oncol Biol Phys 1992;24:747.

60. MacLeod C, Fowler A, Dalrymple C, et al: High-dose-rate brachytherapy in the management of high-grade intraepithelial neoplasia of the vagina. Gynec Oncol 1997;65:74.

61. Ogino I: High-dose rate intracavitary brachytherapy in the management of cervical and vaginal intraepithelial neoplasia. Int J Radiat Oncol Biol Phys 1998;40:881.

62. Barrie JR, Brunschwig A: Late second cancers after apparent successful initial radiation therapy. Am J Roentgenol Ther Nucl Med 1970;108:109.

63. Boice JD, Day NE, Andersen A: Second cancers following treatment for cervical cancer. J Natl Cancer Inst 1985;74:955.

64. Stafl A, Wilkinson EJ, Mattingly RF: Laser treatment of cervical and vaginal intraepithelial neoplasia. Am J Obstet Gynecol 1977; 128:128.

65. Capen CC, Masteerson BJ, Magrina JF, et al: Laser therapy of vaginal intraepithelial neoplasia. Am J Obstet Gynecol 1982;142: 873.

66. Townsend DE, Levine RU, Crum CP, et al: Treatment of vaginal carcinoma in situ with the carbon dioxide laser. Am J Obstet Gynecol 1982;143:565.

67. Jobson VW, Homesley HD: Treatment of vaginal intraepithelial neoplasia with the carbon dioxide laser. Obstet Gynecol 1983; 62:90.

68. Stein S: Carbon dioxide laser surgery of the cervix, vagina and vulva. Surg Clin North Am 1984;885.

69. Woodman CBJ, Jordan JA, Wade-Evans T: The management of VAIN after hysterectomy. Br J Obstet Gynecol 1984;91:707.

70. Curtin JP, Twiggs LB, Julian TM: Treatment of vaginal intraepithelial neoplasia with the carbon dioxide laser. J Reprod Med 1985;30: 942.

71. Stuart GC: Laser vaporization of vaginal intraepithelial neoplasia. Am J Obstet Gynecol 1988;158:240.

72. Sherman AI: Laser therapy for vaginal intraepithelial neoplasia after hysterectomy. J Reprod Med 1990;35:941.

73. Jobson VW, Campion MJ: Vaginal laser surgery. Obstet Gynecol Clin North Am 1991;18:511.

74. Hoffman MS, DeCesare SL: Laser vaporization of grade 3 vaginal intraepithelial neoplasia. Am J Obstet Gynecol 1991;165:134.

75. Volante R, Pasero L, Saraceno L, et al: Carbon dioxide laser surgery in colposcopy for cervicovaginal intraepithelial neoplasia treatment. Ten years experience and failure analysis. Eur J Gynaecol Oncol 1992;13:78.

76. Diakomanolis E, Rodolakis A, Sakellaropoulos G, et al: Conservative management of vaginal intraepithelial neoplasia (VAIN) by carbon dioxide laser. Eur J Gynaecol Oncol 1996;17:389.

77. Benedet JL, Wilson PS, Matisic JP: Epidermal thickness measurements in VAIN. A basis for optimal CO_2 laser vaporization. J Reprod Med 1992;37:809.

78. Spitzer M, Krumholz BA, Seltzer VS, et al: Fevers in patients undergoing vaginal laser surgery. Obstet Gynecol 1988;71:480.

79. Sedlacek TV, Riva JM, Magen AB, et al: Vaginal and vulvar adenosis. An unsuspected side effect of carbon dioxide laser vaporization. J Reprod Med 1990;35:995.

80. Woodruff JD, Parmley TH, Julian CG: Topical 5-fluorouracil in the treatment of vaginal CIS. Gynec Oncol 1975;3:124.

81. Piver MS, Barlow JJ, Tsukada Y, et al: Postirradiation squamous cell carcinoma in situ of the vagina: Treatment by topical 20 percent 5-fluorouracil cream. Am J Obstet Gynecol 1979;135:377.

82. Sillman FH, Boyce JG, Macaset MA, et al: 5-Fluorouracil/chemosurgery for intraepithelial neoplasia of the lower genital tract. Obstet Gynecol 1981;58:356.

83. Ballon SC, Roberts JA, Lagasse LD: Topical 5-fluorouracil in the treatment of intraepithelial neoplasia of the vagina. Obstet Gynecol 1979;54:163.

84. Stokes JM, Sworn MJ, Hawthorne JHR: A new regimen for the treatment of vaginal carcinoma in situ using 5-fluorouracil. Br J Obstet Gynecol 1980;87:920.

85. Bowen-Simpkins P, Hull MGR: Intraepithelial vaginal neoplasia following immunosuppressive therapy treated with topical 5-FU. Obstet Gynecol 1975;43:360.

86. Daly JW, Ellis GF: Treatment of vaginal dysplasia and carcinoma in situ with topical 5-fluorouracil. Obstet Gynecol 1980;55:350.

87. Pride GL, Chuprevich TW: Topical 5-fluorouracil treatment of transformation zone intraepithelial neoplasia of cervix and vagina. Obstet Gynecol 1982;60:467.

88. Caglar H, Hertzog RW, Hreshchyshyn MM: Topical 5-fluorouracil treatment of vaginal intraepithelial neoplasia. Obstet Gynecol 1981; 58:580.

89. Krebs HB: Treatment of VAIN with laser and topical 5-flourouracil. Obstet Gynecol 1989;73:657.

90. Krebs HB, Helmkamp F: Chronic ulceration following topical therapy with 5-fluorouracil for vaginal human papillomavirus–associated lesions. Obstet Gynecol 1991;78:205.

91. Adducci J: Carcinoma in situ of the vagina. Treatment by combined excision and cryosurgery. Geriatrics 1972;121.

92. Jobson VW: Cryotherapy and laser treatment for intraepithelial neoplasia of the cervix, vagina and vulva. Oncology 1991;5:69.

93. Kirwan PH, Smith IR, Naftalin NJ: A study of cryosurgery and the carbon dioxide laser in treatment of CIS of the uterine cervix. Gynecol Oncol 1985;22:195.

94. Guthrie D, Way S: Immunotherapy of non-clinical vaginal cancer. Lancet 1975;2:1242.

95. Mathe G, Busuttil M, Reynes M, et al: Triptorelin in treatment of cervical and vaginal dysplasia related to papillomavirus. Lancet 1988;819.

96. Yliskoski M, Cantell K, Syrjanen K, et al: Topical treatment with human leukocyte interferon of HPV 16 infections associated with cervical and vaginal intraepithelial neoplasias. Gynecol Oncol 1990; 36:353.

97. Peters WA, Kumar NB, Morley GW: Microinvasive carcinoma of the vagina: A distinct clinical entity? Am J Obstet Gynecol 1985; 153:505.

98. Woodruff JFD, Parmley TH: Vaginal tumors, benign and malignant. In Hafez ESE, Evans TN (eds): The Human Vagina. Amsterdam, North-Holland Publishing, 1978, pp 371–381.

99. Scully RE, Bonfiglio TA, Kurman RJ: Vulva. In Scully RE (ed): Histological Typing of Female Genital Tract Tumors, 2nd ed. Berlin, Springer-Verlag, 1994, p 9.

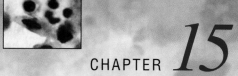

• Lynette Margesson

CHAPTER *15*

Non-neoplastic Epithelial Lesions of the Vulva

Colposcopists have a superb opportunity to recognize and initiate management for women with vulvar disease.

All too commonly, vulvar disorders are missed. They are not seen or are not recognized by caregivers. Cursory histories are taken, quick Papanicolaou (Pap) tests are finished, and the next year's appointment is set. The vulva is hardly seen, and any changes in normal anatomy are not recognized. Colposcopists have a superb opportunity to recognize and initiate management for women with vulvar disease. They are in a perfect position to visualize the vulva, magnify areas as necessary, and biopsy any questionable lesions.

The examiner must be familiar with variations in the normal vulvar anatomy and with vulvar dermatoses. Women often receive little to no education about their external genitalia. Many caregivers also lack education in this area. This chapter will cover briefly the appearance of the normal vulva and the major vulvar dermatoses, with a short review of their management. The focus is on the recognition of these conditions.

NORMAL VULVAR ARCHITECTURE

The lack of a protective keratinized surface in the vulvar vestibule to act as a barrier explains why the tissue is so easily irritated and infected under certain circumstances, such as incontinence.

The vulva is a structure between the thighs bounded laterally by the genitocrural folds, anteriorly by the mons pubis, and posteriorly by the posterior commissure. The main anatomic structures include the mons pubis, labia majora, labia minora, clitoris, vestibule, urethral meatus, hymen, vestibular glands, and Bartholin's glands. The innermost aspect of the vulva is the vestibule; it encompasses the openings of the urinary tract with the urethral meatus and the vagina with the hymenal ring. It is de-

fined as the part of the vulva that extends from the clitoral frenulum, posteriorly to the posterior commissure and laterally to Hart's line, where the nonkeratinized transitional epithelium of the vestibule joins the keratinized squamous epithelium at the base of the medial aspects of the labia minora. The nonkeratinized squamous epithelium in this area contrasts with the keratinized surface of the labia majora and with skin elsewhere and has greater similarity to the mucous membranes of the oropharynx. This explains the similar changes seen in both areas in conditions such as lichen planus and aphthae. The lack of a protective keratinized surface in this tissue to act as a barrier explains why it is so easily irritated and infected under certain circumstances, such as incontinence.

Role of Age and Hormones

At birth, placental estrogen plumps up the hymen and the vestibule. As girls grow into infancy and then childhood, the hymen and the vestibule thin and atrophy, leaving them susceptible to trauma.

The normal appearance of the vulva is variable depending on age and ethnic background. Hormones further modify the size and shape of the labia, the hymenal ring, the degree of pigmentation, and the hair growth. The labia minora vary widely in size, shape, and texture, ranging from small, smooth, and symmetrical to asymmetrical, long, and notched. There can be considerable variation in the appearance of the hymen, from the normal crescentic appearance to a cribriform or imperforate hymen. At birth, placental estrogen plumps up the hymen and the vestibule. Through infancy and then childhood, the hymen and the vestibule thin and atrophy, leaving them susceptible to trauma. In infancy, the labia majora are prominent, the labia minora are small, the vulvar area is hairless, and the hymen is intact. With puberty, hair develops over the labia majora, mons pubis, and perineum, with variable increase in pigmentation of the labia. The labia minora are more prominent, and the vulvar trigone is pink and moist. After menopause, with loss of estrogen, the vulvar vestibule pales, the hair thins and whitens, and the pigmentation fades. The labia majora thin, and the labia minora can exhibit significant atrophy. The clitoris may become more prominent because of the relative increase in androgens. The introitus may be significantly altered, depending on trauma from previous pregnancies and associated weakening of the pelvic floor.[1-4]

Hypoestrogenic atrophy results in loss or alteration of epithelial barrier functions, resulting in increased susceptibility to irritation and infection

Atrophic vulvovaginitis develops with loss of adequate estrogen. Loss of estrogen can result from natural or surgical menopause, antiandrogens, selective estrogen receptor modulators, or ovarian dysfunction. Relative lack of estrogen also develops before menarche, during breastfeeding, and post partum. The result is a thin, relatively dry vulvovaginal epithelium. Epithelial barrier functions are altered, resulting in increased susceptibility to irritation and infection. Patients may complain of vulvar burning, dysuria, pruritus, tenderness, and dyspareunia. On examination of the vulvar trigone and vagina, the epithelium is pale and thinned, and the vaginal folds are smoothed (Fig. 15–1). There may be introital stenosis, petechiae, and fissuring. In severe cases, there may be a heavy, malodorous discharge. Treatment involves avoidance of irritants and topical or systemic replacement of estrogen.

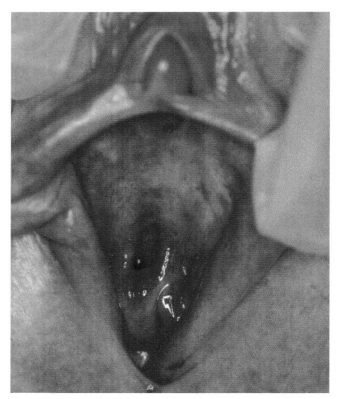

Figure 15–1. Atrophic vulva. Slightly enlarged clitoris owing to loss of estrogen, with a pale, thin vulvar vestibule.

Anatomic Variants

The most frequently misinterpreted vulvar anatomic variations are sebaceous hyperplasia and vulvar papillomatosis.

The most frequently misinterpreted vulvar anatomic variations are sebaceous hyperplasia and vulvar papillomatosis. The sebaceous glands on the inner aspect of the labia minora in some patients may be very prominent, coalescing into yellow, cobbled plaques. They can be confused with neoplasia or rashes. They are harmless glands that cause no symptoms or problems. Reassurance is all that is needed. Around the vulvar vestibule in premenopausal women, vestibular papillae can develop. These are tubular to slightly filiform projections that are symmetrical, soft, and completely asymptomatic. They are easily confused with condylomata. Condylomata are firm, often asymmetrical, filiform papules that are skin colored to reddish. Colposcopy, palpation, or biopsy will differentiate them. Patient reassurance is all that is needed.

History and Physical Examination

Excessive hygiene practices with caustic or highly perfumed products may result in marked irritation.

The clinical evaluation of the patient with vulvar complaints can take time. Many of these patients have chronic symptoms and have had multiple ineffective treatments. It is important to listen patiently and nonjudgementally to these patients. The history should be accurately documented, noting previous treatments, response to treatment, and so on. Note use of over-the-counter preparations and hygiene practices along with the usual menstrual, sexual, and gynecologic history. Excessive hygiene practices with caustic or highly perfumed products may result in marked irritation.

The most common symptoms of vulvar disease are pruritus and pain, alone or in combination. Pain may be manifested as burning. It is important to further characterize the symptoms by noting menstrual association, interventions that relieve or worsen the symptoms, degree of incapacity, when in the menstrual cycle the symptoms occur, and any tendency toward recurrence.

Consider looking elsewhere on the body surface to confirm certain diagnoses, such as examining the oral mucosa to diagnose lichen planus or examining the elbows and knees to confirm that a diffuse, red, scaly rash on the vulva is psoriasis.

During the physical examination, the entire lower genital tract should be examined. The absence of certain anatomic landmarks such as the labia minora should be noted. It is important to check for contracture of the clitoral hood or stenosis of the introitus. Consider looking elsewhere on the body surface to confirm certain diagnoses, such as examining the oral mucosa to diagnose lichen planus or examining the elbows and knees to confirm that a diffuse, red, scaly rash on the vulva is psoriasis. Proper lighting is imperative. It should be bright without glare. Magnification should be used as needed. The signs of vulvar disease are erythema, whiteness, lichenification, purpura, crusting, erosions, ulcerations, exudate, discharge, scarring, and loss of architecture. Questionable areas should be biopsied as needed.[5–7]

With an organized approach and a little training and experience, recognizing vulvar disease can be simplified and can be very rewarding for the patient and the practitioner.

ECZEMA

> **Eczema and dermatitis are synonyms.**

Eczema and dermatitis are synonyms. Eczema is an inflammatory rash on the skin owing to a variety of causes—allergens, irritants, atopy, or seborrhea. Pathologically, all show epidermal spongiosis, with or without acanthosis, and perivascular lymphohistiocytic infiltrates in the dermis. All these conditions can involve the vulva. Other skin or vulvar conditions can be involved secondarily (e.g., irritated lichen sclerosus, lichen sclerosus with an associated allergic contact dermatitis).

ATOPIC DERMATITIS

> **Atopic dermatitis is a very itchy, inflammatory, recurrent dermatosis. It affects up to 20% of the population.**

Atopic dermatitis is a very itchy, inflammatory, recurrent dermatosis. It typically occurs in early childhood in children with a family or personal history of one or more of the following atopic conditions: asthma, hay fever, or eczema. Atopic dermatitis now affects up to 20% of the population. In vulvar patients, it may not be recognized.

> **Atopic dermatitis can be exacerbated by fungal, bacterial, and viral skin infections (most commonly with *Staphylococcus aureus*), directly or with superantigens.**

Atopic patients have an underlying, genetically based, immunoregulatory abnormality. The condition develops as a result of a complex interrelationship among genetic, environmental, immunologic, and pharmacologic factors. Allergic reactions play a role in some patients. In others, (less than 30%) there is disturbance of skin function, infection, and stress. The factors involved in the pathogenesis of atopic dermatitis include the pattern of local cytokine expression, differentiation of helper T cells, multiple roles of immunoglobulin E (IgE), skin-directed cell responses, infectious agents, and superantigens. Cytokines modulate tissue inflammation. The T cells TH1 and TH2, regulated by genetics, cytokines, and pharmacologic factors, play an important role, along with IgE. Skin infections exacerbate and maintain skin inflammation.[8–10] Atopic dermatitis can be exacerbated by fungal, bacterial, and viral skin infections, directly or with superantigens.

Staphylococcus aureus is the most common infectious agent to exacerbate and maintain atopic dermatitis this way.[8, 11–13]

> **Patients with atopic dermatitis have a more permeable skin barrier, with increased water loss resulting in chronically dry skin.**

Epidermal barrier function is defective in atopic patients. These patients have a more permeable skin barrier, with increased water loss resulting in chronically dry skin. This dry skin may provide an entry for allergens, irritants, and skin pathogens.[8]

In atopic patients, inflammation triggers cellular processes, and eczematous lesions are the result. This readily induced, ongoing inflammation and altered skin immune response leads to the secondary changes of xerosis, itching, rubbing, scratching, lichenification, weeping, and secondary infection.[14] Typically, atopic patients react to irritants like soaps, cleansers, perfume products, and even sanitary napkins. As in all itchy rashes, heat, humidity, and stress make the condition worse. Patients then develop an itch-scratch-itch cycle that can result in the development of lichen simplex chronicus.

> **The symptoms of atopic dermatitis are itching and irritation. With excessive scratching, there may be burning, rawness, and even pain.**

Most atopic patients are children with itchy rashes on the limbs and torso. The vulva may be involved, but not commonly. In adults, there is little information about vulvar involvement. The vulva is probably more commonly affected than is realized. The symptoms are itching and irritation. With excessive scratching, there may be burning, rawness, and even pain. There is often a history of a precipitating irritant.

> **On the vulva, the pattern most commonly seen is subacute or chronic atopic dermatitis, with mild redness, dryness, and fine scaling involving the labia majora, inner thighs, and gluteal cleft.**

On physical examination, various stages of atopic dermatitis are seen, depending on the chronicity of the condition. In acute disease, there are ill-defined red papules forming small plaques over erythematous skin. Secondary changes from intense scratching are excoriations, erosions, and weeping, with or without changes of secondary infection. On the vulva, the pattern most commonly seen is subacute or chronic, with mild redness, dryness, and fine scaling, with or without the secondary changes noted above. The area involved includes the labia majora and, variably, the labia minora; the inner thighs; and the gluteal cleft (Fig. 15–2). Changes of lichen simplex chronicus may be seen (see the following discussion). With secondary infection, honey-colored crusting is seen.[15, 16] The diagnosis is made based on the criteria noted earlier plus the clinical pattern on physical examination. A detailed history is needed, with emphasis on family history of atopy, contactants, and so on. Histology is seldom necessary. The differential diagnosis includes contact der-

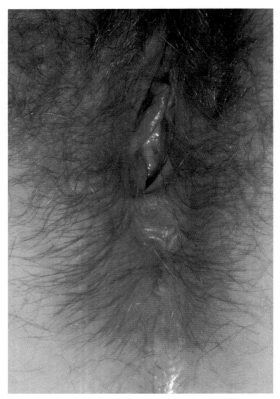

Figure 15–2. Atopic dermatitis. Subacute dermatitis of the vulva and perineum, with mild redness around inferior labia majora, perineum, and perianal area extending to gluteal cleft.

matitis, eczematous candidiasis, psoriasis, and seborrheic dermatitis.

Treatment is directed at preventing inflammation, itching, and secondary problems. The triggering factors must be removed, the skin must be hydrated, and mid-potency corticosteroids are used.

Treatment is directed at preventing inflammation, itching, and secondary problems. The triggering factors must be removed. All irritating soaps, lotions, and hygiene products must no longer be used. Cool, ventilated, loose clothing of natural fibers is best. Stress must be addressed. Allergens should be identified and eliminated if possible. Dry skin must be controlled. Bathing hydrates the skin and soothes open, excoriated areas. During bathing, very little cleanser is necessary—only a mild, unscented soap substitute should be used. After the soak, an ointment must be applied, both as an emollient to retain moisture and as a vehicle for medication. It is best to use a mid-potency corticosteroid like triamcinolone acetonide 0.1% ointment twice a day for 1 to 2 weeks and then intermittently, supplemented with plain petrolatum. Infection must be treated with appropriate antibiotics. Pruritus can be alleviated with antihistamines, local cold packs, and gentle care.[13–15, 17, 18] The new topical immunomodulator ointment, tacrolimus, is safe and effective in children and adults and may prove to be an excellent alternative to topical corticosteroids.[19, 20]

LICHEN SIMPLEX CHRONICUS

Lichen simplex chronicus is the end stage of the itch-scratch-itch cycle. Intense, chronic pruritus results in repetitive rubbing and scratching, thickening, and increased skin markings called lichenification.

Lichen simplex chronicus is the end stage of the itch-scratch-itch cycle. Outdated synonyms for lichen simplex chronicus include neurodermatitis, squamous hyperplasia, and hyperplastic dystrophy. Intense, chronic pruritus results in repetitive rubbing and scratching. The skin responds by thickening, with increased skin markings called lichenification.[21] This lichenified skin develops in previously normal skin, especially in atopic patients. It does, however, also develop as a common end point of several conditions that are chronically scratched (e.g., lichen sclerosus, contact dermatitis).[22] Conditions that may underlie lichen simplex chronicus are listed in Table 15–1. The most important of these are atopic dermatitis, contact dermatitis, and psoriasis.[23]

The defining characteristic of lichen simplex chronicus is relentless pruritus that is worse with heat, stress, and menstruation. The patient has often had years of chronic itch.

Many of the pathophysiologic mechanisms in this condition are the same as those in atopic dermatitis (see previous section). There is an altered barrier function, with involvement of allergens, irritants, and skin pathogens along with altered immunoregulatory processes. Stress plays a major role in this condition, and that further deranges epidermal function.[24] The defining characteristic of lichen simplex chronicus is relentless pruritus that is worse with heat, stress, and menstruation. The patient has often had years of chronic itch. Typically, she states that "nothing helps." Patients wake up at night

▼ Table 15–1

Conditions That May Underlie Lichen Simplex Chronicus

Infections
Candidiasis
Dermatophytosis
Dermatoses
Atopic dermatitis
Lichen sclerosus
Lichen planus
Psoriasis
Metabolic Conditions
Diabetes
Iron-deficiency anemia
Neoplasias
Vulvar intraepithelial neoplasia

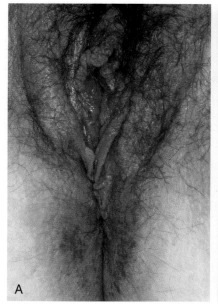
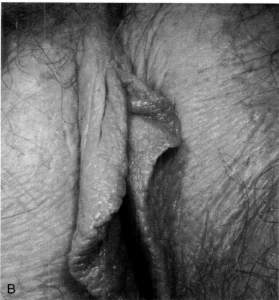

Figure 15–3. *A,* Lichen simplex chronicus. Marked lichenification, erythema, and swelling of labia majora with excoriations, erosions, and perianal crusting. *B,* Lichen simplex chronicus. Lichenification of medial aspects of the labia majora.

scratching. At times, when the vulva is raw, the symptoms change from itch to burning to even frank pain.

> **On physical examination, the vulvar skin is diffusely thickened with increased skin markings or lichenification. The labia may be enlarged and rugose, with variable edema.**

On physical examination, the vulvar skin is diffusely thickened with increased skin markings or lichenification. The labia may be enlarged and rugose, with variable edema. The involvement may be unilateral or bilateral. It may extend widely out onto the labiocrural and inguinal folds. The color is variable with a variety of shades—pink, red, violet, or ruddy brown. There can be hyperpigmentation or hypopigmentation. Scratching results in loss of hair. With continued excoriations, there are open erosions with oozing, fissuring, and honey-colored to serosanguineous crusting[25, 26] (Fig. 15–3).

> **The diagnosis is clinical. A good, extensive history plus a biopsy may be needed to make the diagnosis.**

The diagnosis is clinical. A good, extensive history plus a biopsy may be needed to make the diagnosis and to sort out the underlying conditions listed in Table 15–1. This table shows the spectrum of the differential diagnosis.

> **The treatment aim is to stop the itch-scratch-itch cycle, to restore barrier function, to reduce the inflammation, and to remove the itch.**

The treatment aim is to stop the itch-scratch-itch cycle. To do this, one must restore barrier function, reduce the inflammation, and remove the itch.[27] To restore barrier function, the skin needs a long soak in a sitz bath or a tub with plain water twice a day. No irritating soaps or cleansers should be used.[28] After a soak, a superpotent corticosteroid ointment should be used for a short period of time (1 to 2 weeks), switching to an intermittent treatment schedule or a milder corticosteroid ointment as the condition improves.[29] A short course of oral corticosteroids may be necessary. Intralesional triamcinolone can be used for very thickly lichenified areas.[23] Infection must be treated with an appropriate antibiotic, an anticandidal medication, or both.[30, 31] To control the pruritus, antihistamines should be given during the day and at night (e.g., cetirizine during the day, doxepin at night). Antidepressants like fluoxetine or sertraline can also be useful as antipruritics.

If the condition continues and is difficult to resolve, a contact allergen causing allergic contact dermatitis should be ruled out (see section on contact dermatitis).[28] These patients need a lot of support and ongoing treatment. Relapse is not infrequent.

SEBORRHEIC DERMATITIS

> **Seborrheic dermatitis is a red to yellowish, greasy, dandruff-like, scaling eruption in the hairy areas of the body caused by *Malassezia furfur,* a lipophilic yeast.**

Seborrheic dermatitis is a red to yellowish, greasy, dandruff-like, scaling eruption in the hairy areas of the body. It can involve the vulva in infants and, uncommonly, adult women. The cause of this condition is *Malassezia furfur,* a lipophilic yeast.[32–34] In adults, one sees an increase in this condition with neurologic disease or trauma (e.g., head trauma, spinal injury, Parkinson's disease, stroke), with immunodeficiency (e.g., human immunodeficiency virus [HIV], acquired immunodeficiency syndrome). In these individuals, a change in the epidermal environment with sebum accumulation occurs (often with impaired hygiene), and there is an increase in the *M. furfur* population.

> **With seborrheic dermatitis, there may be no symptoms or just mild irritation. On physical examination, there can be a patchy or diffuse erythematous rash in the hairy area of the vulva.**

With seborrheic dermatitis, there may be no symptoms or just mild irritation. On physical examination, there can be a patchy or diffuse erythematous rash in the hairy area of the vulva. It can extend up into the gluteal cleft and involve the labiocrural and inguinal folds. On the vulva, there is usually a little yellowish scaling, although occasionally it can be slightly psoriasiform. Involvement is often found elsewhere in the more typical areas. The scalp, scalp margins, eyebrows, base of the eyelashes, nasolabial folds and paranasal skin, external ear canals, posterior auricular fold, presternal skin, and upper back are typical areas of involvement with this condition. Here and there are greasy, scaling areas with yellow or red coalescing macules, patches, and papules.[35, 36]

The diagnosis is clinical, because histopathology is nonspecific or psoriasiform. Scraping of the skin may show typical organisms with short hyphae and spores, referred to as "spaghetti and meatballs," in potassium hydroxide preparations. Differential diagnosis includes intertrigo, psoriasis, contact dermatitis, atopic dermatitis, and—less likely—fungal infections. Differentiating this condition from psoriasis may be difficult.[37, 38]

Treatment is with gentle cleansing followed by imidazole cream plus some mild to mid-potency steroid twice a day for 1 to 2 weeks, then maintenance with a low-dose corticosteroid and imidazole cream. Local hygiene is always important to keep the area cool, ventilated, and nonirritated.

CONTACT DERMATITIS

> **Contact dermatitis is an inflammation of the skin resulting from an external agent that acts as an irritant or as an allergen. It is vital to differentiate an irritant from an allergen.**

Contact dermatitis is an inflammation of the skin resulting from an external agent that acts as an irritant or as an allergen. The skin reaction may be acute, subacute, or chronic. It is vital to differentiate an irritant from an allergen.

Primary irritant dermatitis results from repeated exposure to a caustic or physically irritating agent. Anyone exposed to such a product, after enough insult, will react. This is a nonimmunologic reaction. The skin is damaged directly. Examples of such agents are trichloroacetic acid, urine, and feces.[39, 40] Allergic contact dermatitis results from a frank allergic reaction to a low dose of a chemical. This is a type 4 reaction, an immunologic reaction to a sensitizing chemical. Examples of this type of chemical are poison ivy, neomycin, and benzocaine.[41]

The clinical complaints are much the same with both conditions—varying degrees of itch, burning, and irritation that onset acutely or gradually. With an irritant, there is a history of repeated exposure. The condition often presents as a subacute or chronic problem. It is very obvious with patients who are obsessive about personal hygiene. They repeatedly use soaps or deodorizing products. Hygiene issues are difficult for elderly patients. These patients commonly have problems owing to incontinence, with complicating factors of obesity, reduced mobility, and chronic use of pantyliners. They develop, not infrequently, an irritant "diaper dermatitis."[42]

Allergic contact dermatitis is more acute than irritant dermatitis, with sudden onset of symptoms of itching and burning. The patient may be able to identify the offending contactant by this acute onset. The itching is intense, and there may be burning.

> **In a severe acute reaction, there may be erythema, swelling, vesiculation, or even frank bullae. In subacute reactions, there is less swelling, no vesiculation, and more crusting, dryness, or scaling. In chronic contact dermatitis, one sees the same changes as in lichen simplex chronicus.**

On physical examination, the clinical presentation is variable. In a severe acute reaction, there may be erythema, swelling, vesiculation, or even frank bullae. There might be considerable weeping, with scratching and the secondary changes of excoriation, or serosanguineous, honey-colored crusting, with or without infection. In subacute reactions, there is less swelling, no vesiculation, and more crusting, dryness, or scaling (Fig. 15–4). In chronic contact dermatitis, there is a thickening of the skin with increased skin markings (lichenification), induration, erythema, and altered pigmentation (dyspigmentation). These are the same changes one sees in lichen simplex chronicus (see previous section)

The diagnosis is made clinically from the history and physical examination. The allergen may be determined by patch testing. Standard concentrations of known potentially allergenic chemicals are placed on the skin of the back and taped in place for 48 to 72 hours. They are then removed, and the skin is assessed 24 hours later. For some chemicals, a "use test" is set up. The patient puts a small amount of the substance on the skin of the inner arm repeatedly for 3 days. Most dermatologists can perform these tests.[43]

The most common allergens in the vulvar area are benzocaine, fragrance, and neomycin. The potential list of allergens is very long, ranging from rubber products to topical steroids.[44] It is very important to realize that the products patients are using may be contributing to their problems (e.g., a nonresponsive lichen sclerosus patient with allergic reaction to bacitracin).[42, 44] It is also possible that the patient is having problems with both an irritant and an allergen. Pantyliners, soaps, and face cloths are very traumatic to skin. Urine and feces are also very traumatic. Creams may have preservatives, like formalin or imidazolidinyl urea, or perfumes—or the steroid molecule itself may be the allergen. The treatment can be the cause![44–48]

Examples of allergens and irritants in vulvar contact dermatitis are listed in Table 15–2. The differential diagnosis can be very broad and includes eczema, psoriasis, intertrigo, and even bullous pemphigoid. To make a diagnosis, a very specific history is necessary. All products the patient uses must be identified, including medications ingested.[49–51]

The most important treatment is to remove the offending agent or practice and to treat with topical or even systemic corticosteroids and an antihistamine for sedation.

The most important treatment is to remove the offending agent or practice. A dermatologist may be necessary to define allergens. For severe, acute dermatitis, sitz baths may be necessary, followed by bland zinc oxide ointments and topical or even systemic corticosteroids. Antibiotics are necessary for infection. For subacute or chronic eruptions, a mid- to high-potency corticosteroid ointment can be used, such as triamcinolone 0.1% ointment or even clobetasol 0.05% ointment twice a day for 1 to 2 weeks, plus an antihistamine for sedation.[40]

▼ Table 15–2

Examples of Allergens and Irritants in Vulvar Contact Dermatitis

Allergens
Sexual Allergens
Rubber condoms (thiram)
K-Y jelly (propylene glycol)
Quinine hydrochloride (spermicide)
Semen
Metals
Nickel, chromate
Perfumes
Balsam of Peru, cinnamates, citronellol in hygiene products
Medications
Anesthetic (benzocaine)
Antibiotic (neomycin, bacitracin, gentamicin)
Antiseptics (thimerosal, povidone-iodine)
Corticosteroids (tixocortol pivalate, triamcinolone acetonide)
Irritants
Medications (fluorouracil, podophyllotoxin, trichloroacetic acid)
Heat (hot-water bottles, heating pads)
Solvents
Bleach (sodium hypochlorite)
Alcohol
Sweat, urine, and feces
Pantyliners, pads
Frictional trauma

INTERTRIGO

Intertrigo is a mechanical inflammatory dermatosis in the skin folds caused by friction, heat, sweating, and occlusion. This is a very common problem in women with deep skin folds.

Intertrigo is a mechanical inflammatory dermatosis in the skin folds caused by friction, heat, sweating, and occlusion. This is a very common problem in women with deep skin folds. The skin surfaces of the folds rub together, and this friction and the resulting sweat and heat produce maceration. The resulting weeping, dermatitic skin is very susceptible to secondary infection with yeast and bacteria. Humidity; tight, synthetic clothing; and incontinence all make this worse. Obesity significantly compounds the problem. Diabetic patients are particularly susceptible to difficulties.[52] This condition is becoming a common problem for immobile, obese, elderly, and—especially—incontinent women.

Clinically, the symptoms of intertrigo are burning, itching, and irritation, with variable malodor in the labiocrural and inguinal folds, under the abdominal pannus, and in the inframammary area.

Clinically, the symptoms of intertrigo are burning, itching, and irritation, with variable malodor in the labi-

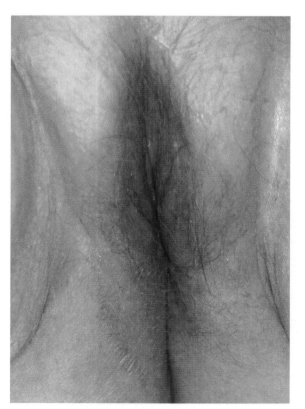

Figure 15–4. Contact dermatitis. Subacute contact dermatitis to benzocaine with erythema, swelling, and scaling of the inferior labia majora extending on the right side of the perineum to the perianal area with minor extension to the right labiocrural fold.

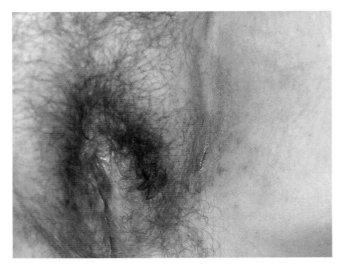

Figure 15–5. Intertrigo. Acute intertrigo with erythema and fissuring in the labiocrural folds in a patient with vulvar lichen planus.

ocrural and inguinal folds, under the abdominal pannus, and in the inframammary area. All are areas where skin surfaces chronically rub together. The physical examination reveals maceration, erythema, fissuring, and weeping in these skin folds. There may be scaly, satellite pustules with secondary candidiasis. The surrounding skin may be acutely inflamed and red or chronically hyperpigmented[53] (Fig. 15–5).

The diagnosis is made clinically. The differential diagnosis includes erythrasma, psoriasis, seborrheic dermatitis, lichen sclerosus, and familial benign pemphigus. Treatment is directed at controlling the precipitating factors. The friction, sweating, and heat must be controlled. Tight, synthetic clothing must be replaced with cool, ventilated clothing of natural fibers. The area should be gently cleansed with a mild soap substitute. For simple cases, a plain powder may be all that is necessary. Efforts should be made to separate the skin folds and keep them from rubbing together. This can be accomplished with strips of soft, thin, cotton laid into the folds. For the rash, a 1% hydrocortisone cream can be used with imidazole cream. It may be best to treat with an antibiotic and antiyeast medication orally for 1 week to control the infectious component.[53–55]

PSORIASIS

Psoriasis is a common, hereditary, papulosquamous disease of the skin characterized by well-defined, reddish papules and plaques with adherent, silvery-white scale.

Psoriasis is a common, hereditary, papulosquamous disease of the skin affecting about 2% of the population. It is characterized, on most of the skin surfaces, by well-defined, reddish papules and plaques with adherent, silvery-white scale. In folds, it is often a more red rash with a fine scale. Typically, it affects the elbows, knees, scalp,

and nails. When it is found in the body folds, it is referred to as *inverse psoriasis* or *flexural psoriasis*. The etiology of psoriasis is a defective or altered immune response in a genetically predisposed individual. T cells interact with an antigen-presenting cell, with a resulting release of cytokines that induce epidermal proliferation. This, in turn, activates T cells in a vicious T cell–mediated, inflammatory sustaining loop.[56, 57]

Psoriasis is triggered by a variety of factors. Trauma to the skin, whether physical (scratching or rubbing), biologic (bacteria or yeast), or chemical (irritating creams, urine, or feces) is important.[58, 59] Drugs such as antimalarials, lithium, and beta blockers flare psoriasis.[60] Stress can play a major factor through the release of substance P. Stress has also been shown to alter epidermal barrier function.[61, 62] Alcohol consumption and smoking are triggers. In the vulva, trauma plays the main role.

Clinically, the patient complains of irritation or itching. This symptom may vary from mild to intense. Scratching spreads the condition and makes the surface open and raw, and the patient may then complain of pain and burning. Symptoms are made worse, as in the eczemas and intertrigo, by stress; heat; humidity; and use of sanitary napkins, tight synthetic clothing, and irritating soaps and lotions. Many simple topical products burn the sensitive tissue of the vulva.

Secondary changes such as excoriation, crusting, and lichenification plus bacterial and yeast infections may further confuse the presentation.

On physical examination, there is a variable picture.[63] Papulosquamous lesions may be dispersed throughout the hairy areas of the mons pubis and labia. These can be thin, scattered, pink lesions of variable size and shape with minor scale (Fig. 15–6). Less commonly, there is a thick, confluent plaque that can be seen forming a horseshoe pattern with a more classic, silvery-white, adherent scale involving all of the hairy area. The inverse form occurs in a bilaterally symmetrical, linear pattern in the folds of the inguinal crease, labiocrural fold, perineum, and

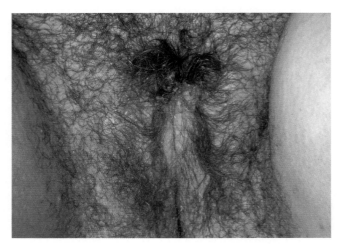

Figure 15–6. Psoriasis. Red, thin plaque of erythema in a horseshoe pattern around the labia majora and mons pubis. No scaling visible.

gluteal cleft. In these areas, there is erythema, maceration, and fissuring. The vulvar mucosa is not involved. Secondary changes such as excoriation, crusting, and lichenification plus bacterial and yeast infections may further confuse the presentation. Very rarely, a pustular presentation is seen as part of a generalized pustular psoriasis.[62–67]

The diagnosis is clinical. It is important to note a history of previous skin rashes and a family history of psoriasis. Check other parts of the skin (scalp, ears, elbows, knees, and nails) for psoriatic changes. Finding typical psoriasis elsewhere on the body confirms the diagnosis. Biopsy is seldom necessary. Differential diagnosis includes seborrheic dermatitis, lichen simplex chronicus, monilial or dermatophyte infection, intertrigo, contact dermatitis, and extramammary Paget's disease.

Treatment depends on severity and extent of disease. Seldom is psoriasis limited to the vulva; it is usually part of a generalized condition. All efforts should be made to stop inflammation, itching, and secondary lesions. In all these conditions, triggering factors must be removed. The same general approach is outlined in atopic dermatitis. Because it spreads this condition, scratching must stop. Systemic medications may be needed. Infection must be treated.

Specific treatments are topical and systemic. For mild to moderate disease, low-dose or intermittent-dose topical steroid ointments can be used for 2 weeks and then tapered to intermittent use. A topical vitamin D derivative ointment can then be alternated with the topical steroid, although at times it can also be irritating. For severe disease, superpotent topical steroid may be necessary for 2 to 3 weeks; then, it too can be alternated with vitamin D/calcipoltriol/calcipoltriene ointment.[68, 69] Long-term use of topical steroids should be avoided. With very extensive, recalcitrant psoriasis, systemic therapy may be necessary. Such treatments include methotrexate, acitretin, hydroxyurea, or cyclosporine. Various forms of ultraviolet light are used. Full discussion of these other options is beyond the scope of this chapter.[70, 71]

LICHEN SCLEROSUS

Lichen sclerosus is the most common chronic vulvar condition seen in vulvar clinics.

Lichen sclerosus is the most common chronic vulvar condition seen in vulvar clinics. This disorder affects both genital skin and other skin. It is variably symptomatic, causing progressive vulvar dysfunction and destruction. The skin and genital lesions show tissue thinning, hypopigmentation, and scarring.

The prevalence of this condition is difficult to estimate, because women may be asymptomatic or may not seek advice about their condition. In one large report, 13.7 of 100,000 women age 50 to 59 years had the condition per year. In another study, 7% of women were affected.[72, 73] It is a condition most commonly reported in white individuals. The average age of onset is difficult to pinpoint. The majority of patients are age 40 to 70 years, but the range is age 6 months to late adulthood.[74, 75]

The etiology of lichen sclerosus is unknown. This condition has been linked to autoimmune diseases, including vitiligo, alopecia areata, thyroid disease, lupus erythematosus, morphea, pernicious anemia, and cicatricial pemphigoid.

The etiology of lichen sclerosus is unknown. Various genetic, autoimmune, infectious, and local factors have been implicated. The cause is probably multifactorial, with genetic and environmental input. Familial cases have been reported. There is an association with class 2 antigen DQ7 in both adult women and children.[74, 76–78] The immunogenetic profile can determine the site of the disorder, the degree of scarring, and the risk of malignant change.[73] Some work indicates persistent, antigen-driven inflammation.[79, 80] Many studies have now focused on immunologic alterations from cytokines to T cell function. This condition has been linked to autoimmune diseases. Up to 40% of patients with lichen sclerosus have thyroid or parietal cell autoantibodies.[81, 82] The autoimmune diseases most often associated with lichen sclerosus are vitiligo, alopecia areata, and thyroid disease. Others include lupus erythematosus, morphea, pernicious anemia, and cicatricial pemphigoid.[83, 84] The relevance of these autoimmune associations is still not clear.

Infection has been linked to lichen sclerosus. The spirochete *Borrelia burgdorferi* has been most often postulated, but it probably is not a causative agent.[85] No other organisms have been found so far.[86] There is no doubt that local factors are important. Any trauma, from scratching to radiation, as in all these vulvar conditions, may trigger lichen sclerosus.[87]

Overall, the most common complaint is pruritus that may be severe and intractable.

The clinical presentation is varied. Too often, there may be little to no obvious symptoms. The patient may complain of late changes of scarring with dyspareunia or even urinary retention. The caregiver may not have noted the loss of normal architecture or hypopigmentation around the vulva. Overall, the most common complaint is pruritus that may be severe and intractable. The patient may wake up at night scratching. A little girl may rub herself all day long. Uncontrollable scratching results in open excoriations, fissures, and secondary infection with pain, dysuria, and dyspareunia.[87] With scratching, the condition flares. If the anal area is involved, defecation can be difficult. Patients are worse during menses, and sanitary napkins cause further irritation. These patients are predictably frustrated and anxious.

On physical examination, there are classic white, atrophic, crinkly papules, plaques in the vulvar area, or both. The skin has a shiny, almost cellophane-like sheen. With continued atrophy, there is a gradual effacement and complete disappearance of the clitoris, the labia minora, or both. In end-stage disease, the introitus is stenosed, and it may be closed.

On physical examination, there are classic white, atrophic, crinkly papules and plaques in the vulvar area, or both. The skin has a shiny, almost cellophane-like sheen. The vulva is involved in 98% of cases, and both vulva and perineum are involved in 48% of cases. There are several patterns.[81] The typical figure-eight pattern is a generalized pattern. It involves the periclitoral area, through the interlabial sulcus and labia minora to the perineum, and it extends in a circle perianally. With continued atrophy, there is a gradual effacement and complete disappearance of the clitoris, the labia minora, or both (Fig. 15–7A). In end-stage disease, the introitus is stenosed, and it may even be completely closed.[88–90] Patchy involvement of the perineum can occur, with just a few white papules here and there or some small white plaques. Other clinical patterns less commonly seen are diffuse erythema with fissures, an overall hypopigmented or vitiliginous pattern, and—rarely—a bullous form. These patterns are not mutually exclusive and can often overlap. Secondary changes are common. Scratching causes purpura and erosions with excoriations. Repeated scratching spreads the condition. The tissue also thickens (lichenification) (Fig. 15–7B). At times, there can be a warty change. Children with lichen sclerosus and torn vulvar tissue, purpura, and scarring are often mistaken for victims of sexual abuse.[91]

The diagnosis is made clinically and confirmed with biopsy. The pathology typically shows epidermal atrophy, edema of the upper dermis, homogenization of the collagen, and an inflammatory infiltrate of mononuclear cells in the underlying stroma.

Up to 20% of patients have lichen sclerosus elsewhere on the skin. Typically, the neck, shoulders, axilla, and breasts are involved. The vagina is spared. There are rare reports of oral lichen sclerosus.[92] The diagnosis is made clinically and confirmed with biopsy. The pathology typically shows epidermal atrophy with orthohyperkeratosis and hydropic degeneration of the basal layer. The upper dermis shows edema and homogenization of the collagen; beneath is an inflammatory infiltrate of mononuclear cells.[93]

The differential diagnosis includes vitiligo, lichen planus, postmenopausal atrophy, cicatricial pemphigoid, pemphigus vulgaris, lichen simplex chronicus, sexual abuse (in children), and extramammary Paget's disease.

In vulvar lichen sclerosus, squamous cell carcinoma can develop in 4% to 5% of cases.

Squamous cell carcinoma can develop in 4% to 5% of cases of lichen sclerosus. This association has been well documented.[94, 95] As a chronically scarring, inflammatory dermatosis, vulvar lichen sclerosus may act as an initiator or promoter of carcinogenesis[96] (Fig. 15–7C).

Topical steroids are the cornerstone of treatment. A superpotent steroid, clobetasol or halobetasol 0.05% ointment, is used twice daily for 2 to 3 months and then intermittently for maintenance one to three times per week.

Treatment can result in dramatic improvement. After a thorough assessment, including a biopsy to confirm the

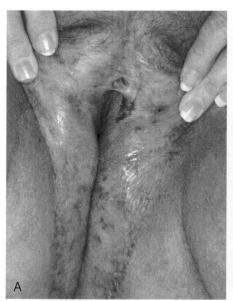
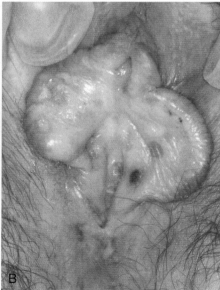
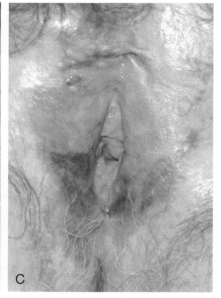

Figure 15–7. *A,* Lichen sclerosus. Figure-eight pattern around the vulva and perianal area with shiny, white, cellophane-like skin, marked purpura, and loss of labia minora and most of the clitoris, plus excoriations, erosions, and crusting. *B,* Swollen, thick, lichenified labia minora with scarring of the clitoris. Very white, shiny color of the inner labia minora and vulvar trigone, with one excoriation and extension of involvement to the edge of the meatus and down through the perineum. *C,* Lichen sclerosus with open areas of squamous cell carcinoma. Very scarred vulva with almost complete loss of clitoris; loss of labia minora; open, slightly thickened, linear erosions beside the clitoris; and open erosions around the right side of the vestibule and posterior fossa, with typical white shiny pattern of lichen sclerosus around the whole area.

diagnosis, general blood testing should be performed to rule out autoimmune diseases such as thyroid disease. Thorough patient education is imperative, because this is a chronic condition requiring long-term care. Topical treatment starts with avoidance of irritants and a regimen of gentle care (see the section on atopic dermatitis). Topical steroids are the cornerstone of treatment. A superpotent steroid, clobetasol or halobetasol 0.05% ointment, is used twice daily for 2 to 3 months and then intermittently for maintenance one to three times per week.[73, 97, 98] By 12 weeks, there is a dramatic improvement, with 77% remission in symptoms. Intermittent superpotent steroids can be used for maintenance.[99] Superpotent steroids can be used efficaciously and safely in children, although they may respond to a mid-potency product.[100, 101] Side effects from topical steroids, when used properly, are rare. For very thick, resistant, hypertrophic lichen sclerosus, intralesional triamcinolone can be helpful.[88, 102] Topical testosterone was recommended in the past but is not very effective and is now not recommended.[103, 104] Retinoids have been used topically and systemically, but with too many side effects.[105, 106]

Surgical management for this condition has been controversial because lichen sclerosus can flare with irritation following surgery. It is, however, very important for specific patient needs such as opening fused labia, dissecting free a buried clitoris, or correcting introital stenosis. It is always necessary for malignant disease.[107]

These patients need to be followed long-term to prevent further scarring and to watch for the small but significant risk of malignancy. Overall, they usually do very well.

LICHEN PLANUS

Lichen planus is typically characterized by a skin eruption of polygonal, pruritic papules and polyhedral plaques that are often shiny with flat tops and show tiny white striae on the surface. The etiology is unknown, although evidence suggests that it is a disorder of cell-mediated immunity.

Lichen planus is typically characterized by a skin eruption of polygonal, pruritic papules and polyhedral plaques that are often shiny with flat tops and show tiny white striae on the surface (Wickham's striae). On the mucous membranes of the mouth or the genitalia, there are thin, lacy, white, patterned lesions. Synonyms for vulvovaginal lichen planus are erosive lichen planus, desquamative inflammatory vaginitis, vulvovaginal-gingival syndrome, and ulcerative lichen planus. The etiology is unknown, although evidence suggests that it is a disorder of cell-mediated immunity in which an exogenous, antigenic stimulus such as a drug, chemical, or superantigen induces cell-mediated immune response in the epithelium, with infiltration of T cells in a genetically predisposed individual. The release of cytokines alters the keratinocytes, triggering an autoimmune reaction with basal keratinocyte destruction.[108–113] Various antigens are known to flare lichen planus. The list of potential drugs is exten-

sive. The commonest are thiazides, nonsteroidal anti-inflammatory drugs, beta blockers, and antimalarials. Environmental metals, from gold in schnapps to mercury in dental fillings, have been implicated. Even some plastics have created problems.[114–116] Infections such as hepatitis B and C and HIV are linked to lichen planus.[117–120]

The disease has three main patterns. The classic presentation is itchy polygonal papules and plaques on wrists and ankles. Vulvar involvement can be part of the generalized rash, with papules on the mons and labia without atrophy or scarring. The vulvovaginal-gingival syndrome is an erosive, destructive form involving the mucous membranes of the mouth, vulva, and even eyes and esophagus, with atrophy and scarring. The last and most rare is the hypertrophic form, with extensive, thick vulvar scarring and variable hyperkeratosis.[121]

Lichen planus of the vulva has been reported and reviewed extensively.[122–131] It is part of a wide spectrum of disease involving the skin, oral mucosa, scalp, nails, eyes, esophagus, bladder, nose, larynx, and anus.[131, 132] The typical patient is 30 to 60 years old.

Eroded, ulcerative lichen planus causes burning and pain that can be chronic and very severe. With vaginal erosion, there is a discharge that can be purulent, malodorous, and copious.

The symptoms are variable. There may be no symptoms in the reticular pattern. Itching may be mild to moderate in the papular form to severe in the hypertrophic form, but these symptoms are not mutually exclusive. Eroded, ulcerative lichen planus causes burning and pain that can be chronic and very severe. With vaginal erosion, there is a discharge that can be purulent, malodorous, and copious. Dyspareunia and apareunia are common.[123–126, 132] With these difficult problems, the patient may experience anger, frustration, and relationship distress. All tend to compromise the therapeutic relationship.[121]

On physical examination, the findings vary depending on the overall pattern. In some patients, the pattern may vary over the years, from a lacy, reticulated pattern to erosive disease. In the classic papulosquamous form, there are small, purple, itchy papules and plaques on the mons pubis, thighs, and labia majora. Reticulated white striae might be seen over the mucous membranes of the vulva, perineum, or perianal area. There may be secondary changes from scratching, and scratching does spread this condition (Fig. 15–8A). In the very hypertrophic form, there is thick, white induration of the vulva with scarring and loss of the labia and clitoral area, as in lichen sclerosus. The introitus may be totally stenosed.

In the erosive form, erosions may be small or large. They may be scattered around the inner labia minora and vulvar trigone. The edges are often white to grayish and exquisitely tender. There is wide variation and loss of normal architecture (Fig. 15–8B and 15–8C). In one series, 70% of women had vaginal involvement.[125] At the edge of the ulcers, one may see the typical lacy pattern. The vaginal changes include acute inflammation and erosion with heavy, thick, seropurulent discharge. There may

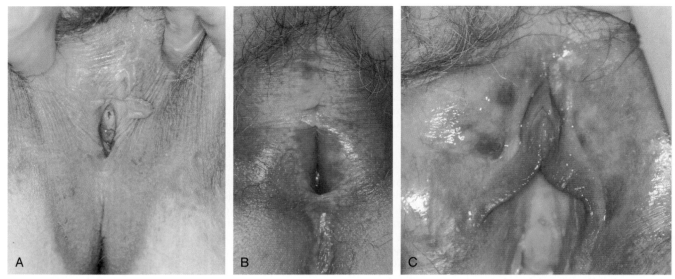

Figure 15–8. *A*, Lichen planus. Diffuse, whitish-pink involvement of the whole vulvar, perineal, perianal area, with extension into the labiocrural area and small erosions secondary to scratching. There is scarring with loss of most of the clitoris and right labium minus in a patient with severe pruritus and secondary candidiasis. *B*, Whitish, scarred vulva with complete loss of the clitoris and labia minora and partial vaginal stenosis. *C*, Periclitoral erosions with surrounding whitish, scarred areas with no loss of architecture.

be a gray pseudomembrane of coagulated serum over the eroded areas. Synechiae can be seen. Stenosis of the vagina is common. With continued disease, the vagina contracts, is foreshortened, and may close completely. Examining a patient with this condition is very difficult. Stenosis may make routine Pap smears impossible. In chronic, noneroded vaginal lichen planus, there may be only loss of rugae and a residual atrophic lining.[121, 133, 134]

Signs of lichen planus may be seen elsewhere on the skin. Seeing these lesions facilitates the diagnosis. In the mouth, a white, lacy pattern on the buccal mucosa and gum margins may be seen. Ulcers and erosions may be present on the tongue and buccal mucosa. In severe involvement of the mouth, there can be scarring. The severity of oral involvement does not correlate with genital disease. On the skin, a fine, red, papulosquamous rash or scattered, itchy, purple papules may be seen. The scalp may show a scarring alopecia. Nails will be thinned, with ridging and even diffuse scarring. To make a diagnosis, it is important to look at all these areas.

The diagnosis is reached on the basis of clinical presentation and biopsy. Immunofluorescence may be needed to differentiate lichen planus from bullous disease.

The diagnosis is reached on the basis of clinical presentation and biopsy. Histopathology typically shows a bandlike lymphocytic infiltrate at the dermoepidermal junction, with a sawtoothed pattern at the rete ridges, acanthosis, hyperkeratosis, and a prominent granular layer.[135] These typical changes are not always seen in the mucosal lesions. The epithelium may be lost. The basal cells may be disorganized and vacuolated. Plasma cells may be

seen.[128, 134] Immunofluorescence may be needed to differentiate lichen planus from bullous disease.

With nonhealing erosions and ulcers, squamous cell carcinoma must be excluded.

The differential diagnosis is mostly between lichen sclerosus and the vesiculobullous diseases, bullous and cicatricial pemphigoid and pemphigus. Behçet's syndrome and lupus erythematosus rarely may present with vulvar ulcers and erosions. Other causes of desquamative vaginitis include genital graft-versus-host disease, severe erythema multiforme, and toxic epidermal necrolysis. Most of these conditions can be differentiated using the clinical pattern and histopathology. Lichen sclerosus and lichen planus may overlap in the same patient, which can be confusing.[136, 137] When the vulva is thick and scratched in hypertrophic vulvar lichen planus, lichen simplex chronicus must be considered, although the patient may have both conditions. With nonhealing erosions and ulcers, squamous cell carcinoma must be excluded. It is not a commonly associated problem but is well recognized.[138-140] The incidence is unknown.[141]

Treatment is challenging. No single agent is universally effective. Topical superpotent steroid ointment like 0.05% clobetasol or halobetasol is used. It may be applied to the vulva or applied intravaginally. Hydrocortisone acetate in a suppository or foam can be effective for vaginal involvement.

Treatment is challenging. No single agent is universally effective. For all types of vulvar lichen planus, it is important to stop irritation and trauma, control symptoms of itching and pain, and treat infections owing to bacteria or yeast, as has already been outlined in the sections on atopic dermatitis and psoriasis. Depression and frustration must be addressed.[131] Topical steroids are still the mainstays of treatment. A topical superpotent steroid ointment like 0.05% clobetasol or halobetasol is used. It may be applied to the vulva or applied intravaginally. Hydrocortisone acetate in a suppository or foam can be effective for vaginal involvement. Effort is made to avoid steroid atrophy. Oral prednisone can be added for 2 to 6 weeks. For limited areas, intralesional triamcinolone can be effective. Vaginal dilators coated with topical steroids can be used to prevent synechiae. Once control is achieved, the use of steroids is tapered.[123, 128]

Many other treatments have been used for this difficult disease. Retinoids in all formulations have been helpful. Oral retinoids have been used to control erosive disease, but little is published on the use of these agents for vulvar disease.[142–144] Azathioprine has been used effectively as a steroid-sparing agent.[143] Cyclosporine systemically and topically has been used with varying success.[145–148] Griseofulvin,[123, 125] dapsone,[123, 125] hydroxychloroquine,[149] and tetracycline with nicotinamide[150, 151] are all potentially helpful. Metronidazole has occasionally been used for generalized disease.[152, 153] Other treatments include thalidomide,[154, 155] interferon,[156] heparin,[156] methotrexate, tacrolimus, and photodynamic therapy.

Surgery may be necessary for vaginal synechiae and for some cases of stenosis. It is always used for malignant change. There is always the potential for rebound flare of lichen planus after surgery, and the use of topical superpotent or systemic steroids may be necessary.

In one series, 38% of vulvar lichen planus patients had complete resolution, 30% with significant resolution; the rest had ongoing problems. Because no one treatment is universally successful, treatments may have to be combined to find a safe and effective program.

SUMMARY OF KEY POINTS

- Colposcopists have a superb opportunity to recognize and initiate management for women with vulvar disease.
- The lack of a protective keratinized surface on the vulvar vestibule to act as a barrier explains why it is so easily irritated and infected under certain circumstances.
- Hypoestrogenic atrophy results in loss or alteration of epithelial barrier functions, resulting in increased susceptibility to irritation and infection.
- The most frequently misinterpreted vulvar anatomic variations are sebaceous hyperplasia and vulvar papillomatosis.
- Examination elsewhere on the body surface may sometimes confirm a vulvar diagnosis.
- Eczema and dermatitis are synonyms.

- Atopic dermatitis is a very itchy, inflammatory, recurrent dermatosis. It affects up to 20% of the population.
- Typically, atopic patients react to irritants like soaps, cleansers, perfume products, and even sanitary napkins with xerosis, itching, rubbing, scratching, lichenification, weeping, and secondary infection.
- Lichen simplex chronicus is the end stage of the itch-scratch-itch cycle.
- Seborrheic dermatitis is a red to yellowish, greasy, dandruff-like, scaling eruption in the hairy areas of the body caused by *M. furfur,* a lipophilic yeast.
- Primary irritant dermatitis results from repeated exposure to a caustic or physically irritating agent, causing direct skin damage.
- Allergic contact dermatitis results from a frank allergic reaction to a low dose of a chemical.
- Intertrigo is a mechanical inflammatory dermatosis in the skin folds caused by friction, heat, sweating, and occlusion.
- Psoriasis is a common hereditary papulosquamous disease of the skin characterized by well-defined, reddish papules and plaques with adherent, silvery-white scale.
- Psoriasis is triggered by physical, biologic, or chemical trauma to the skin; by drugs such as antimalarials, lithium, and beta blockers; by stress; by alcohol consumption; and by smoking.
- Lichen sclerosus is the most common chronic vulvar condition seen in vulvar clinics.
- The etiology of lichen sclerosus is unknown. This condition has been linked to autoimmune diseases including vitiligo, alopecia areata, thyroid disease, lupus erythematosus, morphea, pernicious anemia, and cicatricial pemphigoid.
- On physical examination, lichen sclerosus appears as classic white, atrophic, crinkly papules or plaques in the vulvar area. The skin has a shiny, almost cellophane-like sheen. With continued atrophy, there is a gradual effacement and complete disappearance of the clitoris or the labia minora. In end-stage disease, the introitus is stenosed, and it may be closed.
- The diagnosis of lichen sclerosus is made clinically and confirmed by biopsy.
- In vulvar lichen sclerosus, squamous cell carcinoma can develop in 4% to 5% of cases.
- Topical superpotent steroids are the cornerstone of treatment for lichen sclerosus.
- The diagnosis of lichen planus is reached on the basis of clinical presentation and biopsy. Immunofluorescence may be needed to differentiate lichen planus from bullous disease.

References

1. Margesson LJ: Normal anatomy of the vulva. In Fisher BK, Margesson LJ (eds): Genital Skin Disorders Diagnosis and Treatment. St. Louis, Mosby, 1998, pp 99–107.
2. McLean JM: Anatomy and physiology of the vulva. In Ridley CM, Neill SM (eds): The Vulva, 2nd ed. London, Blackwell Science, 1999, pp 37–63.
3. Lynch PJ, Edwards L: Anatomy. In Lynch PJ, Edwards L (eds): Genital Dermatology. New York, Churchill Livingston, 1994, pp 1–3.
4. DiSaia DJ: Clinical anatomy of the female genital tract. In Scott JR (eds): Danforth's Obstetrics and Gynecology, 7th ed. Philadelphia, Lippincott, 1994, pp 1–8.
5. Margesson LJ: Appendix B. Clinical evaluation of vulvar patients. In Fisher BK, Margesson LJ (eds): Genital Skin Disorders Diagnosis and Treatment. St. Louis, Mosby, 1998, pp 235–236.
6. Lynch PJ, Edwards L: Diagnostic procedures. In Lynch PJ, Edwards L (eds): Genital Dermatology. New York, Churchill Livingston, 1994, pp 7–8.
7. Turner MLC, Marinoff SC: General principles in the diagnosis and treatment of the vulvar diseases. Dermatol Clin 1992;10:275.
8. Leungh DYM, Soter NA: Cellular and immunologic mechanisms in atopic dermatitis. J Am Acad Dermatol 2001;44:S1.
9. Leungh DY: Atopic dermatitis: New insights and opportunities for therapeutic intervention. J Allergy Clin Immunol 2000;105:860.
10. Leungh DY: Pathogenesis of atopic dermatitis. J Allergy Clin Immunol 1999;104:S99.
11. Saloga J, Knop J: Superantigens in skin disease. Eur J Dermatol 1999;9:586.
12. Bunikowski R, Mielke MEA, Skarabis H, et al: Evidence of a disease-promoting effect of Staphylococcus aureus–derived exotoxins in atopic dermatitis. J Allergy Clin Immunol 2001;105:814.
13. Abeck D, Mempel M: Staphylococcus aureus colonization in atopic dermatitis and its therapeutic implications. Br J Dermatol 1998;139(suppl 53):13.
14. Tofle SJ, Hanifin JM: Current management and therapy of atopic dermatitis. J Am Acad Dermatol 2001;44:S13.
15. Margesson LJ: Inflammatory diseases of the vulva. In Fisher BK, Margesson LJ (eds): Genital Skin Disorders Diagnosis and Treatment. St. Louis, Mosby, 1998, pp 154–155.
16. Ball SB, Wojnarowska F: Vulvar dermatoses: Lichen sclerosus, lichen planus, and vulval dermatitis/lichen simplex chronicus. Semin Cutan Med Surg 1998;17:182.
17. Hanifin JM, Chan SC: Biochemical and immunologic mechanisms in atopic dermatitis: New targets for emerging therapies. J Am Acad Dermatol 1999;41:284.
18. Hanifin JM, Tofle SJ: Patient education in the long term management of atopic dermatitis. Dermatol Nurs 1999;11:284.
19. Fleischer AB, Jr: Treatment of atopic dermatitis: Role of tacrolimus ointment as a topical non-corticosteroidal therapy. J Allergy Clin Immunol 1999;104(3 pt 2):S126.
20. Hanifin JM, Ling MR, Langley R, et al: Tacrolimus ointment in the treatment of atopic dermatitis in adult patients: Part I, efficacy. J Amer Acad Dermatol 2001;44:S28.
21. Ridley CM, Neill SM: Non-infective cutaneous conditions of the vulva. In Ridley CM, Neill SM (eds): The Vulva, 2nd ed. London, Blackwell Science, 1999, pp 151–152.
22. Virgili A, Corazza M, Bacilieri S, et al: Contact sensitivity in vulval lichen simplex chronicus. Contact Dermatitis 1997;37:296.
23. Margesson LJ: Inflammatory diseases of the vulva. In Fisher BK, Margesson, LJ (eds): Genital Disorders: Diagnosis and Treatment. St. Louis, Mosby, 1998, pp 157–159.
24. Garg A, Chren MM, Sands LP, et al: Psychological stress perturbs epidermal barrier hemostasis. Arch Dermatol 2001;137:53.
25. Pinkus SH: Vulvar dermatoses and pruritus vulvae. Dermatol Clin 1992;10:297.
26. Lynch PJ, Edwards L: Red plaques with erythematous features. In Lynch PJ, Edwards L: Genital Dermatology. New York, Churchill Livingston, 1994, pp 27–34.
27. Lynch PJ: Epithelial hyperplasia. Presentation of International Society for the Study of Vulvovaginal Diseases (ISSVD). Santa Fe, September 1999.
28. Ball SB, Wojnarowska F: Vulvar dermatoses: Lichen sclerosus, lichen planus and vulval dermatitis/lichen simplex chronicus. Semin Cutan Med Surg 1998;17:182.
29. Brunner N, Yawalkar S: A double-blind, multi-center, parallel-group trial with 0.05% halobetasol propionate ointment vs 0.1% diflucortolone valerate ointment in patients with severe, chronic atopic dermatitis or lichen simplex chronicus. J Am Acad Dermatol 1991;25:1160.
30. Veien NK: The clinician's choice of antibiotics in the treatment of bacterial skin infections. Br J Dermatol 1998;139(Suppl 53):30.
31. Saloga J, Knop J: Super antigens in skin disease. Eur J Dermatol 1999;9:586.
32. Bergbrant IM: Seborrheic dermatitis and pityrosporon yeasts. Cur Top Med Mycol 1995;6:95.
33. Schmidt A: Malassezia furfur: A fungus belonging to the physiological skin flora and its relevance to skin disorders. Cutis 1997;59:21.
34. Faergemann J: Pityrosporon yeasts—what's new? Mycoses 1997;40(suppl 1):29.
35. Ridley CM, Neill SM: Non-infective cutaneous conditions of the vulva. In Ridley CM, Neill SM (eds): The Vulva. 2nd ed. London, Blackwell Science, 1999, pp 1–36.
36. Habif TP, Campbell JL Jr, Quitadamo MJ, et al: Eczema. In Habif TP, Campbell JL Jr, Quitadamo MJ (eds): Skin Disease Diagnosis and Treatment. St. Louis, Mosby, 2001, pp 94–97.
37. Janniger CK, Schwartz RA: Seborrheic dermatitis. Am Fam Physician 1995;52:149.
38. Marinella MA: Erythrasma and seborrheic dermatitis of the groin. Am Fam Physician 1995;52:2012.
39. Denig NI, Hoke AW, Maibach HI: Irritant contact dermatitis. Clues and causes, clinical characteristics and control. Post Grad Med 1998;103:199.
40. Margesson LJ: Inflammatory diseases of the vulva. In Fisher BK, Margesson LJ (eds): Genital Skin Disorders Diagnosis and Treatment. St. Louis, Mosby, 1998, pp 155–157.
41. Lynch PJ, Edwards L: Geriatric problems. In Lynch PJ, Edwards L (eds): Genital Dermatology. New York, Churchill Livingston, 1994, pp 265–266.
42. Pincus SK: Vulvar dermatoses and pruritus vulvae, Dermatol Clin 1992;10:297.
43. Reitschel RL, Fowler JF: Practical aspects of patch testing. In Reitschel RL, Fowler JE (eds): Fisher's Contact Dermatitis. Philadelphia, Lippincott, Williams & Wilkens, 2001, pp 9–26.
44. Corazza M, Mantovani L, Moranini C, et al: Contact sensitization to corticosteroids: Increased risk in long term dermatoses. Eur J Dermatol 2000;10:533.
45. Lewis FM, Shah M, Gawkrodger DJ: Contact sensitivity in pruritus vulvae: Patch test results and clinical outcome. Am J Contact Derm 1999;8:137.
46. Eason LE, Feldman P: Contact dermatitis associated with the use of Always sanitary napkins. Can Med Assoc J 1996;154:1173.
47. Sterry W, Schmoll M: Contact urticaria and dermatitis from self adhesive pads. Contact Derm 1985;13:284.
48. Virgili A, Corazza M, Califano A: Diaper dermatitis in adult, a case of erythema papuloerosive of Sevestre and Jacquet. J Reprod Med 1998;43:949.
49. Bauer A, Geier J, Elsner P: Allergic contact dermatitis in patients with anogenital complaints. J Reprod Med 2000;45:649.
50. Sonnex C: Sexual hypersensitivity. Br J Hosp Med 1988;39:40.
51. Abdul Gaffoor PM: Sexually induced dermatoses. Cutis 1996;57:252.
52. Yosipovitch G, Tur E, Cohen O, et al: Skin surface pH in intertriginous areas in NIDDM patients. Possible correlations to candidal intertrigo. Diabetes Care 1993;16:560.
53. Margesson LJ: Inflammatory disease of the vulva. In Fisher BK, Margesson LJ, (eds): Genital Skin Disorders: Diagnosis and Treatment. St. Louis, Mosby, 1998, p 164.
54. Guitart J, Woodley DT: Intertrigo: A practical approach. Compr Ther 1994;20:402.
55. Hedley K, Tooley P, Williams H: Problems with clinical trials in general practice—a double blind comparison of cream containing miconazole and hydrocortisone with hydrocortisone alone in the treatment of intertrigo. Br J Clin Proct 1990;44:131.
56. Teruit T, Ozawa M, Tagami H: Role of neutrophils in induction of acute inflammation in T-cell-mediated immunodermatosis, psoriasis: A neutrophil-associated inflammation-boosting loop. Exp Dermatol 2000;9:1.
57. Ortonne JP: Recent developments in the understanding of the pathogenesis of psoriasis. Br J Dermatol 1999;140(Suppl 54):1.

58. Rasmussen JE: The relationship between infection with group A beta hemolytic streptococci and the development of psoriasis. Pediatr Infect Dis J 2000;19:153.

59. Saloga J, Knop J: Superantigens in skin disease. Eur J Dermatol 1999;9:586.

60. Wolf R, Ruocco V: Triggering psoriasis. Adv Exp Med Biol 1999; 455:221.

61. Garg A, Chren MM, Sands LP, et al: Psychological stress perturbs epidermal permeability barrier homeostasis. Arch Derm 2001;137: 53.

62. Farber EM, Nall L: Psoriasis: A stress related disease. Cutis 1993; 51:322.

63. Drew GS: Psoriasis. Prim Care 2000;27:385.

64. Margesson LJ: Inflammatory diseases of the vulva. In Fisher BK, Margesson LJ (eds): Genital Skin Disorders: Diagnosis and Treatment. St. Louis, Mosby, 1998, pp 167–169.

65. Lynch PJ, Edwards L: Red plaques with papulosquamous features. In Lynch PJ, Edwards L (eds): Genital Dermatology. New York, Churchill Livingston, 1994, pp 57–61.

66. Pincus SH: Vulvar dermatoses and pruritus vulvae. Dermtol Clin 1992;10:303.

67. Weinraud L, Katz M: Psoriasis vulgaris of the labium majus. Cutis 1986;38:333.

68. Smith KC, Lebwohl M: Topical antipsoriatics. Skin Therapy Lett 2000;5:1.

69. Fogh K, Kragballe K: Recent developments in vitamin D analogs. Curr Pharm Des 2000;6:961.

70. Ashcroft DM, Liwan PO A, Griffiths CE: Therapeutic strategies for psoriasis. J Clin Pharm Ther 2000;25:1.

71. Koo JY: Current consensus and update on psoriasis therapy: A perspective from the US. J Dermatol Clin 1999;26:723.

72. Wakelin SH, Marren P: Lichen sclerosus in women. Clin Dermatol 1997;15:155.

73. Powell JJ, Wojarowska F: Lichen sclerosus. Lancet 1999;353: 1777.

74. Ridley CM: Genital lichen sclerosus (lichen sclerosus et atrophicus) in childhood and adolescence. J R Soc Med 1993;86:69.

75. Thomas RH, Ridley CM, McGibbon DH, et al: Anogenital lichen sclerosus in women. J R Soc Med 1996;89:694.

76. Sahn EE, Bluestein EL, Oliva S: Familial lichen sclerosus et atrophicus in childhood. Pediatr Dermatol 1994;11:160.

77. Cox NH, Michell JNS, Morley WM: Lichen sclerosus et atrophicus in non-identical female twins. Br J Dermatol 1986;115: 743.

78. Powell J, Wojnarowska F, Winsey S, et al: Lichen sclerosus premenarche: Autoimmunity and immunogenetics. Br J Dermatol 2000;142:481.

79. Carlson JA, Grabowski R, Chichester P, et al: Comparative immunophenotypic study of lichen sclerosus: Epidermotrophic CD 57 positive lymphocytes are numerous—implications for pathogenesis. Am J Dermatopathol 2000;22:7.

80. Lubowsky A, Muche JM, Sterry W: Detection of expanded T cell clones in skin biopsy samples of patients with lichen sclerosus et atrophicus by T cell receptor—gamma polymerase chain reaction assay. J Invest Dermatol 2000;115:254.

81. Meyrick Thomas RH, Ridley CM, McGibbon DH, et al: Lichen sclerosus and autoimmunity—a study of 350 women. Br J Dermatol 1988;118:41.

82. Meyrick Thomas RH, Ridley CM, Black MM: The association of lichen sclerosus et atrophicus an autoimmune related disease in males. Br J Dermatol 1998;109:661.

83. Harrington CI, Dunsmore IR: An investigation into the incidence of autoimmune disorders in patients with lichen sclerosus et atrophicus. Br J Dermatol 1981;104:563.

84. Meffert JJ, Davis BM, Grimwood RE: Lichen sclerosus. J Am Acad Dermatol 1995;32:393.

85. Weide B, Walz T, Garbe C: Is morphea caused by *Borrelia burgdorferi*? A review. Br J Dermatol 2000;142:636.

86. Farrell AM, Millard PR, Schomberg KH, et al: An infective aetiology for vulval lichen sclerosus readdressed. Clin Exp Dermatol 1999;24:479.

87. Todd P, Helpern S, Kirby J, et al: Lichen sclerosus and the Koebner phenomenon. Clin Exp Dermatol 1994;19:262.

88. Margesson LJ: Pigmentary changes of the vulva. In Fisher BK, Margesson LJ (eds): Genital Skin Disorders: Diagnosis and Treatment. St. Louis, Mosby, 1998, pp 189–193.

89. Ridley CM, Neill SM: Non-infective cutaneous conditions of the vulva. In Ridley CM, Neill SM (eds): The Vulva, 2nd ed. London, Blackwell Science, 1999, pp 154–164.

90. Lynch PJ, Edwards L: White patches and plaques. In Lynch PJ, Edwards L (eds): Genital Dermatology. New York, Churchill Livingston, 1994, pp 149–158.

91. Warrington SA, deSan Lazaro C: Lichen sclerosus et atrophicus and sexual abuse. Arch Dis Child 1996;75:512.

92. Schulten EA, Starink TM, Vander W: Lichen sclerosus et atrophicus involving the oral mucosa: A report of two cases. J Oral Pathol Med 1993;22:374.

93. Jaworsky C: Connective tissue diseases. In Elder D, Elenitsas R, Jaworsky C, Johnson B Jr (eds): Lever's Histopathology of the Skin, 8th ed. Philadelphia, Lippincott-Raven, 1997, pp 281–282.

94. Scurry JP, Vanin K: Vulvar squamous cell carcinoma and lichen sclerosus. Australas J Dermatol 1997;38(suppl 1):220.

95. Derrick EK, Ridley CM, Kobza-Black A, et al: A clinical study of 23 cases of female anogenital carcinoma. Br J Dermatol 2000;143: 1217.

96. Carlson JA, Ambros R, Malfetano J, et al: Vulvar lichen sclerosus and squamous cell carcinoma: A cohort, case control, and investigational study with histological perspective; implications for chronic inflammation and sclerosis in the development of neoplasia. Hum Pathol 1998;29:932.

97. Dalziel KL, Millard PR, Wornarowska F: Treatment of vulval lichen sclerosus with a very potent topical steroid (clobetasol propionate 0.05%) cream. Br J Dermatol 1991;124:461.

98. Lorenz B, Kaufman RH, Kutzner SK: Lichen sclerosus therapy with clobetasol propionate. J Reprod Med 1998;43:790.

99. Sinha P, Sorinola O, Luesley DM: Lichen sclerosus of the vulva. Long term steroid maintenance therapy. J. Reprod Med 1999;44: 621.

100. Fischer G, Rogers M: Treatment of childhood vulvar lichen sclerosus with potent topical corticosteroid. Pediatr Dermatol 1997;14: 235.

101. Garzon MC, Pallar AS: Ultrapotent topical corticosteroid treatment of childhood genital lichen sclerosus. Arch Derm 1999;135:525.

102. Mazdisnian F, Degregorio F, Masdisnian F, et al: Intralesional injection of triamcinolone in the treatment of lichen sclerosus. J Reprod Med 1999;44:332.

103. Paslin D: Androgens in the topical treatment of lichen sclerosus. Int J Dermatol 1996;35:298.

104. Bornstein J, Heifetz S, Kellner Y, et al: Clobetasol dipropionate 0.05% vs. testosterone propionate 2% topical application for severe vulvar lichen sclerosus. Am J Obstet Gynecol 1998;178:80.

105. Virgili A, Corazza M, Bianchi A, et al: Open study of topical 0.025% tretinoin in the treatment of vulvar lichen sclerosus. One year of therapy. J Reprod Med 1995;40:614.

106. Bousema MT, Romppanen U, Geoger JM, et al: Acitretin in the treatment of severe lichen sclerosus et atrophicus of the vulva: A double blind placebo-controlled study. J Am Acad Dermatol 1994; 30:225.

107. Abramov Y, Elchalal U, Abramov D, et al: Surgical treatment of vulvar lichen sclerosus: A review. Obstet Gynecol Surg 1996;51: 193.

108. Chaiyarit P, Kafrawy AH, Miles DA, et al: Oral lichen planus: An immunohistochemical study of heat shock proteins (HSPs) and cytokeratins (CKs) and a unifying hypothesis of pathogenesis. J Oral Path Med 1999;28:210.

109. Sugarman PB, Satterwhite K, Bigby M: Autocytotoxic T-cell clones in lichen planus. Br J Dermatol 2000;142:449.

110. LaNasa G, Cottani F, Mulargia M, et al: HLA Antigen distribution in different clinical sub-groups demonstrates genetic heterogeneity in lichen planus. Br J Dermatol 1995;132:897.

111. Setterfield J, Neill S, Ridley M, et al: The vulvo-vagino-gingival syndrome is associated with the HLA DQB1*0201 allele. Br J Dermatol 1996;135(suppl 47):43.

112. Ognjenovic M, Kavelovic D, Mikelic M, et al: Oral lichen planus and HLA B. Coll Antropol 1998;22:93.

113. Boyd AS, Neldner KH: Lichen planus. J Amer Acad Dermatol 1991;25:593.

114. Russell MA, King LE, Boyd AS: Lichen planus after consumption of a gold-containing liquor. N Eng J Med 1996;334:603.

115. Laine J, Kalimo K, Hopponen RP: Contact allergy to dental restorative materials in patients with oral lichenoid lesions. Contact Dermatitis 1997;36:141.

116. Yiannias JA, el-Azhary RA, Hand JH, et al: Relevant contact sensitivities in patients with the diagnosis of oral lichen planus. J Amer Acad Dermatol 2000;42(2 pt 1):177.

117. Sanchez-Perez J, DeCastro M, Buezo GF, et al: Lichen planus and hepatitis C: Prevalence and clinical presentation of patients with lichen planus and hepatitis C infection. Br J Dermatol 1996;134:715.

118. Sanchez-Perez, Moreno-Otero R, Borque MJ, et al: Lichen planus and hepatitis C virus infection: A clinical and virologic study. Acta Derm Venereol 1998;78:305.

119. Chuang TY, Stitle L, Brashear R, et al: Hepatitis C virus and lichen planus: A case-control study of 340 patients. J Am Acad Dermatol 1999;41(5 pt 1):787.

120. Fitzgerald E, Purcell SM, Goldman NM: Photo distributed hypertrophic lichen planus in association with acquired immunodeficiency syndrome: A distinct entity. Cutis 1995;55:109.

121. Margesson LJ: Inflammatory diseases of the vulva. In Fisher BK, Margesson LJ (eds): Genital Skin Disorders: Diagnosis and Treatment. St. Louis, Mosby, 1998, pp 169–172.

122. Soper DE, Patterson JW, Hurt WG: Lichen planus of the vulva. Obstet Gynecol 1998;72:74.

123. Edwards L: Vulvar lichen planus. Arch Dermatol 1989;125:1677.

124. Pelisse M: The vulvo-vaginal-gingival syndrome. A new form of erosive lichen planus. Int J Dermatol 1989;28:381.

125. Ridley CM: Chronic erosive vulval disease. Clin Exp Dermatol 1990;15:245.

126. Oates JK, Rowen D: Desquamative inflammatory vaginitis. Genitourin Med 1990;66:275.

127. Bermejo A, Bermejo MD, Roman P, et al: Lichen planus with simultaneous involvement of the oral cavity and genitalia. Oral Surg Oral Med Oral Pathol 1990;69:209.

128. Mann MS, Kaufman RH: Erosive lichen planus of the vulva. Clin Obstet Gynecol 1991;34:605.

129. Eisen D: The vulvovaginal-gingival syndrome of lichen planus. The clinical characteristics of 22 patients. Arch Dermatol 1994;130:1379.

130. Lewis FM, Shah M, Harrington CI: Vulval involvement in lichen planus: A study of 37 women. Br J Dermatol 1996;135:89.

131. Lewis FM: Vulval lichen planus. Br J Dermatol 1998;138:569.

132. Eisen D: The evaluation of cutaneous, genital, scalp, nail, esophageal and ocular involvement in patients with oral lichen planus. Oral Surg Oral Med Oral Pathol Oral Radiol Endod 1999;88:431.

133. Ridley CM, Neill SM: Non-infective cutaneous conditions of the vulva. In Ridley CM, Neill SM (eds): The Vulva, 2nd ed. London, Blackwood Science, 1999, pp 104–107.

134. Lynch PJ, Edwards L: Red plaques with papulosquamous features. In Lynch PJ, Edwards L (eds): Genital Dermatology. New York, Churchill Livingston, 1994, pp 63–72.

135. Toussaint S, Kamino H: Non-infectious, erythematous, papular and squamous diseases. In Elder D, Elenitsas R, Jaworsky C, Johnson B Jr (eds): Lever's Histopathology of the Skin, 8th ed. Philadelphia, Lippincott-Raven, 1997, pp 166–172.

136. Connelly MG, Winkleman RK: Coexistence of lichen sclerosus, morphea and lichen planus. J Am Acad Dermatol 1985;12(5 pt 1):844.

137. Marren P, Millard P, Chia Y, et al: Mucosal lichen sclerosus/lichen planus overlap syndromes. Br J Dermatol 1994;131:118.

138. Lewis FM, Harrington CI: Squamous cell carcinoma arising in vulval lichen planus. Br J Dermatol 1994;131:703.

139. Frank JM, Young AW Jr: Squamous cell carcinoma in situ arising within lichen planus of the vulva. Dermatologic Surg 1995;21:890.

140. Dwyer CM, Kern RE, Millan DW: Squamous carcinoma following lichen planus of the vulva. Clin Exp Dermatol 1995;20:171.

141. Zaki I, Dalzeil KL, Solomonsz FA, et al: The under reporting of skin disease in association with squamous cell carcinoma of the vulva. Clin Exp Dermatol 1996;21:334.

142. Woo TY: Systemic isotretinoin treatment of oral and cutaneous lichen planus. Cutis 1985;35:390.

143. Lear JT, English JSC: Erosive and generalized lichen planus responsive to azathioprine. Br J Dermatol 1996;21:56.

144. Laurberg G, Geiger JM, Hjorth N, et al: Treatment of lichen planus with acitretin. J Am Acad Dermatol 1991;24:434.

145. Borrego L, Rodriguez RR, deFrutos JO, et al: Vulvar lichen planus treated with topical cyclosporine. Arch Dermatol 1993;129:794.

146. Pigatto PD, Chiappino G, Bigardi A, et al: Cyclosporine: For the treatment of severe lichen planus. Br J Dermatol 1999;122:121.

147. Jamec GBE, Baadsgaard O: Effect of cyclosporine on genital psoriasis and lichen planus. J Am Acad Dermatol 1993;29:1048.

148. Becherel PA, Chosidow O, Boisnic S, et al: Topical cyclosporine in the treatment of oral and vulval erosive lichen planus: A blood level monitoring study. Arch Dermatol 1995;131:495.

149. Eisen D: Hydroxychloroquine sulfate improves oral lichen planus. J Am Acad Dermatol 1993;28:609.

150. Sawai, T, Kitazawa K, Danno K, et al: Pemphigus vegetans with esophageal involvement: Successful treatment with minocycline and nicotinamide. Br J Dermatol 1995;132:668.

151. Poskitt L, Wojnarowsky F: Minimizing cicatricial pemphigoid orodynia with minocycline. Br J Dermatol 1995;132:784.

152. Buyuk AY, Karala M: Oral metronidazole treatment of lichen planus. J Am Acad Dermatol 2000;43(2 pt 1):260.

153. Wahba-Yahav AV: Idiopathic lichen planus: Treatment with metronidazole. J Am Acad Dermatol 1995;33(2 pt 1):301.

154. Camisa C, Popovsky JF: Effective treatment of oral erosive lichen planus with thalidomide. Arch Dermatol 2000;136:1442.

155. Popovsky JL, Camisa C: New and emerging therapies for diseases of the oral cavity. Dermatol Clin 2000;18:113.

156. Boyd AS: New and emerging therapies for lichenoid dermatoses. Dermatol Clin 2000;18:21.

157. Reitschel RL, Fowler JF: The role of age, sex and skin color. In Reitschel RL, Fowler JF (eds): Fisher's Contact Dermatitis. Philadelphia, Lippincott, Williams & Wilkins, 2001, pp 41–46.

158. Lynch PJ, Edwards L: Red plaques and eczematous features. In Lynch PJ, Edwards L (eds): Genital Dermatology. New York, Churchill Livingston, 1994, pp 34–41.

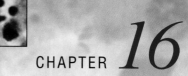

• Alex Ferenczy

CHAPTER *16*

Vulvar Intraepithelial Neoplasia

Since the first report, in 1922, of squamous cell carcinoma in situ of the vulva by French authors Hudelo, Boulanger-Pilet, and Caillau, the disease has taken on increased clinical, pathologic, investigative, and therapeutic interest.[1] During the 1990s, evolutionary changes occurred with respect to the disease's histologic classification and nomenclature, as well as with respect to the understanding of its pathogenic development in relationship with human papillomavirus (HPV) infection. New therapeutic approaches have also been developed.

The term *vulvar intraepithelial neoplasia* has replaced a myriad of traditional and often confusing terms.

In 1987, the Committee on Nomenclature of the International Society for the Study of Vulvar Disease (ISSVD) and the Committee on Histological Classification of Vulvar Tumors and Dystrophies of the International Society of Gynecological Pathologists recommended the use of the unifying generic terms *squamous intraepithelial neoplasia of the vulva* and *vulvar intraepithelial neoplasia* (VIN).[2] Accordingly, VIN has replaced a myriad of traditional and often confusing terms such as leukoplakia, Bowen's disease, bowenoid papulosis, bowenoid dysplasia, bowenoid atypia, erythroplasia of Queyrat, carcinoma simplex, squamous cell carcinoma in situ, and hyperplastic dystrophy with severe atypia. By definition, VIN must be composed of neoplastic cells confined to the boundaries of the squamous epithelium. It may regress, either spontaneously or after incomplete surgical removal; persist; or, if untreated, progress to invasive carcinoma.

The vulvar skin does not present the same morphologic alterations as its cervical counterpart in health and in disease.

The Committee on Histological Classification of Vulvar Tumors and Dystrophies and the Committee on Nomenclature of the ISSVD further recommended classification of VIN into grade 1 (mild dysplasia), grade 2 (moderate dysplasia), and grade 3 (severe dysplasia to carcinoma in situ).[3] The recommended grading of VIN is based solely on the height of the cellular abnormalities within the squamous epithelium. If only the lower third is involved, the VIN is graded 1. If the lower half is affected, the VIN is graded 2, and VIN grade 3 contains abnormal cells in the lower two thirds to the entire epithelium. Histologically, the intraepithelial change is characterized by nuclear hyperchromasia, coarse nuclear chromatin, and disorderly maturation of keratinocytes. Abnormal mitotic figures are seen in VIN 3. The extension of VIN 3 into hair follicles should not be mistaken for invasion. Hair follicles may extend downward 2.8 mm below what appears to be the basement membrane.

It is obvious that this grading system has been extrapolated from that applied to the nonkeratinizing squamous epithelium of the cervix. Unfortunately, there are several problems with grading VIN. First, the vulvar skin does not present the same morphologic alterations as its cervical counterpart in health or in disease; second, cancer pathogenesis in the vulva is different from that operating in the cervix; third, the consensus agreement today is that classifying cervical intraepithelial neoplasia (CIN) on a three-grade continuum is incompatible with current knowledge of the natural history of CIN and is arbitrary, artificial, and nonreproducible. Hence, CIN was reclassified as low-grade and high-grade CIN.[4] At best, VIN could be classified as low-grade and high-grade VIN; however, there has been no compelling epidemiologic, pathologic, and virologic evidence reported in the literature to support either the existence of or the relationship between low-grade and high-grade VIN.

Not a single scientific publication ascribes premalignant potential to VIN 1 or shows that VIN 1 or VIN 2 may progress to VIN 3.

Although the natural history of the so-called VIN 3 lesion is relatively well known, that of VIN 1 is not. Virtually all studies on the clinical, biologic, and morphologic characteristics of VIN have focused on VIN 3. Not a single scientific publication ascribes premalignant potential to VIN 1 or shows that VIN 1 (and, for that matter, VIN 2), may progress to VIN 3. Although occasional reports refer to VIN 1 as either pre-existing (four cases) or associated with invasive squamous cell carcinoma of the vulva, they invariably refer to elderly women with a median age of 71 years.[5] As will be shown later in this chapter, such women share no clinical, demographic, and morphologic similarities with those women who have VIN 3–type lesions. The artificial creation of the VIN grades 1, 2, and 3 classification scheme forces pathologists to make the diagnosis of VIN 1 whenever they face vulvar specimens that contain atypical cells in the lower third of an otherwise normal or hyperplastic squamous epithelium. Such alterations can be seen in a variety of dermatologic conditions, most of which have no relationship to vulvar squamous cell neoplasia (Table 16–1). The clinical implication of diagnosing VIN 1 as being part of the traditional VIN 1 to VIN 3 classification is twofold: (1) patients are wrongfully told that they may have a sexually transmitted disease, which, in turn, may lead to psychosexual distress and (2) patients may be inappropriately treated, often using ablative or excisional means. For example, a young patient with labial micropapillomatosis or vulvovaginitis owing to candidiasis may be inappropriately treated with ablative or even excisional techniques. The worst-case scenario is when young women are subjected to topical 5% fluorouracil (Efudex) treatment for so-called VIN 1. This treatment may result in adverse events, such as severe burning pain associated with extensive epithelial erosions and ulcerations, which, if untreated, may result in *kraurosis vulvae*.

It has been proposed that VIN be divided into two morphologically, clinically, and virologically distinct subsets.

Disease classifications are meaningful if they can be related to pathogenesis, are diagnostically reproducible, and have implications for management. On the basis of currently accumulated data, it has been proposed that VIN be divided into two morphologically, clinically, and virologically distinct subsets. One is characterized histologically by abnormal epithelial growth exhibiting impaired or no cell maturation throughout the epithelium, nuclear aneuploidy, and abnormal mitotic figures.[6] When a lesion is composed of a uniform, undifferentiated, basal cell–type population, it is referred to as basaloid VIN, whereas when a lesion contains a highly pleomorphic cell population with individual cell keratinization, multinucleation, and warty or verrucous, hyperkeratinized surface pattern,

▼ Table 16–1
Vulvar Conditions Referred to As VIN 1

Squamous epithelial hyperplasia
Lichen simplex chronicus
Lichen sclerosus
Hyperplastic dystrophy with atypia
Lichen sclerosus/squamous cell hyperplasia with atypia of repair
Lichen planus
Psoriasis
Seborrheic keratosis
Candidiasis
Micropapillomatosis labialis
Seborrheic/contact dermatitis
Flat/papular condylomata
Condylomata acuminata
Keratosis
Vulvar vestibulitis

VIN, vulvar intraepithelial neoplasia.

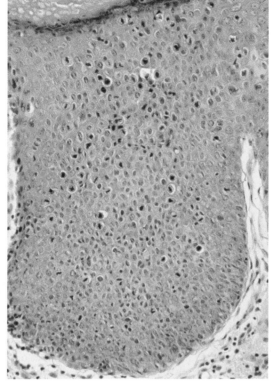

Figure 16–1. Histology of basaloid vulvar intraepithelial neoplasia. Note the transepithelial proliferation of uniform neoplastic cells that resemble basal cells containing numerous mitotic figures.

it is classified as warty VIN[7] (Figs. 16–1 and 16–2). From a clinical viewpoint, distinguishing between these two forms of VIN is not important, because both are often produced by high-risk HPV types, namely types 16 and 18, and are less frequently produced by other high oncogenic risk variants. Both tend to occur in younger women (mean age 30 years), and, in most cases, they are associated with the same demographic and behavioral patterns that are also observed in women with CIN.

Experience suggests that 80% of women with untreated basalo-warty–type VIN may develop invasive disease. Even those women who have been treated carry a 3% to 4% rate of cancer progression.

Typically, both basaloid and warty VINs tend to be multifocal and multicentric, with involvement of the perianal skin and cervical epithelium in approximately 50% of cases.[8] Also, in many cases, both forms coexist, with a direct histologic continuity and the same lesion foci (Figs. 16–3 and 16–4). Both lesions are precursors of basaloid and warty forms of invasive squamous cell carcinoma of the vulva.[9] Experience suggests that 80% of women with untreated basalo-warty–type VIN may develop invasive disease.[10] Even those women who have been treated carry a 3% to 4% rate of cancer progression.[6, 10, 11]

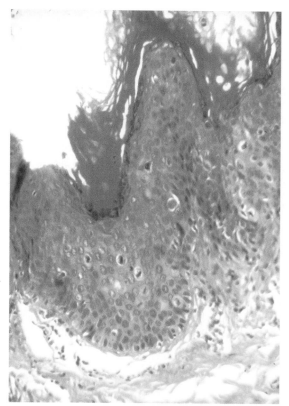

Figure 16–2. Histology of verrucous vulvar intraepithelial neoplasia. Papillary hyperkeratotic surface and pleomorphic neoplastic cells.

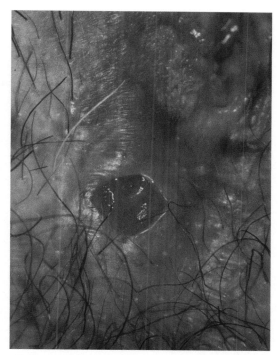

Figure 16–4. Detailed view of invasive carcinoma that developed 9 years after the original diagnosis of vulvar intraepithelial neoplasia.

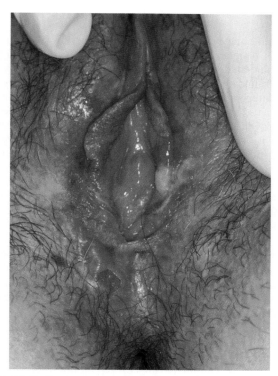

Figure 16–3. Basalo-verrucous form of vulvar intraepithelial neoplasia in a 37-year-old patient who has been a heavy smoker for 20 years. An indurated ulcer is seen in the perineal region at the 7-o'clock position. This is an invasive, basalo-verrucous squamous cell carcinoma with 5-mm dermal invasion.

> **Women with well-differentiated VIN simplex are 10 to 20 years older than and lack the behavioral and demographic risk factors of those with basaloid and warty forms of cancer.**

The second subset of VIN contains nuclear atypia involving only the lower third or the basal cell layer of the squamous epithelium. The inclusion of lesser grades of VIN (VIN 1) among precursor lesions is related to the fact that squamous cell carcinomas of the vulva may arise in association with areas of squamous cell hyperplasia or lichen sclerosus that show only atypia of the lower third of the epithelium. However, the cytonuclear atypia seen in such lesions is similar to that seen in repair-related atypia, with the upper two thirds of the epithelium containing no abnormal cellular features. Because of its extremely well-differentiated morphologic presentation, the term *simplex* has been used by some and the term *differentiated* by others.[7, 8, 12–15] Similar alterations are observed in the epithelium in well-differentiated squamous cell carcinomas of the oral cavity and particularly in lip carcinomas. Moreover, women with well-differentiated VIN simplex are 10 to 20 years older than and lack the behavioral and demographic risk factors of those observed with basaloid and warty forms of cancer.[8, 13, 16]

> **Unlike the poorly differentiated forms of VIN, intraepithelial neoplasia simplex tends to be unifocal, unicentric, and unrelated to HPV infection. It may be related to chronic itch-scratch cycles associated with squamous cell hyperplasia, lichen simplex chronicus, and lichen sclerosus.**

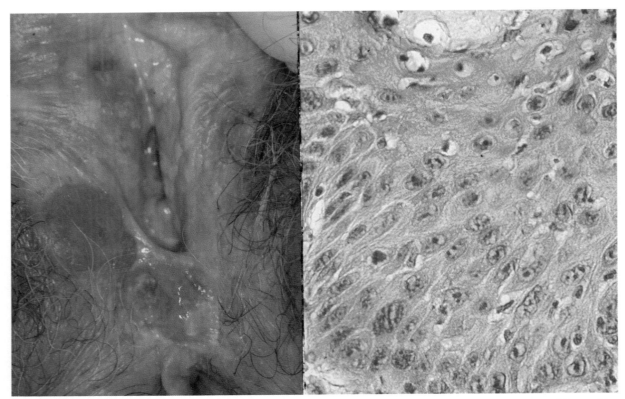

Figure 16-5. *Left,* a well-differentiated, invasive, keratinizing squamous cell carcinoma associated with lichen sclerosus in a 73-year-old woman. *Right,* the histology of vulvar intraepithelial neoplasia "simplex," which was adjacent to the carcinoma. Aside from the large nuclei and prominent nucleoli, cohesion and cellular organization were intact, as was differentiation.

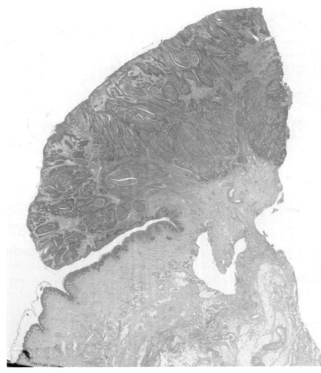

Figure 16-6. Whole mount histologic section of exophytic, keratinizing, well-differentiated invasive squamous cell carcinoma associated with squamous cell hyperplasia in an 89-year-old woman.

Unlike the poorly differentiated forms of VIN, intraepithelial neoplasia simplex tends to be unifocal, unicentric, and unrelated to HPV infection. Rather, its pathogenic background may be related to chronic itch-scratch cycles associated with squamous cell hyperplasia, lichen simplex chronicus, and lichen sclerosus.[17] It is possible, although not proven, that squamous cell hyperplasia in lichen sclerosus is a complication of the latter and may carry an increased malignant potential. The release of unidentified carcinogenic agents, together with the local environment of chronically irritated and inflamed skin, may play a major role in the development of intraepithelial and ultimately invasive, well-differentiated, keratinizing squamous cell carcinoma of the vulva in elderly patients.[18]

About 80% of invasive squamous cell carcinomas of the vulva in elderly patients are associated with untreated, long-standing, symptomatic lichen simplex chronicus, squamous cell hyperplasia, or lichen sclerosus.

Of interest is the clinical observation that, when treated topically with corticosteroid preparations, the lichen simplex chronicus type of symptomatic vulvar dermatosis rarely, if ever, progresses to invasive squamous cell carcinoma.[17] On the other hand, about 80% of invasive squamous cell carcinomas in elderly patients are associated with untreated, long-standing, symptomatic lichen simplex chronicus, squamous cell hyperplasia, or lichen sclerosus[19] (Figs. 16–5 and 16–6). In two series of invasive squamous cell carcinoma of the vulva, the percentage of synchronous VIN 1 was similar to that of squamous cell hyperplasia or lichen sclerosus (i.e., 53% to 59% and 60% to 79%, respectively).[5, 19]

> The basaloid and warty forms are best treated with ablative or excisional techniques, whereas the precursors of the simplex variant—squamous cell hyperplasia, lichen sclerosus, and lichen simplex chronicus—seem to respond well to topical application of potent formulations of corticosteroid cream or ointment.

If it is true that invasive squamous cell carcinomas of the vulva have two different pathogenic characteristics, then logically the nomenclature should reflect their distinctive features. Consequently, it may be time to revise the current classification of vulvar cancer precursors (Table 16–2). The advantage of the proposed classification is that it is based on morphology and currently emerging clinical and virologic data with respect to the two pathogenic origins of squamous cell cancers of the vulvar skin and their precursors. Furthermore, the classification can be related to management schemes. It appears that treating, rather than merely following up, women with vulvar cancer precursors, is the appropriate approach. This approach is likely to reduce the risk of progression to invasion. The basaloid and warty forms are best treated with ablative or excisional techniques, whereas the precursors of the simplex variant—squamous cell hyperplasia, lichen sclerosus, and lichen simplex chronicus—seem to respond well to topical application of potent formulations of corticosteroid cream or ointment. Future therapeutics for basaloid-warty VIN lesions may include immune response modifiers, such as topical 5% imiquimod cream therapy targeting the putative HPV DNA. Those interested in this challenging area of investigation are awaiting results of ongoing clinical trials of women with vulvar cancer precursors treated conservatively with topical formulations of corticosteroids and cell-mediated immune response modifiers.

It is critical to correlate clinical symptoms and signs with histology before embarking on therapy. If correlation is not obtained, review of histology or referral of patients to colleagues with expertise in gynecologic dermatology may be helpful.[20]

▼ Table 16–2

Proposed Classification of Vulvar Squamous Cell Carcinoma Precursors

Vulvar Intraepithelial Neoplasia
Basaloid
Warty
Mixed, basalo-warty
Simplex

Data from Ferenczy A: Intraepithelial neoplasia of the vulva. In Coppleson M (ed): Gynecologic Oncology: Fundamental Principles and Clinical Practice, vol. 1, 3rd ed. London, Churchill Livingstone, 1992, pp 443–463.

SUMMARY OF KEY POINTS

- VIN has replaced a myriad of traditional and often confusing terms.

- The recommended grading of VIN is based solely on the height of the cellular abnormalities within the squamous epithelium.

- The vulvar skin does not present the same morphologic alterations as its cervical counterpart.

- Atypical cells in the lower third of an otherwise normal or hyperplastic squamous epithelium (VIN 1) can be seen in a variety of dermatologic conditions, most of which have no relationship to vulvar squamous cell neoplasia.

- Cancer pathogenesis in the vulva is different from that operating in the cervix.

- There is no evidence that VIN 1 or VIN 2 has premalignant potential.

- There are two forms of vulvar cancer precursors: undifferentiated to poorly differentiated VIN and well-differentiated VIN.

- Undifferentiated to poorly differentiated VIN manifests morphologically as basaloid, warty, or a mixture of both; occurs in younger women; is caused by high–oncogenic risk HPV types; tends to be multifocal and multicentric; and is the precursor of basaloid and verrucous squamous cell carcinomas of the vulvar skin.

- Well-differentiated VIN manifests morphologically as VIN simplex; occurs in women 10 to 20 years older than those in whom undifferentiated to poorly differentiated VIN occurs; tends to be unifocal and unicentric; is unrelated to HPV infection; histologically contains nuclear atypia involving only the lower third or the basal cell layer of the squamous epithelium; may evolve from long-standing, symptomatic vulvar dermatosis; and is the precursor of well-differentiated, keratinizing squamous cell carcinoma of the vulva.

- Experience suggests that 80% of women with untreated basalo-warty type VIN may develop invasive disease. Even those women who have been treated carry a 3% to 4% rate of cancer progression.

- Basaloid and warty VIN lesions tend to involve the perianal skin and cervical epithelium in approximately 50% of cases.

- About 80% of invasive squamous cell carcinomas in elderly patients are associated with untreated, long-standing, symptomatic lichen simplex chronicus, squamous cell hyperplasia, or lichen sclerosus.

- Basaloid and warty forms of VIN are best treated with ablative or excisional techniques.

- The precursors of the simplex variant of VIN,
Continued on following page

squamous cell hyperplasia, lichen sclerosus, and lichen simplex chronicus respond well to topical application of potent formulations of corticosteroid cream or ointment.

References

1. Hudelo M, Boulanger-Pilet M, Caillau M: Erythrokératodermie verruqueuse en nappes symétriques et progressives congénitales. Bull Soc Française Dermatol Syphol 1922;29:45.
2. Colgan TJ: Vulvar intraepithelial neoplasia: A synopsis of recent developments. J Lower Genital Tract Dis 1998;2:31.
3. Report of the Committee on Terminology of the International Society for the Study of Vulvar Disease: New nomenclature for vulvar disease. J Reprod Med 1990;35:483.
4. Wright TC, Kurman RJ, Ferenczy A: Precancerous lesions of the cervix. In Kurman RJ (ed): Blaustein's Pathology of the Female Genital Tract. New York, Springer-Verlag, 1994, pp 229–277.
5. Kagie MJ, Kenter GG, Hermans J, et al: The relevance of various vulvar epithelial changes in the early detection of squamous cell carcinoma of the vulva. Int J Gynecol Cancer 1997;7:50.
6. Crum CP: Carcinoma of the vulva: Epidemiology and pathogenesis. Obstet Gynecol 1992;79:448.
7. Kurman RJ, Toki T, Schiffman MH: Basaloid and warty carcinoma of the vulva. Am J Surg Pathol 1993;17:133.
8. Brinton LA, Nasca PC, Mallin K, et al: Case-control study of cancer of the vulva. Obstet Gynecol 1990;75:863.
9. Jones RW, Rowan DM: Vulvar intraepithelial neoplasia III: A clinical study of the outcome in 113 cases with relation to the later development of invasive vulvar carcinoma. Obstet Gynecol 1994;84:741.
10. Jones RW, Baranyai J, Stables S: Trends in squamous cell carcinoma of the vulva: The influence of vulvar intraepithelial neoplasia. Obstet Gynecol 1997;90:448.
11. Herod JJ, Shafi MI, Rollason TP, et al: Vulval intraepithelial neoplasia: Long term follow up of treated and untreated women. Br J Obstet Gynecol 1996;103:446.
12. Karram M, Tabor B, Smotkin D, et al: Detection of human papillomavirus deoxyribonucleic acid from vulvar dystrophies and vulvar intraepithelial neoplastic lesions. Am J Obstet Gynecol 1988;159:22.
13. Hörding U, Junge J, Daugaard S, et al: Vulvar squamous cell carcinoma and papillomaviruses: Indications for two different etiologies. Gynecol Oncol 1994;52:241.
14. Scurry J, Vanin K, Östör A: Comparison of histological features of vulvar lichen sclerosus with and without adjacent squamous cell carcinoma. Int J Gynecol Cancer 1997;7:392.
15. Leibowitch M, Neill S, Pelisse M: The epithelial changes associated with squamous cell carcinoma of the vulva: A review of the clinical, histological and viral findings in 78 women. Br J Obstet Gynaecol 1990;97:1135.
16. Trimble CL, Hildesheim A, Brinton LA, et al: Heterogeneous etiology of squamous carcinoma of the vulva. Obstet Gynecol 1996;87:59.
17. Scurry J: Does lichen sclerosus play a central role in the pathogenesis of human papillomavirus negative vulvar squamous cell carcinoma? The itch-scratch-lichen sclerosus hypothesis. Int J Gynecol Cancer 1999;9:89.
18. zur Hausen H: Human genital cancer: Synergism between two virus infections or synergism between a virus infection and initiating events. Lancet 1982;2:1370.
19. Zaino RJ, Husseinzadeh N, Hahhas W, et al: Epithelial alterations in proximity to invasive squamous carcinoma of the vulva. Int J Gynecol Pathol 1982;1:173.
20. Ferenczy A: Intraepithelial neoplasia of the vulva. In Coppleson M (ed): Gynecologic Oncology: Fundamental Principles and Clinical Practice, vol. 1, 3rd ed. London, Churchill Livingstone, 1992 pp 443–463.

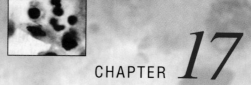

CHAPTER *17*

Vulvar Intraepithelial Neoplasia: Clinical Manifestations

CLINICAL MANIFESTATIONS OF VIN LESIONS

Three types of vulvar intraepithelial neoplasia (VIN) related to human papillomavirus (HPV) are seen by the practicing colposcopist: bowenoid papulosis, classic Bowen's disease, and acetowhite epithelium. Bowen described the diseases that bear his name in 1912. He observed and treated a group of patients 12 to 16 years old and concluded that cautery and curetting were ineffective treatments. He also concluded that these lesions do not lead to cancer except in older individuals with isolated plaquelike lesions.

Bowenoid papulosis appears as pigmented, wartlike growths or papules in younger women, and it almost always has perianal involvement but usually does not have associated vaginal lesions.

Of the three types of VIN 3 seen by the practicing colposcopist, one has been historically referred to as bowenoid papulosis. Although use of this term is discouraged, it does serve to separate clinical forms of VIN 3. Such lesions may increase in frequency and appear as pigmented, wartlike growths or papules. These lesions generally occur in younger women (third to fifth decades of life). Bowenoid papulosis is clinically similar to genital warts in terms of its distribution on vulva (skin and vestibule). The patient with bowenoid papulosis almost always has perianal involvement but usually does not have associated vaginal lesions (Fig. 17–1).

Cases of bowenoid papulosis that progress to invasion are usually extensive lesions and are found in immunocompromised individuals, including smokers.

Bowenoid papulosis contains different HPV types than condyloma acuminatum contains (HPV types 16, 18, 31, and 33 versus HPV types 6 and 11). The high-risk HPV types of bowenoid papulosis, particularly HPV 16, are also associated with an increased risk for cervical intraepithelial neoplasia (CIN) and invasive carcinoma. Bowenoid papulosis shares age of onset (or a slightly later onset) and sexual behavior pattern with condyloma. Bowenoid papulosis is clearly a sexually transmitted disease, and it usually has a benign evolution. Cases of bowenoid papulosis that progress to invasion are usually extensive lesions and are found in immunocompromised individuals, including smokers. Regression of bowenoid papulosis

Figure 17–1. Human papillomavirus infection in a human immunodeficiency virus–positive patient. Histology was condylomata acuminata laterally and vulvar intraepithelial neoplasia grade 3 medially. Human papillomavirus studies were positive.

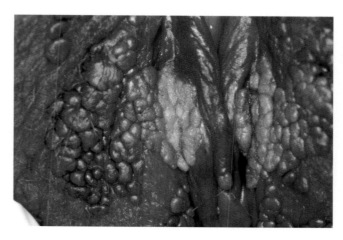

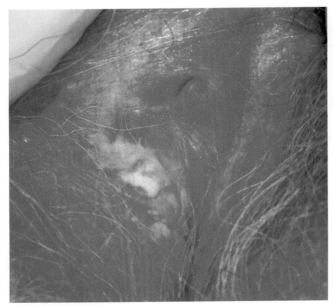

Figure 17-2. Well-differentiated vulvar intraepithelial neoplasia grade 3 associated with lichen sclerosus. Clinically white lesion. Human papillomavirus studies were negative.

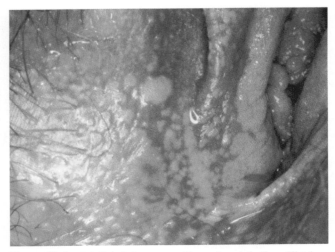

Figure 17-3. Subclinical human papillomavirus infection. Histology showed vulvar intraepithelial neoplasia grade 3. The infection was self-limited and had resolved at 6 months.

has been reported in healthy individuals and in some individuals after pregnancy and cessation of smoking.

Bowen's disease appears as a solitary plaque in older women.

Although Bowen's disease does occur in younger patients, it usually appears as a solitary plaque in older women (sixth decade of life or older) (Fig. 17-2). Unlike other HPV-related VIN lesions, there has not been a reported increase in the incidence of classic Bowen's disease. A study of 75 VIN patients (36 patients with classic Bowen's disease and 39 patients with bowenoid papulosis) demonstrated that these two HPV-related VIN lesions are separable clinically. The age of the onset is later for classic Bowen's disease (55.6 years compared with 33.2 years for bowenoid papulosis). Although classic Bowen's disease and bowenoid papulosis are associated with similar HPV types (types 16, 18, 31, and 33), the risk of invasive carcinoma is much greater with classic Bowen's disease (27.8%) than it is with bowenoid papulosis (2.6%).

Acetowhite VIN lesions appear to coalesce on the mucous membranes of the vestibule but often form small, dome-shaped satellite tumors on the keratinized epithelium across Hart's line.

Acetowhite VIN often appears as a field of acetowhite epithelium that demonstrates small satellite tumors at its periphery. Acetowhite lesions appear to coalesce on the mucous membranes of the vestibule but often form small, dome-shaped satellite tumors on the keratinized epithelium across Hart's line (Fig. 17-3). Although these le-

sions frequently show signs of significant atypia, they often regress. Typing of these lesions in a small number of patients has revealed high-risk types (HPV type 33). It is unknown whether this form of VIN ever progresses.

Role of HPV in VIN

HPV is transmitted by direct contact with site-subtype specificity. Viral VIN 3 is easily diagnosed by biopsy, and lesions are grossly visible (Fig. 17-4); therefore, diagnosis poses little problem. However, treatment proves difficult, most likely because the HPV infection is not limited to visible lesions. The practitioner must also be aware that an even more serious lesion may be present on the cervix in approximately 30% of cases and that HPV DNA is found in more than 80% of cases of VIN 3 and

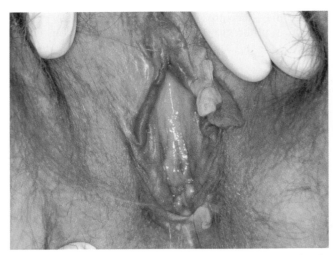

Figure 17-4. Viral vulvar intraepithelial neoplasia grade 3 involving the clitoral prepuce, labia minora, and introitus. Human papillomavirus studies were positive.

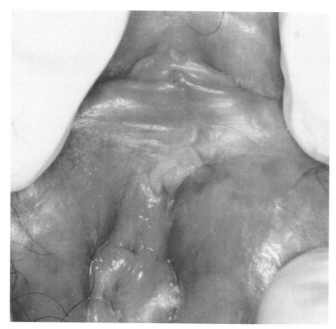

Figure 17–5. Vulvar intraepithelial neoplasia grade 3 in a 30-year-old woman whose husband was treated for external genital warts. Human papillomavirus infection was confirmed, and vulvar intraepithelial neoplasia was diagnosed. The treatment was CO_2 laser vaporization and close follow-up.

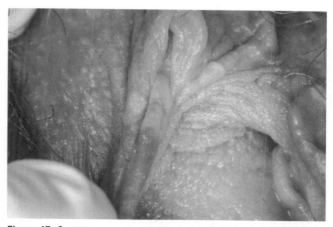

Figure 17–6. Diffuse human papillomavirus infection of the labia minora and vestibule. Histology of the most severe site was vulvar intraepithelial neoplasia grade 3 with signs of human papillomavirus infection. Treatment with imiquimod resulted in complete resolution.

its related cancers (Figs. 17–5 through 17–7). The most common types are HPV 16, 31, and 33.

Despite the tendency for VIN in younger women to be HPV related and for VIN in older women to be related to vulvar dermatoses and to be HPV negative, there is overlap.

Older women with vulvar carcinoma tend to not have HPV-related disease. VIN lesions that are commonly as-sociated with cancer tend to occur in older women and are HPV negative, whereas common, or classic, VIN lesions with koilocytotic atypia, multinucleation, and verrucopapillary morphology generally occur in younger women and are HPV positive. VIN 1 or even VIN 2 found in areas of squamous cell hyperplasia and lichen sclerosus may respond promptly to fluorosteroids, but symptoms (pruritus) and lesions often recur. Lichen sclerosus or squamous cell hyperplasia with significant cytologic atypia may be difficult to manage with topical medication. Persistent symptoms should prompt a search for areas of VIN. However, despite the tendency for VIN in younger women to be HPV related and VIN in older women to be related to vulvar dermatoses and to be HPV negative, there is overlap. Three of six lesions of lichen sclerosus–associated VIN, including one involving invasive carcinoma in an elderly woman, contained HPV nucleic acids; all three lesions exhibited the features of

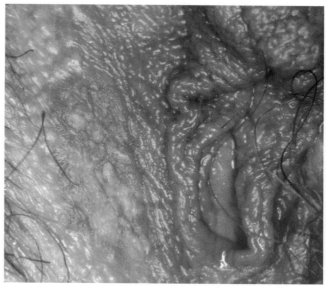

Figure 17–7. Human papillomavirus infection localized to the right labia majora. Histology was vulvar intraepithelial neoplasia grade 3.

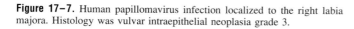

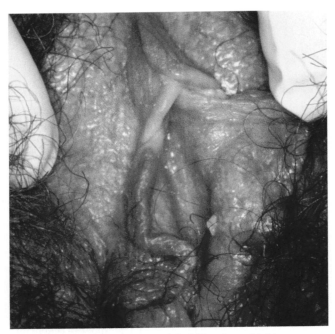

Figure 17–8. Lichen sclerosus on right labia minor with biopsy-proven human papillomavirus–positive lesion on left labia minora.

classic VIN. The finding of HPV across a broad age range suggests that this virus may play a role in vulvar neoplasia at any point in life. HPV in lichen sclerosus–associated VIN links two distinct risk factors to the same neoplasm (Fig. 17–8).

Bowenoid papulosis is treated in a manner similar to that of condylomata acuminata. Persistent VIN in areas of dermatoses is treated with topical, superpotent corticosteroids or with local excision if treatment with corticosteroids fails.

The choice of treatment is determined by lesion type and by grade of the lesion. Bowenoid papulosis is treated in a manner similar to the treatment of condylomata acuminata. Cryosurgery, electrosurgery, laser ablation, topical acids and tretinoin, interferon, and conservative surgical excision have been used successfully. Colposcopically directed laser vaporization is precise and effective and causes little scarring. Plaquelike lesions typical of Bowen's disease are usually removed surgically along with adequate margins (1 to 1.5 cm of contiguous normal-appearing skin) (Fig. 17–9). Persistent VIN in areas of dermatoses (lichen sclerosus and squamous cell hyperplasia) is treated with topical, superpotent corticosteroids or with local excision if treatment with corticosteroids fails.

When VIN involves hair-bearing areas, the disease may extend down the hair shaft for up to 2.8 mm. Eradication of this lesion must use therapy that extends to adequate depth.

When VIN involves hair-bearing areas, the disease may extend down the hair shaft for up to 2.8 mm. Eradi-

cation of this lesion must use therapy that extends to adequate depth (e.g., CO_2 laser vaporization 3.0 mm deep). Patients with HPV-related VIN 3 who are pregnant or are coming off steroids and patients attempting to quit smoking may be observed for a time without treatment. Persistent lesions after the correction of the immunocompromised state require therapy.

Thirty percent of patients with multifocal disease or patients who smoke have a recurrence regardless of method or extent of therapy.

Thirty percent of patients with multifocal disease or patients who smoke have a recurrence regardless of method or extent of therapy (including simple vulvectomy). No treatment for VIN is completely successful; therefore, the most important aspect of therapy is close follow-up of these patients. Patients should be examined with colposcopy every 4 to 6 months, and ongoing therapy should be planned early. Vestibular and perianal recurrences are common without close follow-up examinations, and anal carcinoma is a real risk. Even after 12 disease-free months, 15% to 25% of patients may have recurrence.

Colposcopic Appearance of VIN

Approximately 75% to 85% of VIN lesions are found in non–hair-bearing areas, 30% to 40% of VIN cases are multifocal, and both hair-bearing and non–hair-bearing areas are involved in 15% of cases.

The pigmented papules and plaques of the vulva (bowenoid papulosis and classic Bowen's disease) may involve any site on the vulva and may demonstrate surrounding subclinical HPV infection (Fig. 17-10). HPV-related acetowhite VIN 3 as an isolated finding usually involves the vestibule and extends onto the labia minora. Approximately 75% to 85% of VIN lesions are found in non–hair-bearing areas, 30% to 40% of VIN cases are multifo-

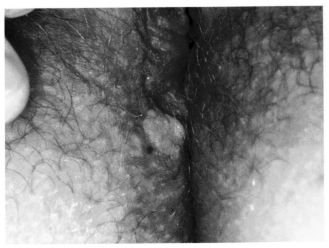

Figure 17–9. A 3 cm × 4 cm plaque of sharply defined vulvar intraepithelial neoplasia grade 3. This condition was formerly referred to as Bowen's disease.

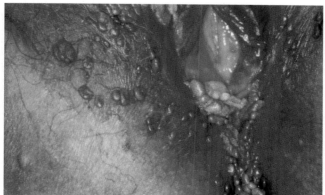

Figure 17–10. Bowenoid papulosis is a viral disease that may resemble genital warts. Note the pigmented papules that tend to coalesce. Frequently, there is contiguous papillary acetowhite epithelium. Histology was vulvar intraepithelial neoplasia grade 3.

cal, and both hair-bearing and non–hair-bearing areas are involved in 15% of cases.

As a general rule, lesions closer to the introitus are less pigmented.

The hair-bearing skin contains more melanocytes than does the mucous membrane, and, as a general rule, lesions closer to the introitus are less pigmented. VIN may be thick, hyperplastic tissue with a raised, often smooth surface, and it may be verrucous or surprisingly macular. Individual lesions may range from a few millimeters to several centimeters in size and have been noted to have sharp borders and even pigmentation (gray to light black lesions or more vascular red lesions).

Almost all VIN, regardless of gross color, will turn acetowhite (to some degree) after application of 3% to 5% acetic acid.

Almost all VIN, regardless of gross color, will turn acetowhite (to some degree) after application of 3% to 5% acetic acid (Fig. 17–11). The colposcopic appearance of VIN is similar to that of condylomata acuminata (i.e., acuminate warts, flat warts, and subclinical papillomavirus infection [acetowhite tissue positive for HPV]). The lesions may be macular with a micropapillary surface contour, or they may be seen only as small, dome-shaped acetowhite tumors. Grossly visible HPV-related VIN might be surrounded by colposcopically visible, subclinical HPV infection of the contiguous skin. Viral involvement of nearby skin contributes to difficulty in treating this condition (Fig. 17–12).

Lesser grades of VIN are more faintly acetowhite. Higher-grade lesions are thicker and more pigmented.

The most common lesion on the labia minora is a micropapillary, flat to slightly elevated, warty lesion.

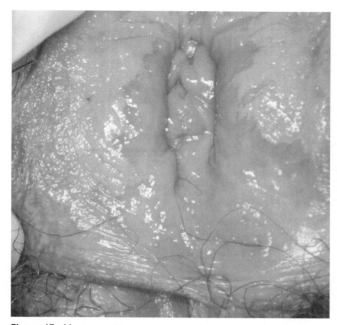

Figure 17–11. Acetowhitening resulting from subacute or chronic inflammation.

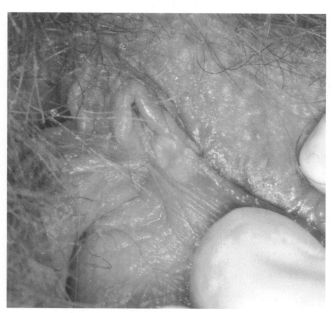

Figure 17–12. Viral vulvar intraepithelial neoplasia grade 3. Digital transmission was suggested by history.

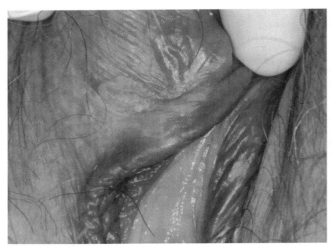

Figure 17–13. Gray-white epithelium forming rounded margins. Histology was vulvar intraepithelial neoplasia grade 3 with viral effects.

Lesser grades of VIN are more faintly acetowhite. Higher-grade lesions are thicker and more pigmented. Lesions may be red, black, white, brown, or gray (Fig. 17–13). Lesions may be sharply demarcated or may fuse with each other. Isolated, pigmented, warty lesions are more common in younger patients, and isolated plaques are more common in older patients. Intra-anal VIN is usually warty and white, but it may be gray or more pigmented. At the anal verge near the rectum, these lesions are often associated with frondlike epithelial papillations, with each frond containing a single-looped capillary (Fig. 17–14). In the more peripheral regions of the vulva, one may note hair shafts protruding from VIN lesions. This finding is commonly associated with involvement of VIN in the hair shaft. These lesions may extend to a depth of 1.5 mm or greater.

Patients with vulvar squamous cell hyperplasia and lichen sclerosus should also be examined colposcopically. VIN appears as areas of thickening or erosion of tissue with a change toward red color but no specific pattern or appearance. With invasion, atypical vessels are visualized. Vascular patterns are generally found on the mucous membranes, because the stromal vessels are more visible in this region. Punctation is the most common colposcopic vascular pattern noted, but mosaic is also seen on occasion.

SUMMARY OF KEY POINTS

- Bowenoid papulosis appears as pigmented, wartlike growths or papules in younger women and almost always has perianal involvement, but it usually does not have associated vaginal lesions.

- Bowenoid papulosis has the same age of onset and sexual behavior pattern as vulvar warts have, is clearly a sexually transmitted disease, and usually has a benign evolution.

- Regression of bowenoid papulosis has been reported in healthy individuals or in individuals after pregnancy and cessation of smoking.

- Cases of bowenoid papulosis that progress to invasion are usually extensive lesions and are found in immunocompromised individuals, including smokers.

- Bowen's disease appears as a solitary plaque in older women.

- The risk of invasive carcinoma is much greater with classic Bowen's disease (27.8%) than it is with bowenoid papulosis (2.6%).

- Acetowhite VIN lesions appear to coalesce on the mucous membranes of the vestibule but often form small, dome-shaped satellite tumors on the keratinized epithelium across Hart's line.

- Although VIN in younger women tends to be HPV related and VIN in older women tends to be related to vulvar dermatoses and to be HPV negative, there is overlap.

- Lichen sclerosus or squamous cell hyperplasia not responsive to treatment with topical medication should prompt a search for areas of VIN.

- Bowenoid papulosis is treated in a manner similar to that of condylomata acuminata.

- Persistent VIN in areas of dermatoses is treated with topical, superpotent corticosteroids or with local excision if treatment with corticosteroids fails.

- When VIN involves hair-bearing areas, the disease may extend down the hair shaft for up to 2.8 mm. Eradication of this lesion must use therapy that extends to adequate depth.

- Patients with HPV-related VIN 3 who are pregnant, coming off steroids, or attempting to quit smoking may be observed for a time without treatment.

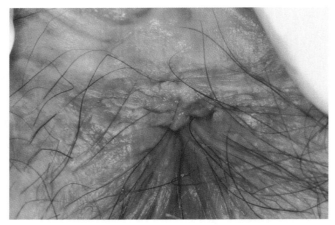

Figure 17–14. Perineal and perianal intraepithelial neoplasia revealing dense white epithelium and frondlike surface. This patient was treated with the CO_2 laser.

- Thirty percent of patients with multifocal disease or patients who smoke have a recurrence regardless of method or extent of therapy.

- Approximately 75% to 85% of VIN lesions are found in non–hair-bearing areas, 30% to 40% of VIN cases are multifocal, and both hair-bearing and non–hair-bearing areas are involved in 15% of cases.

- As a general rule, lesions closer to the introitus are less likely to be pigmented.

- Almost all VIN, regardless of gross color, will turn acetowhite (to some degree) after the application of 3% to 5% acetic acid.

- Lesser grades of VIN are more faintly acetowhite. Higher-grade lesions are thicker and more pigmented.

- Patients with vulvar squamous cell hyperplasia and lichen sclerosus should also be examined colposcopically.

- Punctation is the most common colposcopic vascular pattern noted, but mosaic is also seen on occasion.

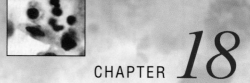
Colposcopy of External Genital Condyloma

Although the colposcope was initially used only to evaluate cervical epithelium, it can also be used to evaluate any accessible surface. First thought of as a "competitor" to exfoliative cytology, the colposcope is now an indispensable tool for evaluation of the entire lower genital tract (cervix, vagina, vulva/perineum, and anus) in women as well as in men.

The normal vulvar epithelium (Fig. 18–1) can be inspected with the unaided eye as well as with the colposcope. The relative lack of active squamous metaplasia in vulvar epithelium minimizes but does not eliminate the possibility of morphologic changes such as punctation and mosaic. Despite this, vulvar abnormalities visible after the application of 3% to 5% acetic acid can still indicate occult disease processes, as is often the case with the cervix. However, the alterations of color, opacity, and surface contour produced by diluted acetic acid application are less consistent and pronounced on the vulvar epithelium than they are on the cervix. One could there-

fore take the position that colposcopy of the vulva is of little practical value unless there is gross alteration of the vulvar skin that is first seen with naked eye examination. This position underestimates the potential value of vulvar colposcopy. The colposcope is an indispensable tool for evaluating the patient with known or suspected vulvar pathology, as well as for evaluating the symptomatic patient with a grossly abnormal-appearing vulva who has an otherwise negative evaluation.

The colposcope is a valuable tool for evaluating the patient with known or suspected vulvar pathology.

Any discussion of the potential value of colposcopy in patients with vulvar condylomata must focus on two distinct groups of patients: those who have gross genital warts and/or preinvasive or invasive lesions and those who have a grossly normal vulvar epithelium but who may have subclinical human papillomavirus (HPV) infection. The usefulness of colposcopy differs for these two groups of patients. Furthermore, there is a well-defined role for colposcopy both during and after treatment of vulvar condylomata.

Women who are otherwise asymptomatic may request treatment for vulvar condylomata because warts are cosmetically unappealing or cause sexual or emotional problems.

CLINICALLY EVIDENT VULVAR CONDYLOMA

The importance of HPV infection in the female population cannot be overestimated. By the year 2000, in the United States alone, there were almost 1.5 million patient visits per year for genital condylomata.[1] Although very few of these genital HPV infections in nonimmunocompromised women ultimately progress to squamous cell carcinoma, HPV infection has contributed to a dramatic increase in the incidence of high-grade vulvar intraepithelial neoplasia, particularly in younger women. Women with HPV who do not have vulvar carcinoma or precur-

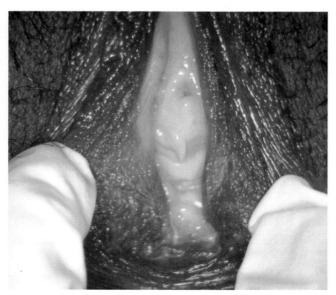

Figure 18–1. Normal vulvar mucosa.

sor lesions may still request or require therapy for genital tract condyloma because it is a cosmetically unappealing condition and may be a cause of emotional and sexual problems, even in women who are otherwise asymptomatic. Although the treatment of external condylomata may not significantly decrease viral transmission to the sexual partner, if it is requested, it should not be denied. HPV is a sexually transmitted disease and may indicate the possible presence of other venereal disease. Condylomatous lesions may also complicate pregnancy outcome.

Some women will be diagnosed with genital condylomata during pregnancy, when the growth of these lesions may accelerate.

Most women with genital tract condylomata will require medical attention either because they have evidence of HPV on the cytologic smear or because they notice the presence of vulvar growths. A smaller number of women will be diagnosed with genital condylomata during pregnancy, when the growth of these lesions may accelerate. It is rare for women to seek medical attention first because they discover genital warts on a sexual partner.

Accurate colposcopic evaluation of the patient with clinical vulvar condylomata is the essential step in both counseling the patient appropriately about the diagnosis and selecting appropriate therapy. Although most patients who present with suspected vulvar warts in fact have vulvar condylomata, this will not always be the case. Mimics of condylomatous lesions can be present, and the colposcopist will need to perform a thorough examination to distinguish among the variants.

Failure to perform colposcopy or magnified examination may result in missing the diagnosis of either verrucous or condylomatous invasive squamous cell carcinoma of the vulva.

Vulvar "warts" should be confirmed to be vulvar condylomata by visual inspection, by colposcopic examination, and by a colposcopically directed biopsy to make an accurate diagnosis. Failure to perform colposcopy or magnified examination may result in missing the diagnosis of either verrucous or condylomatous invasive squamous cell carcinoma of the vulva[2, 3] or in failing to diagnose concomitant vulvar intraepithelial neoplasia or invasion. There is also the possibility of unnecessarily treating patients for normal anatomic variants, such as micropapillomatosis labialis or squamous cell hyperplasia, that may mimic vulvar condylomata. Therefore, it is critical, regardless of how "classic appearing" the vulvar condylomata may be, that the diagnosis of HPV infection be confirmed before any therapeutic intervention.

Regardless of how classic a condyloma may appear, the correct diagnosis must be made before initiation of therapy.

Finally, some colposcopists[4] recommend colposcopic evaluation of the entire lower genital tract, even in the most clinically obvious cases of vulvar condylomata, because many of these women will have HPV-associated disease in other areas, including the perineum, vagina,

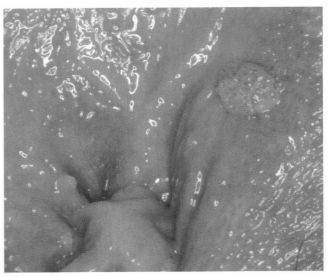

Figure 18-2. Small condylomatous lesions.

and cervix.[5] However, others contend that if the woman has had a recent negative Papanicolaou (Pap) smear, it is not absolutely necessary to immediately proceed to colposcopic examination of the cervix.

The colposcope is the ideal tool to best characterize the morphology of the vulvar lesion, to determine its extent, and to identify additional lesions.

Evaluation of the patient with clinically evident vulvar condylomata begins with gross inspection of the vulva by naked eye examination. Adequate lighting is essential, and inspection of hair-bearing areas must be carried out as well. Once a lesion has been identified (Fig. 18–2), the colposcope is the ideal adjunctive tool to better characterize the morphology of the lesion, to determine its extent, to identify additional lesions, and, if necessary, to evaluate the remainder of the lower genital tract.

The vulva is the most common site of clinically evident HPV infection.

The vulva is the most common site of clinically evident HPV infection. Signs of HPV infection often appear initially as small, warty growths on the labia minora and majora. These growths may extend to the vaginal introitus and perineum, and, in some patients, they may coalesce to form large, confluent, cauliflower-like masses with broad bases (Fig. 18–3). Rapid growth may be particularly pronounced in pregnant patients as well as in patients with immunosuppressive conditions such as uncontrolled diabetes mellitus, inflammatory bowel disease, medical conditions requiring chronic steroid therapy, organ transplantation, and infection with human immunodeficiency virus (HIV).

It is important to rule out verrucous carcinoma in patients who present with massive, ulcerated, cauliflower-like growths on the vulva.

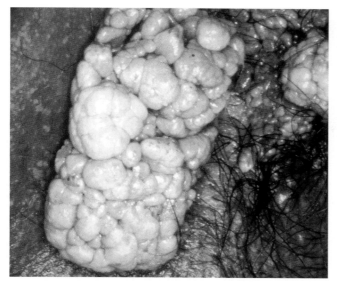

Figure 18–3. Large, cauliflower-like condylomatous growths. Image provided by Dr. Burton Krumholz.

Large, ulcerated, cauliflower-like growths and confluent masses of condylomatous lesions that essentially obliterate the vulva are uncommon (Fig. 18–4). In such cases, biopsies are essential to exclude verrucous carcinoma (Fig. 18–5) and condylomatous squamous cell carcinoma (Fig. 18–6). The individual warty lesion, whether flattened or cauliflower-like, usually has a reassuringly uni-

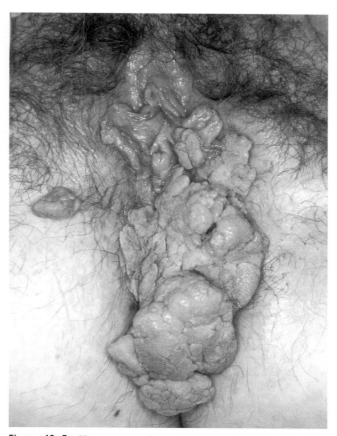

Figure 18–5. Verrucous carcinoma. Image provided by Dr. Alex Ferenczy.

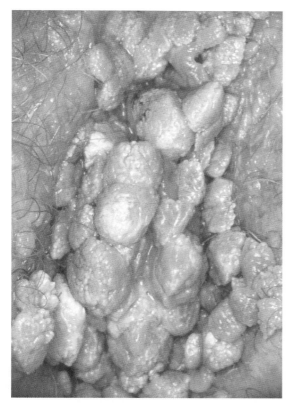

Figure 18–4. Confluent condylomatous growth. Image provided by Dr. Burton Krumholz.

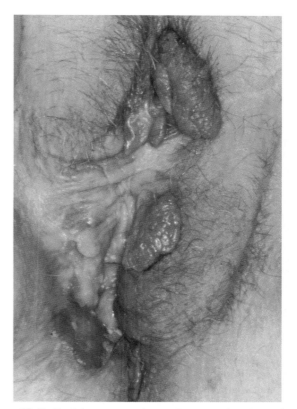

Figure 18–6. Condylomatous carcinoma. Image provided by Dr. Alex Ferenczy.

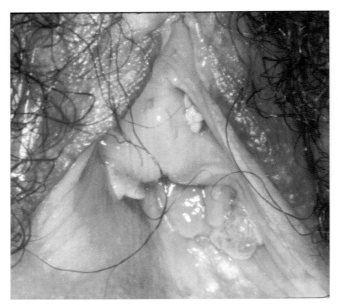

Figure 18-7. Vascular surface of condyloma. Image provided by Dr. Gordon Davis.

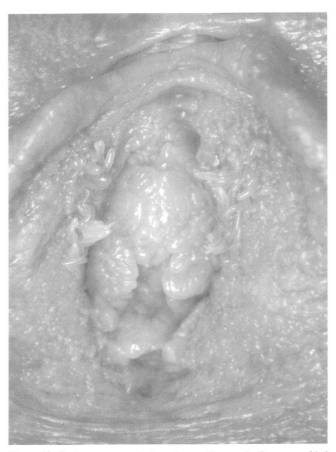

Figure 18-8. Squamous vestibular micropapillomatosis. Image provided by Dr. Burton Krumholz.

form vascular pattern. Occasionally, however, the vascular network may be bizarre or suspicious for invasion, even in otherwise benign-appearing lesions. These changes may be evident only under colposcopic magnification (Fig. 18-7). Selecting the appropriate area for biopsy may be impossible without the aid of a colposcope.

Because HPV is a sexually transmitted disease, any patient with vulvar condylomata is at greater risk of having other sexually transmitted diseases, so she should be screened for chlamydia, gonorrhea, syphilis, hepatitis, and HIV infection. HIV is of particular concern in women who present with massive or very widespread vulvar condylomata (regardless of age), as well as in women with vulvar condylomata that are refractory to any form of therapy. A careful sexual history that includes questions about current and previous sexual partners is essential to counsel patients about potential risks.[6]

The colposcope can help distinguish gross vulvar condylomata from normal anatomic variants such as micropapillomatosis labialis.

Colposcopy is also of value in distinguishing vulvar condylomata from normal anatomic variants, such as vestibular micropapillomatosis labialis,[7] that are of clinical importance only to the extent that they may mimic HPV infection and result in unnecessary treatment (Fig. 18-8). Although the skilled colposcopist will be able to easily distinguish small condylomata from normal anatomic variants, a colposcopically directed biopsy or consultation with another colposcopist may be necessary before instituting or recommending any form of therapy if significant diagnostic doubt exists.

The colposcope can be used to precisely apply topical therapeutic agents to small condylomatous lesions.

Although the diagnosis of overt vulvar condylomata can usually be established by gross visual inspection, the colposcope is of value for close inspection of the remainder of the vulva, particularly the hair-bearing portion, to establish the volume and location of any other HPV-associated disease. The colposcope may also be used occasionally to assist in the precise application of topical therapeutic agents for the treatment of small vulvar warts. Also, large warts may be most effectively treated using surgical or ablative modalities (excision, CO_2 laser, Cavitron ultrasonic surgical aspirator, electrocautery) that are best carried out under colposcopic guidance. This approach maximizes the ability to eradicate all gross disease, to control the depth to which either laser ablative or excision therapy is carried out, and to enhance any treatment by adjunctively treating adjacent, normal-appearing vulvar epithelium. Any vulvar condyloma that appears resistant to either chemical or destructive therapy should be re-evaluated with colposcopy and directed biopsy before instituting alternative therapies.

Any vulvar condyloma that is resistant to chemical or destructive therapy should be re-evaluated with colposcopy before switching therapies.

SUBCLINICAL HPV INFECTION

Subclinical HPV infection is invisible to the naked eye. Three to five minutes after application of 3% to 5% acetic acid to the vulva, distinct, flat, acetowhite areas (Fig. 18–9) or a sharply defined micropapilliferous appearance will be seen. Unlike acetowhite findings on the cervix, the acetowhite reaction on the vulva can be nonspecific and may not be predictive of the normality or abnormality of the epithelium. Finally, in the absence of a biopsy, it is not entirely possible to definitively exclude the presence of vulvar intraepithelial neoplasia by colposcopy alone, because even vulvar intraepithelial neoplasia may have an acetowhite appearance with a spicular or micropapillary surface (Fig. 18–10).

> **Patients with extensive vulvar condylomata should be treated under colposcopic guidance.**

Although colposcopic examination is not necessary before the application of topical therapy to isolated vulvar condylomata, patients with large-volume or confluent vulvar condylomata and those with widespread genital tract disease or confluent plaques of condylomatous vulvar growths should be evaluated and treated under colposcopic guidance. This is necessary to ensure that all gross disease is eradicated, to control the depth of treatment, and to allow for precise "brushing" of clinically normal-appearing vulvar skin surrounding gross condylomata that may harbor latent HPV.[8]

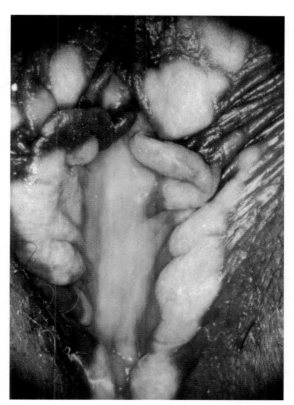

Figure 18–10. Vulvar dysplasia with acetowhite change. Image provided by Dr. Burton Krumholz.

PREGNANT PATIENTS WITH VULVAR CONDYLOMATA

> **It is unknown if treatment of genital condylomata during pregnancy prevents or significantly reduces the development of laryngeal papillomatosis in the newborn.**

An extended discussion of the management of the pregnant patient with HPV-associated disease is covered in Chapter 20. In some women, the diagnosis of genital condylomata is first made during pregnancy. In such cases, the primary concern continues to be possible transmission of HPV from mother to fetus with potential for development of juvenile laryngeal papillomatosis (JLP). It is not known whether transmission primarily occurs before, during, or after labor, whether viral load increases the likelihood of transmission, which source of HPV is of primary importance (vulva, vagina, or cervix), or whether JLP may result from isolated cervical HPV infection.[9] Moreover, for treatment decisions during pregnancy, it is unknown if treatment of genital condylomata during pregnancy significantly lessens the risk of development of JLP in the neonate.

What is clear is that viral growth may be substantial during pregnancy and may be a source of discomfort and bleeding. Because there is no evidence that a cesarean delivery for patients with genital HPV infection prevents JLP, most patients with large-volume condylomata during pregnancy will be faced with the prospect of vaginal

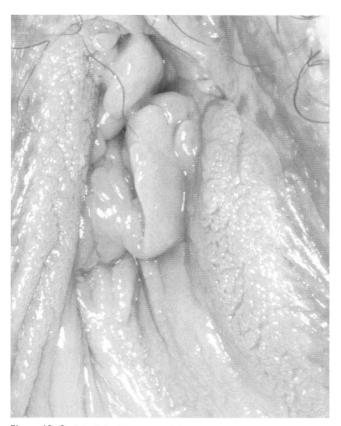

Figure 18–9. Subclinical human papillomavirus with acetowhite change. Image provided by Dr. Vesna Kesic.

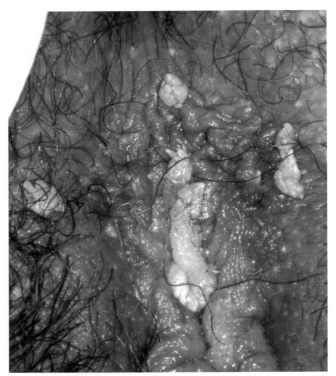

Figure 18–11. Vulvar human papillomavirus in a first trimester pregnancy. Image provided by Dr. Alex Ferenczy.

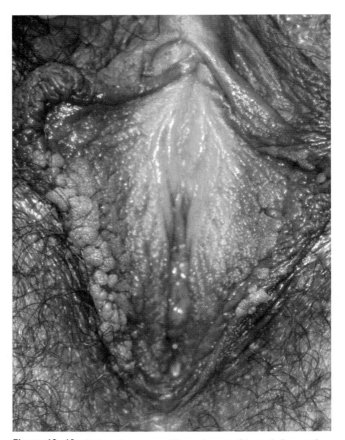

Figure 18–12. Vulvar human papillomavirus at 34 weeks' gestation. Image provided by Dr. Burton Krumholz.

delivery and potential exposure of the fetus to viral inoculation.

Colposcopy is helpful in the evaluation of the pregnant patient with vulvar condylomata to document the presence of vulvar condylomata, to assess the extent of lower genital tract involvement, and to facilitate treatment (by topical agents, CO_2 laser, or other methods) of the vulva before delivery as well as in the postpartum period.[10]

Figures 18–11 and 18–12 illustrate vulvar condylomata in a pregnant patient during the first trimester and at 34 weeks' gestation before laser ablative therapy. Given the increased vascularity of the vulva during pregnancy, the level of precision afforded by the colposcope during laser ablative therapy should help lessen the morbidity of the procedure.

SUMMARY OF KEY POINTS

- Unlike examination of the cervix, colposcopic examination of the cornified vulvar epithelium may not reveal specific vessel patterns and epithelial changes.

- Color, density, and surface contour alterations produced by application of diluted acetic acid are less consistent and pronounced on vulvar epithelium.

- Women with vulvar condylomata who do not have more serious abnormalities may desire treatment for cosmetic reasons or for sexual functioning.

- Although most women who present with a complaint of vulvar warts actually have condylomata, anatomic variants such as micropapillomatosis labialis can be present.

- Colposcopy is an excellent tool to characterize the morphology of the vulvar lesion, to determine its extent, to identify additional lesions, and to potentially evaluate the remainder of the lower genital tract.

- If massive proliferative growths are present on the vulva, verrucous carcinoma and condylomatous squamous cell carcinoma must be ruled out.

- Colposcopy can help identify bizarre or suspicious vessel patterns in otherwise benign-appearing vulvar lesions.

- There is no evidence that treatment of subclinical HPV infection prevents transmission to a sexual partner.

- Colposcopy is not necessary for treatment of small-volume condylomata, although it may assist in precise application of topical agents.

- Following laser ablation of vulvar condylomata, recurrent disease can occur within the treatment field, or new growths can present outside the treated area.

- There is no evidence that treatment of genital condylomata during pregnancy prevents laryngeal papillomatosis in the newborn.

References

1. Buscema J, Naghashfar Z, Sawada E, et al: The predominance of human papillomavirus type 16 in vulvar neoplasia. Obstet Gynecol 1988;71:601.
2. Rando RF, Sedlacek TV, Hunt J, et al: Verrucous carcinoma of the vulva associated with an unusual type 6 human papillomavirus. Obstet Gynecol 1986;67:70S.
3. Rastkar G, Okagaki T, Twiggs LB, Clark BA: Early invasive and in situ warty carcinoma of the vulva: Clinical, histologic, and electron microscopic study with particular reference to viral association. Am J Obstet Gynecol 1982;143:814.
4. Planner RS, Hobbs JB. Intraepithelial and invasive neoplasia of the vulva in association with human papillomavirus infection. J Reprod Med 1988;33:503.
5. Greenberg H, Mann WJ, Chumas J, et al: Cervical and vaginal pathology in women with vulvar condylomata. J Reprod Med 1987; 32:801.
6. Chiasson MA, Ellerbrock TV, Bush TJ, et al: Increased prevalence of vulvovaginal condyloma and vulvar intraepithelial neoplasia in women infected with the human immunodeficiency virus. Obstet Gynecol 1997;89:690.
7. De Deus JM, Focchi J, Stavale JN, De Lima GR: Histologic and biomolecular aspects of papillomatosis of the vulvar vestibule in relation to human papillomavirus. Obstet Gynecol 1995;86:758.
8. Ferenczy A, Mitao M, Nagai N, et al: Latent papillomavirus and recurring genital warts. N Eng J Med 1985;313:784.
9. Patsner B: Human papillomavirus in pregnancy. In Gonik B (ed): Viral Diseases in Pregnancy. Clinical Perspectives in Obstetrics and Gynecology. New York, Springer-Verlag, 1994, pp 185–195.
10. Schwartz D, Greenberg MD, Daoud Y, Reid R: The management of genital condylomas in pregnant women. Obstet Gynecol Clin North Am 1987;14:589.

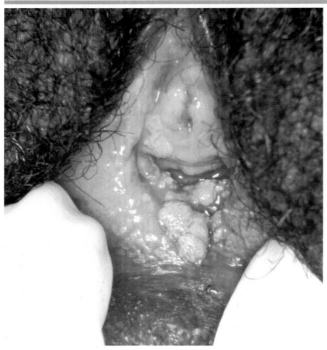

Plate 18-1. Exophytic condyloma of the introitis. Image provided by Dr. Burton Krumholz.

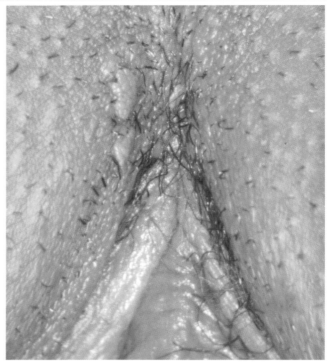

Plate 18-2. Flat condyloma of the mons pubis just above the clitoral hood.

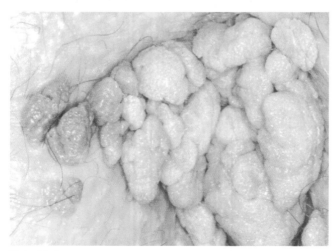

Plate 18-3. Large exophytic condyloma obstructing the introitis. Image provided by Dr. Vesna Kesic.

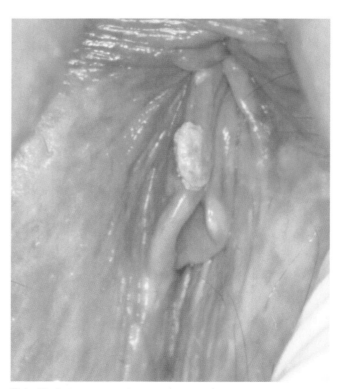

Plate 18-4. Condyloma of the labia minora.

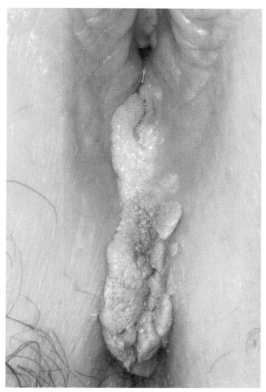

Plate 18-5. Extensive condyloma involvement of the perineum. Image provided by Dr. Vesna Kesic.

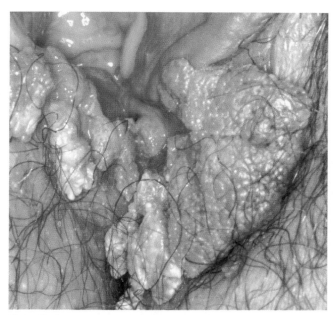

Plate 18-6. Large condyloma of the posterior fourchette. Image provided by Dr. Vesna Kesic.

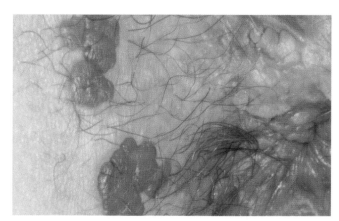

Plate 18-7. Pigmented condyloma of the buttocks and perianal flat condyloma. Image provided by Dr. Vesna Kesic.

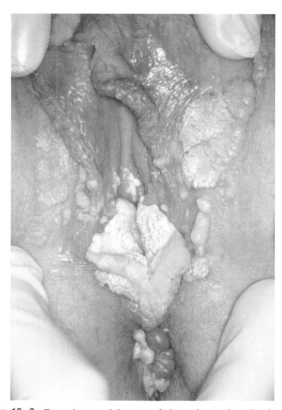

Plate 18-8. Extensive condylomata of the vulva and perianal areas. Image provided by Dr. Gordon Davis.

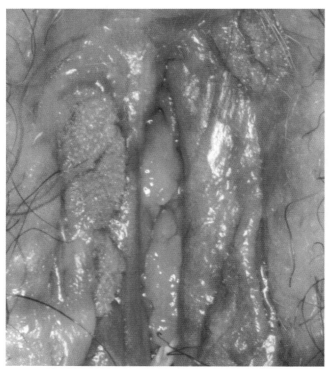

Plate 18-9. Condyloma of the right labia and left periclitoral area. The surface of the condyloma is granular. Image provided by Dr. Burton Krumholz.

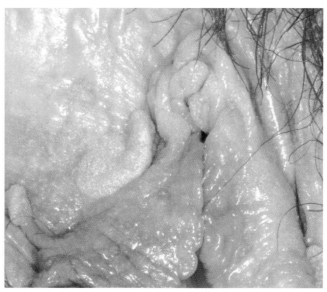

Plate 18-10. Well-circumscribed area of acetowhite epithelium with a granular-surfaced right labia and periclitoral area. Biopsy confirmed a flat condyloma. Image provided by Dr. Vesna Kesic.

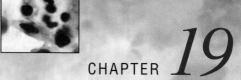

CHAPTER *19*

• Raymond H. Kaufman

Lower Genital Tract Changes Associated with in Utero Exposure to Diethylstilbestrol

In 1971 an association between in utero exposure to diethylstilbestrol and the development of clear cell adenocarcinoma of the vagina and cervix was reported. In some parts of the United States, diethylstilbestrol continued to be prescribed widely through November 1971.

Diethylstilbestrol (DES), a nonsteroidal estrogen, was used from 1941 through 1971 in the United States and through 1978 in Europe in the hope of improving pregnancy outcomes, especially in the woman with prior pregnancy loss and in the diabetic patient. DES was marketed by many companies under more than 70 different names. The peak years of its use were the late 1940s and early 1950s, after which its popularity declined. Despite a report by Deickman[1] in 1953, the medication continued to be used extensively. In some parts of the United States, DES was prescribed widely through November 1971. An estimated 5 to 10 million Americans received DES during pregnancy (DES mothers) or were exposed to the drug in utero (DES daughters and sons). A report by Herbst et al[2] in 1971 demonstrated an association between in utero exposure to DES and development of clear cell adenocarcinoma of the vagina and cervix. Seven of eight women with clear cell adenocarcinoma were delivered of mothers who had received estrogen during their relevant pregnancies. None of 32 normal control women was exposed to DES. After its use was associated with clear cell adenocarcinoma of the vagina and cervix, the drug was banned from use during pregnancy. Since that time, numerous studies have noted the relationship between in utero DES exposure and the presence of other changes in the offspring, including vaginal epithelial changes and structural changes of the cervix and upper genital tract. This review will be limited to those changes noted in the cervix and vagina.

The preponderance of data relating to in utero DES exposure has been obtained from the studies carried out by the National Cooperative Diethylstilbestrol Adenosis (DESAD) project.[3] This multicenter study included Massachusetts General Hospital, the Mayo Clinic, the University of Southern California, and the Baylor College of Medicine. More than 4500 women were followed up prospectively for a period of 10 years with annual examination and since 1984 by questionnaire. The women studied were identified from several sources and included women identified through review of their mothers' pregnancy record and determined to have been exposed to DES and a comparison group of women identified in a similar manner who had no prenatal exposure to DES. Physicians referred additional women to the study clinics, and some women were self-referred for gynecologic examination and follow-up on the basis of documented in utero DES exposure. The least biased of the women entered into the study (40%) were those identified through prenatal record review.

There has been considerable speculation as to the mechanism by which DES may be responsible for the changes identified in the exposed offspring. Walker and Kurth[4] have suggested that DES has a multigenerational effect that is transmitted through the blastocyst, and in fact the authors felt this to be consistent with a fetal germ cell mutation resulting from exposure to DES during pregnancy. It has also been suggested that in utero exposure to DES altered the manner in which the müllerian-derived epithelium was replaced by squamous epithelium advancing up from the urogenital sinus. Hajek et al,[5] using fluorescence in situ hybridization with centromeric probes for chromosomes 1, 7, 11, and 17, noted that there was a frequency of trisomy greater than 5% in the DES-exposed woman. The frequency of trisomy in the control patients was less than 1.5% for all the probes used.

VAGINAL EPITHELIAL CHANGES

The gross findings observed in DES-exposed daughters included columnar epithelium, gland openings, nabothian cysts, white epithelium, mosaic patterns, punctuation, and areas that remain nonstaining after application of Lugol's solution.

Vaginal epithelial changes include those changes observed in the vagina on the basis of colposcopic examination or iodine staining and microscopic changes, including squamous metaplasia and epithelium of müllerian origin (endocervical, endometrial, tubal), in the vagina. The gross findings observed included columnar epithelium, gland openings, nabothian cysts, acetowhite epithelium, mosaic, punctation, and areas that remain nonstaining after the application of Lugol's solution. The microscopic changes included adenosis (columnar cells or their secretory products in the vagina) and squamous metaplasia.

The most frequent location of the vaginal epithelial changes is in the upper third of the vagina, and only a small percentage of women were found to have changes involving the lower third of the vagina.

Studies differed in their estimation of the number of DES-exposed women with adenosis, with estimates ranging from 35% to 90%. Table 19–1 demonstrates the frequency of vaginal epithelial changes in the three study groups exposed in utero to DES.[6] Vaginal epithelial changes were found in 34% of the record review patients, in 59% of the documented walk-in patients, and in 65% of the documented referred patients. This certainly suggests some degree of selection bias in the latter two groups of women. The most frequent location of the vaginal epithelial changes was in the upper third of the vagina, and only a small percentage of women were found to have changes in the lower third of the vagina.

The degree of vaginal epithelial changes is related to the dose and duration of DES exposure and to an early gestational age at first exposure.

Patients with vaginal epithelial changes were found to have been exposed in utero to a higher total dose of DES over a prolonged period of time. Adenosis was observed in 73% of subjects initially exposed during the first 2 months of pregnancy but in only 7% of those initially exposed in the 17th week of pregnancy or later.[7] The frequency of these changes diminished with age, occurring less often among women older than 26 years. Noller

et al[8] suggested that this finding represented a decrease in the frequency of vaginal epithelial changes over time. There was a decrease in the extent of these changes in 29.3% of women followed up over a period of 3 years. Review of biopsy specimens taken at the initial examination of 3339 DES-exposed women revealed that only 45% of the women with vaginal epithelial changes had adenosis. Of significance is the fact that several reports have noted a relationship between clear cell adenocarcinoma and adenosis, primarily the tuboendometrial type.

Careful palpation of the upper vagina may uncover small clear cell adenocarcinomas that are not readily identified on the basis of colposcopic examination.

In evaluating the DES-exposed woman, careful colposcopic and cytologic examinations should be performed. Careful palpation of the upper vagina is extremely important because small clear cell adenocarcinomas may be covered by a normal-appearing squamous epithelium and are not readily identified on the basis of colposcopic examination. Thus, palpation alone may identify submucosal nodules, which require biopsy. In evaluating these women, it is important that a cytologic smear be obtained from the vaginal fornices in addition to one taken from the cervix. Unfortunately, even in the presence of a small clear cell adenocarcinoma, the cytology may be reported as negative.

Colposcopic examination of the DES-exposed woman should include a careful examination of the cervix and the entire vagina.

Colposcopic examination of the DES-exposed woman should include not only careful examination of the cervix but also examination of the entire vagina. Special attention should be paid to the anterior and posterior vaginal walls, which are frequently covered by the blades of the vaginal speculum; these changes may be missed. White epithelium (Fig. 19–1) after the application of 4% to 5% acetic acid most often represents the presence of squamous metaplasia. The presence of punctation and a fine mosaic can occasionally be misleading, because they are most often associated with metaplasia rather than with

▼ Table 19–1

Greatest Extent of Colposcopically Observed Epithelial Change

Most Distal Extent of Change	Participant Classification			
	Record Reviews	*Documented Walk-Ins*	*Documented Referrals*	*Changes, No Documentation*
Vagina	435 (34%)	480 (59%)	473 (65%)	334 (84%)
Upper third	295 (23%)	319 (39%)	305 (42%)	213 (54%)
Middle third	117 (9%)	143 (18%)	134 (18%)	104 (26%)
Lower third	23 (2%)	18 (5%)	34 (5%)	17 (4%)
Total	1275 (100%)	815 (100%)	726 (100%)	396 (100%)

Data from O'Brien PC, Noller KL, Robboy SJ, et al: Vaginal epithelial changes in young women enrolled in the National Cooperative Diethylstilbestrol Adenosis (DESAD) project. Obstet Gynecol 1979;53:300.

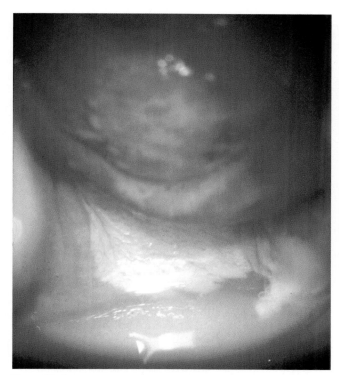

Figure 19–1. Acetowhite epithelium of the posterior vaginal vault area, representing the presence of squamous metaplasia.

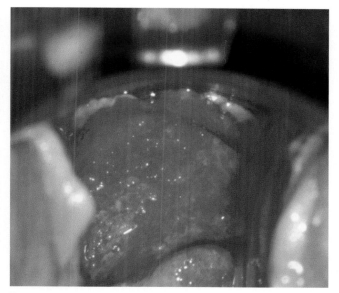

Figure 19–3. Anterior vaginal wall adenosis.

intraepithelial neoplasia. Despite this, such areas should be biopsied. The colposcopic identification of adenosis is usually made on the basis of identification of red, granular-appearing epithelium involving focal or extensive areas of the upper vagina and occasionally the mid- and lower vagina (Figs. 19–2 through 19–4). These foci have

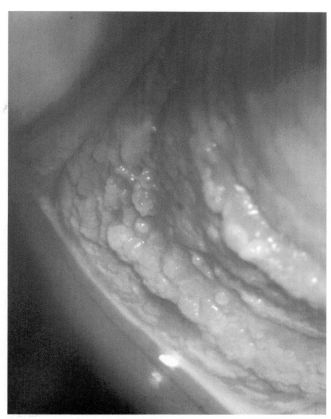

Figure 19–2. Adenosis of the cervicovaginal reflection.

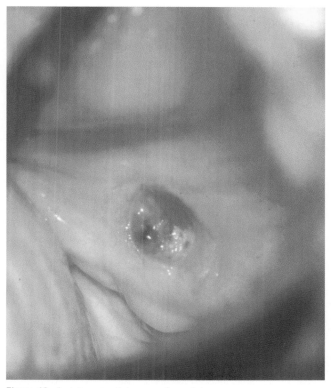

Figure 19–4. Adenosis of the posterior cul-de-sac.

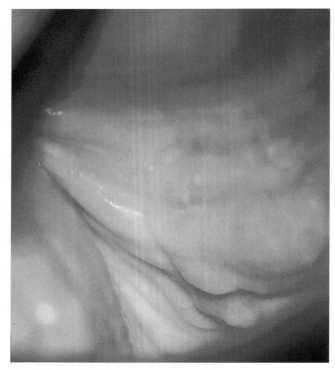

Figure 19–5. Small, submucosal, nabothian cyst.

an appearance similar to columnar epithelium on the exocervix. Not uncommonly, small submucosal nabothian cysts (Fig. 19–5) will be observed, and gland openings may extend onto the surface epithelium. Iodine staining of the vagina often reveals large areas of nonstaining epithelium. These areas frequently have a characteristic appearance (Fig. 19–6).

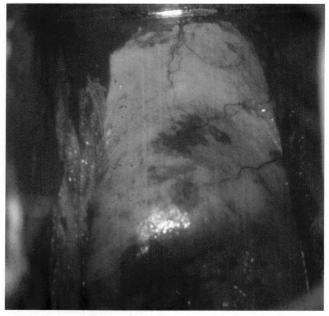

Figure 19–6. Large area of nonstaining epithelium in a diethylstilbestrol-exposed woman.

In a DES-exposed daughter, white epithelium, punctation, and a fine mosaic are most often associated with metaplasia. Despite this, such areas should be biopsied.

STRUCTURAL CHANGES OF THE CERVIX AND VAGINA

The most common structural changes noted in the cervix include cervical collar, coxcomb, pseudopolyp, and hypoplastic cervix. Abnormalities of the vaginal fornix include a shortened fornix, or *vaginal strictures.*

A number of structural changes of the cervix and vagina have been observed in the DES-exposed woman. Some of these changes are so characteristic that their presence strongly suggests that the patient has been exposed to DES even though she does not present with a history of this exposure. The structural defects seen have been reported by Jefferies et al[9] and are listed in Table 19–2. The types and frequency of changes on the entry examination into the DESAD study are presented in Table 19–3.[9] Twenty-five percent of the women identified by record review demonstrated structural changes of the lower genital tract. Similar findings were found in only 2% of nonexposed women. A total of 43% of the walk-in patients were found to have structural changes, and 49% of the referral patients had similar changes. The most

▼ Table 19–2
Structural Defects

Abnormalities of Cervix and Vaginal Fornix	
Coxcomb	
Description	Raised ridge, usually on anterior cervix
Synonym	Hood, transverse ridge of cervix
Collar	
Description	Flat rim involving part to all of circumference of cervix
Synonym	Rim, hood, transverse ridge of cervix
Pseudopolyp	
Description	Polypoid appearance of cervix resulting from circumferential constricting groove, thickening of stroma of anterior or posterior endocervical canal
Synonym	Endocervical stromal hyperplasia
Hypoplastic cervix	
Description	Cervix smaller than 1.5 cm in diameter
Synonym	Immature cervix
Altered fornix of vagina	Absence—complete or partial—of pars vaginalis; abnormality of fornices
	Fusion of cervix to vagina; partial or complete forniceal obliteration

Abnormalities of Vagina Exclusive of Fornix	
Transverse septum, incomplete	
Longitudinal septum, incomplete	

Data from Jefferies JA, Robboy SJ, O'Brien PC, et al: Structural anomalies of the cervix and vagina in women enrolled in the diethylstilbestrol adenosis (DESAD) project. Am J Obstet Gynecol 1984; 148:59.

▼ Table 19–3

Types and Frequencies of Structural Changes Found on Entry Examination

Participant Classification	Structural Changes of Cervix and Vaginal Fornix (%)						
	Any Structural Changes	Any Type	Coxcomb	Collar	Pseudopolyp	Abnormal Fornix	Hypoplastic Cervix
Record review (n = 1655)	25.3	24.8	9.1	13.4	3.4	3.1	3.2
Control (n = 963)	2.3†	2.1†	0.9†	0.8†	0.1†	0.3†	0†
Walk-in (n = 800)	42.6	42.1	14	24.5	1.9	7	9.1
Referral (n = 1089)	48.6	47.8	16.1	30.9	4.5	5.7	6

Data from Jefferies JA, Robboy SJ, O'Brien PC, et al: Structural anomalies of the cervix and vagina in women enrolled in the diethylstilbestrol adenosis (DESAD) project. Am J Obstet Gynecol 1984;148:59.

*Values are percentages of persons in each classification who had the indicated abnormalities. Some participants had more than one.

†Significantly (P < 0.01) less than the record review group (chi square test); two-sided P value = 0.059.

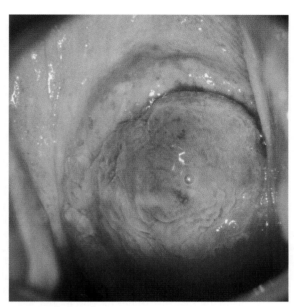

Figure 19–7. Cervical collar.

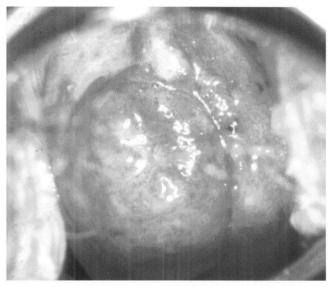

Figure 19–9. Complete cervical collar with pseudopolyp appearance.

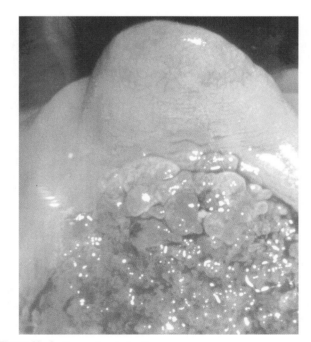

Figure 19–8. Coxcomb anterior lip.

common structural changes noted in the cervix included cervical collar (Fig. 19–7), coxcomb (Fig. 19–8), pseudopolyp (Fig. 19–9), and hypoplastic cervix (Fig. 19–10). Abnormalities of the vaginal fornix were also observed in the record review patients. These latter changes

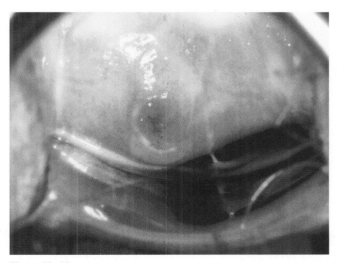

Figure 19–10. Hypoplastic cervix.

included a shortened fornix, or *vaginal strictures*. As the exposed women continue to be followed up, it has been observed that many of these changes disappear over time. Regression of the cervical structural changes was noted in 41% of 361 women. An interesting observation was that regression of these changes occurred most often among women who have experienced a pregnancy.

Intraepithelial Neoplasia and Clear Cell Adenocarcinoma of the Vagina and Cervix

Current data indicate that the occurrence of intraepithelial neoplasia of the vagina and cervix does not appear to be significantly greater in DES-exposed daughters than in an unexposed, comparable group of women.

In 1984, Robboy et al[10] reported that the incidence of intraepithelial neoplasia of the vagina and cervix was significantly higher in women exposed in utero to DES than in an unexposed matched cohort group (15.7 versus 7.9 cases per 1000 person-years of follow-up). For years this concept has persisted, and until the present it was believed to be the absolute truth. However, continued follow-up of this cohort of patients has suggested that this idea may not be the case. The occurrence of intraepithelial neoplasia of the vagina and cervix of DES-exposed women does appear to be greater but not significantly so than that observed in an unexposed, comparable group of women. What must be kept in mind is the fact that the immature metaplasia seen in the DES-exposed individual is often erroneously diagnosed as intraepithelial neoplasia (Fig. 19–11). For this reason, it is advisable to have all such diagnoses reviewed by a pathologist experienced in the interpretation of specimens obtained from the DES-exposed woman.

Despite the potential increased risk for dysplasia, caution is advised when deciding on a mode of treatment. Any mode of surgical treatment (e.g., conization, cautery,

cryosurgery) may be associated with cervical stenosis in a substantial percentage of DES-exposed women, and nearly 30% of DES daughters who underwent cervical cauterization or cryosurgery experienced at least one subsequent pregnancy loss.[11] Treatment of a cervical ectropion for mucorrhea should be discouraged. Treatment with laser vaporization may be less associated with stenosis, but the risk is still present.

Clear Cell Adenocarcinoma of the Vagina and Cervix

Fewer than 1 woman in 1000 exposed in utero to DES develops clear cell adenocarcinoma.

The report of Herbst et al in 1971[2] brought to our attention the association of in utero exposure to DES and development of clear cell adenocarcinoma of the vagina and cervix. Further studies have corroborated their findings. However, the risk of women exposed in utero to DES developing clear cell adenocarcinoma is less than 1 in 1000. The registry for research on hormonal transplacental carcinogenesis at the University of Chicago under the direction of Herbst has reviewed more than 700 cases of adenocarcinoma of the vagina and cervix. Approximately 60% of these women were exposed to DES. The mean age of diagnosis of clear cell adenocarcinoma was 19 years, with the peak incidence occurring in 1975. The frequency of diagnosis has decreased progressively since that time; however, clear cell carcinoma has been diagnosed in DES-exposed women in their early forties. Whether there will be a secondary increase in incidence of this carcinoma in the DES-exposed woman as she enters the years when this type of carcinoma is most often seen (the sixth decade of life and above) is unknown. Thus, continued careful surveillance of these women is necessary.

The mean age of diagnosis of clear cell adenocarcinoma is 19 years, and it has been diagnosed in DES-exposed women as late as their early forties. The peak incidence occurred in 1975.

Herbst et al[12] evaluated the factors related to development of clear cell adenocarcinoma of the vagina and cervix in the DES-exposed woman. Their studies suggested that the relative risk for clear cell adenocarcinoma was greater in those women whose mothers began DES before the 12th week of pregnancy and in those women who were conceived during the winter. A maternal history of at least one spontaneous abortion appeared to increase the risk for the development of carcinoma. More recent data obtained from the follow-up of the DESAD cohort suggest that time of birth may not be related to the development of this carcinoma.

Waggoner et al[13] detected p53 protein in tumors in 14 of 21 cases of clear cell adenocarcinoma. They were unable, however, to identify p53 mutations in any of the cases, suggesting that the tumors contained only wild-type p53. They hypothesized that p53 overexpression in clear cell adenocarcinoma was a response to generalized DNA

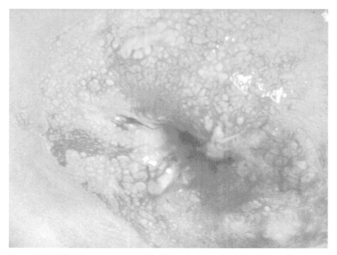

Figure 19–11. Immature metaplasia seen in a diethylstilbestrol-exposed woman.

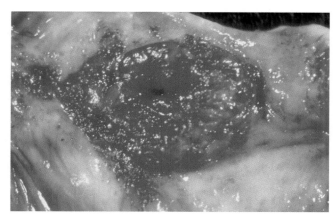

Figure 19–12. Clear cell carcinoma that presented as a firm, granular lesion.

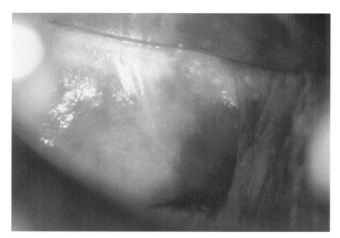

Figure 19–13. Clear cell carcinoma presenting as a small, firm, submucosal nodule.

damage, rather than a result of p53 protein half-life prolongation resulting from mutational inactivation. Waggoner et al suggested that this overexpression of wild-type p53 protein in the clear cell adenocarcinomas might connote a more favorable prognosis compared with that of other gynecologic tumors containing mutated p53 protein.

Clear cell carcinoma may present as a firm granular lesion (Fig. 19–12) that is easily identified; however, it will occasionally present as a small, hemorrhagic nodule or as firm, submucosal nodules (Fig. 19–13). Obviously, biopsy of such areas should be performed.

SUMMARY

Significant changes in the lower genital tract appear to have occurred as a result of in utero exposure to DES. These changes include both structural alterations of the cervix and vagina and epithelial changes that are at times quite confusing to the inexperienced examiner. Although

in utero DES exposure became almost nonexistent after the mid-1970s, there is still a large group of women in their 30s and early 40s who were exposed to this drug. Thus, it is incumbent on the practitioner to be aware of these changes so that these patients can be adequately managed and, more importantly, not overtreated.

SUMMARY OF KEY POINTS

- In some parts of the United States, DES continued to be prescribed widely through November 1971, when the association was reported between in utero exposure to DES and development of clear cell adenocarcinoma of the vagina and cervix.

- Gross vaginal findings observed in DES-exposed daughters include columnar epithelium, gland openings, nabothian cysts, acetowhite epithelium, mosaic, punctation, and areas that remain nonstaining after the application of Lugol's solution.

- The most frequent location of the vaginal epithelial changes is in the upper third of the vagina.

- The degree of vaginal epithelial changes is related to the dose and duration of DES exposure and to an early gestational age at first exposure.

- Careful palpation of the upper vagina may uncover small clear cell adenocarcinomas that are not readily identified on the basis of colposcopic examination.

- The colposcopic examination of the DES-exposed woman should include a careful examination of the cervix and the entire vagina.

- In a DES-exposed daughter, acetowhite epithelium, punctation, and a fine mosaic are most often associated with metaplasia. Despite this, such areas should be biopsied.

- On colposcopy, adenosis is visible as red, granular-appearing epithelium involving focal or extensive areas of the upper vagina, similar to columnar epithelium on the exocervix.

- The most common structural changes noted in the cervix include cervical collar, coxcomb, pseudopolyp, and hypoplastic cervix. Abnormalities of the vaginal fornix include a shortened fornix and vaginal strictures.

- Over time, many of these changes disappear, most often in women who have experienced a pregnancy.

References

1. Dieckman WJ, Davis ME, Ryukiewiez LM, Pottinger RE: Does the administration of diethylstilbestrol during pregnancy have therapeutic value? Am J Obstet Gynecol 1953;66:1062.
2. Herbst AL, Ulfelder H, Poskancer DC: Adenocarcinoma of the vagina: Association of maternal stilbestrol therapy with tumor appearance in young women. N Engl J Med 1971;284:878.

3. LaBarthe D, Adam E, Noller KL, et al: Design and preliminary observation of the National Cooperative Diethylstilbestrol Adenosis (DESAD) project. Obstet Gynecol 1978;51:453.

4. Walker BE, Kurth LA: Multi-generational carcinogenesis from diethylstilbestrol investigated by blastocyst transfers in mice. Int J Cancer 1995;61:249.

5. Hajek RA, Liang JC, Kaufman RH, et al: Does detection of chromosomal abriations by FISK in cervical vaginal biopsies from women exposed to DES in-utero precede clinically evident disease? Proc Am Cancer Res 1995;36:633.

6. O'Brien PC, Noller KL, Robboy SJ, et al: Vaginal epithelial changes in young women enrolled in the National Cooperative Diethylstilbestrol Adenosis (DESAD) project. Obstet Gynecol 1979; 53:300.

7. Herbst AL, Poskanzer DC, Robboy SJ, et al: Prenatal exposure to stilbestrol. N Engl J Med 1975;292:334.

8. Noller KL, Townsend DE, Kaufman RH, et al: Maturation of vaginal and cervical epithelium in women exposed in-utero to diethylstilbestrol (DESAD project). Am J Obstet Gynecol 1983; 146:279.

9. Jefferies JA, Robboy SJ, O'Brien PC, et al: Structural anomalies of the cervix and vagina in women enrolled in the diethylstilbestrol adenosis (DESAD) project. Am J Obstet Gynecol 1984;148:59.

10. Robboy SJ, Noller KL, O'Brien PC, et al: Increased incidence of cervical and vaginal dysplasia in 3,980 diethylstilbestrol-exposed young women. Experience of the National Collaborative Diethylstilbestrol Adenosis project. JAMA 1984;252:2979.

11. Herbst AL, Senekjian EK, Frey KW: Abortion and pregnancy loss among diethylstilbestrol-exposed women. Semin Reprod Endocrinol 1989;7:124.

12. Herbst AL, Anderson S, Hubby MM, et al: Risk factors for the development of diethylstilbestrol-associated clear cell adenocarcinoma: A case controlled study. Am J Obstet Gynecol 1986;154:814.

13. Waggoner SE, Anderson SM, Luce MC, et al. P53 protein expression and gene analysis and clear cell adenocarcinoma of the vagina and cervix. Gynecol Oncol 1996;6:339.

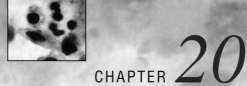

• David G. Weismiller •

CHAPTER *20*

Triage of the Abnormal Papanicolaou Smear and Colposcopy in Pregnancy

The most important function of triage of the abnormal Papanicolaou smear in pregnancy is to exclude invasive disease.

For any woman, an abnormal finding on a Papanicolaou (Pap) smear generates understandable anxiety, particularly because of fear of cancer and possible loss of reproductive function.[1] These concerns are amplified during pregnancy, when worries about possible danger to the fetus may be considerable. The most important function of abnormal Pap smear triage and colposcopy during pregnancy is to exclude invasive cancer. Because of the physiologic, cytologic, histologic, and colposcopic changes of the cervix that normally occur during the gravid state, a significant degree of expertise and experience is required of the colposcopist. Invasive cervical cancer can present as a small, localized, occult lesion, and its appearance may be influenced by these dramatic, but normal, physiologic changes.

Pregnant and nonpregnant women are at similar risk for cervical neoplasia and its precursors, with the incidence of squamous intraepithelial lesions found on cytology during pregnancy reported at 1.26% to 2.2%.

Pregnancy is not a risk factor for the development of cervical intraepithelial neoplasia (CIN). Pregnant and nonpregnant women are at similar risk for cervical neoplasia and its precursors, with the incidence of squamous intraepithelial lesions (SILs) found on cytology during pregnancy reported at 1.26% to 2.2%. Approximately 86% of all SILs identified during pregnancy are classified as low-grade squamous intraepithelial lesions (LSILs). The other 14% are high-grade squamous intraepithelial lesions (HSILs). Histologically diagnosed CIN is found in 0.19% to 0.53% of pregnant patients,[2, 3] but carcinoma of the cervix is uncommon, occurring in only 1 in 3000 pregnancies.

Although rare, cervical cancer is the most common malignancy diagnosed in pregnancy, with a frequency of 1.6 to 10.6 cases per 10,000 pregnancies.[4] The mean age of the pregnant woman at the time of diagnosis of cervical cancer is 31.6 years (range, 31 to 36.5 years).[5] As in nonpregnant patients, the most common histologic type is squamous cell carcinoma, which accounts for more than 80% of all cervical cancers.[6] Of these patients, 70% have early-stage disease, which includes stage 1 and stage 2A lesions.[6–9] Diagnosis at an earlier stage may be due to the fact that pregnant women are seen frequently by health care providers and undergo prenatal examinations and Pap smears. In fact, a third of pregnant patients diagnosed with cervical cancer are asymptomatic.

There appears to be no difference in survival between pregnant and nonpregnant women with cervical cancer when they are matched by age, stage, and year of diagnosis.

Historically, pregnancy was believed to have an adverse effect on the natural history of cervical cancer. More recent studies, however, have shown no difference in survival between pregnant and nonpregnant women with cervical cancer when they are matched by age, stage, and year of diagnosis.[5, 6, 9–12] Pregnancy does not appear to significantly alter the progression or prognosis of cervical cancer.[13] In addition, there is no evidence that CIN progresses more rapidly to an invasive cancer in the pregnant state than in the nonpregnant state.

THE CERVIX IN PREGNANCY

Pregnancy produces dramatic alterations in the gross and colposcopic appearance of the cervix as well as in the cytology and histology of cervical pathology specimens (Table 20–1).

▼ Table 20–1

Alterations in the Cervix in Pregnancy*

Ectocervix

Alterations are mostly the result of the high estrogen status in pregnancy.
Increased vascularity produces a bluish hue.
Acetic acid reaction of the metaplastic epithelium in pregnancy is exaggerated.
There is increase in cervical volume through hypertrophy of the fibromuscular stroma.

Endocervix

Endocervical canal is everted, particularly in the primiparous woman.
There is gaping of the endocervical canal, particularly in the multiparous woman.
Everted epithelium, exposed to the acidity of the vaginal environment, usually results in significant squamous metaplasia.

*Pregnancy produces dramatic alterations in the colposcopic appearance of the cervix. The appearance is determined largely by gestational age.

Physiologic Changes

Most of the physiologic changes of the cervix during pregnancy are due to high estrogen status and include remodeling of the surface contour, increased vascularity, and abundant mucus production.

Most of the physiologic changes of the cervix during pregnancy are due to high estrogen status. Cervical epithelium is highly sensitive to alterations in estrogen levels. There is marked softening and expansion in size. The dimensions of the cervix significantly increase in varying proportions, with associated remodeling of surface contours. Increased vascularity and abundant mucus production are clearly evident. Given the fluctuating estrogen levels associated with pregnancy, the gross appearance of the cervix is determined largely by the gestational age, especially in the primigravida.[14, 15] Increased estrogen content in early pregnancy produces a significant increase in cervical volume through hypertrophy of the fibromuscular stroma. Consequently, the endocervical canal is further everted onto the ectocervix (Fig. 20–1). The extent of eversion varies among individuals and with parity. Eversion of endocervical columnar epithelium is most common and most marked in primiparous gestation. The eversion process begins during the early weeks of pregnancy and is usually clearly apparent in the early second trimester. In subsequent pregnancies, the degree of eversion of the endocervical canal is less significant, but gaping of the endocervical canal may result in a similar exposure of endocervical columnar epithelium to the vaginal environment (Fig. 20–2). The increased vascularity of the cervical epithelium and stroma produces a bluish hue (Chadwick's sign) (Fig. 20–3).

Cytologic Changes

During pregnancy, the endocervical mucosa is everted. This is especially apparent in the second trimester and in the primiparous gestation.

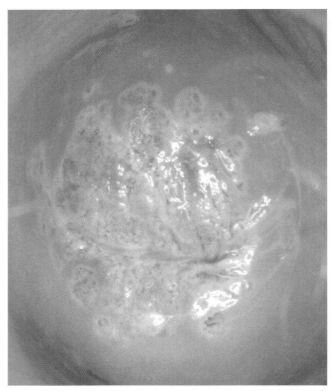

Figure 20–1. Ectropion in the first trimester of pregnancy along with metaplasia.

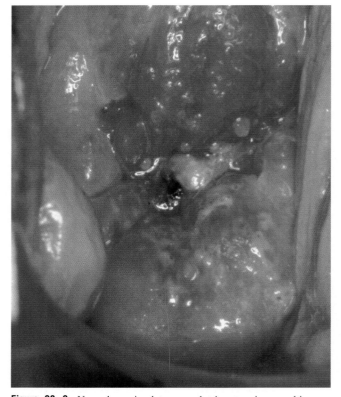

Figure 20–2. Normal cervix, late second trimester, in a multiparous patient.

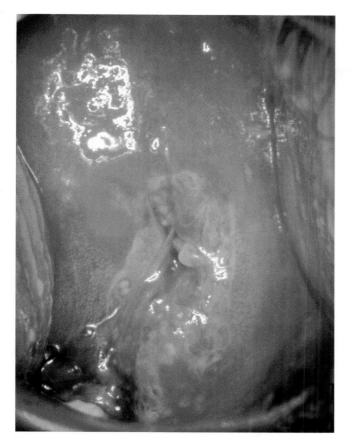

Figure 20–3. Cervix in the second trimester with vascular engorgement leading to the bluish hue called Chadwick's sign. There are also several fine, milia-like, white spots that represent hypertrophy of the stromal cells.

As a result of the physiologic structural changes in the cervix, evaluation and interpretation of cytologic smears is more difficult during pregnancy (Table 20–2). Cellular components are altered in this high-estrogen environment. Basal-cell hyperplasia, immature metaplasia, decidualization of the cervical stroma, and the Arias-Stella reaction may hinder Pap smear interpretation. For the cytopathologist, these factors add to the complexity of the cytologic interpretation. Despite the confusing cellular phenomena, cytometric studies have shown that, morphologically, CIN in the pregnant patient is the same as CIN in the nonpregnant patient.

▼ Table 20–2

Cytologic Assessment in Pregnancy

Papanicolaou smear interpretation is more difficult.
  Immature metaplasia
  Basal cell hyperplasia
  Decidualization
  Arias-Stella reaction
Squamous intraepithelial lesion (SIL) is the same as in the nonpregnant state.

Colposcopic Changes

Colposcopic changes of the cervix in pregnancy, including extensive squamous metaplasia, demand different pattern-recognition skills.

Compared with examination of the cervix in the nonpregnant patient, examination of colposcopic changes of the cervix during pregnancy demands different pattern-recognition skills by the colposcopist (Table 20–3). Serial colpomicrographs of the cervix throughout pregnancy confirm progressive eversion of lower endocervical canal epithelium to an ectocervical position (Fig. 20–4).

▼ Table 20–3

Colposcopic Changes of the Cervix in Pregnancy

Increased prominence of vascular patterns
Decreased prominence of acetowhite epithelium
Immature metaplasia difficult to distinguish from low-grade squamous intraepithelial lesion; acetowhite effect
Decidual—atypical vascular pattern, polypoid, less intense acetowhite staining of abnormal areas
Fine punctation and mosaic pattern within metaplasia, possibly leading to misdiagnosis of lesions

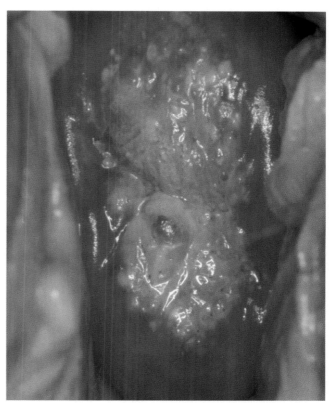

Figure 20–4. Eversion of columnar epithelium in the second trimester of pregnancy. Several small nabothian cysts are present, outlining the peripheral limits of the transformation zone. Acetowhite epithelium is present on the posterior lip of the cervix. Biopsy revealed decidual changes only.

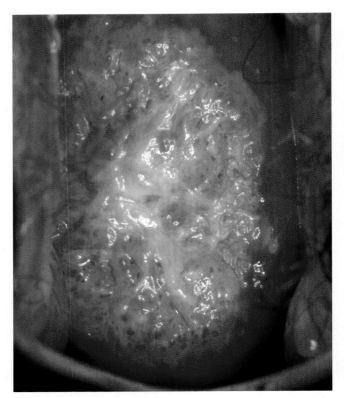

Figure 20-5. Eversion of columnar epithelium onto the portio of the cervix. There is extensive metaplasia and copious thick mucus.

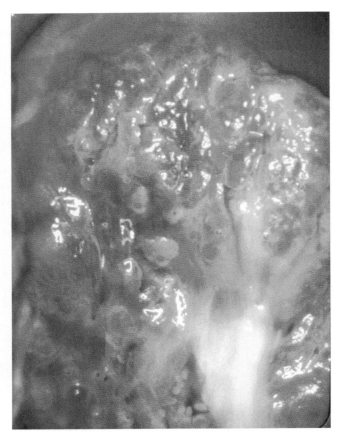

Figure 20-6. Close-up view of columnar epithelium and pregnancy-related metaplasia with fusion of villi. The individual grapelike clusters of the columnar epithelium are no longer evident.

Everted columnar epithelium exposed to the acidity of the vaginal environment, particularly in the first pregnancy, enters a strikingly dynamic phase of squamous metaplasia that progresses throughout the pregnancy (Fig. 20-5). Toward the end of the first trimester, eversion and the resulting metaplasia produce areas of fusion of columnar villi, with islands of immature metaplastic epithelium (Fig. 20-6). This process rapidly progresses through the second trimester, producing a layer of smooth, opaque squamous metaplasia that appears acetowhite after application of 3% to 5% acetic acid (Fig. 20-7). The aceto-white reaction of the immature metaplastic epithelium is exaggerated by the bluish hue secondary to the increased vascularity (Fig. 20-8). The vast expanse of immature metaplasia may be difficult to distinguish from precancerous and cancerous lesions. Tenacious endocervical mucus develops during pregnancy and can hinder colposcopic assessment (Fig. 20-9).

> **Other colposcopic features of the cervix visualized in pregnancy include decidual reaction, increased vascularity, and polypoid surface projections.**

Other colposcopic features can add to the confusion during pregnancy. The decidual changes of the cervix can appear as yellow, raised, and friable lesions. Polypoid surface projections and an atypical vascular pattern contribute to altered morphologic features. The cervical angioarchitecture may lead to colposcopic overgrading of

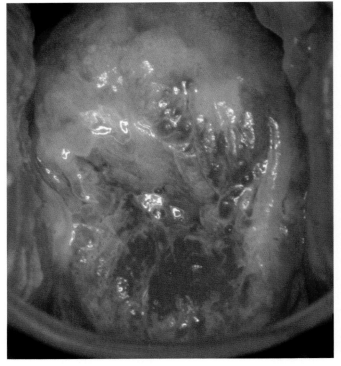

Figure 20-7. Large ectropion with metaplasia.

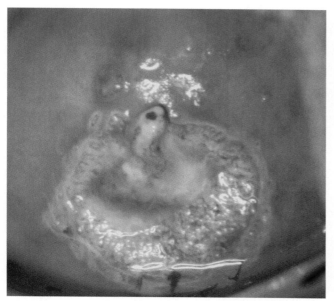

Figure 20–8. Ectropion with metaplasia. There is a mild blue tint to the metaplasia secondary to the increased vascular engorgement of the cervix.

the severity of intraepithelial lesions. However, the pattern of the margins of intraepithelial lesions is the same in the gravid and the nongravid individual and aids in colposcopic assessment.

During pregnancy, the cervical angioarchitecture may lead to colposcopic overgrading of the severity of intraepithelial lesions.

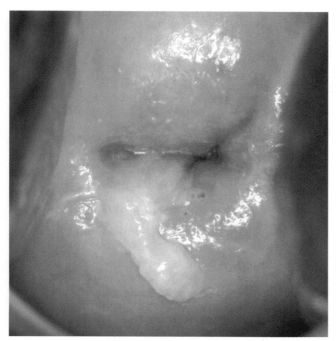

Figure 20–9. Thick mucus and dilated gland openings.

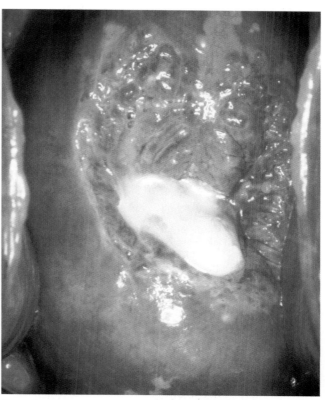

Figure 20–10. Gaping os with eversion of the squamocolumnar junction onto the portio of the cervix. This is a small area of low-grade cervical intraepithelial neoplasia on the anterior lip with a fine mosaic pattern.

In the third trimester, eversion and progressive metaplasia continue until about 36 weeks of gestation and then essentially stop. Usually, the metaplasia is physiologic, but occasionally the metaplastic cells may appear atypical, and the pathologist is forced to distinguish them from CIN. The area of metaplasia persists during the prenatal period and returns to its endocervical position in the puerperium. Alternatively, the metaplasia matures to mature squamous epithelium. In subsequent pregnancies, the preexisting area of metaplasia may again be everted, but not usually as dramatically as in the first pregnancy.

Similar epithelial changes occur in later pregnancies, but to a limited degree. Gaping of the endocervical canal predominates over eversion and is progressive throughout pregnancy, particularly during the third trimester (Fig. 20–10). Squamous metaplasia tends to occur predominantly later in pregnancy. The dynamic phase of squamous metaplasia associated with the first pregnancy is considered critical, representing the stage at greatest risk for initiation of cervical carcinogenesis.

Histologic Changes in Pregnancy

In pregnancy, the cervix is characterized histologically by stromal edema, decidualization, increased vascularity, and enlargement of glandular structures associated with an acute inflammatory response.

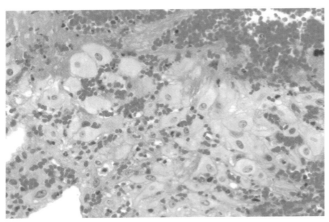

Figure 20–11. Decidual cells in stroma. These cells are large and have poorly defined cell borders. The nuclei are quite uniform, with small nucleoli and a fine chromatin pattern (×400).

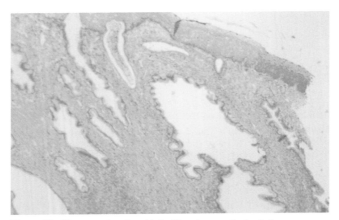

Figure 20–12. Example of multiple dilated stromal glands in pregnancy.

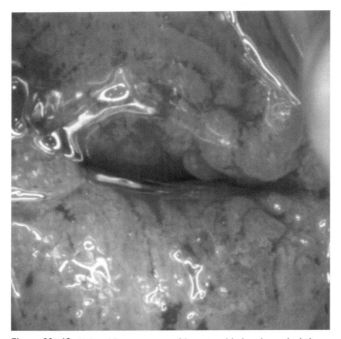

Figure 20–13. Polypoid appearance of hypertrophied endocervical tissue related to pregnancy.

In pregnancy, the cervix is characterized histologically by stromal edema, decidualization, increased vascularity, and enlargement of glandular structures associated with an acute inflammatory response[16] (Fig. 20–11). The enlarged stromal glands are frequently mucus-filled and distort the architecture (Fig. 20–12). Stromal decidualization occurs in the second and third trimesters in approximately 30% of pregnant women. Decidual reactions may produce dramatic changes in the surface contour and may appear clinically suspicious to the inexperienced observer. The endocervical columnar epithelium responds to the estrogen surge by proliferating and folding into polypoid projections (Fig. 20–13). There is an associated increase in mucus production. Hormonal changes may stimulate microglandular hyperplasia.

ABNORMAL CYTOLOGY IN PREGNANCY

An abnormal Pap smear may complicate up to 5% of pregnancies.

The diagnosis of abnormal cervical cytology in pregnancy has become more common because of delayed childbearing and broad cytologic criteria for diagnosis of LSIL. An abnormal Pap smear, including atypical squamous cells of undetermined significance (ASCUS), may complicate up to 5% of pregnancies. This is not unexpected, given that the peak incidence of preinvasive cervical lesions is found in women in their third decade, which is also the time of maximum childbearing activity.[17] Today, although cervical cancer remains rare in pregnancy, the increasing incidence of HSIL and cervical cancer in younger women of childbearing age is troubling. Whenever an invasive cancer is diagnosed post partum, the physician is likely to be challenged for failure to detect the cancer during pregnancy. When that patient had an abnormal Pap smear, and the colposcopic evaluation failed to detect preexisting cancer in the absence of a biopsy, the physician's expertise and judgment are likely to be further challenged.

Because the incidence of invasive cervical cancer is so low and the progression of LSIL to invasive carcinoma is so slow, different triage criteria may be applied to pregnant and nonpregnant patients.[18] Because cytology will underestimate the severity of disease in a small percentage of patients, most authors recommend at least an initial colposcopic examination for a pregnant woman with an abnormal Pap smear.[19, 20] The goal of colposcopic evaluation in pregnancy should be to exclude invasive cervical cancer.

Most pregnant women are referred for colposcopy on the basis of low-grade cytologic abnormalities.

Most pregnant women are referred for colposcopy on the basis of low-grade cytologic abnormalities. Many of these patients have a normal cervix or have minor cervical atypia of little clinical consequence. The initial goal of colposcopy is to exclude invasive cancer. The experience and expertise of the practitioner performing the colposcopy are essential in determining the appropriate management of an individual pregnant woman with an abnormal Pap smear. If, based on the colposcopic impression, the colposcopist cannot exclude the presence of invasive cancer, a directed biopsy should be performed from the area of the most significant abnormality. However, because results of a biopsy are not absolute, close cytologic and colposcopic follow-up is mandatory, with further directed biopsies or a large wedge biopsy if any suspicion of disease progression evolves. If HSIL is confirmed, but the colposcopic impression is not in concordance with the histologic diagnosis, careful colposcopic evaluation of the endocervical canal, vagina, and vulva is mandatory. Definitive diagnostic workup and treatment of precancerous lesions are reserved for the puerperium unless invasive disease is discovered during the prenatal period.

Invasive cancer is rare but can occur in association with only minor cytologic atypia. If any suspicion of invasion exists on cytology, discussion between the colposcopist and the pathologist should ensue before triage decisions are made. A large biopsy specimen is mandatory if colposcopy indicates possible early invasion. If there is genuine suspicion of cancer, wedge biopsy or conization is mandatory to exclude invasive disease and to determine depth of invasion.

> If, on the basis of the colposcopic impression, the colposcopist cannot exclude the presence of invasive cancer, a directed biopsy should be performed from the area of the most significant abnormality.

CYTOLOGIC SAMPLING DURING PREGNANCY

Because the incidences of abnormal cervical cytology and histologically proved CIN are similar among pregnant and nonpregnant women, routine cytologic screening is recommended for pregnant women.[21, 22] Pregnancy presents an opportunity for cervical cancer screening and education. Cytology remains the only currently acceptable screening test for cervical cancer in pregnancy.[23]

> The presence of pregnancy-induced cytologic changes, immature metaplasia, and inflammatory infiltrate may lead to cytologic misdiagnosis.

The presence of pregnancy-induced cytologic changes, immature metaplasia, and inflammatory infiltrate may lead to cytologic misdiagnosis. Hormonally stimulated physiologic changes can be found in cervical cytologic smears. Navicular cells, low karyopyknotic and eosinophilic indexes, and marked cytolysis owing to the abundance of lactobacilli that thrive in the glycogen-rich environment[24, 25] may all lead to diagnostic errors, particularly when the smear is complicated by inflammatory changes or human papillomavirus (HPV) infection (Fig. 20–14). Conversely, actual dysplastic changes could be incorrectly attributed to pregnancy changes, thus leading to false-negative cytology.

Figure 20–14. Papanicolaou smear demonstrating cytolysis. Bare nuclei without cytoplasm are seen with some nuclear irregularities. In the background, relatively large bacterial rods are identified as typical of lactobacilli. These are the features of cytolysis (Döderlein's cytolysis).

COLPOSCOPY IN PREGNANCY

> The patient should be reassured that colposcopic assessment of the cervix during pregnancy will not impair the pregnancy or harm the fetus.

Colposcopy is safe and reliable for the evaluation of abnormal cervical cytology during pregnancy.[2, 14, 15, 18, 20, 26–32] The goal of the colposcopic examination in the pregnant patient with abnormal cervical cytology is to exclude the presence of invasive disease, avoiding the need for cervical conization and allowing treatment to be deferred until the postpartum period. In the nonpregnant patient with an abnormal Pap smear, colposcopically directed biopsy is the standard initial method to identify intraepithelial and occult invasive lesions of the cervix. Controversy surrounds the question as to whether biopsies should be performed during pregnancy in the absence of a colposcopic suspicion of invasive cervical cancer. Some clinicians may be reluctant to perform a biopsy because of the threat of maternal or fetal complications. Several investigators have concluded that biopsy should be performed only if the colposcopic evidence shows invasive carcinoma.[15, 26, 33–35] Others maintain that biopsy should be performed on all cervical lesions detected colposcopically.[29, 30, 36–38] The preponderance of evidence suggests that cervical biopsy during pregnancy should not be deferred if it will assist in making a necessary triage decision.

> The preponderance of evidence suggests that cervical biopsy during pregnancy should not be deferred if it will assist in making an appropriate triage decision.

Colposcopy during pregnancy can be difficult, and interpretation of the colposcopic findings may be challenging. Pattern-recognition skills for the colposcopic evaluation of the cervix of the gravid patient are different from those needed to evaluate the cervix of the nonpregnant patient. The colposcopist must familiarize herself or himself with a new set of normal attributes of the cervix during pregnancy. During pregnancy, some benign changes may cause suspicious colposcopic patterns that mimic severe lesions.[14] For example, cervical ectropion may have a coarse, grapelike appearance; large villi separated by deep longitudinal folds; coarse surface contour; and increased vascularity with confusing angioarchitecture that may result in a suspicious vascular pattern (Fig. 20–15).

Colposcopic examination during pregnancy may provide sufficient documentation of the absence of invasion, so conization can be avoided.

Transient atypical findings associated with active squamous metaplasia may be present on the transformation zone during pregnancy. The new squamous epithelium produced during this active metaplastic transformation, or the extensive immature metaplastic epithelium itself, may exhibit an exaggerated acetowhite appearance (Fig. 20–16). A fine punctation and mosaic pattern may be seen within acetowhite areas of physiologic metaplasia (Fig. 20–17) and may be misinterpreted as disease. The surface contour changes associated with mucus-filled glands and decidual reaction are also confusing. Eversion of the

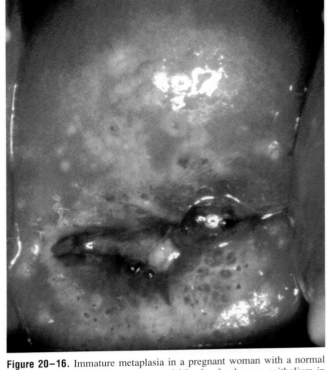

Figure 20–16. Immature metaplasia in a pregnant woman with a normal Papanicolaou smear. There are several islands of columnar epithelium in the field of acetowhite metaplastic epithelium on the posterior lip of the cervix.

endocervical columnar epithelium takes place after the first trimester of pregnancy and tends to be observed more commonly in primigravidas.[39, 40] When prominent vascular changes accompany decidual reaction, the appearance may mimic an invasive cancer. A small focal

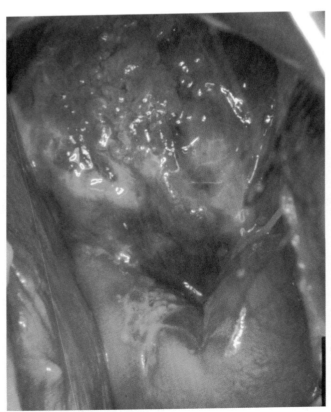

Figure 20–15. Asymmetrical ectropion with increased vascularity, large clefts from hypertrophy of the epithelium, and acetowhite epithelium from metaplasia.

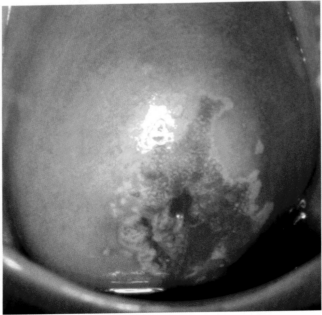

Figure 20–17. Fine mosaic pattern on the anterior lip of the cervix in a pregnant patient with an ectropion and active metaplasia.

area of invasive cancer is sometimes difficult to detect because of the intensity of acetowhite change and the marked increase in vascular abnormalities.

Colposcopy becomes more difficult as gestation advances. The cervix enlarges and becomes hypervascular, and the amount and tenacity of the cervical mucus reaches its maximum. Colposcopy may sometimes fail to detect abnormalities even if great care is taken.

Technique of Colposcopy in Pregnancy

In pregnancy, an unobstructed view of the cervix is mandatory during colposcopy, and the largest vaginal speculum that the patient can tolerate should be used.

In addition to the colposcopic interpretive challenges, physical changes in the lower genital tract make the procedure of colposcopy technically more difficult. The colposcopist is challenged with the increased laxity of the vaginal walls, which produces prolapse through the speculum blades, interfering with proper visualization of the cervix. The use of a lateral wall retractor may help in gaining unhindered access to the cervix. In pregnancy, unobstructed visualization of the cervix is mandatory. A large vaginal speculum will usually be necessary—the largest speculum that the patient can comfortably tolerate. A condom, latex glove finger, or endovaginal ultrasound probe sheath with the tip removed may be rolled onto the speculum for better visualization. Tenacious endocervical

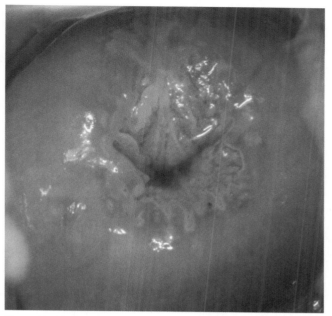

Figure 20–19. Eversion of columnar epithelium onto the portio of the cervix, yielding a satisfactory examination. There is acetowhite epithelium at the 12-o'clock position, representing cervical intraepithelial neoplasia (CIN) 2, and peripherally milder acetowhite epithelium, representing CIN 1.

mucus encountered in pregnancy can be a significant obstacle to adequate visualization (Fig. 20–18). The application of 5% acetic acid to the cervix is mucolytic and will aid in mucus removal. Mucus that cannot be satisfactorily removed may be gently manipulated using cotton-tipped applicators so that the cervix can be systematically examined in quadrants. Careful use of a sponge forceps may be helpful in removing viscous mucus from the ectocervix.

The examination should be gentle, because tissue fragility is more common in pregnancy. If the highly vascular cervical epithelium is traumatized and bleeds, the view can be further compromised.

It is easier to examine the cervix of the gravid patient after 16 to 18 weeks of gestation because of the substantial eversion of the endocervical columnar epithelium.

It is easier to examine the cervix of the gravid patient after 16 to 18 weeks of gestation because of the substantial outfolding or eversion of the endocervical columnar epithelium. As a result of this physiologic eversion, the transformation zone is more accessible for a satisfactory colposcopic examination.[22] The transformation zone is fully visualized in the majority of patients by the 20th week of gestation[28] (Fig. 20–19). For this reason, an unsatisfactory colposcopy occurs less frequently in pregnant patients than in nonpregnant patients.[41] Despite the eversion of the endocervical columnar epithelium in most patients, further instrumentation is sometimes needed to adequately evaluate the endocervical canal and to visualize the entire squamocolumnar junction. An endocervical

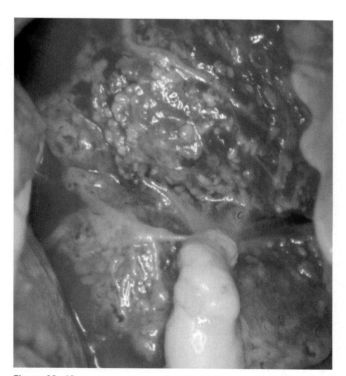

Figure 20–18. Large, normal, early–third trimester cervix demonstrating very active metaplasia, decidualization, and thick mucus. The bumpy acetowhite areas noted (especially on the anterior lip of the cervix) are hypertrophied stromal cells (decidualization reaction).

speculum is often too narrow, especially later in the pregnancy. A ring forceps or two cotton-tipped applicators can be used to evert the epithelium.

Excluding Invasive Disease

> **Treatment deferred until the puerperium implies that no cytologic, colposcopic, or histologic evidence of invasion exists.**

In response to suspicious cytologic or clinical findings, the aim of the colposcopic biopsy is to exclude cancer. The patient may feel anxious about the outcome and worry about possible adverse effects of the examination. Although colposcopic assessment will not impair the pregnancy or harm the fetus, the patient needs reassurance of this fact. If invasive disease is excluded, management of intraepithelial neoplasia will usually consist of conservative follow-up until after delivery. Treatment deferred until the puerperium implies that no cytologic, colposcopic, or histologic evidence of invasion exists. Because a 6- to 12-month delay in the definitive treatment of invasive cancer can have extreme consequences, the importance of accuracy and reliability of triage during pregnancy cannot be overestimated.

> **Most experts agree that the clinical stage, more than the trimester in which the cancer is diagnosed, is probably the most important determinant of prognosis.**

Most experts agree that the clinical stage, more than the trimester in which the cancer is diagnosed, is probably the most important determinant of prognosis.[6] The puerperal state, with its hormonal and vascular changes, does not alter or affect the natural history of invasive cervical cancer, even when it is stratified for stage. Eighty-three percent of cervical cancer during pregnancy is diagnosed as stage 1 disease, 10% as stage 2, 3% as stage 3, and 2% as stage 4. Stage for stage, the prognosis for a pregnant woman with cervical cancer is similar to that of her nonpregnant counterparts.[12] The difficulty in the management of pregnant women relates to the clinical decision on whether to delay therapy to achieve optimal fetal outcome.

TIMING OF BIOPSY AND POTENTIAL COMPLICATIONS

Biopsy is necessary whenever invasive cancer cannot be reliably excluded. Because physiologic changes in pregnancy make colposcopic grading more difficult, biopsy may be necessary to avoid overinterpretation of physiologic changes or underinterpretation of significant lesions.[14, 42–44]

> **Marked edema and vascularity of the cervix during pregnancy may contribute to significant bleeding after punch biopsy, although hemostasis is usually easily attained.**

Colposcopy-directed biopsies may be performed in any trimester of pregnancy, although most colposcopists suggest delaying them until the second trimester. Bleeding is the main concern in obtaining punch biopsies. Marked edema and vascularity of the cervix may contribute to significant bleeding after punch biopsy; however, hemostasis is usually attained without significant difficulty. Because of the increased risk of bleeding during pregnancy, the number of biopsies should be minimized. If possible, one biopsy of the most severe area should be done to establish the histologic diagnosis. The risks of hemorrhage and infection are low, and the risk of premature birth is not increased after a directed biopsy.[37] Authors reporting more than 150 biopsies reported no significant complications related to bleeding,[20, 29, 30, 45, 46] and the procedure may be useful in decreasing the need for conization during pregnancy.[47] Because the rate of false-negative cytology is very high in the presence of invasive disease, it is important to biopsy any suspicious cervical lesion even if the cytology is normal. It is rare that cervical cancer will be undiagnosed during the prenatal period if colposcopy and directed biopsy are used to evaluate abnormal cervical cytology.[30, 41]

> **Colposcopy alone, without directed biopsy, carries a significant risk of underestimating the severity of the cervical lesion.**

Some authors advocate performing biopsies only when expert colposcopic impression indicates high-grade disease.[30] Colposcopy alone, without directed biopsy, carries a significant risk of underestimating the severity of the cervical lesion.[20] In a retrospective study of 612 pregnant women, no cases of invasive cancer were missed when colposcopy was combined with biopsy. However, 14% of colposcopic impressions of low-grade disease were revealed to be histologic CIN 3, and 54% of normal colposcopic impressions were CIN 1 or CIN 2 on histodiagnosis.[9] Histology of colposcopically directed biopsy during pregnancy has been shown to be highly concordant with histology of the surgical specimen at the time of treatment, emphasizing the reliability of biopsy as a diagnostic method. Overestimating the severity of a lesion at histology may result from misinterpreting changes that frequently occur in pregnancy, such as microglandular hyperplasia.[48]

Taking the Biopsy

> **Monsel's solution will interfere with histologic interpretation and should not be applied until after the biopsy is completed.**

A sharp biopsy forceps should always be used. Cotton-tipped applicators soaked in thickened Monsel's solution should be kept immediately at hand. As soon as the specimen is taken with one hand, the Monsel's solution–soaked applicators are pressed firmly onto the bleeding site with the opposite hand. The applicators should be held in place for about 30 seconds. The patient should avoid vigorous activity for approximately 48 hours after the procedure. Occasionally, some bright spotting and discharge may continue for several days. Counseling the patient of these possibilities in advance can help relieve her anxiety.

> **Endocervical curettage should be avoided during pregnancy because of the potential risk of premature rupture of membranes, preterm labor, and uncontrolled bleeding.**

Endocervical biopsy or curettage should not be done during pregnancy owing to the potential risk of premature rupture of membranes, preterm labor, and uncontrolled bleeding.[15]

During pregnancy, diagnostic cervical cone biopsy is restricted to a small, select group of indications. These include the following:

- Minimal stromal invasion on a colposcopically directed biopsy
- Persistent cytologic suggestion of invasive carcinoma on cytology[1, 49, 50] without histologic confirmation of disease

Fortunately, eversion of the squamocolumnar junction during pregnancy improves access to the endocervix and decreases the necessary volume of tissue to be removed.

MANAGEMENT OF ABNORMAL CYTOLOGY IN PREGNANCY

Pregnant patients are unique, in that most cervical dysplasia need not be treated during pregnancy. Management of the pregnant patient with abnormal cervical cytology focuses on documenting the presence of intraepithelial neoplasia while excluding the presence of invasive cancer.[51] Previous investigations have consistently demonstrated the ability of skilled colposcopists to establish the presence of CIN by colposcopically directed biopsy, both before[30] and after birth.[45]

> **The progression rate of CIN to invasion during pregnancy is as low as 0.4%.**

The trend of managing abnormal Pap smears during pregnancy has changed over the decades from an aggressive approach with more liberal use of conization to a more conservative approach of observation. The progression rate of CIN to invasion during pregnancy is as low as 0.4%. Furthermore, the more conservative approach appears to be justified by several studies that document high regression rates of CIN after delivery.[52, 53] Regression rates of 74.1% and 53.8% have been described for CIN 2 and CIN 3, respectively, based on antepartum and postpartum cytologic evaluation.[52] Similarly, up to 65% of untreated low-grade lesions that were followed up sequentially by colposcopy during pregnancy regressed to normal.

> **Although the rate of invasive disease during pregnancy is low, there is no consensus regarding the need for directed biopsy if an intraepithelial lesion is present.**

Most authors recommend a colposcopic examination, with biopsies when indicated, when an SIL is discovered during pregnancy.[18, 20, 29, 37, 41, 54] No agreement exists regarding the need for directed biopsy. During pregnancy, even experts sometimes fail to recognize invasive disease at colposcopy, highlighting the value of directed biopsy. However, it is unclear whether biopsy is more accurate than colposcopy alone.[37] In a review of the literature on colposcopic management of abnormal cervical cytology during pregnancy,[18, 20, 22, 29, 30, 34, 36, 45, 55, 56] cancer was suspected on colposcopy in only 17 of the 25 (68%) patients ultimately found to have invasive cervical cancer, and occult invasive or microinvasive cervical cancer was rare (2 of 753 patients with atypical or mildly dysplastic cytology, 1 of 350 patients with a colposcopic impression consistent with low-grade CIN or lower, and none with both findings).[20, 22, 29, 30, 41, 45, 46, 57] Considering these low rates, biopsy may be omitted safely when neither cytology nor colposcopy suggests high-grade CIN or cancer. The difficulties of colposcopy in pregnancy and the minimal risks of directed biopsy justify biopsy in gravidas whenever the colposcopist cannot confidently exclude cancer based on his or her colposcopic impression. Others, citing a high rate of misdiagnosis when colposcopic evaluation was done without directed biopsies in pregnancy, maintain that biopsy should be performed on all cervical lesions detected colposcopically.[29, 30, 36–38]

> **Pregnant women with cytological abnormalities should be referred to colposcopists with significant experience in the evaluation of pregnant women if there is concern about personal expertise.**

Follow-up of abnormal cytology during pregnancy with repeat smear Pap smears[25, 27] may be inaccurate and unreliable.[41, 54] Pap smears obtained at colposcopy correlate poorly with biopsy diagnoses.[37, 58] This fact, coupled with the difficulty in interpretation of colposcopic findings during pregnancy, argues strongly for the referral of all pregnant women with cytologic abnormalities to colposcopists with extensive experience in the evaluation of pregnant women.

Most patients with preinvasive cervical lesions are able to continue routine obstetric care, and a vaginal delivery can be anticipated. However, many factors must be considered in counseling pregnant patients with invasive cervical carcinoma. These include[38]

1. Patient's desire for continuation of the pregnancy
2. Stage of the disease
3. Number of weeks remaining to achieve fetal viability or lung maturity
4. Effect of the treatment on subsequent fertility or ability to maintain a normal pregnancy

For patients with invasive disease, delay in therapy must be balanced against benefit of improved fetal outcome. Unfortunately, published studies are primarily retrospective, and their conclusions conflict. Progression of early-stage cervical cancer during pregnancy has rarely been reported,[59] and postponing therapy until fetal maturity is achieved does not seem to reduce survival in women receiving standard treatment.[60]

▼ Table 20–4

Abnormalities of the Cervix in Pregnancy

It is rare to find invasive cancer of the uterine cervix in pregnancy.
  The incidence varies from 1.6 to 10.6 cases per 10,000 pregnancies.
  Prognosis is similar to that for nonpregnant patients.
Abnormal Papanicolaou (Pap) smear has become more common.
  It complicates up to 5% of pregnancies.
  Most pregnant women have low-grade disease.
  The most important aspect of the triage of the abnormal Pap smear during pregnancy is excluding invasive cancer.
  A significant degree of expertise and experience is required in the colposcopic triage of the abnormal Pap smear in pregnancy.

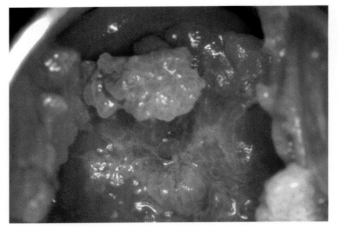

Figure 20–20. Large exophytic condyloma of the anterior cervix in a patient at 20 weeks' gestation.

> **The most common explanation for the high regression rates of CIN following vaginal delivery is cervical trauma that occurs during delivery.**

Contrary to common misconception, the mode of delivery does not seem to have an impact on the patient's outcome.[4, 12] The literature contains conflicting evidence about the influence of route of delivery (vaginal versus cesarean delivery) on regression rates of CIN.[53, 61–63] The most common explanation for high regression rates following vaginal delivery is cervical trauma that occurs at the time of delivery. Trauma may lead to the desquamation of dysplastic cells, followed by subsequent postpartum cervical epithelial repair. Trauma may also occur in women who undergo a cesarean delivery after labor has begun. Other factors may be responsible for the high regression rates in patients undergoing cesarean delivery: (1) the cervix undergoes extensive metaplastic change during pregnancy and post partum, (2) postpartum resolution of immunosuppression is believed to occur during pregnancy, (3) resolution of the enhanced expression of the HPV genome appears to occur during the third trimester, and (4) removal of the lesion or a portion of the lesion by biopsy and the accompanying inflammatory process may enhance the resolution of CIN[61, 63, 64] (Table 20–4).

Minimally Abnormal Pap Smear (ASCUS, LSIL)

It is unlikely that LSIL will progress in pregnancy, and it will often regress completely following delivery. The mother with LSIL should be reassured that neither she nor the baby is at significant risk. Raised, exophytic condylomata of the cervix (Fig. 20–20) could indicate cervical neoplasm, and careful colposcopy is indicated. If there is any doubt, a punch biopsy specimen should be obtained.

> **Pregnant women with cytology indicating LSIL should be evaluated with colposcopy. Histologic confirmation should be necessary only if more significant disease is suspected.**

Pregnant women with cytology indicating LSIL should be evaluated with colposcopy. Histologic confirmation is necessary only if more significant disease is suspected.[41] Considering the low rates of occult invasive and microin-

vasive disease, most authorities agree that biopsy may be safely omitted when neither cytology nor colposcopy suggests a high-grade lesion or invasive cancer. Literature suggests that patients with LSIL or ASCUS during pregnancy do not need serial cytologic or colposcopic evaluation.[65] Many lesions regress spontaneously in the postpartum period. Histologically, these lesions usually represent CIN 1 or squamous metaplasia.[66]

A differing opinion was set forth by Jain et al,[65] who suggested that routine colposcopy for pregnant women with Pap smear indicating ASCUS or LSIL is not necessary. Because none of their patients were found to have carcinoma in situ or invasive carcinoma prenatally, the colposcopic examinations performed during pregnancy did not alter the management of patients. These results are not surprising given the natural history of CIN. Most patients with LSIL have spontaneous regression or persistence of the disease post partum. In untreated patients with LSIL, the progression rate to invasive cancer is approximately 1%.[67] Progression is an extended process. Case-control studies and prospective epidemiologic studies indicate that low-grade lesions take years to develop into invasive cancer.[68] These observations suggest an improbable occurrence of LSIL progressing to cancer during pregnancy. However, those who recommend colposcopy for all these women do so because of concern that the LSIL or ASCUS Pap smear was under-read rather than because of fear that a low-grade lesion will progress rapidly to cancer during the pregnancy.

> **Pregnant patients with LSIL can anticipate a normal vaginal delivery with colposcopic examination in the postpartum period.**

The diagnosis of an intraepithelial lesion is usually made in the first 16 to 18 weeks of pregnancy. Triage guidelines for low-grade cervical lesions in pregnancy are outlined in Table 20–5. These guidelines include examining the patient with colposcopy at least once during the pregnancy. A biopsy is performed if colposcopic findings cannot confidently exclude invasive cancer. A second col-

▼ Table 20–5

Triage of the Abnormal Papanicolaou Smear

Perform colposcopy to confirm abnormal cervical cytology.

Perform a colposcopic-directed biopsy if invasive cancer cannot be confidently excluded on colposcopic grounds; avoid endocervical curettage.

For women with high-grade disease, perform cervical cytology and colposcopy at least once more during the pregnancy; perform biopsy if colposcopy indicates worsening changes.

Perform conization if invasion is suspected and not confirmed by biopsy, if microinvasion or adenocarcinoma in situ of the cervix is found, or in selected patients with high-grade lesions and unsatisfactory colposcopy (individualized).

Anticipate a normal vaginal delivery.

Re-evaluate 3 to 4 months post partum with cervical cytology and colposcopic examination.

Treatment is based on the cytologic, histologic, and colposcopic state of the lesion in the postpartum state.

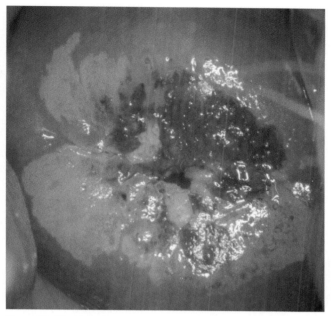

Figure 20–21. Ectropion along with dense acetowhite epithelium at the 9-o'clock position, with some peeling of the margins and subsequent bleeding. There is also a peripheral low-grade lesion present.

poscopic evaluation may be performed at approximately 28 weeks. If there is evidence of disease progression (a change in the colposcopic impression), a biopsy is warranted. For these patients, a normal vaginal delivery is anticipated. If the lesion remains stable, the patient is reviewed for a definitive diagnosis and management approximately 8 to 12 weeks post partum to determine the status of the lesion. If the cytology or colposcopic appearance changes during the follow-up period, a directed biopsy should be obtained. Treatment should be based on regression, persistence, or progression of the lesion at the time of postpartum diagnosis.

These guidelines are not universally accepted. Jain et al[65] offered an alternative management program that would eliminate colposcopy for this group of patients. The authors concluded that pregnant women with a minimally abnormal Pap smear should have a repeat Pap smear post partum. Persistent abnormalities would necessitate a colposcopic evaluation. They concluded that this strategy was safe and resulted in significant cost savings. Further well-designed prospective studies are needed to confirm this recommendation.

HSIL

All pregnant patients with HSIL should be referred for colposcopic examination.

All pregnant patients with HSIL should be referred for colposcopic examination. The colposcopic features of HSIL are usually obvious. The acetowhite epithelium is dense, with distinct margins that are prone to lift and peel in pregnancy (Fig. 20–21). The coarse mosaic and punctation of HSIL can usually be distinguished from anatomic variants (Fig. 20–22). In particular, atypical vessels are not usually produced by physiologic alterations.

All patients with colposcopic features that suggest HSIL, in whom invasive cancer cannot be confidently excluded on colposcopic grounds, should undergo colposcopic-directed biopsy at their initial visit.

In nonpregnant women, HSIL is most commonly surgically excised. This provides the opportunity for histologic examination and for conclusively excluding any stromal invasion. Because of data suggesting complications related to conization during pregnancy, most authors maintain that surgical excision should be avoided during pregnancy and suggest a close follow-up schedule during pregnancy and treatment post partum. Most authorities recommend excisional treatment only if an invasive or microinvasive carcinoma is diagnosed by colposcopic biopsy.

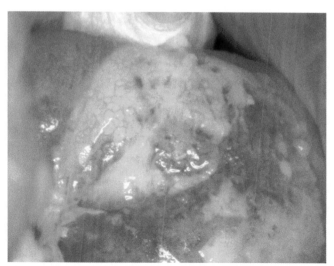

Figure 20–22. High-grade cervical intraepithelial neoplasia with coarse mosaic and dense acetowhite epithelium.

The current guidelines for triage of HSIL during pregnancy should include monitoring colposcopic findings and evaluating lesions closely for the presence of any warning signs of invasion.

All patients with colposcopic features that suggest HSIL, in whom invasive cancer cannot be confidently excluded on colposcopic grounds, should undergo colposcopic-directed biopsy at the initial visit. If invasive disease is not identified, colposcopy and cytology should be repeated in 8 to 12 weeks.[20] Patients with CIN 2 or CIN 3 can be managed conservatively until delivery. If colposcopy shows that the lesion remains stable, additional biopsies may be unnecessary. The patient will have a follow-up appointment for definitive diagnosis and treatment at 8 to 12 weeks post partum.[22] The current guidelines for triage of HSIL during pregnancy include monitoring colposcopic findings and evaluating lesions closely for the presence of any warning signs of cervical cancer. Alternatively, following a confirmatory biopsy during pregnancy, patients may receive a Pap smear every trimester to monitor for progression.[19]

Pap smear with colposcopy appears to be an effective method of monitoring high-grade disease during pregnancy.[69] There is no justification for cone biopsy to treat or evaluate preinvasive disease of any size on the ectocervix when invasive cancer is not suspected.

Because there is a high rate of postpartum regression of cervical disease, even high-grade lesions should be evaluated post partum before treatment.

At the time of postpartum colposcopic assessment, treatment is based on lesion status. Because there is a high rate of postpartum regression of cervical disease, even high-grade lesions should be evaluated post partum before treatment. If the lesion that was evaluated during pregnancy cannot be identified post partum, the patient should be assessed by cytology and colposcopy at 6-month intervals for 2 years before returning to normal cytologic follow-up per published guidelines.

Microinvasive Carcinoma

Even in pregnancy, the diagnosis of microinvasive disease requires histology from a sufficiently large biopsy specimen.

Any indication of invasive disease requires the most conscientious colposcopic, histologic, and cytologic review. The diagnosis of microinvasive carcinoma can be made only on histology of a sufficiently large biopsy specimen. A large wedge biopsy or a cone biopsy is required.[30, 70] A cervical punch biopsy is not confirmatory. Indications for cervical conization during pregnancy are (1) suspected microinvasion on colposcopic examination or colposcopic-directed biopsy or (2) frankly malignant cytology for which invasive cancer cannot be confidently ruled out by colposcopic examination or colposcopic-directed biopsy.

Conization during pregnancy in the presence of suspected microinvasive or invasive disease by cytology or colposcopy is frequently associated with significant morbidity. Data emphasize that conization during pregnancy is associated with a 12% hemorrhagic complication rate, a 5% perinatal mortality rate from preterm labor and maternal chorioamnionitis, and an increase in the rate of preterm labor from 4% to 30%.[71] In addition, up to 50% of pregnant patients have residual CIN after conization. The second trimester seems to be the optimal period for conization to minimize fetal and maternal complications.[20, 30, 72] Even if the procedure is easier, conization is generally avoided during the first trimester because it may cause miscarriage.[73] Others do not share this view.[70] Laser conization has been reported to occur at 27 weeks' gestation without complication.[22] LaPolla et al[18] suggested performing conization during the third trimester, if needed, but only when fetal viability has been achieved, because complications would necessitate immediate delivery.

Microinvasion can be suspected only on colposcopic examination (Fig. 20–23), and even during pregnancy only large wedge biopsy or cervical conization can make the diagnosis, not cervical punch biopsy. Once the diagnosis of microinvasive carcinoma during pregnancy is made by cervical conization with negative margins, the patient may be safely followed up to the point of fetal viability. Depth of invasion and other prognostic features relating to microinvasive disease may influence the timing and route of delivery. There is no convincing evidence that the route of delivery influences the outcome of microinvasive cervical cancer. Patients are usually permitted to deliver vaginally. Microinvasive carcinoma associated with high-risk features (deep stromal invasion, lymphatic

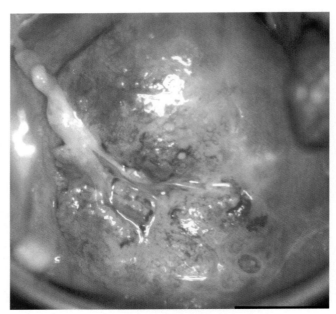

Figure 20–23. Coarse mosaic and atypical blood vessels in a patient with a high-grade squamous intraepithelial lesion. Biopsies revealed microinvasive cancer. A cone biopsy is necessary in such patients to rule out invasive cancer.

or vascular space involvement) may require more radical management (cesarean section and radical hysterectomy).

Invasive Carcinoma

> **If there is no apparent cause for bleeding in pregnancy, a colposcopic examination should be performed to exclude occult cervical cancer.**

Although cervical cancer in pregnancy remains uncommon, it is a clinical dilemma when it does occur. Women with cervical cancer are commonly found to have negative or minimally abnormal Pap smears. Therefore, even in the presence of a negative Pap smear, the implications of misdiagnosed cancer are so important to both mother and fetus that they mandate a high index of suspicion in the presence of symptoms and signs of cervical cancer in pregnant women. If there is no apparent cause for bleeding in pregnancy, a colposcopic examination should be performed to exclude occult cervical cancer. If the cervix feels abnormally firm and indurated or demonstrates an unusual surface contour (Fig. 20–24), colposcopy is indicated to exclude cervical cancer.[4]

> **Progression of early-stage cancer in pregnancy is rare, and to postpone therapy until fetal lung maturity does not seem to reduce survival in women receiving standard treatment.**

The clinical suspicion of cervical cancer during pregnancy requires an appropriate biopsy. If the tumor is visible, a large directed biopsy may be adequate to establish the diagnosis. However, one must be certain that the biopsy contains sufficient stroma to establish the presence of stromal invasion. Usually, a larger tissue sample, either wedge or cone biopsy, is required to establish the depth of involvement.

Pregnant women diagnosed with invasive cervical cancer should be counseled extensively regarding treatment options as well as the impact of treatment on the mother and fetus. Multiple factors should be considered in planning the treatment, including gestational age, tumor size and stage, and the patient's desire to preserve the pregnancy. If invasive cancer is diagnosed early in the pregnancy, a radical hysterectomy with ovarian preservation is normally performed immediately, sacrificing the pregnancy in the maternal interest. In managing small clinical stage 1 cancers during pregnancy, some authors have begun to offer their patients careful observation only until the post partum period. Although the number of patients investigated in this manner thus far has been small,[74, 75] preliminary reports seem to indicate that it may no longer be necessary to sacrifice the pregnancy before fetal viability. A few publications have looked at the effect of delaying definitive therapy until fetal maturity is reached.[7, 9, 74–77] In these reports, treatment delays ranging from 53 to 212 days did not negatively affect maternal survival. However, the number of patients in those series was too small to draw definitive conclusions. Treatment delay seems to be a reasonable option in a patient with early-stage disease who is more than 20 weeks pregnant at the time of

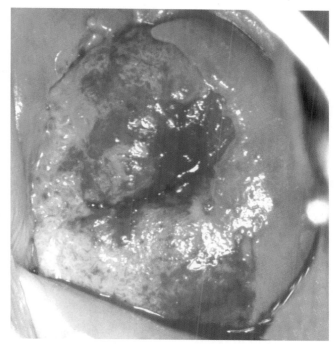

Figure 20–24. This pregnant woman at 20 weeks' gestation had a Papanicolaou smear suggestive of invasive cancer, her cervix felt firm to palpation, and colposcopy revealed dense acetowhite epithelium with atypical vessels involving half of her cervix. Biopsy confirmed invasive cancer.

diagnosis.[77] For patients who elect to continue with the pregnancy and delay treatment, cervical cancer does not seem to affect the fetus adversely; the incidence of intrauterine growth restriction and stillbirth is not increased in those cases.[10]

> **With frankly invasive cancer, concerns relating to intrapartum and postpartum hemorrhage make classic cesarean section followed by radical hysterectomy and node dissection the preferred method of delivery.**

With frankly invasive cancer, concerns relating to intrapartum and postpartum hemorrhage make classic cesarean section followed by a radical hysterectomy and node dissection the preferred method of delivery.[4] There are few reliable data available to determine the impact of vaginal delivery on the outcome of cervical cancer, though there is some suggestion that vaginal delivery may adversely affect maternal survival.[5]

POSTPARTUM ISSUES

> **About 11% of prenatal patients with histologic intraepithelial lesions have normal postpartum cytology.**

Definitive diagnostic evaluation of women with known HSIL during pregnancy should occur 8 to 12 weeks post partum—the time it takes for the cervix to return to a

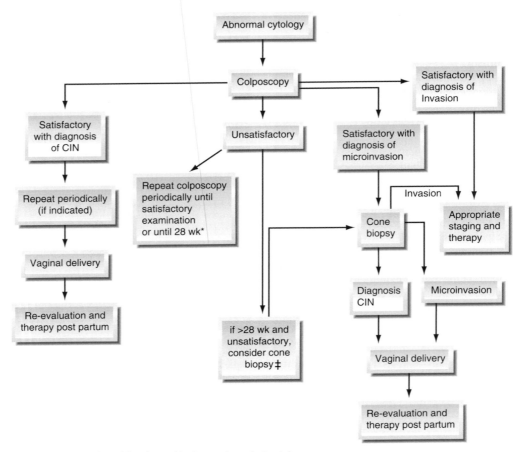

Figure 20–25. Algorithm for triage of gravid patient with abnormal cervical cytology.

normal physiologic state. Even if the postpartum Pap smear is negative, the patient should have a complete colposcopic evaluation, including directed biopsies. About 11.1% of prenatal patients with histologically proven CIN have normal postpartum cytology.[18] Figure 20–25 summarizes the triage of the abnormal Pap smear in pregnancy. The postpartum diagnosis rarely exceeds the diagnosis during pregnancy. Because of the high regression rate of cervical dysplasia in the postpartum period, many colposcopic examinations result in findings of no dysplasia.

LSIL

Women with cytologic and colposcopic evidence of a low-grade lesion during pregnancy (with or without histologic confirmation) should undergo a repeat evaluation about 12 weeks post partum. This should include repeat cytology, colposcopy, and biopsy, if necessary. If a biopsy was done during pregnancy, postpartum histologic reconfirmation of LSIL is not necessary as long as there has been no change in the colposcopic appearance of the lesion and there is no suspicion of more significant disease.

HSIL

HSIL rarely regresses after pregnancy. It has been found that as many as 95% of patients with CIN 3 during pregnancy have residual dysplasia post partum.[69] At a 12-week postpartum evaluation, a complete colposcopic examination with biopsy and endocervical curettage (if indicated) is performed.[20] If the postpartum colposcopy is adequate and normal, cytology and/or colposcopy should be repeated at 6-month intervals for 2 years before returning the patient to routine surveillance. It is estimated that as many as one third of women who have abnormal cytology during pregnancy and normal colposcopy post partum will be found to have CIN within 1 year.[29]

> ## SUMMARY OF KEY POINTS
>
> - The Pap smear is a reliable screening test in pregnancy.
>
> - Approximately 2% of cytology results in pregnancy are abnormal, and invasive disease is rare.

- The goal of colposcopy is to rule out invasive disease and to provide support for conservative observation of intraepithelial lesions.

- The initial triage of abnormal cervical cytology in pregnancy should include colposcopic examination.

- Because of the physiologic alterations of the cervix during pregnancy, colposcopy can be challenging and should be performed by colposcopists who understand the normal and abnormal changes that occur during the prenatal period.

- Most colposcopy during pregnancy is satisfactory because of the eversion of the endocervical columnar epithelium by about 18 weeks' gestation.

- Colposcopically directed biopsies should be performed in pregnancy if the results will appropriately assist in making triage and management decisions.

- Neither preinvasive nor invasive lesions progress more rapidly in pregnancy.

- Management of LSIL in pregnancy includes colposcopic examination followed by repeat colposcopy or cytology if the colposcopist deems it necessary. Vaginal delivery is to be expected, and significant regression of LSIL can occur post partum and obviate the need for follow-up treatment.

- Management of HSIL in pregnancy includes initial colposcopic examination. The need for repeat evaluation later in pregnancy should be individualized to the degree of the patient's disease and the colposcopist's confidence that invasion has been excluded. This is likely to differ depending on the experience and expertise of the colposcopist.

- Vaginal delivery is to be expected, and some regression of HSIL can occur after delivery. Treatment decisions are based on the status of the lesion in the postpartum period.

- Patients with suspected microinvasion should undergo cervical conization. Significant morbidity can occur as a result of conization during pregnancy, including preterm delivery and hemorrhage. There is no convincing evidence that the route of delivery influences the outcome in patients with microinvasion.

- Progression of early-stage cervical cancer in pregnancy is rare, and although reports are few, postponing therapy until fetal lung maturity has been achieved does not seem to reduce survival in women receiving standard therapy. At the time of cesarean delivery, radical hysterectomy with pelvic node dissection is performed.

- Counseling pregnant women is important so they will be reassured that colposcopic assessment will not harm them or the fetus and that complications of directed biopsy are rare and easily managed.

References

1. Joensuu H, Klemi PJ: DNA aneuploidy in adenomas of endocrine organs. Am J Pathol 1988;132:145.
2. Lurain JR, Gallup DG: Management of abnormal Papanicolaou smears in pregnancy. Obstet Gynecol 1979;53:484.
3. Yoonessi M, Wieckowska W, Mariniello D, et al: Cervical intraepithelial neoplasia in pregnancy. Int J Gynaecol Obstet 1982;20:111.
4. Hacker NF, Berek JS, Lagasse LD, et al: Carcinoma of the cervix associated with pregnancy. Obstet Gynecol 1982;59:735.
5. Nevin J, Soeters R, Dehaeck K, et al: Cervical carcinoma associated with pregnancy. Obstet Gynecol Surv 1995;50:228.
6. Jones WB, Shingleton HM, Russell A, et al: Cervical carcinoma and pregnancy. A national patterns of care study of the American College of Surgeons. Cancer 1996;77:1479.
7. Duggan B, Muderspach LI, Roman LD, et al: Cervical cancer in pregnancy: Reporting on planned delay in therapy. Obstet Gynecol 1993;82:598.
8. Greer BE, Easterling TR, McLennan DA, et al: Fetal and maternal consideration in the management of Stage IB cervical cancer during pregnancy. Gynecol Onc 1989;34:61.
9. Hopkins MP, Morley GW: The prognosis and management of cervical cancer associated with pregnancy. Obstet Gynecol 1992;80:9.
10. Baltzer J, Regenbrecht ME, Kopcke W, et al: Carcinoma of the cervix and pregnancy. Int J Obstet Gynecol 1990;31:317.
11. Hannigan EV: Cervical cancer in pregnancy. Clin Obstet Gynecol 1990;33:837.
12. Zemlickis D, Lishner M, Degendorfer P, et al: Maternal and fetal outcome after invasive cervical cancer in pregnancy. J Clin Onc 1991;9:1956.
13. Shivvers SA, Miller DS: Preinvasive breast and cervical cancer prior to or during pregnancy. Clin Perinatol 1997;24:369.
14. Campion MJ, Sedlacek TV: Colposcopy in pregnancy. Obstet Gynecol Clin North Am 1993;20:153.
15. Ostergard DR: The effect of pregnancy on the cervical squamocolumnar junction in patients with abnormal cervical cytology. Am J Obstet Gynecol 1979;134:759.
16. Oliveira A, Keppler M, Luisi A, et al: Comparative evaluation of abnormal cytology, colposcopy and histopathology in preclinical cervical malignancy during pregnancy. Acta Cytol 1982;26:636.
17. Benedet JL, Anderson GH, Simpson ML, et al: Colposcopy, conization, and hysterectomy practices: A current perspective. Obstet Gynecol 1982;60:539.
18. LaPolla JP, O'Neill C, Wetrich D: Colposcopic management of abnormal cervical cytology in pregnancy. J Reprod Med 1988;33:301.
19. Roberts CH, Dinh TV, Hannigan EV, et al: Management of cervical intraepithelial neoplasia during pregnancy: A simplified and cost-effective approach. Lower Genital Tract Dis 1998;2(2):67.
20. Economos K, Veridiano NP, Delke I, et al: Abnormal cervical cytology in pregnancy: A 17-year experience. Obstet Gynecol 1993;81:915.
21. Allen DG, Planner RS, Tang PT, et al: Invasive cervical cancer in pregnancy. Aust N Z J Obstet Gynecol 1995;35:408.
22. Ueki M, Ueda M, Kumagai K, et al: Cervical cytology and conservative management of cervical neoplasia during pregnancy. Int J Obstet Gynecol 1995;14:63.
23. Guerra B, DeSimone P, Gabrielli S, et al: Combined cytology and colposcopy to screen for cervical cancer in pregnancy. J Repro Med 1998;43:647.
24. Dupre-Froment J: Cytologie Gynecologique. Paris, Flammarion Medicine Science, 1974.
25. Meisels A, Morin C: Cytopathology of the Uterine Cervix. Chicago, ASCP Press, 1991.
26. McDonnell JM, Mylotte MJ, Gustafson RC, et al: Colposcopy in pregnancy. A twelve year review. Br J Obstet Gynaecol 1981;88:414.
27. Woodrow N, Permezel M, Butterfield L, et al: Abnormal cervical cytology in pregnancy: Experience of 811 cases. Aust N Z Obstet Gynecol 1998;38:161.
28. Behnam K, Mariano E: The value of colposcopy in evaluating cervical intraepithelial neoplasia during pregnancy. Diagn Gynecol Obstet 1982;4:133.
29. Hellberg D, Axelsson O, Gad A, et al: Conservative management of

the abnormal smear during pregnancy. A long-term follow-up. Acta Obstet Gynecol Scand 1987;66:195.

30. Benedet JL, Selke PA, Nickerson KG: Colposcopic evaluation of abnormal Papanicolaou smears in pregnancy. Am J Obstet Gynecol 1987;157:932.

31. Madej JG Jr: Colposcopy monitoring in pregnancy complicated by CIN and early cervical cancer. Eur J Gynaecol Onc 1996;17:59.

32. Harper DM, Roach MSI: Cervical intraepithelial neoplasia in pregnancy. J Fam Pract 1995;42:79.

33. Stafl A, Mattingly RF: Colposcopic diagnosis of cervical neoplasia. Obstet Gynecol 1973;41:168.

34. DePetrillo AD, Townsend DE, Morrow CP, et al: Colposcopic evaluation of the abnormal Pap test in pregnancy. Am J Obstet Gynecol 1975;121:441.

35. Ferenczy A: HPV-associated lesions in pregnancy and their clinical implications. Clin Obstet Gynecol 1989;32:191.

36. Bakri YN, Akhtar M, Al-Amri A: Carcinoma of the cervix in a pregnant woman with negative Pap smears and colposcopic examination. Acta Obstet Gynecol Scand 1990;69:657.

37. Baldauf JJ, Dreyfus M, Ritter J: Benefits and risks of directed biopsy in pregnancy. J Lower Genital Tract Dis 1997;1:214.

38. Apgar BS, Zoschnick LB: Triage of the abnormal Papanicolaou smear in pregnancy. Prim Care Clin North Am 1998;24:483.

39. Coppleson M, Reid B: The colposcopic study of the cervix during the pregnancy and the puerperium. J Obstet Gynaecol 1966;73:575.

40. Singer A: The uterine cervix from adolescence to the menopause. Br J Obstet Gynaecol 1975;82:81.

41. Baldauf JJ, Dreyfus M, Ritter J, et al: Colposcopy and directed biopsy reliability during pregnancy: A cohort study. Eur J Obstet Gynecol 1995;62:31.

42. Burghardt E: Colposcopy in pregnancy. In Burghardt E (ed): Colposcopy—Cervical Pathology, 2nd ed. New York, Thieme, 1991, p 201.

43. Anderson M, Jordan J, Morse A, Sharp F (eds): A Text and Atlas of Integrated Colposcopy. London, Chapman & Hall Medical, 1992, p 201.

44. Madej JG Jr, Szczudrawa A, Pitynski K: Colposcopy findings of CIN and cancer-like lesions of the cervix in pregnancy. Clin Exp Obstet Gynecol 1992;19:168.

45. Nahhas WA, Clark MA, Brown M: Abnormal Papanicolaou smears and colposcopy in pregnancy: Ante- and post-partum findings. Int J Gynecol Cancer 1993;3:239.

46. Lundvall L: Comparison between abnormal cytology, colposcopy and histopathology during pregnancy. Acta Obstet Gynecol Scand 1989;68:447.

47. Lewandowski GS, Vaccarello L, Copeland LJ: Surgical issues in the management of carcinoma of the cervix in pregnancy. Surg Clin North Am 1995;75:89.

48. Singer A, Monaghan JM: Lower Genital Tract Precancer: Colposcopy, Pathology and Treatment. Boston, Blackwell Scientific, 1994.

49. Choo YC, Chan OLY, Ma HK: Colposcopy in microinvasive carcinoma of the cervix: An enigma of diagnosis. Br J Obstet Gynaecol 1984;92:1156.

50. Hannigan EV, Whitehouse HH, Atkinson WD, et al: Cone biopsy during pregnancy. Obstet Gynecol 1992;60:450.

51. DePetrillo AD: Noninvasive carcinoma of the cervix. In Allen HHA, Nikser JA (eds): Cancer in Pregnancy. Mt Kisco, NY, Futura, 1986, pp 103–111.

52. Kiguchi K, Bibbo M, Hasegawa T, et al: Dysplasia during pregnancy: A cytologic follow-up study. J Reprod Med 1981;26:66.

53. Ahdoot D, Van Nostrand KM, Nguyen NJ, et al: The effect of route of delivery on regression of abnormal cervical cytologic findings in the postpartum period. Am J Obstet Gynecol 1998;178:1116.

54. Kashimura M, Matsuura Y, Shinohara M, et al: Comparative study of cytology and punch biopsy in cervical intraepithelial neoplasia during pregnancy. A preliminary report. Acta Cytol 1991;35:100.

55. Kirkup W, Singer A: Colposcopy in the management of the pregnant patient with abnormal cervical cytology. Br J Obstet Gynaecol 1980;87:322.

56. Giuntoli R, Yeh IT, Bhuett N, et al: Conservative management of cervical intraepithelial neoplasia during pregnancy. Gynecol Oncol 1991;42:68.

57. Kaminski PF, Lyon DS, Sorosky JI, et al: Significance of atypical cervical cytology in pregnancy. Am J Perinatol 1992;9:340.

58. Leiberman RW, Henry MR, Laskin WB, et al: Colposcopy in pregnancy: Directed brush cytology compared with cervical biopsy. Obstet Gynecol 1999;94:198.

59. Dundan RC, Yon JL, Ford JH, et al: Carcinoma of the cervix and pregnancy. Gynecol Oncol 1973;1:283.

60. Sorosky JI, Squatrito R, Ndubisi BU, et al: Stage I squamous cell carcinoma in pregnancy: Planned delay in therapy awaiting fetal maturity. Gynecol Oncol 1995;59:207.

61. Brinton LA, Reeved WC, Brenes MM, et al: Parity as a risk factor for cervical cancer. Am J Epidemiol 1989;130:486.

62. Bosch FX, Munoz N, de Sanjose S, et al: Risk factors for cervical cancer in Columbia and Spain. Int J Cancer 1992;52:750.

63. Yost NP, Santoso JT, McIntire DD, et al: Postpartum regression rates of antepartum cervical intraepithelial neoplasia II and III lesions. Obstet Gynecol 1999;93:359.

64. Rock JD, Thompson JA: Te Linde's Operative Gynecology, 8th ed. Philadelphia, Lippincott-Raven, 1997, p 1403.

65. Jain AG, Higgins RV, Boyle MJ: Management of low-grade squamous intraepithelial lesions during pregnancy. Am J Obstet Gynecol 1997;177:298.

66. Mikhail MS, Anyaegbunam A, Romney SL: Computerized colposcopy and conservative management of cervical intraepithelial neoplasia in pregnancy. Acta Obstet Gynecol Scand 1995;74:76.

67. Garutti P, Segala V, Folegatti MR, et al: Evolution of cervical intraepithelial neoplasia grades I and II: A two-year follow-up of untreated and treated cases. Obstet Gynecol Surv 1992;47:50.

68. Mitchell MF, Schoffenfeld D: The natural history of cervical intraepithelial neoplasia and management of the abnormal Papanicolaou smear. In Rubin SC, Hoskins WJ (eds): Cervical Cancer and Preventive Neoplasia. Philadelphia, Lippincott-Raven, 1996, p 103.

69. Patsner B, Morgan S: Conservative management of cervical intraepithelial neoplasia 3 during pregnancy: Is conization ever indicated? J Lower Gen Tract Dis 1998;2:3.

70. Yandell RB, Hannigan EV, Dinh TV, et al: Avoiding conization for inadequate colposcopy. J Reprod Med 1996;41:135.

71. Hannigan EV, Whitehouse HH, Atkinson WD, et al: Cone biopsy during pregnancy. Obstet Gynecol 1982;60:450.

72. Larsson G, Grunsdell H, Gullberg B, et al: Outcome of pregnancy after conization. Acta Obstet Gynecol Scand 1982;61:461.

73. Doll DC, Ringenberg QS, Yarbro JW: Management of cancer during pregnancy. Arch Intern Med 1988;148:2058.

74. Sorosky JI, Cherouny PH, Podzaski ES, et al: Stage IB cervical carcinoma in pregnancy: Awaiting fetal maturity. J Gynecol Tech 1996;2:155.

75. Sood AK, Sorosky JI, Krogman S, et al: Surgical management of cervical cancer complicating pregnancy: A case-control study. Gynecol Oncol 1996;63:294.

76. Monk BJ, Montz FJ: Invasive cervical cancer complicating intrauterine pregnancy: Treatment with radical hysterectomy. Obstet Gynecol 1992;80:199.

77. Greer BE, Goff BA, Koh WJ, et al: Cancer in the pregnant patient. In Hoskins WJ, Perez CA, Young RC (eds): Principles and Practice of Gynecologic Oncology, 2nd ed. Philadelphia, Lippincott-Raven, 1997, p 463.

Case Study 1 Questions

History

This 30-year-old gravida II, paragravida I, at 20 weeks' gestation, presents with a Pap test showing LSIL. She has never had an abnormal Pap smear before this one. She is sexually active and had seven partners in the past, although she has been with her current partner for 6 years.

Figure 20–26

This is a colpophotograph of her cervix after the application of 5% acetic acid.

- Is the transformation zone fully visualized?
- Describe what you see.
- What is the differential diagnosis for this lesion?
- Is a biopsy necessary?
- Should you perform an endocervical curettage?

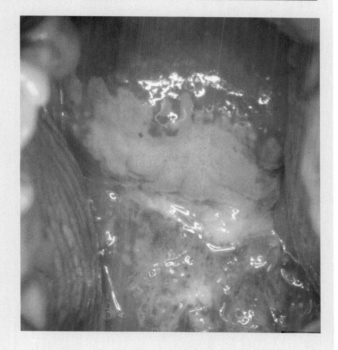

Figure 20–26.

Figure 20–27 is a biopsy of the most severe colposcopic lesion.

- What is your histologic diagnosis?
- What is the next step in this patient's evaluation?

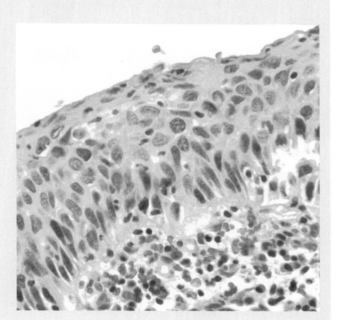

Figure 20–27.

Case Study 1 Answers

Figure 20–26

The cervix is somewhat cyanotic as a result of the pregnancy. In this colpophotograph, the transformation zone is not fully visualized. Although the squamocolumnar junction can be seen on the posterior lip of the cervix, thick mucus in the endocervical canal blocks its view on the anterior lip. It is often possible to manipulate this mucus to visualize the squamocolumnar junction. On the anterior lip of the cervix, there is a flat, acetowhite lesion with a geographic border and no vascular markings. The color is somewhat grayish, but the cyanosis of the cervix can cause the color of the lesion to be undergraded. This is consistent with a low-grade lesion (CIN 1 or condyloma); however, a somewhat higher-grade lesion could not be definitely excluded. A biopsy is not mandatory, and the decision to take one should be based on the comfort level of the colposcopist that she or he has definitely excluded cancer or any other diagnosis that would adversely affect the patient or the pregnancy, should its diagnosis be delayed. Endocervical curettage is definitely contraindicated in pregnancy, because there is a risk that it will result in rupture of the fetal membranes or in hemorrhage.

Figure 20–27

The biopsy shows CIN 3 with crowding and irregularity of the cells along the basal layer and lack of maturation involving the lower two thirds of the epithelium. In a nonpregnant woman, an unsatisfactory colposcopy in association with a high-grade lesion would necessitate conization. However, the risk of complications such as hemorrhage and preterm labor makes conization particularly undesirable in a pregnant patient. Also, the patient's endocervical canal will continue to evert as the pregnancy progresses, raising the possibility that the colposcopy that was unsatisfactory earlier in pregnancy will become satisfactory later. As long as the colposcopist can be confident that the patient does not currently have an invasive cancer, the patient can be followed up through the pregnancy and re-evaluated post partum. If the colposcopist lacks confidence in his or her evaluation, the patient should be referred to a more experienced colleague before resorting to conization.

Key Point of Case 1

As long as the colposcopist can be confident that the patient does not currently have invasive cancer, even a high-grade lesion can be followed up through the pregnancy and re-evaluated post partum.

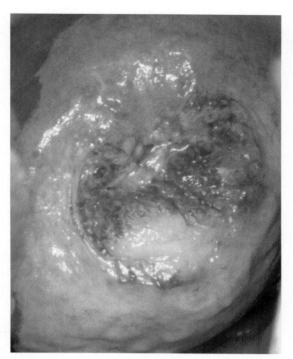

Plate 20-1. Large area of cervical intraepithelial neoplasia (CIN) 1 covering most of the cervix, along with a focal area of dense acetowhite epithelium at the 6-o'clock position. The examination is satisfactory, and there is hypertrophy of the endocervical tissue. A biopsy at 6 o'clock revealed CIN 3.

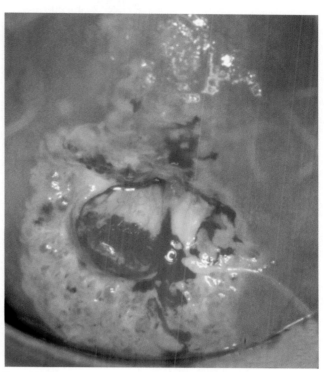

Plate 20-2. Second trimester cervix with a large decidual polyp noted centrally. Metaplasia surrounds the os.

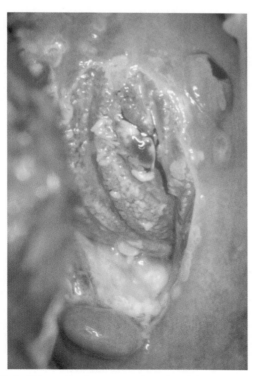

Plate 20-3. This patient has a normal cervix with some distortion of the surface contour from a prior loop electrosurgical excision procedure. Thick mucus is present in the os, and metaplasia has occurred in the area of ectropion on the anterior lip of the cervix.

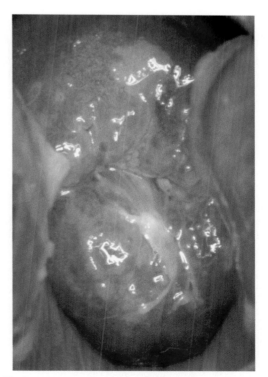

Plate 20-4. Area of cervical intraepithelial neoplasia grade 1 on the anterior lip of a cervix in a woman who is 28 weeks pregnant. The remaining cervix is normal, with thick mucus and increased vascular congestion giving the cervix a blue-violet appearance.

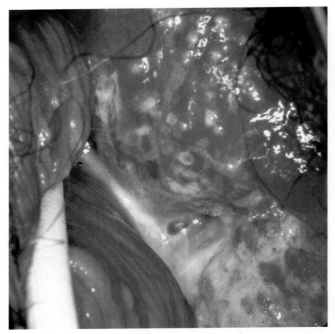

Plate 20-5. Example of normal cervix in the third trimester with violet appearance from vascular engorgement and redundant vaginal walls partially obstructing the view of the cervix.

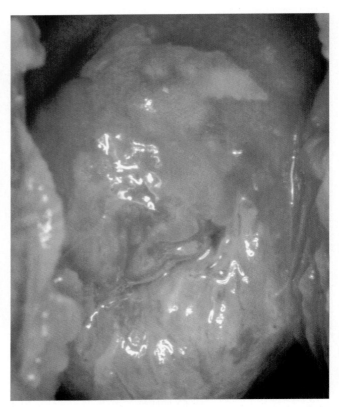

Plate 20-6. Low-grade geographic lesion on the anterior lip of the cervix.

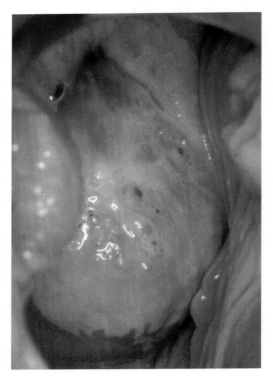

Plate 20-7. Example of a very large low-grade lesion. The transformation zone is extensive and cannot be entirely seen in this view.

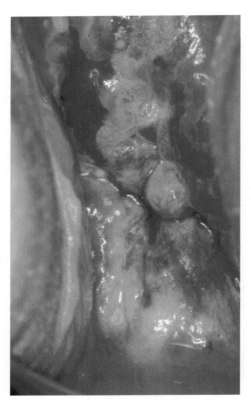

Plate 20-8. Large transformation zone with a fine mosaic pattern at the 12-o'clock position, contact bleeding, and acetowhite epithelium. The squamocolumnar junction cannot be seen in this view. Biopsies were negative.

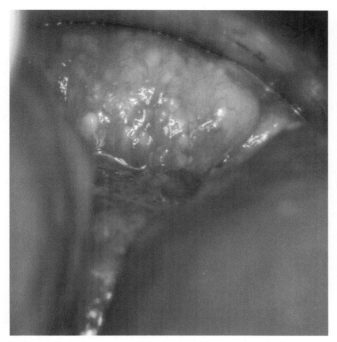

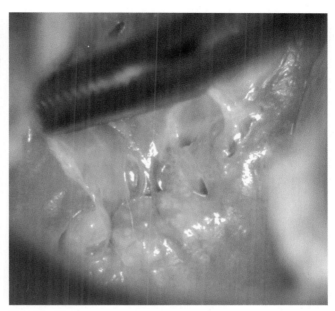

Plate 20–10. Example of dilated gland openings and associated copious mucus production and nabothian cysts.

Plate 20–9. Large transformation zone with multiple nabothian cysts, redundant vaginal walls, and squamocolumnar junction seen on the posterior lip only.

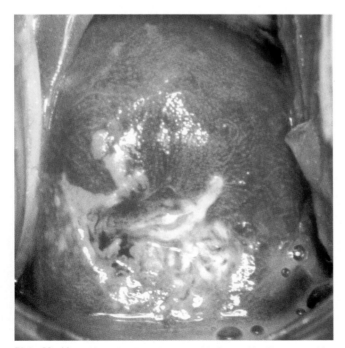

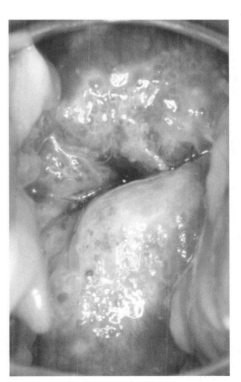

Plate 20–11. Diffuse decidual changes with fine, milia-like, acetowhite areas present. In addition, there is dense acetowhite epithelium present at the 9- to 12-o'clock position. Biopsy revealed cervical intraepithelial neoplasia grade 2.

Plate 20–12. High-grade cervical intraepithelial neoplasia on an early third-trimester cervix. Normal transformation zone components are seen on the anterior lip of the cervix.

- Mark Spitzer
- Anil B. M. Pinto

CHAPTER *21*

Lower Genital Tract Intraepithelial Neoplasia in the Immunocompromised Woman

Since 1993, cervical cancer has been an AIDS–defining condition, and CIN has been an HIV–related condition.

The human immunodeficiency virus (HIV) epidemic first emerged in the 1980s. By 1992, heterosexual transmission of HIV was the primary mode of transmission of the virus to women.[1] The relationship of human papillomavirus (HPV) to cervical cancer and its precursors has also been well established.[2–4] Because both HIV and HPV are sexually transmitted diseases, it is not surprising that many women with HIV infection also harbor HPV. Studies have also shown a high rate of HIV infection among women with HPV-related disease.[5, 6] Since 1993, cervical cancer has been an acquired immunodeficiency syndrome (AIDS)–defining condition, and cervical intraepithelial neoplasia (CIN) has been an HIV-related condition.[7] This chapter will review the relationship of these two diseases and the effect of immune suppression on the manifestation of HPV-related disease. In addition, this chapter will review the literature to determine how to best screen for HPV-related disease in HIV-infected women and how to decide who may need to be screened differently or more intensively. It will also discuss how treatment options may be different for this group of patients as compared with women who have CIN and are not HIV positive, and it will suggest what may be done to improve the cure rate of HIV-positive women undergoing treatment for CIN.

RISK OF CIN IN HIV-INFECTED WOMEN

Independent studies have estimated that the prevalence of CIN in HIV-positive women is between 20% and 77%.

Several studies have found that HIV-infected women are at increased risk of developing CIN.[8–10] HIV-positive women represent perhaps the highest risk group encountered for the development of CIN.[11] Independent studies have estimated the prevalence of CIN in this group to be between 20% and 77%.[8, 12–23] Many studies lack controls and have only a small cohort of patients, making them difficult to compare. Furthermore, their patient populations vary in key areas, such as means of acquisition of HIV infection, duration of illness, patient immune status, and method of diagnosis of HPV-related disease (by cytology or by colposcopy and biopsy). Also, the CIN risk profile, sexual behavior, and HPV status of the patients in some of these studies are not well reported or well controlled, leading to potential bias in some of the studies. The definition of immunodeficiency also varies among studies, making comparison difficult. Consistent definitions are not even used within the same institution, with one definition used in some reports and a different definition used in a later report from the same institution. Immunodeficiency is variously defined as a CD4 count of less than $400/mm^3$ or $500/mm^3$, and severe immunodeficiency is defined as a CD4 count of less than $200/mm^3$. Some studies report their data without describing how many patients were immunosuppressed and to what degree they were immunosuppressed. Because the prevalence of disease and the outcomes vary so widely depending on the degree of immunosuppression, studies that do not "break out" the data are of limited value. Finally, most studies do not address the effect of antiretroviral treatment on the development or recurrence of CIN in HIV-infected women.

It is estimated that the relative risk of CIN in HIV-positive women is almost five times the risk in HIV-negative women.

Mandelblatt[24] reviewed 21 papers published between 1986 and 1990. She identified five well-controlled studies with rigorous methodology. In a meta-analysis, she estimated the relative risk of CIN in HIV-positive women to be almost five times the risk in HIV-negative women. Among those studies combined, 30.7% of HIV-positive women had CIN, compared with 8.3% of HIV-negative controls.

The presence of an oncogenic HPV type is a significant predictor of histologic CIN in HIV-positive women and poses a 7.5-fold increased risk of CIN.

In a large cross-sectional study, Wright[16] colposcopically confirmed CIN in 20% of 398 HIV-positive patients but only 4% of 357 HIV-negative controls (odds ratio, 5.7). However, a more detailed analysis of the data is more revealing. Wright[16] found that most CIN lesions in both HIV-infected and uninfected women were associated with HPV infection and that variables such as smoking history, early age at first intercourse, and number of sexual partners were just surrogate measurements for HPV infection. Moreover, in 52 allograft recipients, Petry[25] showed that without HPV infection, even severely immunodeficient women were free of high-grade CIN. Massad and colleagues[14] found that cervical cytology was abnormal in 38.3% of HIV-infected women compared with 16.2% of similarly high-risk uninfected controls. Finally, in a multivariate analysis of HIV-positive subjects, Maiman and associates[13] found abnormal cytology in 32.9% of their HIV-positive patients and 7.6% of HIV-negative controls. However, further analysis showed that only the presence of an oncogenic HPV type was a significant predictor of CIN on histology, and it posed a 7.5-fold increase in risk.

The higher prevalence of HPV in HIV-positive women may be the result of persistence or reactivation of previously acquired HPV rather than new infection.

Evidence suggests that HIV-positive women have about a fivefold risk of HPV infection and CIN, predominantly owing to the fact that HIV infection is often associated with high-risk behavior, thus increasing the risk for all sexually transmitted infections, including HPV. When the presence of high-risk HPV infection is confirmed, the risk of CIN is even higher. Palefsky et al[26] confirmed the role of traditional risk factors related to HPV positivity in HIV-positive women, but their data also supported the hypothesis that the higher prevalence of HPV in these women was the result of persistence or reactivation of previously acquired HPV rather than new infection. They found that the rate of HPV positivity was highest among those women with the greatest degree of immune compromise (CD4 counts less than 200/mm^3) and lowest among those with the lowest degree of immunocompromise (CD4 counts greater than 500/mm^3 and an HIV viral load less than 4000 copies/mL). When HPV types were grouped into oncogenic risk categories, HPV positivity was more common with increasing immunocompromise in each grouping. HIV-positive women were three times more likely than HIV-negative women to be infected with multiple HPV types (36% versus 12%), and infection with multiple HPV types was increasingly more common in those with lower CD4 counts.[26] These findings confirmed those of an earlier large study by Sun and coworkers.[27] They studied 220 HIV-positive women and 231

HIV-negative controls and found that among women without CIN, HIV-positive women were much more likely to have HPV infection than were HIV-negative controls. Immunosuppressed women (CD4 counts less than 500/mm^3) were most likely to be HPV positive. The cumulative HPV prevalence after four examinations in those women was 95%. HIV-positive women, and especially those who were markedly immunosuppressed (CD4 less than 200/mm^3), were also more likely to have persistent HPV.

HIV-positive women are three times more likely than HIV-negative women to be infected with multiple HPV types, a situation more common in those with lower CD4 counts.

Fink et al[18] found that among HIV-positive women, the proportion of CIN on histology increased from 35% in women with CD4 counts higher than 400/mm^3 to 56% in those with CD4 counts less than 200/mm^3. Schafer and colleagues[28] also found that the risk of CIN closely correlated to the degree of immunosuppression. Significantly, Maiman and associates[13] found that the prevalence of HPV infection, abnormal cytology, and CIN remained relatively constant in the face of increasing immunocompromise until the CD4 count dropped below 200/mm^3, suggesting a biologic threshold for this phenomenon. Heard et al[29] also demonstrated this biologic threshold. They found that women with CD4 counts below 200/mm^3 were twice as likely to have high viral loads. High viral loads, in turn, were associated with high-grade cervical disease (odds ratio, 16.8). Consequently, they found that severely immunosuppressed women (CD4 counts less than 200/mm^3) were 10 times more likely to have cervical disease. However, despite a high degree of immunocompromise, only about half of the women who were HPV positive and had CD4 counts below 200/mm^3 developed CIN.[13] This supports the hypothesis that, even in HIV-positive women, other cofactors play a role in the transition from an oncogenic HPV infection to CIN and cancer.

HIV may act as a cofactor in the transformation of HPV-infected epithelium to intraepithelial neoplasia through T helper 2–mediated cytokine induction in cervical cells.

Klein et al[30] reported that this increased risk of CIN in women with HIV might be due to augmented replication, increased rate of infection, reactivation, or persistence of genital HPV. Molecular interactions between HPV and HIV may also increase the oncogenic potential of cervical HPV infection. Molecular interactions between HIV-1 tat protein and the upstream regulatory region of the HPV genome increase HPV gene transcription.[31] HIV may also act as a cofactor in the transformation of HPV-infected epithelium to intraepithelial neoplasia through T helper 2 (TH2)–2 mediated cytokine induction in cervical cells. By enhancing the expression of viral E6 and E7 oncoproteins, HIV may influence the neoplastic evolution of these lesions.[16, 31] In many studies,[17] the risk of CIN among immunosuppressed HIV-positive patients was almost equal to the risk of CIN in women referred for colposcopy because of Papanicolaou (Pap) smears showing a squamous intraepithelial lesion (SIL). A decrease in the number of Langerhans' cells, a measure of local immunity, has been reported in HIV-positive women in direct correlation with a reduction in the number of CD4 cells.[32]

It has been demonstrated that, in the absence of immunosuppression, there is no significant difference in prevalence of CIN between HIV-positive and HIV-negative women.

The evidence is less clear about the risk of CIN in women who are not immunosuppressed. Some studies[32, 33] have shown diminished local immunity as measured by numbers of Langerhans' cells and macrophages in all HIV-positive patients, including immunocompetent ones. This implies that HIV infection may lead to early impairment of mucosal immunoreactivity because of defective antigen presentation, even in the absence of systemic immunosuppression. Sun and coworkers[34] found that at least part of the promotional effect of HIV positivity on the development of cervical disease occurs even in HIV-infected women whose CD4 counts are greater than 500/mm³. Maiman[35] observed cases of rapidly progressive cervical cancer in asymptomatic HIV-positive patients. In contrast, Smith et al[36] reported an increase in CIN only in immunosuppressed patients. In the absence of immunosuppression, they showed no significant difference in the prevalence of CIN between HIV-positive and HIV-negative patients; however, the number of patients in this study was small. However, in a large multicenter prospective cohort study that evaluated more than 1600 HIV-seropositive women, Massad et al demonstrated that the natural history of cervical disease in immunocompetent HIV-seropositive women was not different from that in HIV-negative controls.[37] In reality, it may be difficult to distinguish the increased risk caused by behavioral patterns in HIV-seropositive women from the increase that may be caused by HIV infection itself.

Although studies suggest that there is an increase in the prevalence of cervical disease in some HIV-positive patients, it is unclear if this represents an increase in low-grade disease, in high-grade disease, or in both. Boardman et al[38] studied women at a colposcopy clinic. HIV-positive women (63% of whom had CD4 counts less than 500/mm³) were compared with controls whose HIV status was either negative or unknown. The HIV-positive women were more likely to have CIN, but the increase was confined exclusively to an increase in low-grade lesions. In a large multicenter study, Massad et al[14] showed that the prevalence of low-grade SIL cytology rose sharply in HIV-infected patients as their CD4 counts declined, whereas the prevalence of ASCUS and high-grade SIL or cancer rose only slightly. Others[25, 39] have shown a similar predominance of low-grade lesions. In contrast, Wright and associates[16, 40] found an increase in both high- and low-grade lesions in HIV-infected women whose cytology showed mild atypia, when they were compared with uninfected women.

Different studies have shown the complete range of disease expression among HIV-positive women, including no increased prevalence of CIN, a disproportionate increase in low-grade lesions, and an increase in all grades of CIN.

In summary, different studies have shown the complete range of disease expression among HIV-positive women. This ranges from some studies that show no increase in the prevalence of CIN, to others that show a disproportionate increase in low-grade lesions, to others that show an increase in all grades of CIN. It is possible that these studies are not contradictory. Because the control groups vary among studies, and some studies lack controls, the studies are very difficult to compare. However, most studies indicate an association between increased immunosuppression and increased grade of CIN. One can postulate that HIV is a marker for the sexual behavior profiles that place a woman at increased risk for acquiring HPV infection. On the basis of this risk factor alone, an HIV-positive woman has a fivefold increased risk for acquiring HPV and CIN. However, if we separate this group of women into those who really did acquire an oncogenic HPV type and those who did not, the HPV-positive group would have a 7.5-fold increased risk, whereas the HPV-negative group would have no increased risk.

In HIV-positive women with oncogenic HPV types, HIV may act synergistically to influence the evolution of CIN 2 and CIN 3, but in the presence of normal immune function, low-grade lesions and overt HPV infections may not be manifested.

When an HIV-negative woman acquires HPV, the infection may progress, resolve, or persist at very low or undetectable levels for a prolonged period of time. Clearance of that active HPV infection is dependent on behavioral, contraceptive, immunologic, and viral factors. Failure to eradicate the infection may influence the development of a preneoplastic lesion.[14] In those with oncogenic HPV subtypes, HIV may also act synergistically to influence the evolution of high-grade CIN lesions. However, in the presence of normal immune function, low-grade lesions and overt HPV infections are not disproportionately manifested. As patients become more immunosuppressed, latent HPV (including low-risk HPV types) is manifested, leading to an increase in low-grade lesions. With longer duration of immunosuppression, and as the CD4 count drops below a threshold level (200/mm³), the prevalence of high-grade lesions increases as well. However, it is also conceivable that the apparent increase in latent HPV and low-grade lesions may be due to bias secondary to an increased surveillance of this population.

Surveillance of HIV-Infected Women

The sensitivity and specificity of cytology in HIV-positive women is comparable to that found in the general population.

Clearly, HIV-positive women require very close surveillance. However, one early report[23] suggested that when compared with colposcopy, cytologic screening was not predictive of CIN in this population. Of the 32 HIV-positive women in this study, 13 had CIN on colposcopically directed biopsy, but only one of these lesions was detected cytologically. A later report from the same hospital confirmed this result,[18] but most of the discrepancy was due to undetected low-grade lesions. Del Priore et al[17] also found that cytologic screening missed a significant number of biopsy-proven CIN lesions (43%). These authors recommended colposcopic surveillance of HIV-positive women. In a subsequent report from the same authors,[13] 248 HIV-infected women and 220 HIV-negative controls all underwent cytology and colposcopy with biopsy. Because all the HIV-positive patients had colposcopy and biopsy, they were able to determine that the sensitivity (0.6) and specificity (0.81) of cytology in this population is comparable to that found in the general population. Subsequent reports by other authors have also shown that the diagnostic sensitivity of Pap smears is not decreased in these women, compared with HIV-negative women.[12, 17, 34, 40] Nevertheless, even if Pap smears in HIV-positive women have the same sensitivity and specificity as those in the general population, the high prevalence of CIN in HIV-positive women means that the false-negative rate would be higher.[13] Consequently, large numbers of high-grade CIN lesions may be missed.[16] Also, because this population has a relatively high non-compliance rate and because of the possibility of accelerated progression of disease in this group of women, accurate initial diagnosis is critical.[11] Therefore, surveillance of these women should be adjusted based on the individual woman's risk for CIN. Women who are not immunosuppressed (CD4 more than 500/mm³) and who have only a slightly increased risk of CIN may be followed up with annual or possibly semiannual Pap smears, although some[13] continue to advocate colposcopic follow-up of these women when resources are readily available. Immunosuppressed women (those with CD4 less than 500/mm³ and especially those with CD4 less than 200/mm³) whose risk of CIN is especially high should be followed up with colposcopy. Because the prevalence of HPV and underlying dysplasia is so high in these women, HPV testing in this group of women is of little clinical value.

Surveillance should be adjusted based on the individual risk of CIN in HIV-positive women; those who are immunocompetent should receive annual cytologic screening, whereas those who are immunosuppressed should be followed with colposcopy.

Natural History

The natural history of HPV lesions in HIV-infected women is unclear. Belafsy et al[42] reported that the progression rate of low-grade lesions in immunocompetent HIV-positive women was about 14%. This rate is about the same as would be expected for HIV-negative women. However, this study was limited in that the initial diagnosis was established cytologically rather than by biopsy in more 90% of patients. Branca et al[20] evaluated women at

risk for HIV. Of the HIV-positive women, 47% had CIN or other HPV-related lesions compared with 23% of HIV-negative women. Over the next 12 months, 37% of those HIV-positive women with CIN 1 or CIN 2 progressed to CIN 3, compared with 17% of HIV-negative controls. Conti et al[43] found that HPV-related disease was four times more likely to progress and three times less likely to regress in HIV-positive women compared with HIV-negative controls. Petry et al[25] found only a 27% regression rate of CIN 1 lesions in immunosuppressed HIV-positive and transplantation patients compared with 62% in immunocompetent controls. These lesions also progressed more rapidly (6.3 months versus 10.5 months) than those in immunocompetent controls. Petry et al[25] found that all patients with CD4 counts less than 400/mm³ or immunosuppression for more than 3 years suffered progression. The authors concluded that HPV-infected women must be immunocompetent to avoid progression of their CIN. Immunosuppression has been associated with higher rates of more oncogenic HPV types and infection with multiple HPV types, which may in turn explain the more aggressive cervical pathology that develops in these women.[11, 23, 34, 44]

Response to Treatment

Not only does untreated HPV-associated disease tend to progress in HIV-positive women, these women also experience a high rate of recurrence and progression even if they undergo conventional treatment.

Not only does untreated disease in HIV-positive women tend to progress, but there is also a tendency toward recurrence and progression in women treated by conventional means. Maiman et al[45] found that disease recurred in 39% of HIV-positive patients who were treated by cryotherapy, laser vaporization, or cold-knife cone biopsy, compared with 9% of HIV-negative controls. They estimated that at 12 months after treatment the recurrence rate for disease in HIV-positive patients was 47% (7% for HIV-negative patients) and at 24 months following treatment was 63% (13% for HIV-negative patients). Eighteen percent of patients with CD4 counts higher than 500/mm³ developed recurrent disease, compared with 45% of those with CD4 counts under 500/mm³. They also found that although cryotherapy seemed an attractive form of treatment for HIV-positive women because of the absence of bleeding and the low risk of iatrogenic transmission of HIV, the cure rate for patients so treated was only 52% compared with 99% for controls. This finding was confirmed by others.[46] Whenever possible, HIV-positive women should be treated using an excisional modality. This is because colposcopically directed biopsies may be poor predictors of disease in these women. Del Priore et al[47] reported that 47% of HIV-positive women with CIN 2 or CIN 3 on cone biopsy had only CIN 1 or HPV on colposcopically directed biopsy, compared with 9% of HIV-negative patients. An earlier study showed that the cure rates using laser therapy and cone biopsy did not differ between HIV-positive patients and HIV-negative controls.[43] However, a later study[48] showed that even cervical conization was not an effective method for eradicating CIN in HIV-positive women and that most patients suffer recurrence even when their surgical margins and the postconization endocervical curettage (ECC) are negative.

> **Because of the low cure rates following cryotherapy, HIV-positive women with CIN should be treated with an excisional modality whenever possible.**

Fruchter et al[49] found that 62% of HIV-positive women treated by a combination of ablative or excisional methods developed recurrence after 36 months, compared with 18% of HIV-negative controls. Most of the recurrences occurred in the first year. Recurrence rates reached 87% at 3 years for women with CD4 counts less than 200/mm^3, compared with 54% for less immunodeficient women. In HIV-positive women, 25% of recurrences also involved progression to a higher-grade lesion at 36 months, compared with 2% of recurrences for HIV-negative women. After a second treatment, 50% of HIV-positive women developed recurrent disease compared with 6% of HIV-negative women. Ten percent of these progressed to a higher lesion. Fifty percent of the remaining six patients had recurrent CIN within 7 months of a third treatment. The vast majority of the HIV-positive women who did not develop recurrent disease had been treated for low-grade lesions.

Wright et al[50] found that 56% of HIV-positive women with all grades of CIN experienced recurrence after treatment with electrosurgical excision, compared with 13% of women with unknown HIV status. HIV-positive women with CD4 counts greater than 500 cells/mm^3 experienced recurrence at a 20% rate, compared with 61% for women whose CD4 count was less than or equal to 500/mm^3. Significantly, among the HIV-positive women, all those with a positive postconization ECC developed recurrence, compared with only half of those with unknown serostatus. Among those with a negative ECC, 48% of HIV-positive women developed a recurrence, compared with 11% of HIV-negative controls. Finally, Cuthill et al[51] reported a significantly higher rate of bleeding and cervicovaginal infections after treatment in HIV-positive women compared with HIV-negative controls.

> **Although HIV-positive women treated for CIN demonstrate high rates of recurrence and progression, aggressive retreatment of recurrence has been successful in preventing progression to invasion.**

Therefore, it seems clear that immunosuppressed HIV-positive women with high-grade CIN are at an extremely high risk for recurrence and progression after treatment. Nevertheless, although the data regarding recurrence and progression after treatment are discouraging, one must recognize that close and meticulous post-therapy follow-up coupled with aggressive retreatment of recurrences has been successful in preventing progression to invasive cancer in these patients and so should not be abandoned.[11] As new medications extend the lives of these women, alternative, more aggressive surveillance, treatment, and maintenance regimens should be considered for those immunosuppressed women with high-grade CIN.[45] 5-Fluorouracil vaginal cream has been used with some success in the care of immunosuppressed women with CIN,[46] and interferon has been used in the treatment of both CIN and HIV-related diseases.[52] One clinical trial used 5-fluorouracil vaginal cream prophylactically every 2 weeks for 6 months after treatment for high-grade cervical disease.[53, 54] This study showed significant benefit from 5-fluorouracil prophylaxis. Only 28% of the treated group developed recurrence after treatment, compared with 47% of the untreated group. Prophylaxis also reduced the likelihood of high-grade recurrences (31% in the untreated group versus 8% in the treated group) and prolonged the time to recurrence.

Finally, there is strong evidence of a dramatic effect of the new, more active antiretroviral medication on the HIV status of these patients. However, the effect of these medications on CIN in these women is not well documented. In a small study, Heard et al[55] showed that although treatment with these new highly active antiretroviral medications did not result in clearance of HPV infections, regression of CIN lesions was seen in these patients. Those with the greatest increases in CD4 counts were most likely to have their CIN regress. Orlando et al[56] also showed regression of CIN in women who responded to antiretroviral therapy with higher CD4 counts while showing progression in those whose CD4 counts failed to respond.

Given the very poor prognosis for such women when they develop cervical cancer, consideration might also be given to vaginal hysterectomy as an alternative to reducing the risk of recurrences, especially in women who have undergone multiple procedures and in whom repeated evaluation has become exceedingly difficult. However, there have been no reports using this approach. Furthermore, when considering this approach, it must be remembered that studies of surgery in immunosuppressed HIV-positive men have shown increased rates of infection and delayed wound healing,[57, 58] and there is a risk of HIV transmission to the surgeon during surgical procedures. Finally, although the woman's risk of cervical neoplasia will be eliminated, she will continue to be at risk for vaginal intraepithelial neoplasia and cancer.

Vaginal and Vulvar Disease

> **High frequencies of vulvar, vaginal, and perianal lesions have been reported in HIV-positive women.**

Finally, specific attention must be directed to the prevalence of vulvar and vaginal neoplasia among HIV-positive women. The study of these lesions is even more limited by the number of available cases than is the study of CIN. High frequencies of vulvar, vaginal, and perianal lesions have been reported in HIV-infected women.[12, 59, 60] These included increased condylomata,[47, 51] vulvar intraepithelial neoplasia (VIN),[12, 60–63] and vulvar cancer.[64] The actual prevalence of VIN among HIV-positive women is difficult to determine because most studies segregate their results by immune status, but estimates range from 5.6% to 37%.[12, 60, 61, 64] Despite lack of detail, evidence seems to indicate that VIN in HIV-positive women is a strong predictor of immunosuppression. Petry et al[64] found that 10 of 11 women with VIN were immunosuppressed (CD4 less than 400/mm³) or had been taking immunosuppressive drugs for more than 10 years. Korn et al found that the mean T cell count among eight HIV-positive women with VIN was 269/mm³, and three of the women had AIDS.[63] They also found recurrence among all five of the HIV-positive women who returned for follow-up, compared with only 4 of 13 controls. Although there has not yet been a sharp increase in vulvar cancers in HIV-positive women, the report by Penn et al[65] of a 100-fold increase in the number of vulvar and vaginal carcinomas in transplant recipients compared with the number in the general population raises great concern. These cancers occurred, on average, 88 months after transplantation, raising concern that as HIV-infected women survive longer in the immunosuppressed state, the number of vulvar cancers will rise. Insufficient data exist on how to best evaluate and treat these women, but until further data are available, colposcopic evaluation and liberal biopsy of vulvar lesions in immunosuppressed women seem prudent.

SUMMARY OF KEY POINTS

- HIV-positive women have at least a fivefold increased risk of acquiring HPV and CIN. Their overall risk is between 30% and 40%.

- HIV-positive women with an oncogenic HPV type have a 7.5-fold increased risk of CIN, whereas those who are HPV negative have no increased risk.

- The risk of CIN rises significantly when the CD4 count falls below 200/mm³.

- The sensitivity and specificity of Pap smears is comparable in HIV-positive women and HIV-negative women.

- Because of the high prevalence of CIN in HIV-infected women, the rate of false-negative cytology may be much higher.

- HIV-positive women with normal immune function should be evaluated semiannually with cytology; immunocompromised HIV-positive women should be evaluated semiannually with cytology and colposcopy.

- The natural history of CIN in HIV-infected women with normal immune function is unclear.

- The rate of progression in immunocompromised women is higher and more rapid than that in women who are not immunocompromised.

- The cure rate for cryotherapy in HIV-positive women is much lower than that for other treatment options.

- In HIV-seropositive women, the recurrence rates 3 years after treatment for CIN may be as high as

54% in women with normal immune function and 87% in women with CD4 counts under 200/mm³.

- Close surveillance and repeated retreatment of recurrence have been able to prevent cancer.

- Prophylactic 5-fluorouracil and highly active antiretroviral therapy have shown promise in reducing recurrence rates after treatment.

References

1. Centers for Disease Control and Prevention: Acquired immunodeficiency syndrome, 1992. MMWR 1993;42:547.
2. Zur Hausen H: Human papillomaviruses in the pathogenesis of anogenital cancer. Virology 1991;184:9.
3. Wright TC, Richart RM: Role of human papillomavirus in the pathogenesis of genital tract warts and cancer. Gynecol Oncol 1990;37:151.
4. Bornstein J, Rahat MA, Abramovici H: Etiology of cervical cancer: Current concepts. Obstet Gynecol Surv 1995;50:146.
5. Spitzer M, Brennessel D, Seltzer VL, et al: Is human papillomavirus-related disease an independent risk factor for human immunodeficiency virus infection? Gynecol Oncol 1993;49:243.
6. Maiman M, Fruchter RG, Serur E, Boyce JG: Prevalence of human immunodeficiency virus in a colposcopy clinic. JAMA 1988;260:2214.
7. Centers for Disease Control and Prevention: 1993. Revised classification system for HIV infection and expanded surveillance case definition for AIDS among adolescents and adults. MMWR 1992;41:1.
8. Schrager LK, Friedland GH, Maude D, et al: Cervical and vaginal squamous cell abnormalities in women infected with human immunodeficiency virus. J Acquir Immune Defic Syndr 1989;2:570.
9. Schafer, Friedland W, Mielke H, et al: Increased frequency of cervical dysplasia/neoplasia in HIV-infected women is related to the extent of immunosuppression. Am J Obstet Gynecol 1991;164:593.
10. Vermund SH, Kelley KF, Klein RS, et al: High risk of human papillomavirus infection and squamous intraepithelial lesions among women with symptomatic human immunodeficiency virus infection. Am J Obstet Gynecol 1992;165:392.
11. Maiman M: Management of cervical neoplasia in human immunodeficiency virus-infected women. Monogr Natl Cancer Inst 1998;23:43.
12. Korn AP, Autry M, DeRemer PA, Tan W: Sensitivity of the Papanicolaou smear in human immunodeficiency virus-infected women. Obstet Gynecol 1994;83:401.
13. Maiman M, Fruchter RG, Sedlis A, et al: Prevalence, risk factors and accuracy of cytologic screening for cervical intraepithelial neoplasia in women with human immunodeficiency virus. Gynecol Oncol 1998;68:233.
14. Massad LS, Reister KA, Anastos KM, et al: Prevalence and predictors of squamous cell abnormalities in Papanicolaou smears from women infected with HIV-1. J AIDS 1999;21:33.
15. Feingold AR, Vermund SH, Kelley KF, Schreiber LK, Munk G, Friedland GH, et al. Cervical cytological abnormalities and papillomavirus in women infected with HIV. J Acquir Immune Defic Syndr 1990;3:896.
16. Wright TC, Ellerbrock TV, Chiasson MA, et al: CIN in women infected with HIV: Prevalence, risk factors, and validity of Papanicolaou smears. Obstet Gynecol 1994;591.
17. Del Priore G, Maag T, Bhattacharya M, et al: The value of cervical cytology in HIV-infected women. Gynecol Oncol 1995;56:395.
18. Fink MJ, Fruchter RG, Maiman M, et al: The adequacy of cytology and colposcopy in diagnosing cervical neoplasia in HIV-seropositive women. Gynecol Oncol 1994;55:133.
19. Murphy M, Pomeroy L, Tynan M, et al: Cervical cytological screening in HIV-infected women in Dublin—a six year review. Int J STD AIDS 1995;6:262.
20. Branca M, Delfino A, Rossi E, et al: Cervical intraepithelial neoplasia and human papillomavirus related lesions of the genital tract in

HIV positive and negative women. Eur J Gynaec Oncol 1995;16: 410.

21. Drapkin AL, Livingston EG, Dodge R, et al: Cervical intraepithelial neoplasia in HIV-infected women in a southeastern U.S. population. South Med J 1997;90:893.

22. Johnson JC, Burnett AF, Willet GD, et al: High frequency of latent and clinical human papillomavirus cervical infections in immunocompromised human immunodeficiency virus infected women. Obstet Gynecol 1992;79:321.

23. Maiman M, Fruchter RG, Serur E, et al: Colposcopic evaluation of human immunodeficiency virus seropositive women. Obstet Gynecol 1991;78:84.

24. Mandelbatt JS, Fahs M, Garibaldi K, et al: Association between HIV infection and cervical neoplasia: Implications for clinical care of women at risk for both conditions. AIDS 1992;6:173.

25. Petry KU, Scheffel D, Bode U, et al: Cellular immunodeficiency enhances progression of human papillomavirus-associated cervical lesions. Int J Cancer 1994;57:836.

26. Palefsky JM, Minkoff H, Kalish LA, et al: Cervicovaginal human papillomavirus infection in human immunodeficiency virus-1 (HIV)-positive and high-risk HIV-negative women. J Natl Cancer Inst 1999;91:226.

27. Sun XW, Kuhn L, Ellerbrock TV, et al: Human papillomavirus infection in women infected with the human immunodeficiency virus. N Engl J Med 1997;337:1343.

28. Schafer A, Friedmann W, Mielke M, et al: The increased frequency of cervical dysplasia-neoplasia in women infected with human immunodeficiency virus is related to the degree of immunosuppression. Am J Obstet Gynecol 1991;164:593.

29. Heard I, Tassie JM, Schmitz V, et al: Increased risk of cervical disease among human immunodeficiency virus–infected women with severe immunosuppression and high human papillomavirus load. Obstet Gynecol 2000; 96:403.

30. Klein RS, Ho GYF, Vermund SH, et al: Risk factors for squamous intraepithelial lesions on Pap smear in women at risk for human immunodeficiency virus infection. J Inf Dis 1994;170:1404.

31. Vernon SD, Hart CE, Reeves WC, Icenogle JP: The HIV-1 tat protein enhances E2-dependent human papillomavirus 16 transcription. Virus Res 1993;27:133.

32. Spinillo A, Tenti P, Zappatore R, et al: Langerhans' cell counts and cervical intraepithelial neoplasia in women with human immunodeficiency virus infection. Gynecol Oncol 1993;48:210.

33. Rosini S, Catagirone S, Tallini G, et al: Depletion of stromal and intraepithelial antigen-presenting cells in cervical neoplasia in human immunodeficiency virus infection. Hum Pathol 1996;27:834.

34. Sun XW, Ellerbrock TV, Lungu O, et al: Human papillomavirus infection in human immunodeficiency virus seropositive women. Obstet Gynecol 1995;85:680.

35. Maiman M, Fruchter RG, Serur E, et al: Human immunodeficiency virus infection and cervical neoplasia. Gynecol Oncol 1990;38:377.

36. Smith JR, Kitchen VS, Butcherby M, et al: Is HIV infection associated with an increase in the prevalence of cervical neoplasia. Br J Obstet Gynaecol 1993;100:149.

37. Massad LS, Ahdieh L, Benning L, et al: Evolution of cervical abnormalities among women with HIV-1: Evidence from surveillance cytology in The Women's Interagency HIV study. J AIDS, accepted for publication.

38. Boardman LA, Peipert JF, Cooper AS, et al: Cytologic-histologic discrepancy in human immunodeficiency virus positive women referred to a colposcopy clinic. Obstet Gynecol 1994;84:1016.

39. Strigle SM, Walts AE: Underutilization of the Papanicolaou smear in human immunodeficiency virus positive women. J Acquir Immune Defic Syndr 1995;9:206.

40. Wright TC, Moscarelli RD, Dole P, et al: Significance of mild cytologic atypia in women infected with human immunodeficiency virus. Obstet Gynecol 1996;87:515.

41. Heard I, Bergeron C, Jeannel D, et al: Papanicolaou smears in human immunodeficiency virus seropositive women during follow-up. Gynecol Oncol 1995;86:749.

42. Belafsky P, Clark RA, Kissinger P, Torres J: Natural history of low grade squamous intraepithelial lesions in women infected with human papillomavirus virus. J Acquir Immune Defic Syndr 1996;11:511.

43. Conti M: Prevalence and risk of progression of genital intraepithelial neoplasia in women with human immunodeficiency virus infection. Adv Gynecol Obstet Res 1991;3:283.

44. Laga M, Icenogle JP, Marsella R, et al: Genital papillomavirus infection and cervical dysplasia-opportunistic complications of HIV infection. Int J Cancer 1992;50:45.

45. Maiman M, Fruchter RG, Serur E, et al: Recurrent cervical intraepithelial neoplasia in human immunodeficiency virus-seropositive women. Obstet Gynecol 1993;82:170.

46. Sillman FH, Sedlis A, Boyce JG: A review of lower genital intraepithelial neoplasia and the use of tropical 5-fluorouracil. Obstet Gynecol Surv 1985;40:190.

47. Del Priore G, Gilmore PR, Maag T, et al: Colposcopic biopsies versus loop electrosurgical excision procedure histology in human immunodeficiency virus-positive women. J Reprod Med 1996;41:653.

48. Holcomb K, Matthews RP, Chapman JE, et al: The efficacy of cervical conization in the treatment of cervical intraepithelial neoplasia in HIV-positive women. Gynecol Oncol 1999;74:428.

49. Fruchter RG, Maiman M, Sedlis A, et al: Multiple recurrences of cervical intraepithelial neoplasia in women with the human immunodeficiency virus. Obstet Gynecol 1996;87:338.

50. Wright TC, Koulos J, Schnoll F, et al: Cervical intraepithelial neoplasia in women infected with the human immunodeficiency virus: Outcome after loop electrosurgical excision. Gynecol Oncol 1994;55:253.

51. Cuthill S, Maiman M, Fruchter RG, et al: Complications after treatment of cervical intraepithelial neoplasia in women infected with human immunodeficiency virus. J Reprod Med 1995;40:823.

52. Yliskoski M, Cantell K, Syrjanen K, Syrjanen S: Topical treatment with human leukocyte interferon of HPV-16 infections associated with cervical and vaginal intraepithelial neoplasias. Gynecol Oncol 1990;36:353.

53. Maiman M, Fruchter R: Cervical neoplasia and the human immunodeficiency virus. In Rubin SC, Hoskins WJ (eds): Cervical Cancer and Preinvasive Neoplasia. Philadelphia, Lippincott-Raven, 1996, pp 405–416.

54. Maiman M, Watts H, Anderson J, et al: Vaginal 5-fluorouracil for high-grade cervical dysplasia in human immunodeficiency virus infection: A randomized trial. Obstet Gynecol 1999;94:954.

55. Heard I, Schmitz V, Costagliola D, et al: Early regression of cervical lesions in HIV-seropositive women receiving highly active antiretroviral therapy. AIDS 1998;12:1459.

56. Orlando G, Fasolo MM, Schiavini M, et al: Role of highly active antiretroviral therapy in human papillomavirus-induced genital dysplasia in HIV-1-infected patients. AIDS 1999;13:424.

57. Wakeman R, Johnson CD, Wastell C: Surgical procedures in patients at risk of human immunodeficiency virus infection. J R Soc Med 1990;83:315.

58. Burke EC, Orloff SL, Freise CE, et al: Wound healing after anorectal surgery in HIV-infected patients. Arch Surg 1991;1267.

59. Adachi A, Fleming I, Burk RD, et al: Women with human immunodeficiency virus infection and abnormal Pap smears: A prospective study of colposcopy and clinical outcome. Obstet Gynecol 1993;81:372.

60. Chiasson MA, Ellerbrock TV, Bush TJ, et al: Increased prevalence of vulvovaginal condyloma and vulvar intraepithelial neoplasia in women infected with the human immunodeficiency virus. Obstet Gynecol 1997;89:690.

61. Fruchter RG, Maiman M, Sillman FH, et al: Characteristics of cervical intraepithelial neoplasia in women infected with the human immunodeficiency virus. Am J Obstet Gynecol 1994;171:531.

62. Byrne MA, Taylor-Robinson D, Munday PE, Harris JRW: The common occurrence of human papillomavirus infection and intraepithelial neoplasia in women infected by HIV. AIDS 1989;3:379.

63. Korn AP, Abercrombie PD, Foster A: Vulvar intraepithelial neoplasia in women infected with human immunodeficiency virus-1. Gynecol Oncol 1996;61:384.

64. Petry KU, Kochel H, Bode U, et al: Human papillomavirus is associated with the frequent detection of warty and basaloid high grade neoplasia of the vulva and cervical neoplasia among immunocompromised women. Gynecol Oncol 1996;60:30.

65. Penn I: Cancers of the anogenital region in renal transplant recipients. Cancer 1986;58:611.

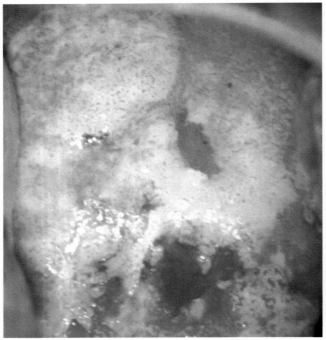

Plate 21–1. Extensive disease in an immunosuppressed, human immunodeficiency virus–positive woman. Dense acetowhite epithelium with punctations is seen extending all the way to the portio vaginalis at the 11-o'clock position. Atypical vessels are seen.

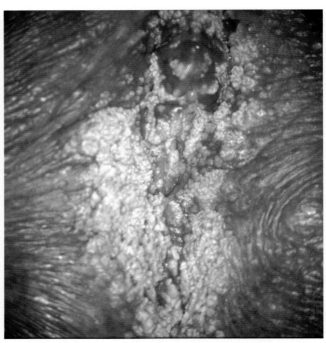

Plate 21–2. Chronic perianal warts in an immunosuppressed, human immunodeficiency virus–positive patient.

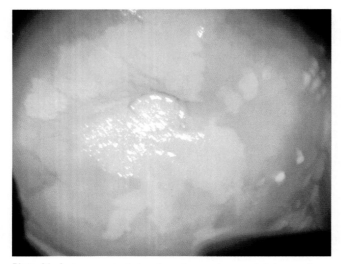

Plate 21–3. Low-grade lesion in a human immunodeficiency virus–positive patient. The lesion is large and has a geographic border. Satellite lesions extend onto the portio.

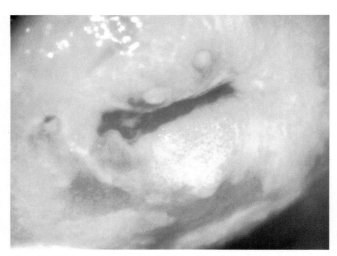

Plate 21–4. Immunosuppressed, human immunodeficiency virus–positive patient. Dense acetowhite epithelium with coarse punctation is seen at the external os and extending toward the portio.

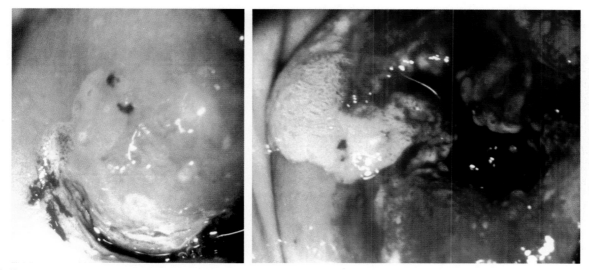

Plate 21–5. *Left,* Colpophotograph of an immunosuppressed, human immunodeficiency virus–positive patient. She was found to have acetowhite epithelium with coarse punctation at the 10-o'clock position. Biopsy showed cervical intraepithelial neoplasia grade 3. *Right,* The same patient, who was lost to follow-up and returned 14 months later. She was found to have a raised acetowhite lesion with atypical vessels in the same 10-o'clock position. Biopsy revealed invasive cancer.

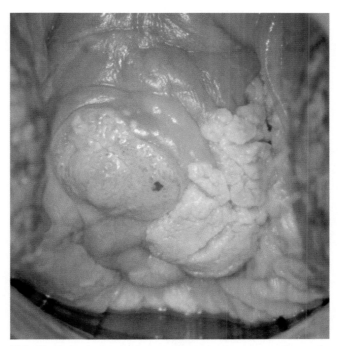

Plate 21–6. A raised, spiked, acetowhite lesion is seen extending to the portio of the cervix and onto the vagina. The squamocolumnar junction is not seen. In addition, there is an area of lesser acetowhite epithelium at the 12-o'clock position associated with small, atypical blood vessels. Biopsy of the bright acetowhite epithelium revealed condyloma, and biopsy at the 12-o'clock position showed cervical intraepithelial neoplasia grade 3. Such extensive lesions are common in immunosuppressed women and make adequate treatment with negative margins very difficult.

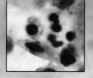

• John L. Pfenninger

CHAPTER *22*

Androscopy: Examination of the Male Partner

Human papillomavirus infection accounts for less than 1% of malignancies in men.

The human papillomavirus (HPV) infects both male and female genitalia.[1] Although penile HPV infection is very common and oncogenic HPV types are associated with penile cancer, the male is not at particularly high risk for developing cancer of the penis.[2, 3] In the United States, HPV infection is associated with less than 1% of malignancies in men.[4] The primary risk factors for penile carcinoma appear to be infection with HPV, sex outside a monogamous relationship, smoking, and lack of hygiene.[5] The absolute number of sexual partners alone is not a high-risk indicator.[6, 7] In other cultures, where a man may be "monogamous" with four or five wives, there is no increased risk of cancer of the cervix or penis.[8-10] Immunosuppression, such as occurs with human immunodeficiency virus (HIV) infection, increases the risk of development of more severe disease.[11]

Homosexual men who have anal-receptive intercourse are at markedly increased risk for anal and rectal carcinoma.[12-14] Cancer of the anal canal in women and in homosexual men is more likely to be associated with HPV.[15] The mechanism seems to involve HPV infection of the dentate or pectinate line in the rectum, which is analogous to the squamocolumnar junction (SCJ) of the cervix.[16, 17] Some experts have advocated cytologic sampling of the anal canal to detect preinvasive and invasive lesions.

Sexual partners of women with genital warts or with preinvasive or invasive disease of the lower genital tract are invariably HPV-infected themselves.[18-20] Women who have sex with men whose previous female partners had high-grade cervical lesions have a much higher incidence of cervical dysplasia and cancer.[21] The profile of a high-risk male is noted in Table 22-1.[22]

One of the major goals of treatment of the male partner is to inform him of the risks of HPV transmission and the benefits of eliminating high-risk behaviors.

Although men have a much lower risk of developing HPV-related cancer than their female partners have, men often act as unknowing vectors in the transmission of HPV infection. Therefore, one of the major goals of "treatment" of the male partner is to inform him of the risks of HPV transmission and the benefits of eliminating high-risk behaviors.[23]

There are several clinical manifestations of HPV infection in men. Condylomata may exist on the penis, scrotum, anus, or suprapubic area and in the urethral meatus (Figs. 22-1 to 22-5).[24] The lesions may be acuminate and visible to the naked eye, or they may be flat and visible only after application of 5% acetic acid. The virus may also be latent, with no clinical signs.

It may be difficult to predict the histology of a penile lesion even when it is observed under magnification.

▼ Table 22-1

High-Risk Conditions for HPV Infection in Males

Multiple sexual partners (>3)
Homosexual or bisexual orientation
Current or past HPV infections, lesions
Sex with a female who has had high-grade SIL, condyloma
Current or past history of other sexually transmitted diseases
IV drug use

HPV, human papillomavirus; IV, intravenous; SIL, squamous intraepithelial lesion.

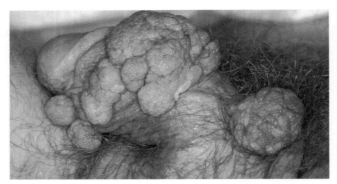
Figure 22–1. Several large condylomata acuminata of the penis.

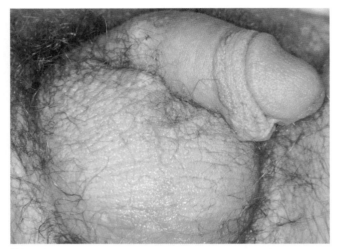
Figure 22–2. White scrotum syndrome—diffuse acetowhite epithelium from human papillomavirus.

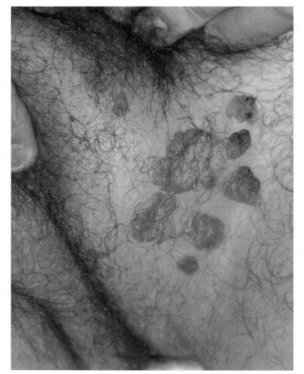
Figure 22–3. Pigmented condyloma.

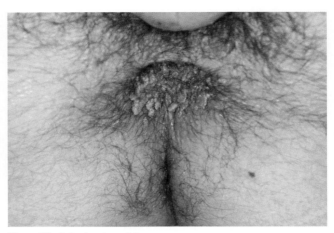
Figure 22–4. Perianal condyloma.

Unlike a lesion on the cervix, the histology of a penile lesion is difficult to predict even when it is observed under magnification. Some lesions with the appearance of classic condylomata are actually squamous intraepithelial lesions (SILs) or bowenoid carcinoma in situ. Others that appear dysplastic are simply genital warts. The lesions can be differentiated only by biopsy.[24]

The differential diagnosis of penile lesions is outlined in Table 22–2. Because patients may be embarrassed about discussing genital lesions, their chief complaints can be misleading. It is only after clinical examination and possibly biopsy that a definitive diagnosis can be made.

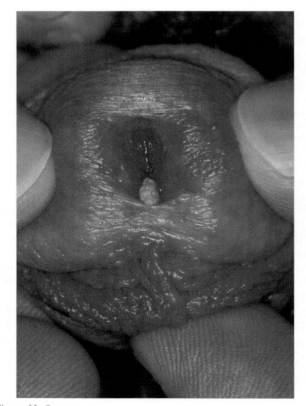
Figure 22–5. Condyloma of the penile meatus.

▼ Table 22–2

Differential Diagnosis of Anogenital Lesions in Men

Infectious Lesions

Condylomata acuminata
Herpetic lesions (herpes simplex virus)
Molluscum contagiosum
Syphilis
   Chancre
   Condylomata lata
Tinea pubis

Noninfectious Benign Lesions and Conditions (Including Normal Variants)

Anal polyp
Contact dermatitis
Cysts
Nevus
Normal variant papular lesions of the frenulum and corona
   (Pearly penile papules)
Seborrheic keratosis
Sentinel "polyp" on a chronic fissure
Skin tags

Preneoplastic and Neoplastic Lesions

Penile intraepithelial neoplasia
   Erythroplasia of Queyrat
   Bowen's disease
   Bowenoid papulosis
Cancer (squamous cell carcinoma of the penis and anus, prolapsing adenocarcinoma of the rectum)

▼ Table 22–3

Indications for Androscopy (Evaluation and Education of the Male Regarding HPV)

Identification of the presence or absence of anogenital skin lesions
Identification of the most severe lesions, allowing directed biopsy of these lesions
Reassurance of both partners
Medical-legal indications—documentation in child abuse cases
Recurrent disease in the female partner
Providing of patient education and reinforcement of a change in high-risk sexual and personal habits
Chronic pruritus/irritation

HPV, human papillomavirus.

ANDROSCOPY

Early papers described the procedure of "colposcopy of the penis" to identify HPV lesions in men. Later, the terms *penoscopy* and *androscopy* were applied.[25–29] The procedure involves applying 5% acetic acid to the penis, scrotum, perineum, and anal areas and then visualizing these areas under magnification with illumination. As in colposcopy, the purpose of androscopy is to identify the most severe lesions, allowing directed biopsy and treatment of those lesions; to reassure the man regarding the extent of the infection (or lack thereof); and to provide an opportunity for patient education.[30]

Androscopy is the examination of the male genitalia after staining with 5% acetic acid using magnification and illumination to identify the most severe lesions.

Indications for Androscopy

The indications for androscopy are noted in Table 22–3.[25, 29] It is not essential that every man with condyloma undergo androscopy. When a partner is found to have HPV-related disease, the role of androscopy is controversial. Some experts question the value of androscopy in men without grossly visible lesions,[31] whereas others suggest that men whose partners have HPV-related disease should be screened.[32] However, when male genitalia are examined without magnification, only 20% of lesions

are identified.[23, 27, 33] Even when no lesions are found on initial visual inspection, if androscopy is performed repeatedly over 1 year, 85% of men exposed to HPV are eventually found to have a biopsy-proved infection.

Men often present requesting evaluation for the presence of infection after being exposed to HPV. Those exposed to HPV will almost always have contracted the virus even if a condom was used. HPV is highly contagious.[29] Even in the absence of visible lesions, men can transmit the virus to their sexual partners. The U.S. Food and Drug Administration (FDA) has been petitioned to require condom manufacturers to state on packages that condoms do not offer protection from infection with HPV.

Treatment of HPV infection in men as a method to reduce recurrence of disease in their female partners has also been a source on controversy.[34, 35] Although some experts initially recommended that all male partners of infected females be examined and treated, this approach may be of little value.[36] Studies do not support the suggestions that large or multiple lesions in the male may shed more virus and that some females may be more susceptible to high HPV numbers.[37]

Patient History

Men are rarely queried about their history of sexual abuse, and the responses to specific questions can be surprising.

Before the first visit, the patient should receive patient education materials regarding HPV and the role of the male partner in transmitting infection.[38] The purpose of the history is to assess risk status. Smoking increases risk of dysplasia and cancer by decreasing immune function in the skin.[39] Age at first intercourse helps define possible length of exposure to HPV. A history of sexual abuse should be ascertained. Men are rarely queried about sexual abuse, and their responses can be surprising.

History of genital warts, how they were treated, recurrences, and partners with HPV infection should be discussed. If a previous partner had cervical cancer, then the patient may have a high-risk HPV type, and his current partner(s) should be considered at increased risk.

All patients should be queried about exposure to any other sexually transmitted diseases. The patient should be encouraged to be tested for HIV and should be offered screening for other sexually transmitted diseases, including syphilis.

Equipment

> **Punch biopsy instruments such as Keyes' dermatologic punches are generally not indicated for biopsy of penile, scrotal, or anal lesions.**

Materials and equipment for performing androscopy are listed in Table 22–4.

It is vitally important to have sharp, high-quality tissue scissors (i.e., small, curved Metzenbaum scissors). Low-quality instruments may pinch or crush tissue rather than cut it sharply. Punch biopsy instruments such as Keyes' dermatologic punches are generally not indicated for biopsy of penile, scrotal, or anal lesions. Even perineal lesions can be biopsied with a scalpel blade using a shave technique or scissors excision. Warts are very superficial, so deep biopsies are unnecessary.

Rather than use a colposcope for magnification, some clinicians prefer to wear loupes or to use a handheld lens. The colposcopic technique of examination of the male genitalia, however, is easy to learn if the instrument is available.

Technique of Androscopy

In the examination room, the patient is instructed on how to saturate the entire penis, scrotum, perineum, and anal area using a spray bottle of warm 5% acetic acid (vinegar). The genitalia are soaked for least 5 minutes, and then the process is repeated, resulting in two thorough soakings.

During the 5-minute interval while the genitalia are being soaked, the clinician may use the opportunity to review the history and explain the procedure to the patient. No informed consent is necessary. The patient is asked to assume the dorsal lithotomy position with his feet in stirrups so the genitals are positioned at the end of the table, similar to the position for a pelvic examination. The entire genital area is moistened with 5% acetic acid once again and examined, first with the naked eye and then with the colposcope on low power (×3.5 to ×5).[40]

The technique of androscopy is slightly different from that of colposcopy. When the cervix is visualized with a colposcope, the depth of field is quite shallow. Also, because the cervix is stationary, it is unnecessary to adjust the colposcope frequently to maintain the focus. In the male, the area examined (glans penis to suprapubic and anal area) is larger, and the distance from the colposcope to the genitalia varies considerably, so the colposcope must be focused more frequently. It may be easier to keep the colposcope stationary and to move the area to be examined into the plane of focus.

The genitals are kept saturated with 5% acetic acid during the entire examination. The penis, urethral meatus, scrotum, suprapubic area, perineum, and perianal tissues are examined. Lesions in the hair-bearing areas are often difficult to detect. It is best to palpate these areas to ensure that no lesions are missed.

Anoscopy is not indicated on a routine basis, and a digital examination is not performed unless there are other indications. If external perianal lesions are identified, treating these lesions first will avoid trauma from insertion of the anoscope and reduce the theoretical risk of tracking HPV infection intra-anally. If only a few lesions are present, they can be excised or cauterized at the same time as the examination. If a digital examination is essential, it should be performed at the time of anoscopic inspection. Some lesions in the anus are not easily palpable because they are small or filamentous, whereas others may be concealed in mucosal folds. Using both methods of examination will decrease the likelihood of missing any lesions.

> **Although some bladder cancers have been associated with HPV, routine cystoscopy is not recommended for patients with genital warts.**

In the past, cystoscopy was recommended to rule out urethral or bladder lesions caused by HPV. Although some bladder cancers have been associated with HPV,[41] routine cystoscopy is not currently recommended for patients with genital warts because of concern that the trauma of the procedure may increase the risk of proximal infection.

Although the entire visit can take as little as 15 minutes, additional time should be scheduled to allow an opportunity to obtain a patient history, to treat limited lesions, and to educate the patient. If more extensive lesions are present, another appointment may be required. A follow-up androscopic examination is usually scheduled for 1 month later if lesions were treated to ensure that none have returned.

Clinical Findings

The differential diagnosis of penile lesions is listed in Table 22–2.

▼ Table 22–4

Materials and Equipment for Androscopy

Examination table with stirrups (preferably a power table)
5% acetic acid (vinegar) in a spray bottle
2% lidocaine without epinephrine in a 5-mL syringe, 30-gauge needle
Colposcope with low power of ×3.5 to ×5 or a quality magnification lens or loupe
Quality tissue scissors (small, curved Metzenbaum)
#5 surgical blade (blade handle optional)
Toothed forceps
Formalin jar for tissue specimens
4 × 4 gauze pads
Monsel's solution
Cotton-tipped applicators
Antibiotic ointment or petroleum jelly
Ive's slotted anoscope
Radiofrequency (electrosurgical) unit

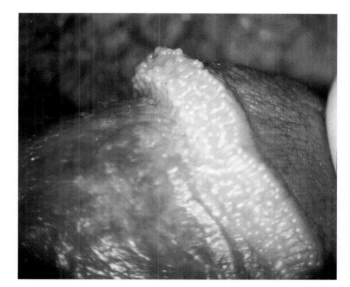

Figure 22-6. Pearly penile papules along the corona of the penis.

As with female genitalia, HPV lesions on male genitalia turn white after the application of 5% acetic acid. The lesions may be totally flat or raised (acuminate). Inflammation in the groin area may also turn white. At times, the entire scrotum will exhibit a faint acetowhite reaction (white scrotum syndrome).[33] Biopsies and DNA typing confirm HPV infection. However, carcinoma of the scrotum is extremely rare.[42] Inflammation of the scrotum and groin area can turn it white, which is more commonly seen.

Krebs evaluated 155 men with androscopy and found lesions between 1 mm and 45 mm in diameter (median, 3 mm).[23] Eighty-seven percent had lesions on the penile prepuce near the frenulum, 42% had involvement of the penile shaft, 20% had lesions on the glans, 11% had lesions on the corona, 6% had lesions on the urethral meatus, 6% had lesions on the urethra, 5% had lesions on the scrotum, 2% had lesions along the crural fold, 1% had lesions on the symphysis pubis, and 3% had lesions in the anus.

There is no lesion in the male genital area that is analogous with leukoplakia in the female genital area. Occasionally, chronic perianal dermatitis in men can become lichenified and appear white before the application of 5% acetic acid. However, the process is more diffuse and generalized rather than focal, as leukoplakia is in women.

Pearly penile papules are usually located on the glans corona and can be misinterpreted as condylomata.

Pearly penile papules (PPPs), frequently observed around the glans corona, are 1- to 3-mm excrescences that may be misinterpreted as condylomata acuminata by patients and clinicians (Fig. 22-6). Unlike condylomata, PPPs are smooth and white before application of 5% acetic acid. The frenulum may also exhibit papular lesions that appear wartlike. When in doubt, a biopsy should be performed. Biopsies may also be done to reassure patients and to satisfy their desire for a definitive diagnosis.

There are few reliable colposcopic signs to differentiate dysplastic lesions from simple HPV lesions in men.

Unlike colposcopy in the female, there are few reliable colposcopic signs to differentiate dysplastic lesions from simple HPV lesions in men.[43] Leukoplakia and mosaic are virtually never observed. Classic punctation is also rarely seen, and on the male genitalia it more closely resembles the punctate vascularity seen with verrucae of the hands and feet. SILs of the male genitalia are likely to be slightly hyperpigmented or inflamed. The only reliable way to define the nature of penile lesions is by biopsy. Bowen's disease (squamous cell carcinoma in situ or penile intraepithelial neoplasia) is generally indistinguishable from a classic wart (Fig. 22-7). Bowenoid papulosis lesions are multiple and erythematous and occur on a thin, scaly base. In patients younger than 40 years, this disease is usually considered benign and self-limited. In patients older than 40 years, bowenoid papulosis is considered a cancer precursor. The diagnosis can be made only by biopsy.[44]

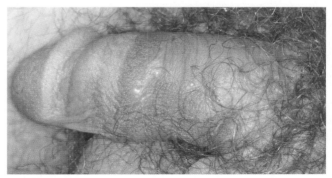

Figure 22-7. Penile intraepithelial neoplasia grade 3.

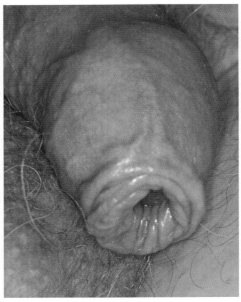

Figure 22–8. Erythroplasia of Queyrat before foreskin retracted.

Erythroplasia of Queyrat is carcinoma in situ that generally occurs under the foreskin (Figs. 22–8 and 22–9). Although the lesions may have been present for years and may be similar in appearance to benign condylomata acuminata, the presence of friability and ulceration should make one suspect penile carcinoma. Penile carcinoma can resemble a wart.

Biopsy of a lesion on the male genitalia is obtained with sharp tissue scissors, a scalpel blade, a dermal curette, or a radiofrequency loop electrode.

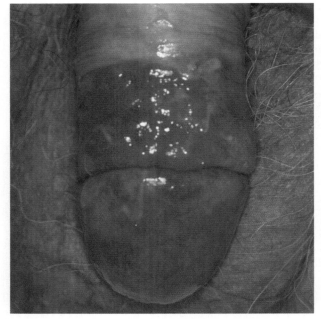

Figure 22–9. Erythroplasia of Queyrat visible after foreskin retracted.

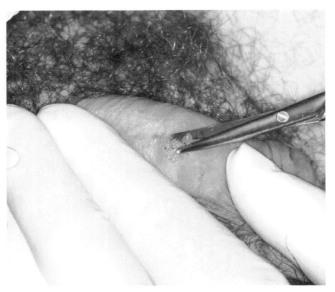

Figure 22–10. Excisional biopsy of a penile shaft condyloma with sharp tissue scissors.

BIOPSY

It is not necessary to biopsy a typical condyloma before treatment.

Biopsy of a male genital lesion is obtained using sharp tissue scissors (small, curved Metzenbaum scissors), a scalpel blade, a dermal curette, or a radiofrequency loop electrode (Fig. 22–10). It is not necessary to biopsy a typical condyloma before treatment, but lesions that do not resolve after two treatment sessions should be biopsied to differentiate them from verrucous carcinoma or condylomata lata (secondary syphilis).

Most biopsies of the penis, scrotum, perineum, and perianal areas are readily obtained. First, the involved skin is pinched between the thumb and the index finger to tent the tissue and the lesion. Next, 0.1 to 0.2 mL of 2% lidocaine without epinephrine is injected with a 30-g needle. The lesion is then simply snipped off with scissors or shaved off with a scalpel blade. A 3-mm tissue sample is sufficient for histologic diagnosis. With large lesions, radiofrequency excision is preferred. Bleeding is generally minimal and may be controlled with either direct pressure or application of Monsel's solution.

A biopsy obtained with a dermatologic punch biopsy instrument or a cervical biopsy forceps may excise too deep a sample on the male genitalia. Intra-anal lesions, on the other hand, are most readily biopsied or excised using a small cervical biopsy forceps. Urethral meatal lesions are generally not biopsied unless they fail to respond to treatment.

TREATMENT

In placebo-controlled studies, genital warts clear spontaneously in 20% to 30% of patients within 3 months.[37]

▼ Table 22-5

Treatment of Condyloma in the Male (Methods and Reported Efficacy)

Medical	Efficacy
Caustic	
Trichloroacetic acid, 85%	81%
Podofilox, 0.5% liquid/gel	45–50%
Podophyllin, 10–25% liquid	22–77%
Immune enhancing	
Imiquimod cream	52%
Interferon injection	19–62%

Surgical	Efficacy
Cryotherapy	63–88%
Electrodesiccation	94%
Surgical removal (radiofrequency, curettage, shave)	93%
Laser	31–94%
Infrared coagulation	50–76%

> **Asymptomatic, flat, faintly acetowhite changes on the male genitalia do not require treatment and rarely need biopsy for diagnostic confirmation.**

There is little benefit to attempting to eradicate all mildly acetowhite findings on the male genitalia. Asymptomatic, flat, faintly acetowhite changes on the male genitalia do not require treatment and rarely need biopsy for diagnostic confirmation. The goal of treatment in men should be to eliminate visible or symptomatic lesions, to educate the patient about the disease process, and to discuss methods to prevent recurrence and spread. Examination with magnification allows recognition of small lesions, making them easier to treat. It also ensures removal of entire lesions. However, studies have shown that even after the most aggressive treatments, residual HPV DNA can be detected.[45] Therefore, the eradication of HPV should not be a goal of treatment.[46]

Methods of treatment in men are similar to those in women (Table 22–5).[47–49] If only a few small lesions are present, it is quicker and more cost-effective to remove them by a method similar to that described for biopsy.

TOPICAL THERAPIES (PATIENT APPLIED)

Imiquimod and podofilox have approximately a 50% to 60% efficacy rate and cost around $120 per month for treating average-sized lesions. Patients can apply these preparations themselves, thus reducing the number of office visits. Imiquimod is an immune enhancer and works through a different mechanism than that of podofilox, which is a caustic agent and the purified active ingredient of podophyllin.[37, 50, 51]

Use of 5-fluorouracil cream has been described in three situations: use for lesions of the urethral meatus, use for perianal lesions, and prophylactic use to reduce recurrence following treatment with other modalities. The main side effect of topical fluorouracil is mild to severe local inflammation. With lesions of the urethral meatus, a small amount of fluorouracil is placed on the end of a cotton-tipped applicator and then applied to the lesions twice daily for 7 to 10 days. Fluorouracil cream may also be applied once or twice weekly for up to 6 to 8 weeks to treat large perianal condylomata. If fluorouracil is well tolerated by the patient, the frequency of application may be increased, but the patient must be monitored carefully because of the risk of ulceration. As a prophylactic agent to prevent recurrent disease on any of the anogenital areas, fluorouracil can be used once per month for 6 months. However, imiquimod may prove to be a better agent for this indication, with fewer side effects.

TOPICAL THERAPIES (CLINICIAN APPLIED)

Another effective treatment for condylomata is 85% trichloroacetic acid (TCA). The preparation is inexpensive but must be applied by the clinician every 1 to 3 weeks. For small lesions, the wooden end of a cotton-tipped applicator is dipped in TCA solution and then applied to the lesions. For larger areas, the cotton-tipped end of the applicator is used. On application, the tissue immediately turns a snow-white color (Fig. 22–11). The application site may burn intensely for 5 minutes. Applying TCA quickly to all lesions may minimize the discomfort. Use of topical anesthesia before treatment with TCA should be discouraged because it may actually protect the warts from the effects of therapy. TCA does not need to be neutralized or removed after treatment, and the area may be washed after the patient arrives home without decreasing efficacy. The destruction of viable tissue occurs almost immediately, and sloughing occurs in a few days. The efficacy of treatment is approximately 80%, depending on number and size of lesions present.

> **Use of topical anesthesia before treatment with trichloroacetic acid should be discouraged because it may actually protect the warts from the effects of therapy.**

Interferon is rarely used except when all other modalities have failed. Drawbacks include its cost and frequent side effects.[37]

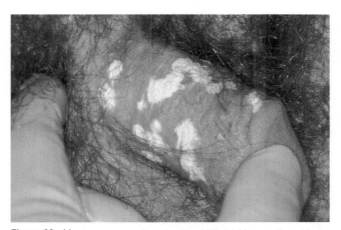

Figure 22–11. Appearance of penis after 85% trichloroacetic acid was applied.

Most lesions may also be treated with cryotherapy using a close-tipped nitrous oxide unit or with liquid nitrogen. The close-tipped cryotherapy provides more control, but the liquid nitrogen is quicker. The latter can be applied with a small nozzle and a spray gun (Brymil or Wallach) or by dipping a cotton-tipped applicator into the liquid nitrogen and then applying it to the wart. For the treatment to be effective, an ice ball must form at least 3 mm beyond the lesion. After the treated area thaws, immediate retreatment will enhance effectiveness. Depending on the amount of tissue to be treated, topical or injectable local anesthesia is used. Scarring is rare, and the patient's potential to have and maintain an erection is not compromised. Some hypopigmentation may result. After treatment, the area may become edematous, and bullae may form. The bullae may later slough, producing an open lesion. The bullae may be left intact or removed. The efficacy of treatment is approximately 75% but varies among reported studies.

SURGICAL TREATMENT

Condylomata may also be removed using any one of a number of surgical approaches. Before the application of any of these modalities, the skin must be anesthetized. Two percent lidocaine without epinephrine is injected superficially with a 30-g needle just beneath each lesion. For extensive penile lesions, a dorsal penile block or ring block may be used. Additional anesthesia is used at the frenulum, because this area is particularly difficult to anesthetize.

Laser ablation of external lesions is highly effective when properly used and has excellent cosmetic results. Drawbacks include the high cost of equipment and the need for greater operator expertise. HPV and HIV have been documented in laser smoke plumes, so suction filter devices are essential if this modality is selected for treatment.[52, 53]

> **Electrodesiccation and surgical excision using radiofrequency current may be the treatments of choice for warts on male external genitalia.**

Electrodesiccation and surgical excision using radiofrequency current may be the treatments of choice for lesions on male external genitalia. Success rates approach 90%. The equipment is less expensive, and the technique is easier to master than is laser. With the electrosurgical unit (ESU) set at coagulation mode, all lesions are merely touched with a 3- to 5-mm ball electrode. The warts desiccate and can be wiped away. Any residual tissue can be identified with magnification and then cauterized. Electrodesiccation works best for small lesions. Larger lesions may require a radiofrequency excision technique.

Radiofrequency excision is best performed under direct colposcopic guidance. The area is anesthetized as discussed previously. The high-frequency ESU is set in "cutting" mode at 15 to 20 watts. A short shank dermatological loop electrode is used to excise the lesion. The skin on the penis is very thin, and care must be taken to maintain a very superficial excisional plane and to not

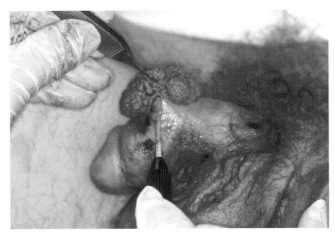

Figure 22–12. Large penile condyloma being removed with radiofrequency surgery.

penetrate too deeply. Only the smallest lesion should be removed with a single pass. The excision should proceed slowly, layer by layer. Initially, the condylomata may bleed significantly, especially when they are large. But as all the abnormal tissue is removed, bleeding stops. Monsel's solution can be used to control any residual bleeding that is not controlled with pressure (Figs. 22–12 and 22–13).

Although condylomata may be removed surgically using sharp tissue scissors or by shaving them with a scalpel, the tendency is to go too deep unless the lesions are small. Surgical excision with suture closure is almost never indicated for simple wart treatment.

A device called the infrared coagulator (CooperSurgical, Redfield Corporation) has received FDA approval for treatment of external lesions. The treatment uses an intense beam of light. The automatic timer controls depth of penetration. The usual setting is 0.75 to 1 second. The unit tip is simply applied to the lesion, and the trigger is pulled. Several applications may be needed to treat an entire lesion if it is large. The treated area immediately turns white and eventually sloughs. Reported

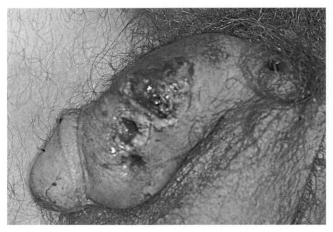

Figure 22–13. Postradiofrequency surgery of large penile condyloma.

efficacy is 70% to 80%, and there is little, if any, residual scarring. Postoperative treatment is the same as for other destructive modalities.

Penile intraepithelial neoplasia does not always require treatment unless it is severe (penile intraepithelial neoplasia grade 3). When it must be treated, any of the previously noted methods may be used. Penile intraepithelial neoplasia grade 3 is not as aggressive and difficult to control as vulvar intraepithelial neoplasia grade 3.

POSTOPERATIVE INSTRUCTIONS

It is very important to maintain a moist healing environment with use of antibiotic ointments or petroleum jelly.

Topical anesthetics (e.g., 5% lidocaine ointment) are effective for treatment of postoperative discomfort. It is very important to maintain a moist healing environment with use of over-the-counter antibiotic ointments (e.g., Bacitracin) or petroleum jelly. The treated (denuded) area should be washed three to four times daily with mild soap and water, followed by application of ointment as often as needed to keep the area moist. Ointment also helps prevent clothing from adhering to the tissue. If the patient complains of itching and redness with vesicle formation, a neomycin allergy should be suspected and the patient should be switched to an antibiotic ointment without neomycin.

It is best to schedule a follow-up examination in 2 to 4 weeks to ensure that all lesions have resolved and to treat any lesions that may have appeared in the interim. Patients with severe lesions should be re-examined after 4 months and then after 12 months to check for recurrence.

Counseling

Counseling and advice for male patients are noted in Table 22–6. Patients should be discouraged from smoking. The relationship among smoking, cervical dysplasia, and cervical cancer is well documented;[39, 54] smoking also increases the risk of penile cancer.[5] Women whose partners smoke have a higher rate of cervical dysplasia. Three mechanisms have been postulated: passive smoking effects, agents in tobacco smoke that adhere to the male's fingers and are introduced into vaginal mucus during vaginal and clitoral stimulation using the fingers, and contaminated semen and/or seminal fluid.[55–58]

Monogamy prevents new exposure to other HPV types. Patients infected with less aggressive HPV types (HPV 6 or HPV 11) risk exposure to higher-risk HPV types (HPV 16 or HPV 18) with each new sexual contact.

Some studies have suggested that a diet high in folic acid and other nutrients may reduce the incidence of cervical dysplasia in women. Similar studies have not been performed in men, but they may benefit similarly.[59, 60]

Patients may feel embarrassment, guilt, anger, and frustration about HPV infection.

▼ Table 22–6

Counseling and Advice for Men with HPV Infection

Do not smoke, and your partner should not smoke.
Practice monogamy.
Notify female partners of any HPV exposure so they can obtain a routine cytologic screening.
Eat a healthy diet, including five helpings of fruits and vegetables per day.
Consider taking a multivitamin daily.
Consult your clinician for recurrent lesions in the anogenital area.
Obtain colorectal screenings per recommended guidelines.
Use condoms to reduce the risk of transmission of STDs.

HPV, human papillomavirus; STD, sexually transmitted disease.

It is important to deal with the psychosocial aspects of HPV-related disease.[61] Patients may feel embarrassment, guilt, anger, and frustration. Studies show that patients are more receptive to the sexually transmitted disease aspects of HPV infection when they are addressed directly.[62]

Condom use should be discussed with the patient, but it is important to note that because HPV is a multicentric disease in both men and women, a condom is not fully protective. However, it should be stressed that condoms will protect against other sexually transmitted diseases, including syphilis, HIV, and gonorrhea, while providing contraceptive benefits.[63–65] It is unknown if use of nonoxynol-9 prevents the spread of HPV. Mutually monogamous partners do not need to continue to use condoms for HPV "protection."

Once unprotected sexual intercourse has occurred, women with documented HPV infection often ask if their male partner should be examined. If no obvious lesions are seen on the male genitalia, and if the male partner has reviewed pertinent information and understands the significance of the disease, a clinical examination (androscopy) is not necessary. If any lesions are seen, or if there are questions, an appointment should be made.

Many women express concern that unless the male partner is examined and treated, they will suffer a recurrence after treatment. It is important to explain that the goals of therapy are to make a diagnosis, reduce symptoms, remove any obvious lesions, and provide patient education. Treating the male partner has little effect on recurrence of disease in the female.[36]

SUMMARY OF KEY POINTS

- Men are not at high risk of developing cancer of the genitalia, and in the United States, HPV infection is associated with less than 1% of malignancies in men.

- Genital warts in men can occur on the penis, scrotum, anus, and suprapubic areas or in the urethral meatus.

- Androscopy is examination of the male genitalia under magnification after 5% acetic acid has been applied.

Continued on following page

- It is critically important to have sharp, high-quality surgical instruments available for biopsy of male genitalia.

- Neither anoscopy nor cystoscopy is routinely performed on male patients with genital warts.

- Care should be taken to avoid misinterpreting acetowhite findings on the male genitalia as HPV infection.

- Few colposcopic findings on the male genitalia reliably differentiate between benign and preinvasive lesions. Biopsy may be the only way to accurately make a diagnosis.

- Most lesions on male genitalia are biopsied by pinching the involved skin to tent the tissue so the lesion can be snipped off with scissors or shaved off with a scalpel blade.

- Treatments for genital warts can be initially effective, although recurrences are common.

- Electrodesiccation and surgical excision with radiofrequency current are the treatments of choice for genital warts in men, although topical therapy can produce successful results.

- Postoperative maintenance of a moist healing environment minimizes discomfort and aids healing.

Acknowledgments

The author wishes to thank Pat Wolfgram (librarian, Mid-Michigan Medical Center) for research and assistance and Kay Pfenninger for secretarial support.

All photographs courtesy of the National Procedures Institute, copyright 2001.

References

1. Krogh G: Clinical relevance and evaluation of genito-anal papillomavirus infections in the male. Semin Dermatol 1992;11:229.
2. Fine RM: The penial condyloma-cancer connection. Int J Dermatol 1987;26:289.
3. Weiner JS, Liu ET, Walther PJ: Oncogenic human papillomavirus type 16 in association with squamous cell cancer of the male urethra. Cancer Res 1992;52:5018.
4. Noel JC, Vancenbossche M, Peny MO: Verrucous carcinoma of the penis: Importance of human papilloma typing for diagnosis and therapeutic decisions. Eur Urol 1992;22:83.
5. Malek RS, Goellner JR, Smith T, et al: Human papillomavirus infection and intraepithelial-in-situ, and invasive carcinoma of the penis. Urology 1993;42:159.
6. Bosch FG, Castellsague X, Munoz N, et al: Male sexual behavior and human papilloma DNA. J Natl Cancer Inst 1996;88:1060.
7. Munoz N, Castellsague, Bosch FG, et al: Difficulty in elucidating the male role in cervical cancer in Columbia, a high risk area for the disease. J Natl Cancer Inst 1996;88:1068.
8. Boon ME, Susanti I, Tache MJ: Human papillomavirus (HPV): Association of male and female genital carcinoma in a Hindu population. Cancer 1989;64:559.
9. Brinton LA, Jun-Yao L, Shon-De R, et al: Risk factors for penile cancer: Results from a case control study in China. Int J Cancer 1991;47:504.
10. Scinicariello F, Rady P, Saltzstein D, et al: Human papillomavirus 16 exhibits a similar integration pattern in primary squamous cell carcinomas of the penis and in its metastases. Cancer 1992;70:2143.
11. Poblet E, Alfaro L, Ferdander-Segoviano P, et al: Human papillomavirus associated with penile squamous cell carcinoma in HIV-positive patients. Am J Surg Path 1999;23:1119.
12. Palefsky JM: Anal cancer and its precursors: An HIV-related disease. Hosp Phys 1993;1:35.
13. Daling JR, Weiss NS, Klopfenstein, et al: Correlates of homosexual behavior and the incidence of anal cancer. JAMA 1982;247:1988.
14. Xi LF, Critchlow CW, Wheeler CM, et al: Risk of anal carcinoma-in-situ in relation to human papillomavirus type 16 variants. Cancer Res 1998;58:3839.
15. Frisch M, Fenger C, Vanden Brule AJ, et al: Variants of squamous cell carcinoma: Cancer of the anal canal and perianal skin and their relation to human papillomavirus. Cancer Res 1999;59:753.
16. Noffsinger A, Witte D, Fenoglio-Preiser CM: The relationship of human papillomaviruses to anorectal neoplasia. Cancer 1992;70:1276.
17. Goldie SJ, Kuntz KM, Weinstein MC: The clinical effectiveness and cost-effectiveness of screening for anal squamous intraepithelial lesions in homosexual and bisexual HIV-positive men. JAMA 1999;281:1822.
18. Barasso R, DeBruge J, Croissant O, et al: High prevalence of papilloma-associated penile intraepithelial neoplasia in sexual partners of women with cervical intraepithelial neoplasia. N Engl J Med 1987;317:916.
19. Zabbo A, Stein BS: Penile intraepithelial neoplasia in patients examined for exposure to human papillomavirus. J Urol 1993;41:24.
20. Schneider A, Sarvada E, Gissman L, et al: Human papillomavirus in women with a history of abnormal Papanicolaou smears and in their male partners. Obstet Gynecol 1987;69:554.
21. Blythe JG, Cheval MJ: Colposcopy of condylomatous men. Missouri Med 1989;86:31.
22. Cannistra SA, Niloff JM: Cancer of the uterine cervix. N Engl J Med 1996;334:1030.
23. Krebs HB: Management of human papillomavirus-associated genital lesions in men. Obstet Gynecol 1989;73:312.
24. Wikström A, Hedblad MA, Johasson B, et al: The acetic acid test in evaluation of subclinical genital infection: A competence study on penoscopy, histopathology, virology and scanning electron microscopy findings. Genitourinary Med 1992;68:90.
25. Pfenninger JL: Androscopy: A technique for examining men for condyloma. J Fam Pract 1989;29:286.
26. Sedlacek TV, Cunname M, Carpineilla V: Colposcopy in the diagnosis of penile condyloma. Am J Obstet Gynecol 1986;154:494.
27. Epperson WJ: Androscopy for anogenital HPV. J Fam Pract 1991;33:143.
28. Epperson WJ: Preventing cervical cancer by treating genital warts in men: Why male sex partners need androscopy. Postgrad Med 1990;88:229.
29. Newkirk GR, Grannath BD: Teaching colposcopy and androscopy in family practice residencies. J Fam Pract 1990;31:171.
30. Pfenninger JL: Letter to the editor. J Fam Pract 1991;33:566.
31. Patton D, Rodney WM: Androscopy of unproven benefit. J Fam Pract 1991;33:135.
32. Strand A, Rylander E, Wilander E, et al: HPV infections in women with squamous intraepithelial neoplasia and/or high risk HPV. Acta Derm Venereol 1995;75:312.
33. Rosemburg SK, Greenburg MD, Reid R: Sexually-transmitted papillomavirus in men. Obstet Gynecol Clin North Am 1987;14:495.
34. Krebs HB, Helmkamp B: Treatment failure of genital condyloma acuminata in women: Role of the male sexual partner. Am J Obstet Gynecol 1991;169:337.
35. Comite SL, Castadot MJ: Colposcopic evaluation of men with genital warts. J Am Acad Dermatol 1988;18:1274.
36. Krebs HB, Helmkamp B: Does the treatment of genital condyloma in men decrease the treatment failure rate of cervical dysplasia in the female sexual partner? Obstet Gynecol 1990;76:660.
37. Human papillomavirus infections. MMWR 1993;42:83.
38. Stewart DE, Lickrish GM, Sierra S, et al: The effect of educational brochures on knowledge and emotional distress in women with abnormal Papanicolaou smears. Obstet Gynecol 1993;81:280.
39. Slattery ML, Robinson LM, Schuman K, et al: Cigarette smoking and exposure to passive smoke are risk factors for cervical cancer. JAMA 1989;261:1593.
40. Pfenninger JL: Androscopy. In Pfenninger JL, Fowler GC (eds): Procedures for Primary Care Physicians. St. Louis, Mosby, 1994, pp 514–519.

41. Gazzaniga P, Vercillo R, Gradilone AT, et al: Prevalence of papillomavirus, Epstein-Barr virus, cytomegalovirus, and herpes simplex virus type 2 in urinary bladder cancer. J Med Virol 1998;55:262.
42. Burmer GG, True LD, Kriegar JN: Squamous cell carcinoma of the scrotum associated with human papillomavirus. J Urol 1993;149:374.
43. Demeter LM, Stoler MH, Bonnez W, et al: Penile intraepithelial neoplasia: Clinical presentation and an analysis of the physical state of human papilloma DNA. J Infect Dis 1993;168:38.
44. Habif TP: Pre-malignant and malignant non-melanoma skin tumors and sexually-transmitted viral infections. In Habif TB (ed): Clinical Dermatology: A Color Guide to Diagnosis and Therapy, 3rd ed. St. Louis, Mosby, 1996, pp 297–345, 649–687.
45. Riva JM, Sedlacek TV, Cunnane MF, et al: Extended carbon dioxide laser vaporization in the treatment of subclinical papillomavirus infections of the lower genital tract. Obstet Gynecol 1989;73:25.
46. Richart R: Men and HPV. Prim Care 1995;8:5.
47. Ling MR: Therapy of genital human papillomavirus infections. Part I: Indications for the justification of therapy. Int J Dermatol 1992;31:682.
48. Kling A: Genital warts—therapy. Semin Dermatol 1992;11:247.
49. Maw RD: Treatment of anogenital warts. Dermatol Clin 1998;16:829.
50. Beutner KR, Tyring SK, Trofatter KF Jr, et al: Imiquimod, a patient-applied immune-response modifier for treatment of external genital warts. Antimicrob Agents Chemother 1998;42:789.
51. Kraus SJ, Stone KM: Management of genital infections caused by human papillomavirus. Rev Infect Dis 1990;6:5620.
52. Garden JM, O'Banian K, Shelnitz LS, et al: Papillomavirus in the vapor of carbon dioxide laser-treated verrucae. JAMA 1988;259:1199.
53. Baggish MS, Polesz BJ, Joret D, et al: Presence of human immunodeficiency virus DNA in laser smoke. Lasers Surg Med 1991;11:197.
54. Szarewski A, Jarvis MJ, Sasieni P, et al: Effect of smoking cessation on cervical lesion size. Lancet 1996;347:941.
55. Tokudome S: Semen of smokers and cervical cancer risk [letter]. J Natl Cancer Inst 1997;89:96.
56. Vincent CE, Vincent B, Griess FC, et al: Some marital-sexual concomitants of carcinoma of the cervix. South Med J 1975;68:552.
57. Brown DC, Pereira L, Garner JB: Cancer of the cervix and the smoking husband. Can Fam Physician 1982;28:499.
58. Whidden P: Cigarette smoking and cervical cancer [letter]. Int J Epidemiol 1994;23:1099.
59. Butterworth CE, Hatch KD, Macaluso M, et al: Folate deficiency and cervical dysplasia. JAMA 1992;267:528.
60. Kwasniewska A: Dietary factors in women with dysplasia. Nutr Cancer 1998;30:39.
61. Campion MJ, Brown JR, McCance DJ, et al: Psychosexual trauma of an abnormal cervical smear. Br J Obstet Gynecol 1988;95:175.
62. Reed BD, Ruffin MT, Garenflo DW, et al: The psycho-sexual impact of human papillomavirus cervical infections. Am J Med 1997;102:3.
63. Daling JR, Weiss NS: Are barrier methods protective against cervical cancer? Epidemiol 1990;1:261.
64. Hildesheim A, Brinton LA, Mallin K, et al: Barrier and spermicidal contraceptive methods and risk of invasive cervical cancer. Epidemiol 1990;1:266.
65. Thomas I, Wright G, Ward B: The effect of condom use on cervical intraepithelial neoplasia grade I (CIN I). Aust N Z J Obstet Gynecol 1990;30:236.

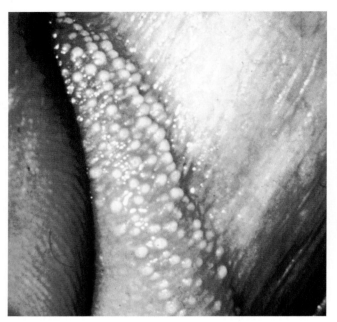

Plate 22-1. Pearly penile papules of the corona of the penis.

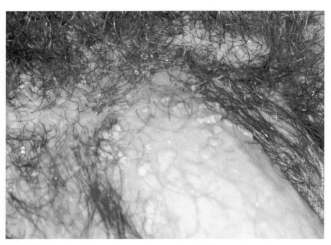

Plate 22-2. Condylomata acuminata of penile base and pubis.

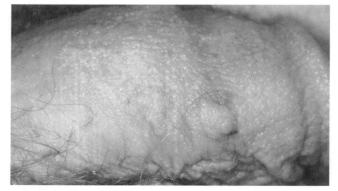

Plate 22-3. Single condyloma of the shaft; also, flat condyloma seen only after the application of 5% acetic acid.

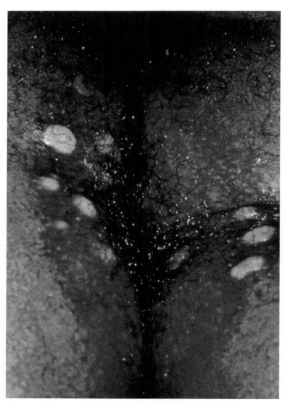

Plate 22-4. Condyloma latum.

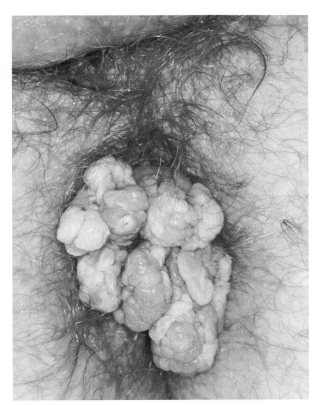

Plate 22-5. Large condylomata of the perianal area.

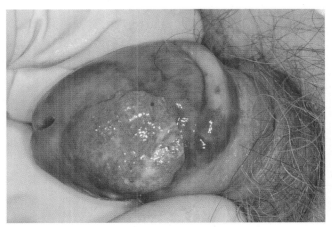

Plate 22-6. Large penile cancer of the glans.

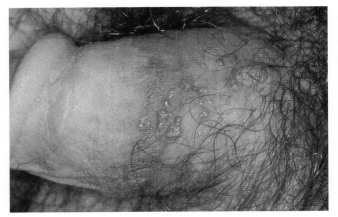

Plate 22-7. Condylomata acuminata of penis.

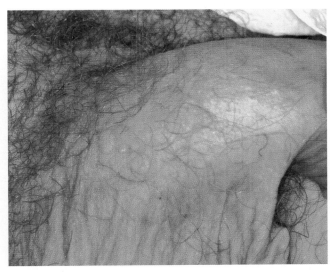

Plate 22-8. Condylomata acuminata of penis.

- Dennis J. Butler
- Gregory L. Brotzman

CHAPTER *23*

Psychosocial Aspects of Colposcopy

It is now clearly documented that a variety of complicated psychological reactions can occur in the process of screening, diagnostic procedures, and treatment.

Advances in the detection and treatment of the preclinical manifestations of cervical cancer have dramatically reduced the incidence and mortality of cervical cancer. This decline has been accompanied by an increase in the recognition of precancerous conditions. As this progress has been achieved, increased attention has been focused on the psychological and emotional reactions of women with abnormal cervical smears and those referred for colposcopy. It is now clearly documented that in the process of screening, diagnostic procedures, and treatment, a variety of complicated psychological reactions can occur.

Furthermore, individual patient reactions have been found to play a determining role in adherence with follow-up. Although rates vary, current estimates suggest that in some settings, up to 45% of women with an abnormal cervical Papanicolaou (Pap) smear do not return for colposcopy or surveillance as recommended.[1, 2] Because the morbidity and mortality of cervical cancer can be significantly reduced with appropriate monitoring and treatment, it is essential to identify and overcome barriers to obtaining medical care.

When informed of an abnormal Pap result, patients experience a heightened sense of vulnerability, uncertainty, fear, and anxiety.[3] The physician and other health care professionals have the responsibility to reduce patient anxiety. However, many patients are not adequately counseled about abnormal smears and the specifics of diagnostic follow-up. Well-designed patient information systems not only can defuse anxiety, but also can increase patient participation and facilitate adherence to follow-up. A comprehensive perspective is essential, because the barriers to compliance are multicausal and include psychological, educational, logistical, and medical care dimensions.

This chapter reviews the nature and types of reactions that women have to abnormal Pap smears and then examines preparation for colposcopy. At each step of medical care, anticipatory and strategic interventions are identified and evaluated for appropriateness to those women who

are at risk for psychological distress. A longitudinal approach is encouraged and should emphasize prevention of distressing reactions to abnormal Pap smears, preparation for colposcopy, and ongoing care.

IMPACT OF THE ABNORMAL PAP SMEAR RESULT

Although the cervical smear is, in practice, a routine and common screening test for sexually active women, it is a procedure that can have a profound psychological impact. There is well-established evidence of a broad range of potential emotional, psychological, behavioral, and social disruptions in the lives of women and their families following an abnormal Pap smear. From these reports have come recommendations for physician anticipation of such reactions, strategies for enhancing patient follow-up, methods for patient education, and suggestions for reassurance and support. Health care professionals can clearly play a role in modifying the impact that a seemingly minor diagnosis of an abnormal cervical smear has on patients and their partners.

The predominant emotion experienced by women on learning of an abnormal Pap smear is anxiety or a heightened state of apprehension.

When a woman learns of an abnormal Pap smear, the predominant emotion she experiences is anxiety, a heightened state of apprehension that has cognitive, emotional, and behavioral components.[3, 4] At its most basic level, anxiety is a feeling of increased vulnerability and a sense of loss of control. It serves to alert the individual to a threat and to mobilize coping skills. A reasonable amount of anxiety is considered appropriate and healthy if it motivates an individual to develop a plan of action. Excessive anxiety and intrusive worrying, however, result in such reactions as denial, avoidance, and indecisiveness, all of which interfere with compliance.

Stressful or threatening medical situations result in two types of anxiety. Outcome anxiety is "results related" and refers to patients' apprehension about their medical condition and its potential consequences. Procedure anxiety is "examination related" and refers to patients' distress about the medical tests and procedures they expect to experience. Outcome anxiety tends to surface with the report of an abnormal finding, and procedure anxiety commonly increases as the patient gets closer to the colposcopic examination.

Women with abnormal Pap smears have been found to experience significantly greater anxiety compared with controls.[3] In some cases, their anxiety has been found to be greater than that among patients awaiting breast biopsy results and to be similar in severity to that of women after an abnormal serum screening test for fetal anomalies.[5, 6] Patients awaiting colposcopy have also been found to have significantly greater anxiety than nonreferred (surveillance) patients.[4, 7] Although levels of anxiety are heightened and significant, they do not typically meet the criteria for psychiatric diagnosis.[8]

> **Women tend to expect a normal Pap smear result, and an abnormal finding causes an alteration in their self-perception, making "patients" of individuals who are asymptomatic and feel well.**

One element that can serve to intensify anxiety about an abnormal result is the routine nature of the Pap smear. Women tend to expect a normal result, and an abnormal finding causes an alteration in their self-perception, making "patients" of people who are asymptomatic and feel well.[9] The disclosure of an abnormal smear can precipitate reactions of depersonalization ("This isn't happening to me!") marked by disbelief and mild-to-moderate dissociative reactions.

Common outcome fears experienced by women with abnormal Pap smears have been extensively documented and verified in multiple investigations.[10–12] The most common fear is of having cancer—in particular, cervical cancer. A second predominant fear is the belief that an abnormal smear is an indication of infertility or reduced reproductive ability. Another common concern or distressing reaction is that there will be a loss of sexual response or functioning whether treatment is indicated or not.

Although those outcome fears are somewhat anticipated and more accessible to disclosure, other concerns can be present. Because of the sensitivity of these concerns, they can be difficult to recognize and elicit. The patient may experience feelings of guilt that stem from a belief that the abnormal Pap smear is a punishment for sexual promiscuity or other perceived indiscretions.[13] Other women react with the belief that they are infectious and that they may have somehow infected sexual partners or, indirectly, family members.[14] Patients have also attributed abnormal smears to chance, early sexual activity, oral contraceptive usage, pregnancy, and previous infections.[8]

> **When confronted with an abnormal Pap smear result, patients experience a disturbance in self-image, resulting in a reduction in their confidence to confront what will be required for further evaluation.**

In-depth interviews with patients informed of an abnormal smear have uncovered a deeper psychological im-

pact. Patients report an experience of biographical disruption best described as a feeling of "bodily betrayal."[15] This can be understood as a disturbance in the patient's self-image resulting in a reduction in her confidence to confront the demands of the abnormal findings. Common self-descriptions include viewing oneself as less attractive, tarnished, unclean, or "let down" by one's body.[8, 13] As part of this disruption of self-image, women also report a diminished view of their sexual attractiveness. This change in self-perception is further complicated by their uncertainty as to whether they are ill, have cancer, or can be cured. The feeling of bodily betrayal creates an internal tension that can manifest as anger and depression. For the first time in their lives, many women must confront their own mortality.

Initial reactions to the news of an abnormal Pap result can be difficult to identify because they are suppressed by the shock of an unexpected result, because they develop over time, and because the emotional reactions are often displaced or overshadowed by logistical and informational needs. Symptomatic reactions may be more accessible on direct inquiry. Among symptoms documented in women with abnormal smears are sleep disturbance, irritability, depressed affect, crying episodes, anger outbursts, weight change, loss of interest in sexual activity, and disruption in sexual relationships.[10, 11] Patients interviewed about their reactions typically used such affective terms as worried, nervous, fearful, upset, shocked, panicked, horrified, or "feeling alone." Symptomatic reactions are prevalent, with up to 25% of women reporting impairment in daily activities, 50% reporting impairment in sexual interest, and 40% reporting disruption in sleep patterns.[10] One fifth of patients with abnormal results have been found to report distressing levels of anxiety until the time of colposcopy.

Reactions may also be difficult to identify because patients may be reluctant to disclose the extent of their anxiety.[16] Their reluctance to disclose their anxiety may be related to their reactions to how they were told of the abnormal result.[17] Patients will disclose less if they perceived the manner of the physician as impersonal. Thus, when making an assessment of a woman's emotional state or level of understanding, the clinician should be careful not to assume that a nonanxious response is adaptive. A nonanxious response can be doubly deceptive because intense internal anxiety interferes with processing and integrating of the factual information and logistical details necessary for follow-up.

> **The clinician should be careful not to assume that a nonanxious response to the Pap smear result is adaptive when making an assessment of a woman's emotional health or understanding.**

The intensity of patient reactions cannot always be viewed as a direct response to the news of an abnormal Pap smear. Patients may have existing risk factors that intensify reactions, including a history of psychiatric difficulties or patterns of disrupted relationships.[8] Concurrent stressors such as work, family, additional health problems, school responsibilities, financial difficulties, or limited social support can complicate the reaction to an abnormal smear as well. The news of an abnormal smear has also been found to have a reciprocal effect in that the distress of the abnormal Pap result reactivates or intensifies concurrent stressors.[3, 11]

The impact of an abnormal Pap test has also been shown to have potentially persistent effects. Three months following an abnormal smear, some patients continue to report elevated levels of generalized anxiety, fear of cancer, and impairment in mood, activity, sexual interest, and sleep patterns.[10]

INTERVENTIONS

The physician's primary clinical task with the patient who has an abnormal cervical smear is to acknowledge patient distress and encourage appropriate follow-up. Noncompliance with follow-up is a critical concern and is found among all groups of patients but is highest among younger, unmarried, less educated women of lower socioeconomic status.[18] Unfortunately, those at greatest risk for precancerous cervical disease not only are the least likely to have an initial Pap smear but also are less likely to adhere to recommended diagnostic procedures if an abnormality is detected.[2] Patients' involvement in their care is associated with improved adherence, greater satisfaction with providers, better understanding of medical details, improved coping, and improved quality of life. Noncompliance may create a self-defeating cycle in which failure to comply sustains uncertainty and distress, which, in turn, contributes to delay in follow-up.

> **Noncompliance with follow-up is a critical concern and is found among all groups of patients but is highest among younger, unmarried, less educated women of lower socioeconomic status.**

Because Pap smears are routine and usually normal, physicians and patients often have a low expectation of vulnerability or a false sense of reassurance before the examination.[16] It may be helpful to provide anticipatory guidance through the process of foreshadowing, in which patients are alerted that results can be abnormal but that effective interventions are available.[8] It is also important to inform patients that abnormal smears infrequently imply cancer and that most patients can be managed with surveillance or other low-impact interventions. Identifying support personnel within the physician's office can also provide reassurance in the event of an unexpected result. Forewarning can reduce the initial reactions of shock, disbelief, and sense of catastrophe that occur when a patient first learns that her Pap smear is abnormal.

Patient Education

Reducing outcome and procedure anxiety can be accomplished by providing information, education, support, and reassurance. In general, to alleviate anxiety, it is useful to focus on the objective features of the threat, such as the risk factors, and the reasons for further diagnostic steps or treatment options. Although it is not productive to focus exclusively on emotional responses, eliciting the patient's reaction and acknowledging her distress in a supportive manner are critical.[2]

Information provided to patients should highlight the specific areas of patient concern that have been identified as impeding compliance. These include fear of cancer, fear of losing sexual or reproductive functioning, and aversion to medical procedures. Written patient education materials have been found to be cost-effective, to reduce anxiety, and to encourage positive attitudes.[19] This effect extends to even low-effort interventions. For example, women receiving an informational booklet by mail reported less anxiety than those not receiving this information.[17] However, on a cautionary note, providing information may increase knowledge but not reduce anxiety. Providing information best reduces anxiety if it fosters a sense of control over outcomes. Variables to be considered in supplied information about abnormal Pap smears include amount of information, ease of reading, extent of focus on procedures, and extent to which the disease process is highlighted. Brief, simple information may be most effective in reducing anxiety.[6]

> **Brief, simple information may be most effective in reducing anxiety.**

Providing information should be approached cautiously and preceded by assessment in three critical areas: How much does the patient know, how much would she like to know, and how much does she want to be involved?[20] Some patients prefer avoidance and distraction as means of coping with stressful situations. Thus, the provision of informative material is no guarantee that it will be read, that it will be understood, or that it will help reassure the patient.[21] In some cases, it may be counterproductive.[22]

Preparatory information is most beneficial when a patient's preference for information and involvement is matched with the amount and degree of specificity of supplied information. Women with higher preferences for information tend to ask more questions during visits, and women who request written information tend to prefer more involvement in their care.[23] It has been found that those women who asked more questions reported higher levels of confidence in their care after the examination. However, educational level and differences in social status affect the balance of the physician-patient interaction. Patients with lower educational levels have been found to ask fewer questions and be less assertive during visits in which their Pap results were discussed.[23]

Patients will have difficulty understanding the information they receive if health care professionals fail to give clear recommendations or use unfamiliar and vague terms. Even terms such as *colposcopy* and *precancerous,* which are quite common among professionals, have been misunderstood or misinterpreted by patients. For example, patients have interpreted "precancerous" as meaning they have an early form of cancer and will eventually die from it.[2] Other research has discovered that patients are confused by procedures and believe that they had a colposcopy when the speculum was inserted for a normal examination or that they had a colposcopy when the Pap smear was done.[24] Thus, patients should be encouraged to ask questions, but this may not be sufficient to ensure that they understand key information. It is the clinician's responsibility to clearly indicate that an abnormal smear is not a confirmation of cancer but simply indicates a finding that requires further investigation.

The success of interventions that provide information about cervical cancer has been documented primarily with higher socioeconomic groups. More intensive, specialized efforts are necessary for groups at high risk for noncompliance. Studies of nonadherent groups have found that the barriers to follow-up care extend well beyond a lack of understandable information about results and procedures. These additional barriers include fatalism and hopelessness about cancer, forgetting, transportation difficulties, child care needs, time constraints, conflicting health beliefs, and cultural differences.[2] Many patients in the high-risk, noncompliance group have also had multiple impersonal, disrupted, or dissatisfying experiences with the health care system and have turned to self-care.

An intervention that has proved successful in modifying poor compliance rates is the implementation of structured telephone counseling.[25] Low-income minority women who had missed a scheduled initial colposcopy appointment received a telephone call that addressed informational, psychological, and logistical barriers to keeping appointments. This 15-minute contact proved highly effective in addressing the barriers and improved adherence to follow-up. A telephone counseling intervention with high-risk groups is better than telephone confirmation, which is in turn better than standard reminders.[25, 26]

> **A telephone counseling intervention with high-risk groups is better than telephone confirmation, which is in turn better than standard reminders.**

Although clearly a multifactorial process, a self-reported tendency to forget appointments is an especially powerful predictor of noncompliance.[25, 27] Research suggests that efforts to identify forgetful patients and provide telephone or mailed reminders can reduce rates of nonadherence. The clinician can ask patients directly if they tend to be forgetful or if they can predict their likelihood of compliance. Once patients have specified the likely impediments to follow-up, problem-solving strategies can be individually tailored. For example, with one group of patients, once the impediment of transportation difficulty was identified, providing transportation assistance was the most successful intervention for improving attendance at colposcopy appointments.[27]

Social support also plays a role in managing the distressing emotions that arise when a patient is told that a cervical smear is abnormal.[12] Support can be of four types: emotional, instrumental (resources), providing information, or providing appraisal (offering advice). For many medical conditions, patients turn to their usual reference groups for support, but in studies of patients with abnormal Pap results, family or partners are not universally viewed as resources for social support.[4] Elements that inhibit seeking of support include the absence of a close partner; perceived stigma; embarrassment at discussing anatomy; fear of sexual rejection; and view of the male partner as disinterested, uninformed, or unable to understand. Failure to inform partners has been reported by more than one fourth of patients. However, when informed, partners have been noted to report an increase in worry, to seek further information, and to encourage the patient to follow through with colposcopy. This sug-

gests that clinicians should address the issue by encouraging patients with abnormal Pap smears to consider disclosure to trusted partners, friends, or family.

> **Clinicians should encourage patients with abnormal Pap smears to consider disclosure to trusted partners, family, or friends.**

COLPOSCOPY

Although concerted educational efforts have improved awareness of the need for annual Pap smears, women remain less informed about the nature and purpose of colposcopy. When women's sources of information about colposcopy were examined, it was found that although friends and family were a source of information about Pap smears, they were significantly less informed about colposcopy.[28] Most patients reported that their limited information about colposcopy came exclusively from physicians or nurses during brief office encounters. Thus, they attend appointments with many unanswered questions.

Qualitative research relying on individual interviews suggests that there is a complex interaction of four major themes among patients referred for colposcopy. Patients had a general sense of something wrong with their health, they were apprehensive about the procedure, they experienced persistent uncertainty about the meaning of an abnormal smear, and they were confused about the process of referral.[29] In studies of minority women, one fourth had no idea what colposcopy was, and more than half did not know what having an abnormal Pap smear meant or what could be found by colposcopy.[24, 28]

Additional investigations suggest that informational deficits are further complicated by patients' lack of understanding of the basic anatomic features associated with colposcopy. High numbers of women referred for colposcopy do not know the location of the cervix or the site of the Pap smear.[24] Many were unaware that there might be more than one biopsy, that an examination of the labia was involved, or that the colposcope did not enter the vagina.

Patients have expressed uncertainty about what will happen during the procedure and, in particular, have expressed concern about pain or discomfort. They subsequently reported feeling worried about loss of sexual functioning or reproductive ability as a result of the procedure.[25] Their questions included what would be done physically, how long would it last, how much it would hurt, and if it would involve specific actions such as scraping.[29] They also asked questions about the use of the colposcope.

Although colposcopy has not been found to be a significantly painful experience, it involves mild-to-moderate discomfort and transient pain. Nearly 50% of women who underwent colposcopy reported having been tense and having experienced a fair amount of physical discomfort during the procedure.[30] However, few studies have systematically examined the issue of pain. In a study of adolescents, they were observed to exhibit three to five behavior expressions of pain during the colposcopy.[31] Self-rated pain scores were found in another study to be significantly lowered with use of a nonsteroidal anti-inflammatory medication, but all subjects reported tolerating the procedure well.[32]

Concern has been expressed that waiting time for the colposcopic examination may increase anxiety and reduce compliance.[3, 33] In one longitudinal study, one fourth of patients were reassured by the long wait, believing that it indicated that they did not have a serious problem. However, another fourth expressed impatience and anger at delays in follow-up. Almost a year after their colposcopy, a third of patients continued to express dissatisfaction with the waiting time they had experienced. The clinic involved in the study subsequently reduced wait times for colposcopy to 2 weeks after referral.[8] In general, an appointment within a few weeks to a month is recommended to foster compliance. Appointments immediately after an abnormal Pap smear result are likely to be helpful and increase patient satisfaction, whereas longer waits allow intervening variables to interfere with follow-up.

> **Appointments immediately after an abnormal Pap smear are likely to be helpful and increase patient satisfaction, whereas longer waits allow intervening variables that may foster noncompliance.**

The completion of the colposcopic examination has been found to be particularly effective in reducing patient anxiety.[4] However, some caution in this regard is warranted. Reductions in anxiety may reflect reduced concern about the procedure itself but may not reflect reduction in concerns or fears about cancer. Improvements in mood might be attributed to immediate relief after termination of a stressful medical procedure. Research indicates that up to one fifth of patients remain highly anxious after colposcopy and that others experience heightened levels of anger, distressing thoughts, and avoidance.[34]

Guidance and Education

As previously noted, when information about colposcopy is provided, anxiety declines and compliance improves. However, the timing of information sharing is an important variable. Providing patient education at the colposcopy appointment can be time-consuming and ineffective. There is a great amount of information to be shared, and patients are known to have a multitude of concerns and questions. Thus, anticipatory education and guidance are recommended.

The question of when patients prefer to receive information about colposcopy has been examined. The majority of women preferred to be told details about colposcopy at the time they received the results of their abnormal Pap smears.[24] One third of patients indicated they would prefer to receive educational materials and information between the time the results were discussed and the time the procedure was performed. When those patients with significantly elevated levels of anxiety were told about colposcopy at the time the appointment was first scheduled, less than one tenth had elevated levels of anxiety at the time of the procedure.[35]

The source of information about colposcopy is also a relevant consideration. For many patients, an abnormal Pap smear as the result of an annual examination with a primary care physician results in referral to a specialist. When referral is involved, patients often express a strong preference to receive colposcopy information from their family physician.[24]

Not all information about colposcopy is most effective when provided in advance. Procedural information is useful to answer patient questions about the length, timing, and technical aspects of colposcopy. Such information is most effective when provided in advance because it allows the patient to assess the situation and formulate questions.[36]

At the time of the examination, sensory and behavioral information should be emphasized. Sensory information prepares the patient by orienting her to the physical sensations that accompany the colposcopy procedure—what is seen, heard, touched, tasted, or smelled.[36] Behavioral information consists of advice about how the patient can make herself more comfortable or reduce discomfort during the procedure. Both sensory information and behavioral information should follow procedural information and are optimally effective when shared at the time of colposcopy. The importance of orienting patients to the sensory experience of colposcopy has been supported by extensive patient interviews. First-time colposcopy patients have not previously experienced similar physical sensations and lack an objective physical orientation to the physician's activities.

> **The importance of orienting patients to the sensory experience of colposcopy has been supported by extensive patient interviews.**

The experiences of women who have had a colposcopy have also been examined immediately after the procedure. Particular attention has been devoted to soliciting their views on how to modify or improve the experience. Their responses are especially noteworthy in that they reflected little on the experience of the procedure but emphasized the need to modify interactional components. They strongly desired more time to talk with the physician about their concerns.[4, 24] On a related topic, they would have liked more effort on the part of the physician to be supportive and provide more individualized care. Further, patients felt they would have benefited if more understandable terms had been used. Finally, they thought the entire process could be improved if the results of the colposcopy could have been reported personally rather than by mail or telephone message.

Because it is often emotionally difficult and logistically complicated to raise the issue of the patient's psychological reaction to an abnormal Pap smear and to colposcopy, clinicians should consider the use of an available patient self-report inventory. The Psychosocial Effects of Abnormal Pap Smears Questionnaire (PEAPS-Q) consists of 14 items that focus on four areas of distress: reaction to the colposcopy procedure, beliefs or feelings about the abnormal smear and alterations in self-perception, worry about infertility, and effect on sexual relationships.[37] This instrument can provide a nonthreatening way to address sensitive concerns. Further, by identifying the areas of distress, the clinician can target appropriate counseling and patient education.[30] Because the PEAPS-Q measures reactions after colposcopy, the responses can be used as a type of debriefing to alleviate persistent anxiety, concerns, or misinformation.

Developing Effective Tracking Systems

Most attention to the psychosocial aspects of the abnormal Pap smear and the colposcopy experience has focused on patient variables (knowledge, anxiety, compliance), physician-patient relationships, or environmental influences. From a systems perspective, two other considerations emerge. The first involves having an active, formalized tracking system for practice management. The second highlights the value of a collaborative, multidisciplinary approach to the patient.

The positive results of reminders and telephone counseling strategies that target noncompliant patients are deceiving in that such approaches first require a reliable, organized practice plan. Although clinicians recognize the importance of early intervention and scheduled surveillance, in a busy multiphysician environment, many variables can challenge the intention to consistently follow up patients. Thus, developing a formalized care algorithm and designing a systematic response are fundamental. By identifying the flow of care and including multiple professionals from the clinic, "critical checkpoints" can be created to facilitate the assessment of the patient's progress.[38] Because of the complexity of the process, it may be necessary to develop a computerized tracking system that reminds patients to return and prompts clinicians to respond with specific information and actions at each visit. It has been suggested that published noncompliance rates for colposcopy may actually be misleading because of the limited tracking systems of practices. Patients may follow up at a better rate than reported, but not within the physicians' recommendations.[39]

A tracking system that reminds patients to return and prompts clinicians to respond with specific information and actions at each visit is fundamental to colposcopic practice.

Using a Team Approach

Needs for education, reassurance, counseling, and support for the colposcopy patient can arise from the time of the Pap smear through the time colposcopy results are obtained. Because of the time and effort involved, it is unreasonable for an individual clinician to be available to provide all such dimensions of care. Specialized nurses, patient educators, and counselors have proved effective in improving patient satisfaction and addressing patient concerns. When such personnel have been identified as available on a routine or per-need basis, their use has increased, nonscheduled contacts with the physician have decreased, patient anxiety has declined, and compliance with care plans has improved.[40]

The use of specific anxiety-reducing techniques such as progressive muscle relaxation or visual imaging has been considered for especially distressed patients. Teaching these techniques generally requires additional support, training, and time. There have been no systematic efforts

▼ Table 23–1

Goals for the Clinician Who Evaluates an Abnormal Papanicolaou Smear

To provide accurate information (or to correct misinformation) about abnormal Papanicolaou smears

To anticipate and address patient fears and concerns (e.g., cancer, infectivity)

To reassure patients and to decrease negative expectations

To stress the importance of follow-up and to problem-solve factors that contribute to noncompliance

To develop collaborative relationships with other supportive health care providers

to determine if such techniques would be cost-effective in reducing patient anxiety related to colposcopy. The use of a structured cognitive-behavioral approach has been examined, with equivocal results.[21] Although no significant differences were found for typically anxious patients, there was an indication that cognitive-behavioral training may have helped the most distressed patients.

Table 23–1 summarizes the goals of the clinician who provides evaluation of the abnormal Pap smear.

SUMMARY OF KEY POINTS

- Attention to the psychological needs of the patient presenting for colposcopy is an essential component of care.

- The process, from the initial notification of the abnormal Pap smear result to the colposcopy procedure, involves a complex array of reactions that require the patient to sequentially cope with anxiety-arousing information and experiences.

- A longitudinal, comprehensive, multidisciplinary approach is indicated to achieve effective patient care and compliance with follow-up guidelines.

- When informed of an abnormal Pap smear result, patients experience a heightened sense of vulnerability, uncertainty, fear, and anxiety.

- Excessive anxiety and intrusive worrying manifest with such reactions as denial, avoidance, and indecisiveness, all of which interfere with compliance.

- The most common fear experienced by a woman with an abnormal Pap smear is fear of cancer—in particular, cervical cancer.

- Initial reactions to the news of an abnormal Pap result can be difficult to identify because they are suppressed by the shock of an unexpected result, because they develop over time, and because the emotional reactions are often displaced or overshadowed by logistical or informational needs.

- Noncompliance is highest among younger, unmarried, less educated women of lower socioeconomic status.

- Information provided to patients should highlight the specific areas of patient concern that could impede compliance, such as fear of cancer, fear of losing sexual or reproductive functioning, and aversion to medical procedures.

- Because some patients prefer avoidance and distraction as mean of coping with stressful situations, providing informational material is no guarantee that it will be read or understood by the patient.

- It is the clinician's responsibility to clearly indicate that an abnormal Pap smear is not a confirmation of cancer but rather is an indication of a need for further investigation.

- A 15-minute telephone consultation to low-income minority women has been highly effective in addressing barriers to compliance and has therefore improved compliance to follow-up.

- Elements that inhibit support during this time include absence of a close partner, perceived stigma, embarrassment at discussing anatomy, fear of sexual rejection, and view of the male partner as disinterested, uninformed, or unable to understand.

- Women presenting for colposcopy may not have any idea what is involved in the procedure, may not understand the anatomic structures, and are worried about pain or discomfort. Most women prefer to be told details about colposcopy at the time the results of the abnormal Pap smear are relayed.

- Up to a year after colposcopy, a third of patients continued to express dissatisfaction with the waiting times they experienced before the colposcopy appointment day.

- Patients prefer to receive the results of the colposcopic examination in person rather than by mail or by telephone message.

- Because of the complexity of developing a systematic approach to patient care, it may be necessary to develop a computerized tracking system that reminds patients to return and prompts clinicians to respond with specific information and actions at each visit.

- The inclusion of a specialized nurse, patient educator, or counselor has proved effective in improving patient satisfaction and addressing patient concerns.

References

1. Lane DS: Compliance with referrals from a cancer-screening project. J Fam Pract 1983;17:811.
2. Miller S, Mishel W, O'Leary A, et al: From human papillomavirus (HPV) to cervical cancer: Psychosocial processes in infection, detection and control. Ann Behav Med 1996;18:219.
3. Nugent LS, Tamlyn-Leaman K, Isa N: Anxiety and the colposcopy experience. Clin Nurs Res 1993;2:267.
4. Bell S, Porter M, Kitchner H, et al: Psychological response to cervical screening. Prev Med 1995;24:610.
5. Scott DW: Anxiety, critical thinking and information processing during and after breast biopsy. Nurs Res 1983;32:24.
6. Marteau TM, Kidd J, Cuddleford L: Reducing anxiety in women referred for colposcopy using an information booklet. Br J Health Psych 1996;1:181.
7. Jones MH, Singer A, Jenkins D: The mildly abnormal cervical smear: Patient anxiety and choice of management. J Royal Soc Med 1996;89:257.
8. Gath DH, Hallam N, Mynors-Wallis L, et al: Emotional reactions in women attending a UK colposcopy clinic. J Epidemiol Community Health 1995;49:79.
9. Posner T: Ethical issues and the individual woman in cancer screening programmes. J Adv Health Nurs Care 1993;2:55.
10. Lerman C, Miller S, Scarborough R, et al: Adverse psychological consequences of positive cytologic cervical screening. Am J Obstet Gynecol 1991;165:658.
11. Beresford J, Gervaize P: The emotional impact of abnormal Pap smears on patients' referral for colposcopy. Colposcopy Gynecol Laser Surg 1986;2:83.
12. Lauver R, Baggot A, Kruse K: Women's experiences in coping with abnormal Papanicolaou results and follow up colposcopy. J Obstet Gynecol Neonatal Nurs 1999;28:283.
13. Lehr S, Lee M: The psychosocial and sexual trauma of a genital HPV infection. Nurs Pract Forum 1990;1:25.
14. McDonald TW, Neutens JJ, Fischer LM, et al: Impact of cervical intraepithelial neoplasia diagnosis. Gynecol Oncol 1989;34:345.
15. Rajoram S, Hill J, Rave C, et al: A biographical disruption: The case of an abnormal Pap smear. Health Care Women Internat 1997;18:521.
16. Somerset M, Peters TJ: Intervening to reduce anxiety for women with mild dyskaryosis: Do we know what works and why? J Adv Nurs 1998;28:563.
17. Wilkinson C, Jones JM, McBride J: Anxiety caused by abnormal results of cervical smear tests: A controlled trial. Br Med J 1990;300:440.
18. Michielutte R, Disecker RA, Young LD, et al: Non compliance in screening follow up among family planning clinic patients with cervical dysplasia. Prev Med 1985;14:248.
19. Paskett ED, White E, Carter WB, et al: Improving follow-up after an abnormal Pap smear: A randomized controlled trial. Prev Med 1990;19:630.
20. Buckman R: How to Break the Bad News. Baltimore, Johns Hopkins University Press, 1992.
21. Richardson PH, Doherty I, Wolfe CD, et al: Evaluation of cognitive-behavioral counseling for the distress associated with an abnormal cervical smear result. Br J Health Psych 1997;2:327.
22. Miller S, Roussi P, Altman D, et al: Effects of coping style on psychological reactions of low income minority women to colposcopy. J Reprod Med 1994;9:711.
23. Barsevick AM, Johnson JE: Preference for information and involvement, information seeking and emotional responses of women undergoing colposcopy. Res Nurs Health 1990;13:1.
24. Nugent LS, Tamlyn-Leaman K: The colposcopy experience: What do women know? J Adv Nurs 1992;17:514.
25. Miller SM, Siejak KK, Schroeder CM, et al: Enhancing adherence following abnormal Pap smears among low-income minority women: A preventive telephone counseling strategy. J Natl Cancer Inst 1997;89:703.
26. Lerman C, Hanjani P, Caputo C, et al: Telephone counseling improves adherence to colposcopy among lower-income minority women. J Clin Oncol 1992;10:330.
27. Marcus AC, Crave LA, Kaplan CP, et al: Improving adherence to screening follow-up among women with abnormal Pap smears: Results of a large clinic-based trial of three intervention strategies. Med Care 1992;30:216.
28. Massad LS, Meyer P, Hobbs J: Knowledge of cervical cancer screening among women attending urban colposcopy clinics. Cancer Detect Prevent 1997;21:103.
29. Tomaino-Brunner C, Freda MC, Runowicz CD: "I hope I don't have cancer": Colposcopy and minority women. Oncol Nurs Forum 1996;23:39.
30. Stinnet BA: Use of the Psychosocial Effects of Abnormal Pap Smears Questionnaire (PEAPS-Q) in a community hospital colposcopy clinic. J Lower Genital Tract Dis 2000;4:34.

31. Rickert VI, Kozlowski KJ, Warren AM: Adolescents and colposcopy: The use of different procedures to reduce anxiety. Am J Obstet Gynecol 1994;170:504.

32. Rodney WM, Huff M, Euans D, et al: Colposcopy in family practice: Pilot studies of pain prophylaxis and patient volume. Fam Pract Res J 1992;12:91.

33. Jones MH, Singer A, Jenkins D: The mildly abnormal cervical smear: Patient anxiety and choice of management. J Royal Soc Med 1996;89:257.

34. Palmer AG, Tucker S, Warren R, et al: Understanding women's response to treatment for cervical intraepithelial neoplasia. Br J Clin Psych 1993;32:101.

35. Boag FC, Dillon AM, Catalan J, et al: Assessment of psychiatric morbidity in-patients in a colposcopy clinic situated in a genitourinary clinic. Genitourinary Med 1991;67:481.

36. Barsevick AM, Lauver D: Women's informational needs about colposcopy. Image 1990;22:23.

37. Bennetts A, Irwig L, Oldenburg B, et al: PEAPS-Q: A questionnaire to measure the psychosocial effects of having an abnormal Pap smear. J Clin Epidemiol 1995;48:1235.

38. Block B, Branham RA: Efforts to improve the follow-up of patients with abnormal Papanicolaou test results. J Am Board Fam Pract 1998;11:1.

39. Patterson T, Roworth M, Hill M: An investigation into the default rate at the Fife clinic: Implications for target setting. J Public Health Med 1995;17:65.

40. Baxter K, Peters TJ, Somerset M, et al: Anxiety among women with mild dyskaryosis: Costs of an educational intervention. Fam Pract 1999;16:353.

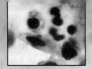

- Mark Spitzer
- Gregory L. Brotzman
- Barbara S. Apgar

CHAPTER *24*

Practical Therapeutic Options for Treatment of Cervical Intraepithelial Neoplasia

ELECTROSURGICAL LOOP EXCISION

Electrosurgical loop excision of the cervix is known by two names: loop electrosurgical excision procedure and large loop excision of the transformation zone.

Electrosurgical loop excision, also known as the loop electrosurgical excision procedure (LEEP) and large loop excision of the transformation zone, has become one of the most common ways to treat cervical intraepithelial neoplasia (CIN), both in the United States and in the rest of the world. Modern electrosurgical units (ESUs) incorporate many advances that allow the surgeon to excise large specimens with a minimal amount of thermal damage and with a minimal risk of bleeding and other complications. Because it is cheaper, faster, and easier to learn and perform, LEEP has replaced laser surgery as the principal method for treating high-grade CIN.

LEEP was first developed in England as a substitute for ablative treatments of the cervix.[1] It was indicated in women who met the criteria for satisfactory colposcopy and therefore were candidates for ablative treatments of the cervix.[2, 3] The ease with which LEEP can be done and the fact that it is easily done under local anesthesia with few short-term complications make it an ideal outpatient procedure.[2–4] Early proponents of LEEP recognized that removal of the entire transformation zone was theoretically less subject to false-negative results than colposcopy, which might be subject to a misdirected biopsy. In fact, early reports indicated that 1% to 2% of women undergoing LEEP were found to have microinvasive or invasive cancer where none was suspected before the procedure.[2–5] This result, combined with the ease of the procedure, the high patient acceptability, and the low morbidity rate, fostered initial enthusiasm for using a "see and treat" approach rather than colposcopy for all women with abnormal Papanicolaou (Pap) smears.[2, 3, 6] In this approach, women with abnormal Pap smears were evaluated with LEEP rather than with colposcopy and directed biopsy. Unfortunately, early reports of this approach

showed that many women had either very minor abnormalities on their LEEP specimens or only negative metaplastic or inflammatory changes.[7, 8] In the United States today, most clinicians use LEEP only after first confirming the histologic grade of disease with a colposcopically directed biopsy.[4, 7, 9] In England, LEEP is reserved for women whose smears show a high-grade squamous intraepithelial lesion (HSIL) or who have a significant colposcopic lesion extending into the endocervical canal.

Electrosurgical Physics

Modern ESUs apply an alternating current to tissue at frequencies above those that cause nerve and muscle stimulation.

Modern ESUs must be distinguished from older Bovie units that treated cervical disease by heating and cauterizing the tissue. ESUs apply an alternating current to tissue. Common household current alternates at 60 Hz. Stimulation of nerve and muscle by an alternating current (termed *faradic effects*) occur maximally at frequencies between 10 and 100 Hz. These faradic effects cause muscular tetany and may result in electrocution. However, at frequencies above 2500 Hz, these effects gradually diminish, and above 300 kHz, they are essentially absent. This is why modern ESUs operate at a frequency between 500 kHz and 4 million Hz and are known as radiofrequency generators.

Unlike older ESUs that transmitted electricity directly from an electrical outlet to ground, modern ESUs isolate the main power by passing it through a transformer, eliminating the risk of alternative pathway burns.

All electrical current flows in a closed circuit, and the electrical current always seeks to return to its source. Older ESUs transmitted electricity directly from an electrical outlet and returned it to that outlet (return to ground). Such units placed the patient at risk for alternative pathway burns when the electricity flowing from the

ESU through the patient found an alternative path to ground through a conductive substance that inadvertently became grounded (such as a dangling piece of jewelry or an electrocardiogram lead). The electrical current could become focused in that area, causing a burn. In modern ESUs, passing the main power through a transformer isolates it. In such isolated units, "grounding" the patient does not close the electrical circuit, and there is no alternative pathway through which electricity can flow, eliminating the risk of alternative pathway burns. Only ESUs with such isolated circuitry should be used.

Desiccation occurs when the electrode is in direct contact with the tissue.

To properly use electrosurgery, it is important to understand the types of electrosurgical effects one is likely to see. *Desiccation* occurs when the electrode is in direct contact with the tissue. The temperature within the cells rises slowly to less than 100°C. Water evaporates from the cells, and cellular proteins coagulate. Hemostasis results from the drying of blood and the contraction of small blood vessels.

As the tissue is vaporized during the LEEP, the steam from the exploding cells forms a steam envelope around the loop electrode that prevents direct contact between the electrode and the tissue.

Cutting occurs when the temperature within the cells rises quickly to more than 100°C. The water in the cells rapidly boils, and the cells explode. This requires very high and continuous current density, meaning that the current produced by the ESU must be focused in a very small area. This occurs principally when the electrode is not in physical contact with the tissue and the electric current is traversing the gap between the electrode and the tissue (traveling in an *arc*). LEEP is ideally started with the electrode not in contact with the tissue. As the tissue is vaporized, steam from the exploding cells forms a *steam envelope* around the loop. The steam envelope prevents contact between the electrode and the tissue and, combined with ionization of the steam in the electric field, facilitates formation of an arc. Moving the loop too quickly collapses the steam envelope and places the electrode in direct contact with the tissue. This reduces the power density, and the electrosurgical effect reverts to desiccation rather than cutting. The loop stops cutting, and thermal tissue damage occurs. The observed effect is that the loop drags through the tissue and bends. Proper technique requires that the loop be moved slowly and continuously through the tissue being cut.

During spray coagulation, the current is interrupted rather than continuous, resulting in dissipation of the steam envelope and in protein coagulation, hemostasis, and destruction of lesional tissue.

The final electrosurgical effect is *spray coagulation*. In this form of coagulation, the electrode does not make contact with the tissue, similar to electrosurgical cutting.

But because the current is interrupted rather than continuous, the steam envelope dissipates, resulting in protein coagulation, hemostasis, and destruction of lesional tissue. Tissue that has been subjected to spray coagulation cannot be used for histopathologic evaluation.

During LEEP, electricity passes from the electrosurgical loop electrode through the body, back to the grounding pad, and then back to the ESU.

During LEEP, the ESU is used in a monopolar arrangement. This means that the electricity passes from the electrosurgical loop through the body, back to the grounding pad or dispersive electrode, and then back to the ESU. Reducing the distance that the electricity needs to travel through the patient reduces the resistance encountered and minimizes the amount of electrical current needed to create the desired effects. Therefore, the dispersive pad should be positioned as close as possible to the surgical site. The ideal site to place the dispersive pad during LEEP is on the upper thigh.

The amount of electricity flowing during LEEP is the same at the loop electrode and at the dispersive pad. However, because the surface area at the dispersive pad is much larger, the power density (PD) is lower, and no electrosurgical effects occur at the dispersive pad. Previous-generation dispersive pads that become partially detached pose a risk of electrosurgical burns at that area. Modern ESUs do not operate if the dispersive pad is partially detached.

Equipment

As a safety precaution, the ESU should be equipped with isolated circuitry, and the dispersive pad should prevent current from flowing if the pad is not properly applied.

The equipment required for LEEP is listed in Table 24–1. One should ensure that the ESU is a newer one with isolated circuitry and that the dispersive pad is of the type that prevents current from flowing if it is not

▼ Table 24–1

Equipment Needed for Electrosurgical Loop Excision

Electrosurgical generator
Patient grounding (dispersive) pad
Various sizes and shapes of loop electrodes
Ball electrodes (3- and 5-mm sizes)
Insulated electrode handle
Nonconductive speculum with smoke-evacuator port
Nonconductive vaginal sidewall retractor
Smoke evacuator and filter system
Colposcope
3% to 5% acetic acid or vinegar
Aqueous Lugol's solution (half strength)
Large cotton swabs
Local anesthetic with vasopressin (in the ratio of 10 units of vasopressin in 30 mL of 1% lidocaine)
Dental-type syringe with 27-gauge needles, 1.5 inches in length
Monsel's paste or gel
Specimen bottles with 10% neutral-buffered formalin
12-inch needle holder and 2–0 resorbable suture material

properly applied. These are important safety precautions that prevent unintended burns. The electrosurgical loop is made of a thin, flexible wire connected to an insulated traverse bar. The loop is fixed into a pencil-type holder. Current is activated either by pressing a button on the holder or by depressing a foot pedal. A thin wire allows a higher PD than a thicker wire allows, and it produces less thermal damage to the tissue. Although, intuitively, a thicker and more rigid wire might be more desirable to prevent bending of the wire as it passes through the tissue, in fact, the wire should not be making contact with the tissue at all. If the loop is seen to bend, it indicates that the operator is pushing the loop through the tissue too rapidly, causing the steam envelope to collapse and desiccating rather than cutting the tissue. Thicker loops also cause more thermal damage to the tissue. The insulated traverse bar prevents thermal damage to the surface epithelium as it is traversed by the loop. Loops are available in various sizes so that the size of the loop can be individualized to the width and depth of the lesion and the transformation zone. The traverse bar also limits the depth of excision.

The ball electrode used for cautery hemostasis also comes in varying sizes; usually 3 mm and 5 mm in diameter. The larger the electrode, the lower the PD. The electrode should be chosen on the basis of the desired effect.

The use of a nonconductive, rather than a metal, speculum prevents transmission of current from the electrode to the unanesthetized vagina.

The use of a nonconductive, rather than a metal, speculum prevents transmission of current from the electrode to the unanesthetized vagina. It is important to realize that although contact with a metal speculum will cause a brief shock to the patient, the large surface area of the speculum will likely disperse the current and prevent any burns. Even brief shocks are not desirable, however, because they may cause the patient to jump or move during the excision. The nonconductive speculum includes a smoke-evaluator port. Plastic tubing is placed in the port and then attached to the smoke evacuator unit. The evacuator unit removes the smoke generated in the vagina as the loop excision is performed. Without smoke evacuation, the operator cannot visualize the cervix during the excision.

Technique

As with all surgical procedures for CIN, LEEP is contraindicated in women with active cervical, vaginal, or pelvic infections and in women with known, frankly invasive cervical cancer. It should be used only with caution in women who are pregnant[10] or who have a known bleeding disorder. After informed consent is obtained, the patient is placed in the dorsal lithotomy position, and a nonconductive, coated speculum with smoke evacuation capability is placed into the vagina. Ideally, a vaginal sidewall retractor will help protect the vaginal sidewall from inadvertent contact with the electrosurgical loop. However, if the vaginal walls are sufficiently distant from the cervix, a sidewall retractor may not be necessary.

Three percent to 5% acetic acid is then applied to the cervix, and colposcopy is used to delineate the limits of the lesion. Because the acetic acid effect may be obscured by the injection of a local anesthetic, some have advocated painting the cervix with Lugol's solution to delineate the limits of the lesion before LEEP.

The size of the loop chosen should depend on the lateral extent of the transformation zone and how far the lesion extends into the endocervical canal.

Once the lesion is visualized, an appropriately sized loop is chosen. The size of the loop chosen should depend on the lateral extent of the transformation zone and how far the lesion extends into the endocervical canal. Ideally, the entire transformation zone should be removed in one piece. However, when the transformation zone is very large and extends onto the portio of the cervix, this may not be possible without unnecessarily removing too much cervical stroma. In such cases, the central portion of the transformation zone can be removed with a single sweep, and the remaining anterior and posterior segments of the transformation zone can be removed with a second, shallower sweep. If the colposcopist can confidently exclude invasion in the peripheral portions of the transformation zone, these areas can be desiccated or spray coagulated using the ball electrode after the removal of the central conization specimen.

The dispersive pad is attached to the patient's upper thigh and to the ESU, and smoke evacuator tubing is attached to the speculum and smoke evacuator. Up to 10 mL of local anesthetic (in a ratio of 10 units of vasopressin in 30 mL of 1% lidocaine) is injected circumferentially into the cervix using a fine needle (27 gauge or finer). The injection should be superficial (only a few millimeters) and should cause the injection site to blanch (Fig. 24–1).

Lower power settings minimize thermal damage to the tissue, making the pathology specimen easier to interpret and reducing patient discomfort.

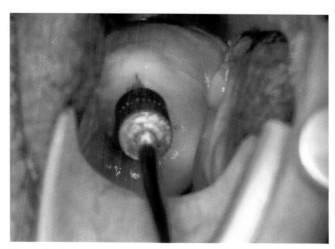

Figure 24–1. Injection of local anesthetic before cervical electrosurgical loop excision or laser surgery.

The power setting needed to perform LEEP varies with the size of the loop chosen, the placement of the dispersive electrode, and the technique used. Furthermore, the settings on many ESUs (especially older ones) do not provide accurate representation of the unit's power output during a procedure. In general, the lowest power setting should be used that will allow the clinician to easily perform the procedure. Lower power settings minimize thermal effects to the tissue, making the pathology specimen easier to interpret, and also reduce the discomfort experienced by the patient.

The procedure is always done under direct colposcopic guidance. The choice as to which direction to pass the loop relates to the size and shape of the transformation zone, the position of the cervix, the amount of room in the vagina, and the laxity of the vaginal walls. The loop should be passed in the direction that makes the procedure easiest. The specimen can then be removed by one of two techniques. One may begin by placing the tip of the loop approximately 3 to 5 mm beyond the peripheral margin of the transformation zone and not quite in contact with the cervical tissue (Fig. 24–2). After the power is activated, electrical sparks can be seen arcing at the tip of the loop. The loop is then slowly plunged into the cervical stroma to the desired depth. When the colposcopy is satisfactory, the LEEP specimen needs to be 5 mm to 8 mm in depth. When the lesion or the transformation zone extends into the endocervical canal, or when the endocervical curettage is positive, a deeper LEEP conization should be performed (discussed later). The loop is then brought underneath the transformation zone (Fig. 24–3) and pulled out 3 to 5 mm beyond the peripheral margin of the transformation zone on the opposite side. The second possible technique begins by laying the loop over the transformation zone so that it encompasses the lesion, bending the loop slightly in the process. The power is then turned on. After a few seconds, the loop cuts into the cervix. When the wire straightens out, the loop is then brought under the remainder of the transfor-

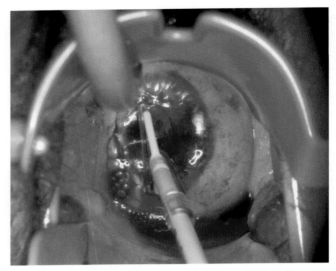

Figure 24–3. An electrosurgical loop excision as the loop is passed under the transformation zone.

mation zone and out the opposite side. Although this technique is a little easier, the fact that the loop initially makes contact with the cervix causes it to desiccate the tissue and causes more thermal damage at the ectocervical margin.

> **The "top hat" technique removes less stroma than a cone biopsy removes, but the specimens may suffer extensive thermal damage and be uninterpretable in the laboratory.**

In cases where the transformation zone is not fully visualized, the lesion extends into the endocervical canal, or the endocervical curettage result is positive, a cone biopsy is indicated. LEEP can be used as a substitute.[4, 11, 12] In this case, a larger (deeper) loop may be used. Alternatively, a shallow, superficial specimen can be obtained, followed by excision of a smaller endocervical specimen. This so-called top hat technique has the advantage of removing less stroma than a large LEEP conization removes. However, the small endocervical specimen frequently suffers from extensive thermal damage and may be uninterpretable histologically.

Another approach to electrosurgical conization is the use of a device called a Fisher cone rather than a wire loop. In the Fisher cone, a fine wire is passed between the insulated stem and the insulated base of the device. The device comes in several sizes, and the angle that the wire makes with the central stem, coupled with the depth to which the device is pushed into the cervix, dictates the depth and width of the cone. In using the Fisher cone, one must take great care to ensure that the right size cone is chosen. If not, the specimen may be too deep or insufficiently wide to remove the entire transformation zone. The procedure for electrosurgical conization using the Fisher cone is as follows: After the power is turned on, the wire is plunged into the cervix to its desired depth. The Fisher cone is rotated 360 degrees using the central

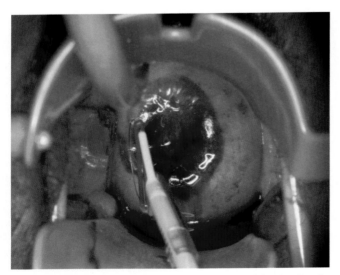

Figure 24–2. An electrosurgical loop excision is started by plunging the loop into the cervix just lateral to the transformation zone.

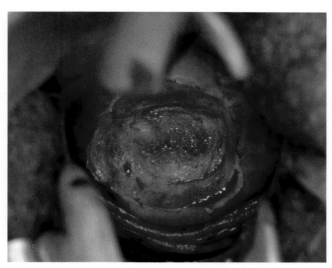

Figure 24—4. Appearance of the cone bed after the electrosurgical loop excision specimen has been removed.

stem as a guide to follow the inner aspect of the endocervical canal. One disadvantage of the Fisher cone is that when the shape of the cervix or the transformation zone is irregular, the Fisher cone may remove too much or not enough tissue. Also, if the procedure must be momentarily interrupted because it is difficult to complete the rotation in one motion, restarting the current while the wire is within the cervical stroma may result in additional thermal injury to the specimen.

> **Bleeding is controlled with use of the ball electrode or with thickened Monsel's paste or gel.**

Once the cone specimen has been removed with a forceps (Fig. 24–4), the defect is carefully cauterized using the ball electrode. Most of the bleeding is usually found along the ectocervical edge. For additional hemostasis, thickened Monsel's paste or gel may be applied to the base of the defect.

When fine wire loops are used, the cone specimen exhibits little thermal damage.[13–15] The cure rate for women treated with LEEP is comparable to that for women treated with laser or cold knife conization (CKC) and depends on whether the conization margins are positive or negative. If the margins are negative, a cure rate of approximately 95% can be expected.[1–4, 6, 16, 17] With positive endocervical margins, the cure rate is approximately 70%.[4]

Complications

> **Complications occur in 1% to 2% of LEEP cases and include heavy bleeding and infection.**

After LEEP, the patient can expect a heavy, brown, and sometimes malodorous discharge for up to 2 to 3 weeks.[3, 18, 19] Immediate complications occur in 1% to 2% of cases and include heavy vaginal bleeding and infec-

tion.[2–4, 6, 16, 17] A higher rate of hemorrhagic complications occurs when greater amounts of cervical tissue are removed.[3, 20, 21] Because hemostasis is usually more tenuous immediately after a LEEP, the patient should avoid any heavy lifting or strenuous activity for at least 2 weeks after the procedure and should avoid inserting anything into the vagina for 4 weeks. Because the procedure removes a portion of the endocervical canal, blood flow during the first menses after the procedure may be much heavier than the patient is accustomed to. To avoid alarm on the part of the patient, the procedure should be scheduled for immediately after menses, allowing maximal healing before the next menses, and the patient should be alerted to the possibility of heavy bleeding. Bleeding that comes at the time of the expected period should be managed expectantly. Heavy bleeding not associated with menses (heavier than the patient's normal menstrual flow) may need to be treated. If the patient is not hemorrhaging, she should reduce her degree of physical activity. If the bleeding persists, the patient should be examined, and any bleeding sites may be treated with electrocautery or with thickened Monsel's solution. Clots adherent to the base of the crater *should not* be removed. They likely represent a vessel that was the source of the bleeding and has now clotted. Removing the clot will just cause the bleeding to resume.

> **Clots adherent to the base of the crater should not be removed because they likely represent a vessel that was the source of the bleeding and has now clotted.**

Postprocedure infection may present as malodorous discharge.[22] However, because discharge is very common in all women undergoing this procedure, distinguishing between a normal discharge and an infection may be difficult. The first indication of cervical infection may be delayed bleeding or delayed healing.

> **A small percentage of patients suffer late complications, including delayed bleeding and cervical stenosis.**

Later complications include delayed bleeding and cervical stenosis. An unsatisfactory colposcopy occurs in 1.3% to 9% of women after LEEP, and cervical stenosis occurs in 1.3% to 3.8%.[3, 6, 16, 18] An extreme example of cervical stenosis can be found in postmenopausal women undergoing LEEP, in women undergoing a second LEEP, or in those for whom the LEEP excision is very deep.[23] Cervical stenosis is avoided by having endocervical cells that are stimulated by estrogen. In each of these cases, a necessary element is missing. In postmenopausal women not taking hormone replacement therapy, the endocervical cells are not stimulated because of the hypoestrogenic state. Women undergoing deep conization or repeat conization are at risk for removal of all of their endocervix, leaving nothing to be stimulated by estrogen.[23] In both cases, these women are at risk for cervical os obliteration. When some endocervix remains, stenosis might be prevented by daily application of vaginal estrogen for up to 1 month after surgery.[23] Little can be done to prevent cervical stenosis in the last case. The fertility of women is probably unaffected after a single LEEP.[24–27] However, large LEEP or repetitive LEEPs procedures may increase the risk of infertility related to cervical factors, such as cervical stenosis or poor-quality or scanty cervical mucus.

CARBON DIOXIDE LASER

> **Carbon dioxide laser is used for specific situations in which its versatility offers advantages over LEEP.**

Throughout the 1980s, the carbon dioxide (CO_2) laser became an increasingly more popular modality for treatment of cervical disease. Until the advent of LEEP, the CO_2 laser represented the most versatile and effective tool available for the treatment of CIN. It offered the advantages of a high cure rate,[28, 29] an ability to treat almost any extent and grade of disease, an ability to vaporize or excise tissue as needed, excellent healing, and a low complication rate.[30, 31] The major disadvantages of the CO_2 laser were the cost of equipment and the need for more extensive physician training. These disadvantages led to diminished use of the CO_2 laser once LEEP became available. Today, most clinicians reserve CO_2 laser for specific cases where its versatility offers advantages over LEEP.

The term *laser* is an acronym for light amplification by stimulated emission of radiation. The CO_2 laser produces a monochromatic beam of light in the infrared portion of the spectrum that is coherent (all waves are exactly in phase with one another) and collimated (all rays are parallel to one another). This allows the beam to be focused through the use of a series of lenses and mirrors. At its focal point, the energy produced by the laser beam is sufficient to instantaneously boil the intracellular water of any tissue with which it comes into contact. The tissue is thus vaporized, producing a crater at the point of contact.

Laser Physics

> **The amount of energy applied to the tissue is a product of the energy output of the laser and the size of the laser spot.**

The amount of energy applied to the tissue is a product of the relationship of two factors. One factor is the energy output of the laser, measured in watts (w). The other factor is the size of the laser spot, measured in square centimeters. The PD is the unit used to measure the energy that the laser applies to a given area of tissue. The PD is calculated with the formula $PD = 100 \times w/cm^2$. At low PD, the tissue is heated more slowly, and heat is conducted to adjacent tissue, resulting in thermal injury. The amount of heat conducted to the adjacent tissue is directly related to the amount of time that the laser is applied to the tissue. Because a laser used at a lower PD needs more time to achieve its desired effect, it also allows more time for the heat to be conducted to the adjacent tissue and for that tissue to be damaged by the heat. In tissue that has been irreversibly damaged by the heat but not vaporized by the laser, the appearance of cell

death is delayed. However, the heat generated by the laser at lower PD also has advantages. It helps achieve hemostasis by coagulating blood and tissue proteins and contracting and sclerosing smaller vessels. The use of a lower PD also allows the operator greater control over the depth of vaporization.

> **The use of a lower PD allows the operator greater control over the depth of vaporization at the expense of greater thermal damage.**

When tissue is subjected to high PD, the tissue will instantaneously vaporize, allowing little time for heat to be conducted to adjacent tissue and minimizing the zone of thermal injury. However, at higher PD, the laser vaporizes tissue very rapidly, forcing the operator to keep the beam in constant rapid motion to avoid the inadvertent creation of deep craters. The use of lower PD allows the operator greater control over the depth of vaporization. The challenge to the clinician is to use the laser at the highest possible PD that will still allow control of the effects of the beam. Clinicians with greater experience and skill are able to use higher PD and to achieve better and more predictable results.

Three zones of tissue injury are described when tissue is subjected to laser vaporization. In the innermost zone of the vaporization crater, the tissue has been vaporized. In the next layer, the tissue has been heated and subjected to lethal thermal injury but not vaporized. This tissue will eventually slough. It is this zone that is of greatest concern to the clinician because the extent of devitalized tissue is not apparent at the time of surgery and becomes apparent only later. In the most peripheral zone, the tissue has suffered nonlethal thermal injury. Although the extent of damage is not immediately apparent at the time of surgery, this tissue will recover. The main challenge of CO_2 laser surgery is to minimize the zone of lethal thermal injury and, to some extent, the zone of nonlethal thermal injury, while maintaining control of the depth of laser vaporization.

Equipment

> **When treating lower genital tract lesions with the CO_2 laser, colposcopic magnification and guidance should be employed and a micromanipulator should be used.**

Today, most CO_2 lasers are completely self-contained portable units that may be used in the hospital or in the office. The size and price of the machine usually relate to the amount of power it is able to generate, but most lower genital tract procedures can be done with machines generating between 20 and 40 w. Because the wavelength of the beam is 10.6 μm (in the invisible infrared portion of the electromagnetic spectrum), CO_2 lasers must have an additional aiming beam. This is usually a second, very low power, helium-neon aiming laser beam. The beams are produced by the lasers in the base cabinet and are transferred via a series of mirrors and lenses through an articulated arm to the colposcope. A micromanipulator is attached to the colposcope and allows the clinician to

▼ Table 24–2

Equipment Needed for CO_2 Laser Surgery

CO_2 laser
Micromanipulator with variable spot size
Blackened nonreflective speculum with smoke-evacuator port
Blackened nonreflective vaginal sidewall retractor
Smoke evacuator and filter system
Right-angle skin hook
Colposcope
3% to 5% acetic acid or vinegar
Aqueous Lugol's solution (half strength)
Large cotton swabs
Local anesthetic with vasopressin (in the ratio of 10 units of vasopressin in 30 mL of 1% lidocaine)
Dental-type syringe with 27-gauge needles, 1.5 inches in length
Monsel's paste or gel
Specimen bottles with 10% neutral-buffered formalin
12-inch needle holder and 2–0 resorbable suture material

CO_2, carbon dioxide.

view the laser beam through the colposcope and to control it via a joystick apparatus. When treating lower genital tract lesions with the CO_2 laser, one must always use colposcopic magnification and guidance and a micromanipulator. It is inappropriate to use the laser as a handheld device in this application because this approach deprives the clinician of the control necessary to obtain optimal results.

One important feature of the micromanipulator is its ability to vary the spot size of the laser.

One important feature of the micromanipulator is its ability to vary the spot size of the laser. The clinician is able to raise the PD by narrowing the spot size and to lower the PD by using a larger spot size. This ability allows the clinician to easily balance the extent of thermal injury, the speed at which the tissue is being vaporized, and his or her degree of control by using the visible effect on the tissue as a guide.

The equipment required for a laser surgical procedure is listed in Table 24–2. Because of the smoke generated by laser procedures, they should always be done in a well-ventilated room, using a high-efficiency smoke evacuation and filtration device. Before vaporizing tissue, the laser must first vaporize any liquid covering the tissue, so moist gauze pads may be used to protect the area surrounding the operative field from inadvertent laser injury. However, because all laser surgery in this area is done under direct colposcopic guidance, many experienced laser surgeons do not find this precaution necessary. Because the laser beam will be reflected by any shiny surface, laser instruments (speculums, retractors, and manipulators) should all be blackened and nonreflective. For manipulating the cervix, a manipulator with a short, right-angle hook is most effective. Curved hooks are more difficult to use.

Technique

At high PD, tissue vaporization is very rapid, and there is little thermal injury but also little hemostatic effect.

The CO_2 laser can be used as either a vaporization tool or a cutting tool. For a vaporization tool, larger spot sizes are used. The laser is usually set at a high power setting, and the spot size used is the largest one that will still allow a good balance among tissue vaporization, thermal injury, and control of the laser. In the cutting mode, the spot size is reduced to its narrowest diameter, allowing use of very high PD, even though the overall power output by the laser may be somewhat lower. At such high PD, tissue vaporization is very rapid, and there is little thermal injury but also little hemostatic effect. Control is often achieved by operating the laser in short bursts, manipulating the tissue, and then operating the laser again. Newer and more expensive lasers may have a super-pulse or ultra-pulse mode. In this mode, the laser generates very high power output for brief millisecond bursts, followed by a millisecond period of rest. The high power outage allows for vaporization and cutting of tissue with minimal thermal injury, whereas the rest allows the small amount of heat generated to dissipate and gives the operator greater control over the beam.

If the transformation zone is not fully visualized, the laser is used to cut a cone-shaped specimen.

Three techniques are commonly used to treat cervical disease with the laser. When the transformation zone and the lesion are fully visualized, they may be vaporized, usually to a depth of 7 to 10 mm. When the transformation zone is not fully visualized or the disease extends into the endocervical canal, a laser conization is done, using the laser to cut a cone-shaped specimen to be submitted for histologic evaluation. The width and depth of the cone are tailored to the degree and extent of disease. When the disease extends well onto the portio of the cervix *and* into the endocervical canal, a combination conization is the ideal technique. The central portion of the transformation zone is excised to an appropriate depth as a CO_2 laser conization while the peripheral portion of the transformation zone, which usually contains lower-grade disease, is vaporized. This approach preserves cervical tissue and minimizes both long-term and short-term complications.

Most laser procedures can be done using a local anesthetic, and experienced laser surgeons can do these procedures in the office setting. Only in rare instances, when the patient is extremely uncooperative or when the anatomy necessitates extreme amounts of manipulation, is it necessary to do such procedures with the patient under general anesthesia. Some clinicians premedicate the patient with ibuprofen before the procedure; however, this is not absolutely necessary.

Because the blood must be vaporized by the laser before the bleeding vessel can be sclerosed, it is somewhat difficult to control brisk bleeding with the laser.

As with all surgical procedures for CIN, laser surgery is contraindicated in women with active cervical, vaginal, or pelvic infections and in women with known, frankly invasive cervical cancer. It should also be used with caution in women who are pregnant or who have a known bleeding disorder, because blood, just like any other liquid, will interfere with the clinician's ability to achieve the desired tissue effect with the laser. When bleeding is encountered, the blood dissipates the laser energy, preventing it from reaching its intended target. Because the fluid must be vaporized by the laser before it can sclerose the bleeding vessel, it is somewhat difficult to control brisk bleeding with the laser. To control such bleeding, all excess blood is removed while a cotton-tipped applicator is used to control the bleeding by direct tamponade of the bleeding vessel. The laser is then used at the lower PD settings to vaporize and coagulate the tissue around the bleeding vessel. The cotton-tipped applicator is slowly rolled away as the laser beam is applied to the tissue and the underlying vessel. When the bleeding is brisk and difficult to temporarily control with focal tamponade, completion of the procedure with the CO_2 laser becomes increasingly difficult.

Laser Procedure

After informed consent is obtained, the patient is placed in the dorsal lithotomy position, and a black, nonreflective speculum with smoke evacuation capability is placed into the vagina. Diluted acetic acid is applied to the cervix, and colposcopy is used to delineate the limits of the lesion. Because the acetic acid effect may be obscured by the injection of local anesthetic, some have advocated painting the cervix with Lugol's solution to delineate the limits of the lesion. After injecting the local anesthetic (in a ratio of 10 units of vasopressin in 30 mL of 1% lidocaine) (see Fig. 24–1), the laser is used at low PD to outline the areas to be vaporized or excised (Fig. 24–5). Beginners may find it helpful to do this by tracing a

series of dots using short bursts of the laser and then connecting the dots. More experienced laser surgeons will simply outline this area initially.

Technique for Vaporization

> **When vaporized at the appropriate PD, the tissue in the crater should be mostly white, with small, well-dispersed flecks of black char.**

The spot size is set at the largest spot that will allow the laser to generate between 500 and 1000 w/cm^2 and still permit the laser surgeon control to vaporize only the areas desired. Ideally, this can be estimated by observing the effects of the laser on the tissue. When vaporized at an appropriate PD, the tissue in the crater should be mostly white, with small, well-dispersed flecks of black char (Fig. 24–6). The more black char that is seen, the lower the PD and the greater the thermal damage to the tissue. A complete absence of char means that the PD is very high, and the operator may find it difficult to control the laser or may have difficulty achieving hemostasis.

Every laser surgeon develops her or his own method for controlling the effects of the laser. Some use small, slow, overlapping, circular motions of the beam, whereas others use rapid, back-and-forth oscillations of the beam. However it is achieved, the desired result is to avoid leaving the beam in any one spot for an extended period of time, because this will create a deep crater in the tissue, and any bleeding at the base of this hole will be very difficult to control. The transformation zone is vaporized until a barrel-shaped defect 7 to 10 mm deep is achieved. The depth is measured by use of a rod-shaped measuring device. A laser surgeon may vaporize the stroma immediately surrounding the endocervix to a shallow depth. This will cause the endocervical mucosa to

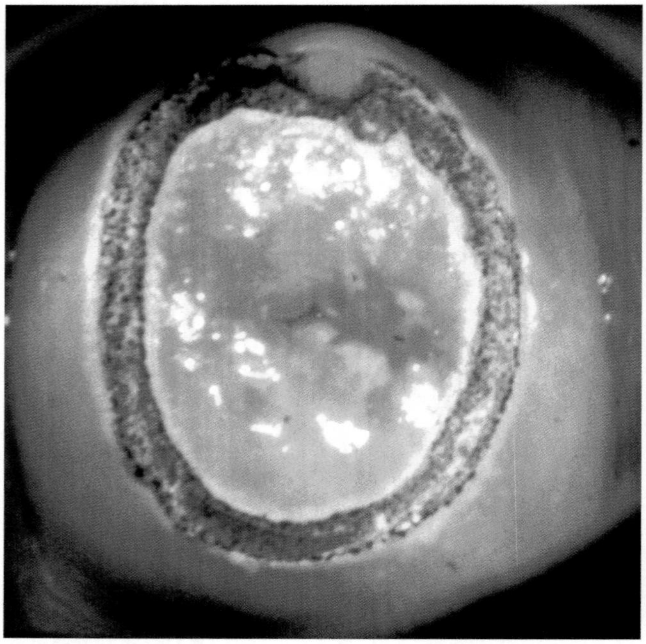

Figure 24–5. Circumference of a laser vaporization (or conization) as it is delineated by the laser.

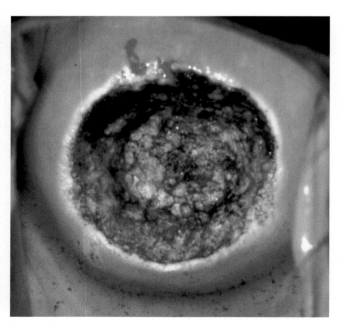

Figure 24–6. Appearance of the cone bed after completion of laser vaporization.

evert (*buttoning*). The laser surgeon may then continue to vaporize 2 to 3 mm more of endocervix (*clipping*). This allows the laser surgeon to exercise some degree of control as to where the squamocolumnar junction (SCJ) will ultimately be located. The laser surgeon can locate the SCJ farther out onto the ectocervix by clipping less of the endocervix or can locate it more in the endocervical canal by clipping more. After the vaporization is complete, excess char is gently swabbed out of the crater with large cotton swabs soaked in diluted acetic acid.

Technique for Excisional Conization

> **After the peripheral margin of the cone is outlined with the CO_2 laser, the laser is set at 800 to 1200 w/cm^2 with the smallest possible spot size.**

After the peripheral margin of the cone is outlined with the CO_2 laser, the laser is set at 800 to 1200 w/cm^2 with the smallest possible spot size. The cervix is incised with the laser along the margin of the cone, to a depth of 3 to 5 mm. In narrower and deeper cones, this incision may need to be deeper. Wider and shallower cones may need a shallower incision. Traction is applied to the cut edge of the cone in one direction using a right-angle hook, and the laser beam is directed at the inner margin of the base of the incision (Fig. 24–7). This procedure is repeated as traction is applied to the cervical cone sequentially in all directions, gradually undercutting the cone specimen. In an effort to minimize thermal damage to the endocervical portion of the cone, some authors have advocated making the last cut at the endocervical margin with a scalpel or scissors. Others, however, have found it acceptable to cut this margin with the laser at high power.[32]

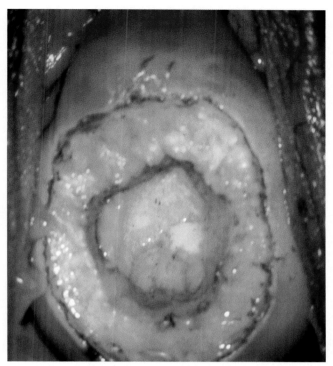

Figure 24–8. Combination laser conization. The laser has vaporized the outer aspect of the transformation zone. The inner cone specimen will be excised.

Some authors follow excision of the cone specimen with endocervical curettage or an endocervical biopsy of the canal beyond the cone specimen. However, this practice is not shared by all. Creation of an endocervical button and clipping of the endocervical tissue may be done as described in the section on laser vaporization.

Combination Laser Cone Biopsy

> **If the transformation zone or lesion extends deep into the endocervical canal *and* out onto the portio, a combination excision/vaporization cone biopsy can be performed.**

In instances where the transformation zone or cervical lesion extends deep into the canal *and* out onto the portio, some have advocated doing a combination excision/vaporization cone biopsy. This procedure uses aspects of both procedures described previously. The central portion of the transformation zone is excised as a laser excision cone biopsy, and the outer portion of the lesion or transformation zone is vaporized as a laser vaporization cone. This minimizes the amount of tissue lost in the procedure (Fig. 24–8).

Complications

> **The rate of bleeding with laser surgery is less than that with CKC and comparable to that expected with LEEP.**

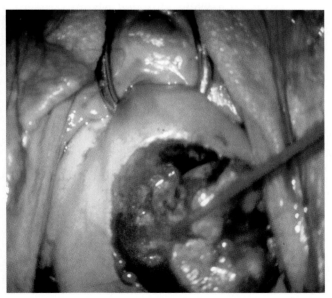

Figure 24–7. Laser excisional conization. The hook is retracting the cone specimen laterally so that the laser can excise it.

The immediate postoperative problems seen with laser surgery of the cervix are the same as those seen with any other operative procedures and include bleeding and infection. The rate of bleeding with laser surgery is less than that with CKC[34, 35] and comparable to that expected with LEEP.

As with LEEP, after laser surgery the patient can expect a heavy, brown, and sometimes malodorous discharge for up to 2 to 3 weeks. Immediate complications occur in 1% to 2% of cases and include heavy vaginal bleeding and infection. As with the instructions for immediately after a LEEP, the patient should avoid any heavy lifting or strenuous activity for at least 2 weeks after the procedure and should avoid inserting anything into the vagina for 4 weeks. Blood flow during the first menses after the procedure may be much heavier than normal. Ideally, the procedure should be scheduled for immediately after menses, allowing maximal healing before the next menses, and the patient should be alerted to the possibility of heavy bleeding. At first, any bleeding other than hemorrhage should be managed expectantly. The patient should reduce her degree of physical activity, and if the bleeding continues the patient should be examined; any bleeding sites may be treated with Monsel's paste or gel. Clots adherent to the base of the crater *should not* be removed. They likely represent a vessel that was the source of the bleeding and is now clotted. Removing the clot will just cause the bleeding to resume.

Postconization cervical stenosis in postmenopausal women might be prevented by the use of vaginal estrogen cream.

Postprocedure infection may present as a malodorous discharge. However, because discharge is very common in all women undergoing this procedure, distinguishing a normal discharge from an infection may be difficult. Later complications include delayed bleeding and cervical stenosis. Postmenopausal women or women undergoing a second procedure are at risk of cervical stenosis.[35] This may be prevented by treating the women with vaginal estrogen cream.[23] The fertility of women is probably unaffected following a single laser procedure.[36, 37] However, large or repetitive laser procedures may increase the risk of infertility related to cervical factors, such as cervical stenosis or poor-quality or scanty cervical mucus.[37]

CRYOTHERAPY

In well-selected patients, cryotherapy is an effective therapeutic option for the treatment of CIN.

Even in the midst of newer technologies such as laser and loop electrosurgical excision for the treatment of CIN, cryotherapy remains an effective therapeutic option for treatment of CIN in many patients. Cryotherapy has been used for more than half a century and has a proven efficacy and safety record.[38–43] In well-selected patients who fit the criteria for ablative therapy, cryotherapy can effectively treat all grades of CIN. The critical point in the effective application of cryotherapy for treatment of

CIN is complete understanding of its limitations. Only patients in whom a high rate of cure can be expected should be treated with cryotherapy, whereas the others should be treated with alternative modalities such as LEEP and laser surgery.

Cryotherapy Physics

The lethal zone is under the probe at the center of the ice ball and extends to a point 2 mm proximal to the margin of the ice ball.

Cryotherapy involves the cooling of tissue (usually with nitrous oxide) until cryonecrosis has occurred. Freezing of the tissue followed by thawing leads to formation of intracellular ice crystals, expansion of intracellular material, and rupture of the cells with subsequent denaturation of cell proteins. During cryotherapy, freezing of tissue results after formation of an ice ball. When nitrous oxide is used, the temperature at the tip of the cryoprobe is between $-65°C$ and $-85°C$. Cell death occurs at $-20°C$. At the margin of the ice ball, the temperature is $0°C$. The lethal zone is under the probe at the center of the ice ball and extends to a point 2 mm proximal to the margin of the ice ball. Distal from that point to the margin of the ice ball is a recovery zone where the temperature of the ice ball is between $0°C$ and $-20°C$. The extent of the lateral spread of the ice ball also gives a good approximation of the depth of the freeze. An ice ball that forms 7 mm lateral to the probe can be expected to have frozen the tissue about 7 mm deep to the probe. However, because the freeze is nonlethal in the last 2 mm, the freeze cannot be assumed to have treated disease any deeper than 5 mm.

Patient Selection

Destruction to a depth of 7 mm should eradicate involved crypts in more than 99% of cases.

Histologic evaluations of cervical tissue have shown that the mean depth to which cervical glandular crypts are involved with dysplasia is 1.24 mm. This means that most of the time, when there is extension of dysplasia into the cervical glandular crypts, the disease will be within the depth that can be effectively treated with cryotherapy. However, some dysplasia involves glandular crypts that are deeper. Destruction to a depth of 7 mm should eradicate involved crypts in more than 99% of cases. It is for this reason that most authorities recommend treatment of dysplasia be at least 7 mm deep to maximize the cure rate. Cryotherapy does not reliably treat tissue to that depth. Although cryotherapy is usually effective in the management of CIN, because it usually destroys to a depth of 5 mm as well as 5 mm lateral to the edge of the cryoprobe,[44, 45] others have demonstrated that the cure rate for high-grade disease may be lower. In one study,[46] tissue temperatures during cryotherapy were measured, and it was found that use of a small, flat probe could not eradicate disease located deep within glandular crypts. Because crypt involvement is a characteristic of high-grade lesions such as CIN 3, the study's author advocated that such cases be managed with excision rather than cryotherapy.

> **Cure rates may be reduced when cryotherapy is used to treat women whose cervix is large or whose lesion is large or extends into the endocervical canal.**

The location of lesional tissue may also play a role in the effectiveness of cryotherapy. Lesions at the 3- and 9-o'clock positions on the cervix have an increased blood supply from the cervical branches of the uterine artery. The blood flowing through the area warms the tissue and makes it slightly more resistant to reaching the critical lethal temperature with freezing. This reduces the cure rate.[47] Finally, a large lesion (greater than two quadrants), a large cervix (greater than 3 to 3.5 cm), and extension of disease into the endocervical canal all result in a reduced cure rate with cryotherapy. It is not the grade of the lesion that determines effectiveness of therapy, but the size of the lesion being treated.[38, 39, 41] It has been demonstrated that if disease in the endocervical canal is treated with cryotherapy, the failure rate is higher.[39, 48] In each case, the higher failure rate is related to the inability of the probe to freeze all the diseased tissue down to the critical lethal temperature.

Equipment

> **Use of a flat cryoprobe or one with a small central nipple diminishes the possibility of cervical stenosis.**

The equipment required for cryotherapy is listed in Table 24–3. There are several types of cryosurgical units, with the basic components consisting of a tank of nitrous oxide with a pressure gauge, a handle, and a probe to apply to the cervix. Ferris and Ho reviewed the various cryotherapy units available in 1992.[49] The choice of a cryoprobe to be used depends on the size of the lesion and the morphology of the transformation zone. Use of a flat cryoprobe or one with a small central nipple diminishes the possibility of cervical stenosis (Fig. 24–9). This type of probe will also be less likely to cause the SCJ to recess into the endocervical canal resulting in an unsatisfactory colposcopy on follow-up examination.[50–53] Large probes should be avoided on cervices with a portio diameter of less than 3 to 3.5 cm. It is important to use a

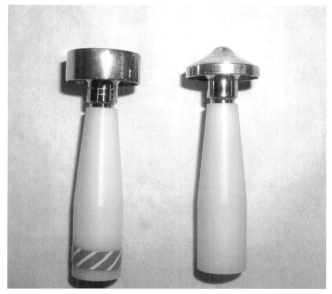

Figure 24–9. Flat probe and probe with a shallow central tip.

large nitrous oxide tank with a pressure gauge and at least 20 pounds of pressure. This will allow for a faster and more effective freeze. With smaller tanks, the pressure may drop below the critical level in the middle of the procedure, making it impossible to achieve an adequate size ice ball. It is also important to have several cryoprobe tips available to choose from, including an assortment of shapes and sizes. This will allow the clinician to choose the appropriate size and maximize the chances of cure.

Technique

> **The best time to perform cryosurgery is 1 week after the start of the menses.**

The best time to perform cryosurgery is 1 week after start of the patient's menses. This ensures that the patient is not pregnant and allows the cervix to heal before the next menses. When cryosurgery is performed immediately before menses, the cervix may swell and block the menstrual outflow, causing cramping. If there is a possibility that the patient is pregnant, a pregnancy test should be performed before the procedure.

The patient is placed in the dorsal lithotomy position, and an intravaginal speculum is inserted. If the vaginal sidewalls prevent adequate visualization of the cervix, or if they are lax and overlap the cervix, a vaginal sidewall retractor should be used. This prevents inadvertent freezing of the vagina. Colposcopy is performed to confirm the absence of invasive disease. The nitrous oxide tank is activated, and the clinician should check the pressure gauge to confirm that the pressure in the tank is sufficient (at least 20 pounds with the indicator in the green zone) before starting the procedure. If the pressure is inadequate, the treatment will not be successful. A properly sized and shaped cryoprobe is selected, placed on the cryogun, and screwed tightly in place. An improperly

▼ Table 24–3

Equipment Needed for Cryosurgery

Cryogun
Large nitrous oxide tank with a pressure gauge and at least 20 psi of pressure in the tank
Various sizes and shapes of cryotips
Water-soluble lubricating gel
Vaginal speculum
Colposcope
3% to 5% acetic acid or vinegar
Vaginal wall retractors
Disinfectant for cryoprobes

secured probe tip can become a projectile when it is subjected to high pressure once the probe is activated. The gun is activated, and the O-ring on the stem is checked. If gas escapes around the contact area between the probe and the stem of the cryogun, the O-ring should be replaced.

The cryoprobe should cover the transformation zone but not contact the vaginal sidewalls.

The cryogun with the probe attached is inserted into the vagina and applied to the transformation zone to check if the size of probe is adequate. The probe should cover the transformation zone but not touch the vaginal sidewalls. When treating a very large transformation zone, overlapping treatments may be needed. After the correct size of probe is determined, the cryogun is removed from the vagina, and a thin layer of lubricating gel is applied to the cryoprobe to effect a sufficient seal with the cervix. The cryogun is placed on cervix again and is activated to allow gas to flow into the unit. The patient should be warned that she will hear a pop and hiss as the cryogun is activated. The freeze should continue until at least a 7- to 10-mm ice ball is present outside the probe. Time is not as critical as formation of the ice ball, because each cervix requires a different time to create the 7- to 10-mm ice ball formation. If the nitrous oxide tank has sufficient pressure at the start of the procedure, a sufficient freeze should be achieved in 3 to 5 minutes, with the time being somewhat less for the second freeze. Freezing for more than 5 minutes does not appreciably increase the size of the ice ball or improve outcome.[47] However, it is important to recognize that the total ice ball lateral spread of freeze of 7 to 10 mm is necessary to ensure a freeze depth of 5 mm. Although this size of ice ball is ideal, the ice ball should be no less than 5 mm beyond the edge of the cryoprobe to ensure an adequate freeze. The less the lateral spread of the ice ball, the less the depth of the treatment (Figs. 24–10 and 24–11).

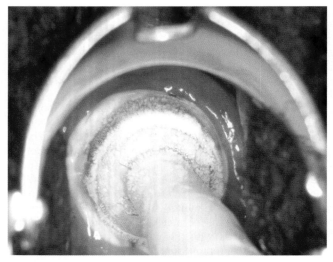

Figure 24–10. Probe applied to the cervical transformation zone. The ice ball can be seen forming peripheral to the edge of the probe.

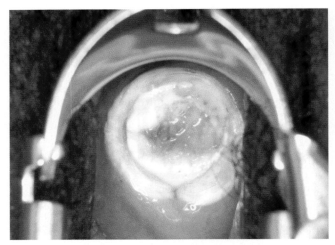

Figure 24–11. Appearance of the cervix after the cryoprobe is removed.

After the ice ball is sufficiently formed, the cryogun is deactivated, and the cervix is allowed to thaw for approximately 4 to 5 minutes. During thawing, the central zone under the probe tip becomes soft. It is important not to remove the probe tip from the cervix until it is defrosted. Pulling the probe off the cervix before it is defrosted produces pain and bleeding. Although there is controversy over whether a single freeze or a double freeze is more effective, in general, a freeze-thaw-freeze regimen is recommended.[47, 54] If a freeze-thaw-freeze regimen is selected, the cryoprobe is again placed on cervix, and another freeze is performed. This freeze should also be sufficiently long for a 7-mm ice ball to form. A 10-mm ice ball is ideal but is rarely achieved. Once the cervix has thawed, the cryoprobe is removed from the vagina.

Re-epithelialization is complete 6 weeks post treatment in 47% of patients and in all patients by 3 months.

On the day of the procedure, the tissue demonstrates erythema and hyperemia. Within the next 24 to 48 hours, bullae or vesicles form with associated edema. The tissue then sloughs. The eschar corresponds to the depth of the freeze. Cervices heal by granulation and re-epithelialization. Re-epithelialization is complete in 47% of patients 6 weeks post treatment and in all patients by 3 months[55] (Fig. 24–12).

Side Effects and Complications of Treatment

Patients will experience a profuse, watery discharge for 2 to 3 weeks after cryotherapy of the cervix.

Cryotherapy of the cervix is usually accompanied by pain and cramping of varying degrees.[56] These cramps are produced by release of prostaglandins and are relieved by nonsteroidal anti-inflammatory agents. Some advocate for

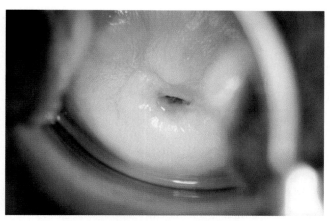

Figure 24–12. Appearance of cervix 3 months after cryotherapy. Note the hypertrophic appearance of the cervix and the paleness, especially near the os. This represents posttreatment stromal fibrosis.

use of local anesthesia at the time of cryotherapy to reduce pain associated with the procedure. About 3% of patients experience cramps severe enough to warrant stronger drugs. About 20% of patients experience flushing and lightheadedness; therefore, patients should rise slowly from the examination table after the procedure. Patients will experience a profuse, watery discharge for 2 to 3 weeks after the cryotherapy.[55] There are some who believe the discharge may be decreased by the use of Amino-Cerv twice daily for 14 days. Removal of the eschar 2 days after the procedure does not significantly reduce the amount of discharge.[57] Cryotherapy is contraindicated in pregnancy; if there is a suspicion for cancer; if there is a discrepancy among the colposcopy, cytology, and histology results; or if an active cervical, vaginal, or pelvic infection exists.

There is no evidence that cryotherapy negatively affects future fertility or pregnancy outcome.

Some individuals advocate that adolescents be tested for gonorrhea and chlamydia within 2 weeks of therapy.[51] Cervical stenosis sufficient to prevent passage of the cytobrush is rare. To minimize the risk of cervical stenosis, the external os should be probed at each follow-up visit. Serious complications related to cryotherapy are rare.[42] Possible complications include vasovagal episodes, infection, mucometria, infection, and bleeding. There is no evidence that cryotherapy has any adverse impact on fertility or pregnancy outcome.[58]

COLD KNIFE CONIZATION

For many years, and even before the popularity of colposcopy, CKC was the standard treatment for treating CIN when uterine conservation was the desired outcome. In more recent years, the ease with which laser conization and LEEP conization may be done, the fact that these procedures can be performed in outpatient settings, and their reduced morbidity relative to CKC have combined to create a trend whereby these newer procedures frequently replace CKC. Many practitioners have limited the

use of CKC to situations in which very large conizations are needed or in which evaluation of the histology is critical and the risk of even a small possibility of cautery artifact at the margins cannot be tolerated. Such instances include cases where invasive or microinvasive carcinoma is suspected or cases of adenocarcinoma in situ of the cervix. However, even with these indications, some feel that, in the hands of an experienced practitioner, laser conization or electrosurgical loop conization can provide an adequate specimen with respect to size and histologic quality.

The risk of intraoperative bleeding and the need for surgical assistance mean that CKC is almost always done in the operating room.

Although some have suggested that CKC can be done with local anesthesia, the risk of intraoperative bleeding and the need for surgical assistance (retraction) mean that this procedure is almost always done in the operating room.

Technique

The patient is placed in the dorsal lithotomy position, and a speculum is inserted into the vagina, exposing the cervix. The transformation zone and the lesion are then delineated. If a colposcope is available, the procedure is done under direct colposcopic guidance, but if one is not available, the cervix is painted with Lugol's iodine to identify the limits of the transformation zone and the limits of the lesion.

A variety of techniques have been used in an attempt to limit blood loss during CKC, including placement of lateral hemostatic sutures and use of vasoconstrictive agents.

A variety of techniques have been used in an attempt to limit blood loss during CKC. The most popular of these involves laterally placed hemostatic sutures at the proximal portion of the cervix to ligate the descending cervical branches of the uterine artery. Another approach is to inject a vasopressor agent directly into the substance of the cervix in a manner similar to that used in laser and LEEP conization. Many clinicians use both techniques. A circumferential incision is then made at the periphery of the transformation zone as delineated by colposcopy or Lugol's staining. The incision need not be circular and can follow the border of the transformation zone and lesion. The incision is then continued deeper, gradually tapering toward the endocervical canal until the specimen is removed. The size and shape of the specimen and the extent of the taper are all determined by the location and extent of disease. Grasping the cone specimen with a tissue forceps facilitates traction and manipulation of the specimen. However, because this may cause trauma that will denude the cervical epithelium and make it impossible to adequately evaluate the cone histologically, some surgeons place traction sutures into the cone specimen at the start of the procedure and use these sutures to manipulate the specimen. Some of these sutures can be left in place at the conclusion of the procedure to help the pathologist identify the 12-o'clock position on the specimen.

After removal of the specimen, a variety of techniques can be used to achieve hemostasis of the cone bed. The traditional Sturmdorf suture is a vertical mattress suture that folds the remaining ectocervical epithelium into the conization bed and tamponades the bleeding vessels. Although effective at achieving hemostasis, this technique distorts the cervical anatomy and makes it very difficult to adequately visualize the transformation zone in the future. As a result, most authorities now advocate that bleeding in the conization bed be controlled by electrocautery, simple sutures, or even Monsel's paste, rather than by Sturmdorf sutures.

Complications

CKC has the highest complication rate of any of the treatments for CIN.

CKC has the highest complication rate of any of the treatments for CIN. Short-term and long-term complications include primary and secondary hemorrhage, infection, cervical stenosis, and increased pregnancy wastage. The incidence of significant bleeding after CKC is between 5% and 10%.[59] Should bleeding develop, it is important to evaluate the patient under ideal conditions. This involves visualization of the cervix to identify any bleeding site and treating the bleeding point with cautery or simple suturing. Generalized oozing can be treated with Monsel's paste or gel. In rare cases, a tight pack should be inserted into the vagina and the patient observed in the hospital for 24 hours. Despite significant bleeding, blood transfusion is rarely necessary.

Cervical stenosis occurs in 2% to 3% of patients who undergo CKC,[59] although this is a relatively rare problem. It is more common that the entire transformation zone cannot be visualized after CKC, and this may represent a problem in follow-up.

It is likely that the incidence of infertility and pregnancy wastage after CKC is directly related to the size of the cone itself.

The question of fertility after CKC is controversial;[60-62] however, in all likelihood, the incidence of infertility and pregnancy wastage after CKC is directly related to the size of the cone itself.[63] The larger the cone, the greater the incidence of infertility and preterm labor.

SUMMARY OF KEY POINTS

- LEEP excises the transformation zone with high-frequency (radiofrequency) current using a thin electrode.
- Modern ESUs used in LEEP incorporate many advances that allow the operator to excise large specimens with a minimal amount of thermal damage and a minimal risk of bleeding and other complications.

- Cutting during LEEP requires very high and continuous current density so that the water in the cell rapidly boils and the cell explodes. To accomplish this, the electrode must not come in direct contact with the tissue.
- A steam envelope that forms around the loop is critical to achieving the power density necessary to cut with LEEP. If the loop is moved too quickly, the steam envelope collapses and places the electrode in direct contact with the tissue. Instead of the tissue being cut, desiccation occurs and thermal damage ensues.
- The size and shape of the loop used should be tailored to the size and extent of the transformation zone and its extension into the endocervical canal.
- Complications of LEEP include intraoperative and postoperative bleeding or infection. An unsatisfactory colposcopy occurs in 1.3% to 9% of women after LEEP, and cervical stenosis occurs in 1.3% to 3.85% of treated women.
- The CO_2 laser produces a monochromatic beam of light in the infrared portion of the spectrum that is coherent and collimated. At its focal point, the energy produced by the laser beam is sufficient to instantaneously boil the intracellular water of the tissue.
- A micromanipulator is attached to the colposcope and allows the operator to view the laser beam through the colposcope and to control it via a joystick, to vary the spot size of the laser and raise or lower the power density.
- In well-selected patients who are candidates for ablative therapy, cryotherapy can effectively treat all grades of CIN.
- Cryotherapy involves the cooling of tissue, usually with nitrous oxide, until cryonecrosis has occurred. Freezing of the tissue followed by thawing leads to formation of intracellular ice crystals, expansion of intracellular material, and rupture of the cells with subsequent denaturation of cell proteins.
- Freezing of the tissue with cryotherapy results after formation of an ice ball. The lethal zone of cellular death is under the cryoprobe at the center of the ice ball and extends to a point 2 mm proximal to the margin of the ice ball.
- Cervical dysplasia involving gland crypts may be too deep for adequate cellular destruction with cryotherapy.
- Reasons for lower-than-expected cure rates of cryotherapy include failure to perform a freeze-thaw-freeze technique, a large cervix (3 cm to 3.5 cm), a lesion larger than two quadrants, and extension of disease into the endocervical canal.
- Cryotherapy should be performed 1 week after

menses to avoid edema that could block menstrual flow, causing cramping.

- To ensure an adequate freeze, the ice ball formation should be no less than 5 mm beyond the edge of the cryoprobe.

- Cryotherapy may be accompanied by cramping of varying degrees. Most patients will experience a profuse, watery discharge for 2 to 3 weeks after the procedure. Cervical stenosis as a result of the procedure is rare.

- There is no evidence that cryotherapy, laser surgery, or LEEP has an adverse impact on fertility or pregnancy outcome.

- CKC is usually performed when large specimens are needed or when evaluation of the histology is critical and any thermal damage is not acceptable. Such instances include cases of suspected microinvasive carcinoma or adenocarcinoma in situ.

- Complications of CKC include intraoperative and postoperative hemorrhage, cervical stenosis, and increased pregnancy wastage.

References

1. Prendiville W, Cullimore J, Norman S: Large loop excision of the transformation zone (LLETZ). A new method of management for women with cervical intraepithelial neoplasia. Br J Obstet Gynaecol 1989;96:1054.
2. Bigrigg MA, Codling BW, Pearson P, et al: Colposcopic diagnosis and treatment of cervical dysplasia at a single clinic visit: Experience of low-voltage diathermy loop in 1000 patients. Lancet 1990; 336:229.
3. Luesley DM, Cullimore J, Redman CWE, et al: Loop diathermy excision of the cervical transformation zone in patients with abnormal cervical smears. BMJ 1990;300:1690.
4. Spitzer M, Chernys AE, Seltzer VL: The use of large-loop excision of the transformation zone in an inner-city population. Obstet Gynecol 1993;82:731.
5. Gunasekera C, Phipps JH, Lewis BV: Large loop excision of the transformation zone (LLETZ) compared to carbon dioxide laser in the treatment of CIN: A superior mode of treatment. Br J Obstet Gynaecol 1990;97:995.
6. Hallam NF, West J, Harper C, et al: Large loop excision of the transformation zone (LLETZ) as an alternative to both local ablative and cone biopsy treatment: A series of 1000 patients. J Gynecol Surg 1993;9:77.
7. Alvarez RD, Helm CW, Edwards RP, et al: Prospective randomized trial of LLETZ versus laser ablation in patients with cervical intraepithelial neoplasia. Gynecol Oncol 1994;52:175.
8. Brady JL, Fish ANJ, Woolas RP, et al: Large loop diathermy of the transformation zone: Is 'see and treat' an acceptable option for the management of women with abnormal cervical smears? J Obstet Gynecol 1994;14:44.
9. Wright TC, Richart RM, Ferenczy AF: Electrosurgery for HPV-Related Lesions of the Anogenital Tract. New York, Arthur Vision, 1992.
10. Robinson WR, Webb S, Tirpack J, et al: Management of cervical intraepithelial neoplasia during pregnancy with loop excision. Gynecol Oncol 1997;64:153.
11. Oyesanya O, Amerasinghe C, Manning EAD: A comparison between loop diathermy conization and cold-knife conization for management of cervical dysplasia associated with unsatisfactory colposcopy. Gynecol Oncol 1993;50:84.
12. Mor-Yosef S, Lopes A, Pearson S, et al: Loop diathermy cone biopsy. Obstet Gynecol 1990;775:884.
13. Baggish MS, Barash F, Nowl Y, Brooks M: Comparison of the thermal injury zones in loop electrical and laser cervical excisional conization. Am J Obstet Gynecol 1992;166:545.
14. Wright TC, Richart RM, Ferenczy A, Koulos J: Comparison of specimens removed by CO_2 laser conization and loop electrosurgical excision procedures. Obstet Gynecol 1992;79:147.
15. Turner RJ, Cohen RA, Voet RL, et al: Analysis of tissue margins of cone biopsy specimens obtained with 'cold-knife', CO_2 and Nd:YAG lasers and a radio frequency surgical unit. J Reprod Med 1992;37:607.
16. Wright TC, Gagnon MD, Richart RM, Ferenczy A: Treatment of cervical intraepithelial neoplasia using the loop electrosurgical excision procedure. Obstet Gynecol 1992;79:173.
17. Keijser KG, Kenemans P, van der Zanden PH, et al: Diathermy loop excision in the management of cervical intraepithelial neoplasia: Diagnosis and treatment in one procedure. Am J Obstet Gynecol 1992;166:1281.
18. Murdoch JB, Grimshaw RN, Monaghan JM: Loop diathermy excision of the abnormal cervical transformation zone. Int J Gynecol Cancer 1991;1:105.
19. Lopes A, Pearson SE, Mor-Yosef S, et al: Is it time for a reconsideration of the criteria for cone biopsy? Br J Obstet Gynaecol 1989; 96:1345.
20. Doyle M, Warwick A, Redman C, et al: Does application of Monsel's solution after loop diathermy excision of the transformation zone reduce post-operative discharge? Results of a prospective randomized controlled trial. Br J Obstet Gynaecol 1992;99:1023.
21. Whiteley PF, Olah KS: Treatment of cervical intraepithelial neoplasia: Experience with the low-voltage diathermy loop. Am J Obstet Gynecol 1990;162:1272.
22. Cullimore J: Management of complication from LLETZ. In Prendiville W (ed): Large Loop Excision of the Transformation Zone: A Practical Guide to LLETZ. London, Chapman and Hall Medical, 1993, pp 88–91.
23. Spitzer M: Vaginal estrogen administration to prevent cervical os obliteration following cervical conization in women with amenorrhea. J Lower Genital Tract Dis 1997;1:53.
24. Cruickshank ME, Flannelly G, Campbell DM, Kitchener HC: Fertility and pregnancy outcome following large loop excision of the cervical transformation zone. Br J Obstet Gynaecol 1995;102:467.
25. Bigrigg A, Haffenden DK, Sheehan AL, et al: Efficacy and safety of large-loop excision of the transformation zone. Lancet 1994;343:32.
26. Bloomfield PI, Buxton J, Dunn J, Luesley DM: Pregnancy outcome after large loop excision of the cervical transformation zone. Am J Obstet Gynecol 1993;169:620.
27. Haffenden DK, Bigrigg A, Codling BW, Read MD: Pregnancy following large loop excision of the transformation zone. Br J Obstet Gynaecol 1993;100:1059.
28. Anderson MC: Treatment of cervical intraepithelial neoplasia with the carbon dioxide laser. Report of 543 patients. Obstet Gynecol 1982;59:720.
29. Wright VC, Davies E, Riopelle MA: Laser surgery for cervical intraepithelial neoplasia: Principles and results. Am J Obstet Gynecol 1983;145:181.
30. Baggish MS: Laser management of cervical intraepithelial neoplasia. Clin Obstet Gynecol 1983;26:980.
31. Baggish MS: Complications associated with carbon dioxide laser surgery in gynecology. Am J Obstet Gynecol 1981;139:568.
32. Baggish MS, Dorsey JH, Adelson M: A ten-year experience treating cervical intraepithelial neoplasia with the CO_2. Am J Obstet Gynecol 1989;161:60.
33. Larsson G, Alm P, Grundsell H: Laser conization versus cold knife conization. Surg Gynecol Obstet 1982;154:59.
34. Fenton DW, Soutter WP, Sharp F, James C: A comparison of knife and CO_2 excisional biopsies. In Sharp F, Jordan JA (eds): Gynecological Laser Surgery. New York, Perinatology Press, 1986, pp 77–84.
35. Spitzer M, Krumholz BA, Seltzer VL: Cervical os obliteration after laser surgery in patients with amenorrhea. Obstet Gynecol 1990;76:97.
36. Spitzer M, Herman J, Krumholz BA, Lesser H: The fertility of women after cervical laser surgery. Obstet Gynecol 1995;86:304.
37. Spitzer M: Fertility and pregnancy outcome after treatment of cervical intraepithelial neoplasia. J Lower Genital Tract Dis 1998;2:225.

38. Richart R, Townsend D, Crisp W, et al: An analysis of "long term" followup results in patients with cervical intraepithelial neoplasia treated with cryosurgery. Am J Obstet Gynecol 1980;137:8236.

39. Arof H, Gerbie M, Smeltzer J: Cryosurgical treatment of cervical intraepithelial neoplasia: Four year experience. Am J Obstet Gynecol 1984;150:865.

40. Einerth Y: Cryosurgical treatment of CIN III. A long term study. Acta Obstet Gynecol Scan 1988;67:62730.

41. Mitchell MF, Tortolero-Luna G, Cook E, et al: A randomized clinical trial of cryotherapy, laser vaporization, and loop electrosurgical excision for treatment of squamous intraepithelial lesions of the cervix. Obstet Gynecol 1998;92:737.

42. Nuovo J, Melnikow J, Willan A, Chan B: Treatment outcomes for squamous intraepithelial lesions. Int J Gynacol Obstet 2000;68:25.

43. Martin-Hirsch PL, Paraskevaidis E, Kitchener H: Surgery for cervical intraepithelial neoplasia. Cochrane Database of Systematic Reviews [computer file]. (2):CD001318, 2000.

44. Anderson M, Hartley R: Cervical crypt involvement by intraepithelial neoplasia. Obstet Gynecol 1980;55:546.

45. Boonstra H, Aalders J, Koudstaal J, et al: Minimum extension and appropriate topographic position of tissue destruction for treatment of cervical intraepithelial neoplasia. Obstet Gynecol 1990;75:227.

46. Ferris DG: Lethal tissue temperature during cervical cryotherapy with a small flat cryoprobe. J Fam Pract 1994;38:153.

47. Boonstra H, Koudstaal J, Oosterhuis J, et al: Analysis of cryolesions in the uterine cervix: Application techniques, extensions and failures. Obstet Gynecol 1990;75:232.

48. Ferency A: Comparison of cryo and carbon dioxide laser therapy for cervical intraepithelial neoplasia. Obstet Gynecol 1985;66:7938.

49. Ferris D, Ho J: Cryosurgical equipment: A critical review. J Fam Pract 1992;35:185.

50. Draeby-Kristiansen J, Garsaae M, Bruun M, et al: Ten years after cryosurgical treatment of cervical intraepithelial neoplasia. Am J Obstet Gynecol 1991;165:43.

51. Hillard P, Biro F, Wildey L: Complications of cervical cryotherapy in adolescents. J Reprod Med 1991;36:711.

52. Berget A, Andreasson B, Bock J: Laser and cryosurgery for intraepithelial neoplasia. A randomized trial with long term follow-up. Acta Obstet Gynecol 1991;70:231.

53. Stienstra KA, Brewer BE, Franklin LA: A comparison of flat and shallow conical tips for cervical cryotherapy. J Am Board Fam Pract 1999;12:360.

54. Bryson S, Lenehan P, Lickrish G: The treatment of grade 3 cervical intraepithelial neoplasia with cryotherapy: An 11-year experience. Am J Obstet Gynecol 1985;151:201.

55. Townsend D, Richart R: Cryotherapy and carbon dioxide laser management of cervical intraepithelial neoplasia: A controlled comparison. Obstet Gynecol 1983;61:75.

56. Harper DM: Pain and cramping associated with cryosurgery. J Fam Pract 1994;39:551.

57. Harper DM, Mayeaux EJ, Daaleman TP, et al: The natural history of cervical cryosurgical healing. The minimal effect of debridement of the cervical eschar. J Fam Pract 2000;49:694.

58. Montz FJ: Impact of therapy for cervical intraepithelial neoplasia on fertility. Am J Obstet Gynecol 1996;175:1129.

59. Jones HW: Cone biopsy and hysterectomy in the management of cervical intraepithelial neoplasia. Clin Obstet Gynecol 1995;9:221.

60. Weber T, Obel EB: Pregnancy complications following conization of the uterine cervix. Acta Obstet Gynecol Scand 1979;58:347.

61. Bjerre B, Eliasson G, Linell F, et al: Conization as only treatment of carcinoma in situ of the uterine cervix. Am J Obstet Gynecol 1976;125:143.

62. Jones JM, Sweetnam P, Hibbard BM: The outcome of pregnancy after cone biopsy of the cervix: A case controlled study. Br J Obstet Gynecol 1979;86:913.

63. Leiman G, Harrison NA, Rubin A: Pregnancy following conization of the cervix: Complications related to cone size. Am J Obstet Gynecol 1980;136:14.

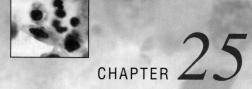

CHAPTER *25*

Management Scenarios

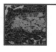

• Mark H. Stoler

A

Management of Abnormal Squamous Cells of Undetermined Significance and Low-Grade Squamous Abnormalities of the Uterine Cervix

The variability of a diagnosis of atypical squamous cells of undetermined significance represents a combination of factors, including evolving cytologic definitions; poor interobserver reproducibility among cytopathologists; and issues of sampling, cellular preservation, and microscopic observation.

The management of low-grade squamous epithelial abnormalities detected on cervical cytology is a common problem for health care providers.[1-4] Although cervical cancer is the second or third most common malignancy affecting women worldwide, in the United States, there are only 12,800 cases of carcinoma annually, resulting in about 4600 deaths. Despite the fact that the United States has a highly screened population, each year only 50 million Papanicolaou (Pap) smears are performed of the 100 million that are potentially needed. Approximately 0.6% (300,000) of the 50 million Pap smears performed each year yield a high-grade squamous intraepithelial lesion (HSIL). The management of this category of cytologic abnormality is not controversial. The standard of care is to detect and eradicate this abnormality. In comparison

with the prevalence of HSIL, approximately 2% to 3% of smears yield a diagnosis of low-grade squamous intraepithelial lesion (LSIL). Although somewhat more variable, a similar number of women are also diagnosed as having atypical squamous cells of undetermined significance (ASCUS). The variability of an ASCUS diagnosis represents a combination of factors, including evolving cytologic definitions; poor interobserver reproducibility among cytopathologists; and issues relating to problems of sampling, cellular preservation, and microscopic observation. These technical and interpretive problems combine to contribute to this heterogeneity. The diagnostic accuracy of ASCUS smears is limited because, by definition, they are either equivocal or nondiagnostic for either squamous intraepithelial lesion or some other well-defined benign entity.

The management of ASCUS/LSIL is of concern because a small but important minority of these women have HSIL or even carcinoma on colposcopy and biopsy.

Through the mid-1990s, there was no universal agreement as to how to best manage women with a cytologic diagnosis of LSIL or ASCUS.[5] It seems clear from retrospective data that most low-grade lesions regress spontaneously and that many equivocal lesions are shown to be benign. This is particularly true in younger women in whom the ASCUS/LSIL diagnosis most commonly represents the recent acquisition of a human papillomavirus (HPV) infection that usually proves to be pathologically and clinically transient.[6–11] However, the management of ASCUS/LSIL is of concern because a small but important minority of these women are found to have HSIL or even carcinoma on colposcopy and biopsy.[2, 12–14] Thus, the critical question in the management of a woman presenting with an ASCUS or LSIL Pap smear is her risk for having invasive carcinoma or one of its proximate precursors (e.g., HSIL). Until the 1990s, hard data addressing this question were lacking.

> **Immediate colposcopy for women with ASCUS/LSIL in a population where the prevalence of HSIL is low can be a very expensive option, resulting in many unnecessary colposcopies and overtreatment of a significant number of women.**

Given these concerns, clinicians have been operating under guidelines that promote any of three possible strategies for the management of ASCUS/LSIL.[5] The most aggressive strategy is immediate colposcopy. Assuming an adequate and skilled colposcopic assessment, this strategy has the advantage of being highly sensitive for the detection of prevalent HSIL. However, if the prevalence of HSIL in the population is low, this can be a very expensive option, resulting in many unnecessary colposcopies and overtreatment of a significant number of women. In contrast, conservative management usually takes the form of cytologic follow-up for low-grade abnormalities. In the limited and retrospective literature available, this option is often found to be safe and effective, particularly for young individuals in whom the short-term risk of developing invasive cancer is very low. Unfortunately, the societal expectation of "perfect" prevention of cervical cancer has increased the pressure on the clinician to do "everything possible" to prevent cervical cancer. Also, women are often unwilling to wait for the outcome of long-term cytologic observation. Thus, some clinicians and patients may be uncomfortable with conservative management. An intermediate strategy would be highly attractive if it limited the proportion of colposcopic referrals while effectively finding almost all the women with HSIL among those presenting with either LSIL or ASCUS on cytology. Such a strategy could potentially clarify management guidelines for women with ASCUS and LSIL. Several large clinical trials have started to attempt to address this question.

THE ASCUS/LSIL TRIAGE STUDY

The National Cancer Institute initiated the ASCUS/LSIL triage study (ALTS) in the late 1990s. ALTS is a multi-center, randomized clinical trial designed to evaluate three alternative methods for the management of women presenting with low-grade squamous abnormalities on Pap smear. Those methods are immediate colposcopy, cytologic follow-up, and triage with HPV DNA testing.[4] The background and rationale for this trial take into account improvements in our knowledge of the biology of LSIL and the relationship of HPV infection to the development of squamous intraepithelial lesion and cervical cancer.

> **ALTS was designed to evaluate the three strategies for triage of mild cervical cytologic abnormalities: immediate colposcopy, cytologic follow-up, and triage using HPV DNA testing.**

At the time of the second Bethesda Workshop in 1991, participants disagreed strongly on the proper management of ASCUS and LSIL.[15, 16] However, they did agree on what the main management strategies might be: immediate colposcopy, cytologic follow-up, and triage using HPV DNA testing. Over the decade of the 1990s, advances in HPV testing finally produced an accurate and reproducible HPV assay system.[17–24] Accurate HPV DNA testing could be helpful in the management of ASCUS/LSIL in two ways. First, the risk of HSIL is strongly associated with the patient's HPV type. This association might help predict the natural history of low-grade lesions. More importantly, with a sensitive assay, the presence or absence of high-risk HPV types might help define the accuracy of the original cytologic diagnosis, in that HPV-negative patients are more likely to have had a false-positive cytologic diagnosis. Therefore, ALTS was designed to evaluate the three strategies for triage of mild cervical cytologic abnormalities. The main end point of the study is the detection of all cases of histopathologically defined cervical intraepithelial neoplasia (CIN) grade 3 using a strict *truth determination* algorithm.[4] Immediate colposcopic assessment was used as the reference standard for sensitivity. The specific objectives of the trial were as follows:

1. To determine the effectiveness of cytologic follow-up of ASCUS and LSIL. Patients were followed at 6-month intervals for a period of 2 years.
2. To assess whether the addition of one-time HPV testing provides accurate, cost-effective triage for patients with a Pap smear diagnosis of ASCUS or LSIL. The assay used was the commercially available Hybrid Capture II (HCII) test at a 1-pg/mL cutoff level.

Women 18 years and older with no known history of ablative or excisional therapy of the cervix were invited to participate in ALTS. After a community referral diagnosis of ASCUS or LSIL, eligible women underwent an enrollment evaluation that included pelvic examination, collection of cervical specimens for a liquid-based (ThinPrep) cytologic evaluation, and HPV DNA testing for high-risk HPV types out of the ThinPrep collection vial. The patients were randomized to one of three arms. Women in the immediate colposcopy (IC) arm were referred for colposcopy immediately or within 3 weeks of enrollment. Women in the conservative management arm

(CM) were referred for colposcopy only for a cytologic diagnosis of HSIL or carcinoma. Women randomized to HPV triage were sent for colposcopy when the enrollment test was HPV DNA positive for cancer-associated HPV types or, rarely, when it was missing or inadequate. Regardless of the arm into which they were randomized, all women were followed at 6-month intervals for 2 years. At each 6-month follow-up visit, enrollees had a pelvic examination and repeat collection of a ThinPrep specimen for both masked HPV testing and cytologic evaluation. Those patients whose cytologic diagnosis during follow-up was HSIL or carcinoma were immediately referred for colposcopic examination. At the 24-month exit visit, all women were scheduled for a colposcopic examination. The preferred management of any identified lesions was the loop electrocautery excision procedure (LEEP) so that a definitive pathologic assessment could be made. A detailed description of this clinical trial, including the multi-layered quality assurance assessments and safety net structures, has been published.[4]

High-Risk HPV Types in LSIL

> **Most women with LSIL are positive for cancer-associated HPV types. Because of this finding, the potential for this assay to effectively triage a population of women with an LSIL diagnosis is obviously limited.**

> **Most of these "high-risk" HPV viral infections produce only low-grade lesions that are transient and not productive of high-grade dysplasia.**

Before discussing management strategies for mildly dysplastic (LSIL) Pap smears as compared with ASCUS Pap smears, it is pertinent to review some of the data from the enrollment phase of the ALTS. As noted previously, the central question of the ALTS trial was whether a high-quality HPV test can be useful in the triage of women with either of these cytologic diagnoses. Several cross-sectional clinical studies have used HPV testing in the triage of women with mild abnormalities on their Pap smear.[19, 25, 26] These studies suggested that cancer-associated HPV DNA testing is highly sensitive for histologically confirmed HSIL, and that HPV testing of women with LSIL would be most useful if cancer-associated HPV types were not detected in the great majority of women with LSIL. If most women with LSIL were positive for cancer-associated HPV types, HPV DNA testing would not be useful in the triage of LSIL. Indeed, the ALTS enrollment data showed that the latter is the case.[27] An early analysis of the enrollment database before completion of enrollment demonstrated that of 642 women with an LSIL diagnosis who had analyzable HPV (HCII) results, 82.9% of the women (95% confidence interval [CI] = 79.7% to 85.7%) tested positive for the high-risk probe mix used in the HCII assay. This high frequency of high-risk HPV positivity was confirmed by independent polymerase chain reaction assays on a subset of 210 of these patients with a very high concordance. Because of this finding, the potential for this assay to effectively

triage a population of women with an LSIL diagnosis is obviously limited. This study supports a growing consensus that earlier reports, which suggested that low-grade dysplasias were highly associated with low-risk HPV viral types, were incorrect. Most of the mucosotropic viral infections that occur in the uterine cervix are high-risk viral types. Furthermore, most of these "high-risk" viral infections produce only low-grade lesions that are transient and not productive of high-grade dysplasia. Thus, the term *high-risk* or *oncogenic HPV* is a relative misnomer.[1, 7, 10]

Correlation of HPV Testing in the ASCUS Population

> **Based on the *truth-determined* diagnoses, 55% of the ASCUS diagnoses for the enrollment referral cytologies were confirmed, 31% of cases were downgraded to negative/reactive, and 14% were upgraded to squamous intraepithelial lesion (11% LSIL and 3% HSIL).**

Because of the findings in the population of women with LSIL, the HPV enrollment arm for the LSIL subset in the ALTS was closed and the other arms of the trial were enriched with additional ASCUS patients. This led to a final enrollment of 3488 women with a referral diagnosis of ASCUS randomized equally among the three arms of the trial. In addition, 1572 LSIL patients completed the enrollment data set of 5060 women.[28] Based on the *truth-determined* diagnoses, 55% of the ASCUS diagnoses for the enrollment referral cytologies were confirmed, 31% of cases were downgraded to negative/reactive, and 14% were upgraded to squamous intraepithelial lesion (11% LSIL and 3% HSIL). Virtually all of these were conventional Pap smears. For the correlated ThinPrep smears collected at the enrollment examination, 44.9% were negative; 32.5% were ASCUS; 18.1% were LSIL, and, most significantly, only 7% were diagnosed as HSIL. By protocol, all patients in the IC arm, all patients with an absent or positive HPV HCII test result in the HPV arm, and all patients with an HSIL cytologic diagnosis in the CM arm were referred for an immediate colposcopic examination. Biopsies were taken of any colposcopically suspected squamous intraepithelial lesion. If the biopsy results at the clinical center showed CIN 2 or worse, a LEEP was performed. Final case definitions were based on the pathology quality control group diagnoses. The most severe histologic finding for a woman was considered her enrollment final diagnosis.

> **Of the 1149 women with ASCUS smears on enrollment in the immediate colposcopy arm of the ALTS, the combined prevalence of HSIL was 11.4%. In contrast, when the threshold used for cytologic triage to colposcopy was HSIL, on the repeat cytology the prevalence of high-grade disease was only 4.8%.**

Assuming that the colposcopically directed biopsy provided virtually complete ascertainment of disease, then the immediate colposcopy arm reflected the prevalence of disease among those patients enrolled in the ASCUS trial. Of the 1149 women in this arm, 25.4% had no lesion identified at colposcopy, 46.9% had no pathologic lesion on biopsy, 14.5% had CIN 1, 6.3% had CIN 2, and 5.1% had CIN 3. Thus, overall, the combined CIN 2 plus CIN 3 (HSIL+) prevalence was 11.4%. There was no statistical difference between the prevalence of HSIL+ in the HPV triage arm and that in the IC arm. This strongly suggests that HPV triage captures all the high-grade disease. In contrast, when the threshold used for cytologic triage to colposcopy was repeat cytology with a diagnosis of HSIL, the prevalence of high-grade disease was much lower in the CM arm. Specifically, 56 of 1164 (4.8%) cases of CIN 2+ were identified in the CM arm using the HSIL+ cytologic referral threshold, as compared with 267 of 2324 (11.5%) in the combined IC + HPV arm. This deficit was highly statistically significant (p < 0.001).

> **In patients presenting with an ASCUS cytology, management with repeat cytology using a threshold of ASCUS or greater is nearly equivalent to a highly sensitive HPV test in selecting patients for referral to colposcopy.**

In summary, at the clinically relevant threshold of HSIL (CIN 2+), HPV testing as performed in the ALTS had a sensitivity of 95% (CI 92% to 97%).[28] This resulted in referral to colposcopy of 55% of patients with a positive predictive value of 20% and a negative predictive value of 99%. In other words, women could be 99% sure that they did not have a high-grade CIN lesion (CIN 2+) if their HPV test for high-risk HPV types was negative. The triage arm using the conservative HSIL+ cytology threshold had a sensitivity of 35% (CI 29% to 41%) while referring 7% of the patients to colposcopy. It had a positive predictive value of 58% and a negative predictive value of 92%. However, lowering the cytology referral threshold to any squamous abnormality (i.e., ASCUS+) improved the sensitivity to 85% (CI 80% to 89%) but resulted in 58% of the patients being referred to colposcopy. It had a positive predictive value of 17% and a negative predictive value of 96%. Thus, in patients presenting with an ASCUS cytology, management with repeat cytology using a threshold of ASCUS or greater is nearly equivalent to using a highly sensitive HPV test in selecting patients for referral to colposcopy. The implications of this finding will be discussed further.

Interobserver Reproducibility of Cervical Cytologic and Histologic Diagnosis

> **The reproducibility of biopsy diagnosis is at least as variable and problematic as that of cytologic diagnosis. The evolution of diagnostic classifications, the amount of experience that a colposcopist may have in recognizing abnormalities, the quality and location of colposcopic biopsy, and the experience of the pathologist with the spectrum of biopsies presented are all sources of diagnostic variability.**

Some additional contextual information is necessary. The interaction between the clinician and the pathologist is critical to the management of cervical neoplasia. Clear communication between the parties regarding the clinical and pathologic findings allows optimal management while minimizing patient morbidity. From the clinician's standpoint, it is of paramount importance to know how well his or her clinical and colposcopic impressions correlate with the pathologist's cytologic and histologic diagnoses. Patient management is entirely predicated on the pathologist's diagnosis. Variability in diagnostic interpretation of any given smear or biopsy may lead to radically different patient management decisions. Inherent in the colposcopy-biopsy management strategy is the assumption that the colposcopically directed cervical biopsy is an accurate representation of what is found on the patient's cervix. The clinician often assumes that the results of the biopsy taken under colposcopic guidance accurately represent the severity of the pathology visualized through the colposcope. In addition, it is a common clinical assumption that it is easier for the pathologist to arrive at a biopsy-based pathologic diagnosis than a cytologic diagnosis and that this diagnosis is more reproducible. However, examination of literature underlying these assumptions suggests that the reproducibility of biopsy diagnosis is at least as variable and problematic as that of cytologic diagnosis. As far back as the mid-1960s, Ashley stated that any competent pathologist should be able to accurately diagnose carcinoma in situ of the cervix; the literature has failed to support such a statement.[29–46] Furthermore, the evolution of diagnostic classifications may hinder, rather than improve, communication between pathologists and clinicians. Other sources of diagnostic variability include the amount of experience that a colposcopist has in recognizing abnormalities, the quality and location of colposcopic biopsy, and the experience of the pathologist with the spectrum of biopsies presented for routine diagnosis.[47–50]

Clearly, diagnostic reproducibility is critical to the practice of pathology as well as to the clinical management of pathologically diagnosed cervical cancer and its precursors. Previous studies on the reproducibility of cervical neoplasia diagnosis are best characterized as limited in size and, for the most part, statistically inadequate. The controversy in the United States over the proper evaluation and management of LSIL and equivocal (ASCUS) cervical cytologic diagnoses was the primary reason for the development of the ALTS. The ALTS was designed in part to compare reproducibility of both cytologic and histologic diagnoses of the pathologist at the clinical center and the central pathology quality assurance group. Careful statistical design and multiple data correlations, including HPV testing, provide the ideal database for evaluating reproducibility of both cervical cytology and histologic diagnosis.[51]

> **Regardless of specimen type, there was only moderate interobserver reproducibility between the pathologist at the clinical center and the quality control pathology group, with quality control pathologists tending to give less severe interpretations of all three types of specimens.**

As noted previously, during enrollment in the ALTS, the clinical centers interpreted 4948 ThinPreps and 2237 colposcopic biopsies. Both groups also independently reviewed 535 LEEP specimens. The comparisons between the clinical center and the quality control groups were performed in a completely masked manner. All pathologists were masked to each other's diagnosis as well as to the colposcopic data and the HPV DNA test results. To quantify the extent of diagnostic agreement, kappa values were calculated to test the level of interobserver agreement in diagnoses. The conclusion of these analyses was that, regardless of specimen type, there was only moderate interobserver reproducibility between the pathologist at the clinical center and the quality control pathology group. There was significant asymmetry in each class of comparison, suggesting that there was a systematic pattern of disagreement between the clinical center and the quality control pathologists, with quality control pathologists tending to give less severe interpretations in all three types of specimens.

Specifically, for thin-layer cytology, the overall kappa was 0.46. Of 1473 original diagnoses of ASCUS, only 43% of those diagnoses were concordant with the quality control group final diagnosis. Most of the rest were downgraded to normal by the quality control pathology group. There was also significant variation among HSIL, for which concordance was only 47% (47.1%, with 27% and 22.6% of diagnoses downgraded to LSIL or ASCUS, respectively, by the quality control reviewers). Thus, the overall kappa for enrollment ThinPrep cytology in the ALTS was 0.46 (CI 0.44 to 0.48), and, not surprisingly, the equivocal classification (ASCUS) was the source of most interobserver disagreement.

Diagnostic reproducibility on colposcopic biopsies was no better than cytologic reproducibility and derived largely from disagreements about the morphologic criteria for mild dysplasia/CIN 1/LSIL. Having more abundant tissue (i.e., LEEP specimens) did not significantly improve interobserver reproducibility.

Overall, diagnostic reproducibility on colposcopic biopsies was no better than cytologic reproducibility. The kappa values for colposcopic biopsy were virtually identical for the 2237 biopsies in the analysis. However, the histologic variability derived largely from disagreements about the morphologic criteria for mild dysplasia/CIN 1/LSIL (including koilocytotic atypia). The diagnosis of CIN 1 at the clinical centers was corroborated by the quality control group in only 42.6% of 887 biopsies. Of originally diagnosed CIN 1 biopsies, the pathology quality control group called 41% negative. Equivocal diagnoses on histology were exceptionally rare (8.2% and 3.5% of the clinical center versus quality control diagnoses, respectively). As expected, there was much better concordance at the extremes of diagnosis, with totally normal histologic specimens and HSIL demonstrating concordance in 90.8% and 76.9% of cases, respectively. Having more abundant tissue (i.e., LEEP specimens) did not significantly improve interobserver reproducibility.

Although these data support the concept that even among experts there is no better than moderate interobserver reproducibility, the question of how to best determine the true diagnosis in problematic cases of disagreement still needs to be addressed. Potentially, HPV testing can address this issue. If one accepts the thesis that all women with squamous intraepithelial lesions are HPV positive, then the correlation between cytologic diagnosis and HPV positivity may provide independent quality assurance of diagnostic certainty.[7, 9, 52–55] In a 1994 study, Sherman et al suggested this linear relationship between diagnostic certainty and HPV positivity in a population of 200 women with atypical Pap smears.[46] In that study, very few women whose consensus cytology was normal were high-risk HPV positive. In contrast, those patients whose consensus cytology was squamous intraepithelial lesion were HPV positive in more than 90% of cases. Cases of diagnostic uncertainty (i.e., ASCUS) had an intermediate rate of HPV positivity related to the variables that produce the ASCUS diagnosis. This relationship has been abundantly validated through the data generated in the enrollment population of the ALTS.[27, 28, 51] On thin-layer cytology, concordant normal diagnoses are HPV positive in approximately 30% of cases. In contrast, concordant squamous intraepithelial lesion diagnoses are HPV positive in 89% of LSIL and 96% of HSIL cases. Equivocal cytologic diagnoses are 60% HPV positive, representing the heterogeneity inherent in this group. Clinical center diagnoses that are revised downward from ASCUS to negative have HPV-positivity rates that are much more similar to concordant negative diagnoses (37% versus 31%, respectively). Similarly, the HPV-positivity rates for clinical center LSIL diagnoses downgraded to normal/negative were similar to the HPV positivity in concordant negative biopsies. This suggests that in the ALTS database, the systematic differences between the clinical centers and the quality control pathology groups reflect somewhat valid differences of opinion.

Clinicians need to be aware of the relatively low degree of reproducibility in diagnosis even among expert pathologists as well as the compounding variability that may be present owing to variations in clinicians' experience in colposcopic assessment and biopsy placement.

The major implications of these data are that diagnostic variability is substantial for all types of histologic specimens and that histopathologic diagnosis of cervical biopsies is not appreciably more reproducible than thin-layer cytology. It is important that clinicians be aware of the relatively low degree of reproducibility that exists even among expert pathologists as well as the compounding variability that may be present owing to differences in clinicians' experience at colposcopic assessment and biopsy placement. Because of this, objective independent methods of assessing diagnostic accuracy such as HPV testing may assume a more prominent role in the management of patients with mild squamous abnormality on Pap smear.

MANAGEMENT OF LSIL AND ASCUS

> **Because the follow-up phase of the ALTS has not yet been completed or analyzed, the tripartite strategy suggested in 1994 still remains valid. But the ALTS data presented thus far predict that an HPV testing strategy may be clinically effective in reducing the rate of colposcopic referral with little or no risk to the patient.**

Given the limited reproducibility of histologic, cytologic, and colposcopic diagnoses, what can one recommend as an improved management strategy for a patient presenting with a cytologic diagnosis of ASCUS or LSIL? The 1994 *JAMA* recommendations did not have the data to strongly support one management strategy over another. In addition, the HPV testing modalities available at that time were significantly less sensitive and specific. Furthermore, despite the previously stated problems with interobserver reproducibility, since the initiation and revision of the Bethesda System there appears to be significant improvement in cytopathologic diagnostic specificity.[28, 51] Because of this, and because the follow-up phase of the ALTS has not yet been completed or analyzed, the tripartite strategy suggested in 1994 still remains valid. Based on the ALTS data presented thus far, both cytologic follow-up and HPV testing strategies are similarly effective in reducing the rate of colposcopic referral with little or no risk to the patient. However, because of their relatively similar effectiveness, a detailed cost-effectiveness analysis between these two strategies will be both complex and very necessary to clearly promote one strategy over another.

> **Approximately 5% to 10% of ASCUS patients and 10% to 15% of LSIL patients, respectively, will have an existent HSIL.**

It is somewhat reassuring that the data generated in the ALTS agree very well with the majority of the retrospective data regarding the prevalence of HSIL in patients with ASCUS or LSIL Pap smears.[2, 3, 8, 12–14, 56] Approximately 5% to 10% of women with ASCUS smears and 10% to 15% of women with LSIL smears, respectively, will have an existent HSIL.[28, 57] These general statements should be tempered by two additional considerations: the age of the patient and any descriptors modifying the ASCUS diagnosis.

> **The positive predictive value for HSIL is low for young women with minor cytologic abnormalities and those in the perimenopausal and postmenopausal age group but higher in women age 30 to 45 years.**

The overall goal of patient management is to minimize the risk of developing cervical cancer or its most likely proximate precursor, HSIL. The age-related prevalence of the latter and the natural history and prevalence of its low-grade precursors are important considerations. Simply, ASCUS and LSIL diagnoses are very common in young women, whereas invasive squamous cell carcinoma is very rare. As best as can be determined, the natural history of cervical carcinogenesis spans at least 1 if not 2 decades (albeit with a broad distribution).[10, 11, 58–60] Because of this, the likelihood that women with an LSIL or ASCUS diagnosis have HSIL on biopsy (positive predictive value) is very low, particularly if they are younger than 25 years. Because of its relatively lower prevalence, a similar abnormality in a woman age 30 to 45 years will have a higher positive predictive value of finding HSIL on biopsy, especially if it is associated with HPV positivity for high-risk HPV types. Similarly, in the perimenopausal and postmenopausal age group, mild cytologic abnormality is quite common, but it is often much harder for the cytopathologist to relate it to squamous intraepithelial lesion diagnosis.[61, 62] Atypia in this age group has a lower positive predictive value because of the morphologic overlap among benign age-related changes; LSIL; and, more rarely, HSIL. Yet the relative prevalence of HSIL and cervical cancer is much higher. Therefore, an independent test (e.g., HPV) that might clarify the morphologic diagnosis could be very useful.

> **Smears with changes having so-called atypical squamous cells of immature metaplastic type have approximately a fivefold to tenfold higher risk of having an existing HSIL on follow-up, compared with ASCUS with more mature cytoplasm, which yields a squamous intraepithelial lesion diagnosis in only 5% to 10% of cases.**

In addition, data suggest that despite the lack of interobserver reproducibility, the ASCUS category can be logically split on morphologic grounds into subgroups that predict risk of existing LSIL versus HSIL.[13, 14, 56, 63, 64] Atypical squamous changes can be subclassified based on whether the cytoplasm of the cells in question is mature and differentiated with a polygonal configuration or whether it has an immature, metaplastic-appearing cytoplasm. Patients with the latter type of ASCUS (so-called atypical squamous cells of immature metaplastic type) have approximately a fivefold to tenfold higher risk of having an existing HSIL on follow-up, compared with the former type of ASCUS, which yields a squamous intraepithelial lesion diagnosis in only 5% to 10% of cases. Thus, it may be possible and preferable to qualify the ASCUS diagnosis into ASCUS—rule out LSIL for the former and ASCUS—rule out HSIL for the latter.

LSIL Management

> **In patients with an LSIL diagnosis on Pap smear, there does not seem to be a role for HPV testing because 85% to 90% of these patients are high-risk HPV positive.**

Thus, there does not seem to be a role for HPV testing in patients with a cytologic diagnosis of LSIL because 85% to 90% of these patients are high-risk HPV positive.[27] Triage using this management scheme is obviously ineffective in this case. The clinician is faced with the choice of cytologic follow-up, which in most young individuals will probably result in resolution of the lesion over the course of 1 to 2 years. The only alternative is immediate colposcopy. Approximately 90% of those colposcopies will not yield an HSIL lesion. Depending on clinical factors, such as the age of the patient and the patient's sexual history, the prevalence of LSIL decreases markedly over the third to fourth decades of life, with a corresponding increase in relative prevalence of HSIL. This suggests that at some point, a diagnosis of LSIL might predict an existing HSIL with a high enough frequency to make colposcopic assessment worthwhile. In the absence of hard data, this line is crossed somewhere between the ages of 35 and 45 years. Similar to HPV testing, persistent low-grade abnormalities on subsequent Pap smears strongly predict a higher risk of identifying HSIL on colposcopic assessment in an age-related manner.[65–67] This reflects the fact that HPV persistence is a major risk factor for the progression of cervical preneoplasia.

ASCUS Management

HPV testing is an effective triage method for women with ASCUS cytology.

Not surprisingly, for women with ASCUS, similar considerations apply, although the utility of HPV testing to effectively triage this group seems highly likely. The ability to use conservative management to follow an ASCUS diagnosis is based on the belief that serial independent cytologic testing will effectively find high-grade lesions before cancer develops.[8, 26, 48, 68] As mentioned previously, the risk of a high-grade lesion in these women is an age-related phenomenon. Some may be alarmed at the fact that 10% to 15% of the patients in the ALTS and similar trials have a prevalent HSIL, but these studies were mostly studies of young individuals. Furthermore, preliminary data suggest that the high-grade lesions detected in young women with an ASCUS smear are probably smaller and more difficult to detect cytologically than are dysplasias of similar grade that present with a more definitive cytologic diagnosis of HSIL. This suggests that, over time, many small, early, high-grade lesions will grow to be more readily detectable. Indeed, this is why the follow-up phase of the ALTS is so critical and is what distinguishes the ALTS from virtually all other studies to date. These points need to be kept in mind when evaluating the relative deficit of detection of HSIL captured by conservative cytologic follow-up compared with immediate HPV triage by HCII high-risk DNA testing. On the other hand, compared with 1994 data, the data from several studies clearly demonstrate that the sensitivity of the current generation of HPV tests effectively identifies patients at risk for existent HSIL with an efficacy similar to that of colposcopic evaluation of the entire population.[24, 26, 28, 69] A single repeat abnormal Pap smear closely approximates but does not meet this level of sensitivity. Either strategy effectively eliminates the need for colposcopy in approximately 40% to 50% of the population. Therefore, the decision to use conservative management versus HPV testing is reduced to an evaluation of available resources, patient wishes, and relative cost-effectiveness.

SUMMARY OF KEY POINTS

- The management of ASCUS/LSIL is of concern because a small but important minority of these women have HSIL or even carcinoma on colposcopy and biopsy.

- Approximately 5% to 10% of ASCUS patients and 10% to 15% of LSIL patients, respectively, have an existent HSIL.

- Immediate colposcopy for women with ASCUS/LSIL in a population where the prevalence of HSIL is low can be a very expensive option, resulting in many unnecessary colposcopies and overtreatment of a significant number of women.

- ALTS was designed to evaluate the three strategies for the triage of mild cervical cytological abnormalities: immediate colposcopy, cytologic follow-up, and triage using HPV DNA testing.

- Most women with LSIL are positive for cancer-associated HPV types. Because of this finding, the potential for this assay to effectively triage women with an LSIL diagnosis is obviously limited.

- Most of these "high-risk" HPV viral infections produce only low-grade lesions that are transient and not productive of high-grade dysplasia.

- When subjected to expert cytopathology review, only half of ASCUS diagnoses are confirmed, a third are downgraded to negative/reactive, and a sixth are upgraded to squamous intraepithelial lesion.

- Expert pathologists tend to give less severe interpretations of cytologic and histologic specimens.

- Histologic diagnosis is no more reliable or reproducible than cytologic diagnosis.

- Diagnostic reproducibility on colposcopic biopsies was no better than cytologic reproducibility and derived largely from disagreements about the morphologic criteria for mild dysplasia/CIN 1/LSIL.

- Of the women with ASCUS smears who were subjected to immediate colposcopy, 11.4% were found to have HSIL. In contrast, when triage to colposcopy was by repeat cytology with a threshold of HSIL, high-grade disease was found in only 4.8%. Among patients with ASCUS cytology, management with repeat cytology using a threshold of ASCUS or greater is nearly equivalent to a highly sensitive HPV test in selecting patients for referral to colposcopy.

- In the evolution of diagnostic classifications (as in the Bethesda System), the amount of experience that a colposcopist may have in recognizing abnor-

Continued on following page

malities, the quality and location of colposcopic biopsy, and the experience of the pathologist with the spectrum of biopsies presented are all sources of diagnostic variability.

- Because the follow-up phase of the ALTS has not yet been completed or analyzed, the tripartite strategy suggested in 1994 still remains valid. But the ALTS data presented thus far predict that an HPV testing strategy may be clinically effective in reducing the rate of colposcopic referral with little or no risk to the patient.

- The positive predictive value for HSIL is low for young women with minor cytologic abnormalities and those in the perimenopausal and postmenopausal age group but higher in women age 30 to 45 years.

- Smears with changes having so-called atypical squamous cells of immature metaplastic type have approximately a fivefold to tenfold higher risk of having an existing HSIL on follow-up, compared with ASCUS with more mature cytoplasm, which yields a squamous intraepithelial lesion diagnosis in only 5% to 10% of cases.

- Among patients with an LSIL diagnosis on Pap smear, there does not seem to be a role for HPV testing because 85% to 90% of these patients are high-risk HPV positive. HPV testing is an effective triage method for women with ASCUS cytology.

References

1. Stoler MH: Advances in cervical screening technology. Mod Pathol 2000;13:275.
2. Stoler MH: Does every little cell count? Don't "ASCUS." Cancer 1999;87:45.
3. Wilbur DC: Atypical squamous cells of undetermined significance. Is help on the way? Am J Clin Pathol 1996;105:661.
4. Schiffman M, Adrianza ME: ASCUS-LSIL Triage Study. Design, methods and characteristics of trial participants. Acta Cytol 2000; 44:726.
5. Kurman RJ, Henson DE, Herbst AL, et al: Interim guidelines for the management of abnormal cervical cytology. JAMA 1994;271: 1866–69.
6. Ostor AG, Mulvany N: The pathology of cervical neoplasia. Curr Opin Obstet Gynecol 1996;8:69.
7. Stoler MH: Human papillomaviruses and cervical neoplasia: A model for carcinogenesis. Int J Gynecol Pathol 2000;19:16.
8. Solomon D, Frable WJ, Vooijs GP, et al: ASCUS and AGUS criteria. International Academy of Cytology Task Force summary. Diagnostic cytology towards the 21st century: An international expert conference and tutorial. Acta Cytol 1998;42:16.
9. Schiffman MH: New epidemiology of human papillomavirus infection and cervical neoplasia. J Natl Cancer Inst 1995;87:1345.
10. Richart RM, Masood S, Syrjanen KJ, et al: Human papillomavirus. International Academy of Cytology Task Force summary. Diagnostic cytology towards the 21st century: An international expert conference and tutorial. Acta Cytol 1998;42:50.
11. Pinto AP, Crum CP: Natural history of cervical neoplasia: Defining progression and its consequence. Clin Obstet Gynecol 2000;43:352.
12. Wilbur DC, Stanley F, Patten MD Jr: Atypical cells of squamous type. Cancer 1997;81:327.
13. Sheils LA, Wilbur DC: Atypical squamous cells of undetermined significance. Stratification of the risk of association with, or progression to, squamous intraepithelial lesions based on morphologic subcategorization. Acta Cytol 1997;41:1065.
14. Sherman ME, Tabbara SO, Scott DR, et al: "ASCUS, rule out HSIL": Cytologic features, histologic correlates, and human papillomavirus detection. Mod Pathol 1999;12:335.
15. Kurman RJ, Solomon D: The Bethesda System for Reporting Cervical/Vaginal Cytologic Diagnoses: Definitions, Criteria and Explanatory Notes for Terminology and Specimen Adequacy. New York, Springer-Verlag, 1994.
16. Sherman ME, Schiffman MH, Erozan YS, et al: The Bethesda System. A proposal for reporting abnormal cervical smears based on the reproducibility of cytopathologic diagnoses. Arch Pathol Lab Med 1992;116:1155.
17. Cavuslu S, Mant C, Starkey WG, et al: Analytic sensitivities of hybrid-capture, consensus and type-specific polymerase chain reactions for the detection of human papillomavirus type 16 DNA. J Med Virol 1996;49:319.
18. Cope JU, Hildesheim A, Schiffman MH, et al: Comparison of the hybrid capture tube test and PCR for detection of human papillomavirus DNA in cervical specimens. J Clin Microbiol 1997;35:2262.
19. Cox JT: Evaluating the role of HPV testing for women with equivocal Papanicolaou test findings. JAMA 1999;281:1645.
20. Cox JT, Lorincz AT, Schiffman MH, et al: Human papillomavirus testing by hybrid capture appears to be useful in triaging women with a cytologic diagnosis of atypical squamous cells of undetermined significance. Am J Obstet Gynecol 1995;172:946.
21. Lorincz AT: Hybrid Capture method for detection of human papillomavirus DNA in clinical specimens: A tool for clinical management of equivocal Pap smears and for population screening. J Obstet Gynaecol Res 1996;22:629.
22. Schiffman MH, Schatzkin A: Test reliability is critically important to molecular epidemiology: An example from studies of human papillomavirus infection and cervical neoplasia. Cancer Res 1994; 54:1944.
23. Schiffman MH, Kiviat NB, Burk RD, et al: Accuracy and interlaboratory reliability of human papillomavirus DNA testing by hybrid capture. J Clin Microbiol 1995;33:545.
24. Schiffman M, Herrero R, Hildesheim A, et al: HPV DNA testing in cervical cancer screening: Results from women in a high-risk province of Costa Rica. JAMA 2000;283:87.
25. Cox JT: HPV testing: Is it useful in triage of minor Pap abnormalities? J Fam Pract 1998;46:121.
26. Manos MM, Kinney WK, Hurley LB, et al: Identifying women with cervical neoplasia: Using human papillomavirus DNA testing for equivocal Papanicolaou results. JAMA 1999;281:1605.
27. Human papillomavirus testing for triage of women with cytologic evidence of low-grade squamous intraepithelial lesions: Baseline data from a randomized trial. The Atypical Squamous Cells of Undetermined Significance/Low-Grade Squamous Intraepithelial Lesions Triage Study (ALTS) Group. J Natl Cancer Inst 2000;92:397.
28. Solomon D, Schiffman M, Tarone RE: Comparison of HPV testing, repeat cytology and immediate colposcopy in ASCUS triage: Baseline results from a randomized trial (ALTS). J Natl Cancer Inst 2001;93(4):293.
29. Cocker J, Fox H, Langley FA: Consistency in the histological diagnosis of epithelial abnormalities of the cervix uteri. J Clin Path 1968;21:67.
30. Confortini M, Biggeri A, Cariaggi MP, et al: Intralaboratory reproducibility in cervical cytology. Results of the application of a 100-slide set. Acta Cytologica 1993;37:49.
31. Creagh T, Bridger JE, Kupek E, et al: Pathologist variation in reporting cervical borderline epithelial abnormalities and cervical intraepithelial neoplasia. J Clin Pathol 1995;48:59.
32. de Vet HC, Koudstaal J, Kwee WS, et al: Efforts to improve interobserver agreement in histopathological grading. J Clin Epidemiol 1995;48:869.
33. Doornewaard H, van der Schouw YT, van der Graaf Y, et al: Observer variation in cytologic grading for cervical dysplasia of Papanicolaou smears with the PAPNET testing system. Cancer 1999;87:178.
34. Evans DMD, Shelley G, Cleary B, Baldwin Y: Observer variation and quality control of cytodiagnosis. J Clin Path 1974;27:945.
35. Genest DR, Stein L, Cibas E, et al: A binary (Bethesda) system for classifying cervical cancer precursors: criteria, reproducibility, and viral correlates. Hum Pathol 1993;24:730.

36. Horn PL, Lowell DM, LiVolsi VA, Boyle CA: Reproducibility of the cytologic diagnosis of human papillomavirus infection. Acta Cytol 1985;29:692.

37. Ismail SM, Colclough AB, Dinnen JS, et al: Observer variation in histopathological diagnosis and grading of cervical intraepithelial neoplasia. Br Med J 1989;298:707.

38. Jones S, Thomas GD, Williamson P: Observer variation in the assessment of adequacy and neoplasia in cervical cytology. Acta Cytol 1996;40:226.

39. Joste NE, Rushing L, Granados R, et al: Bethesda classification of cervicovaginal smears: Reproducibility and viral correlates. Hum Pathol 1996;27:581.

40. Lee KR, Minter LJ, Crum CP: Koilocytotic atypia in Papanicolaou smears. Reproducibility and biopsy correlations. Cancer 1997;81:10.

41. McCluggage WG, Bharucha H, Caughley LM, et al. Interobserver variation in the reporting of cervical colposcopic biopsy specimens: Comparison of grading systems. J Clin Pathol 1996;49:833.

42. Siegler EE: Microdiagnosis of carcinoma in situ of the uterine cervix: A comparative study of pathologists' diagnoses. Cancer 1956;9:463.

43. Yobs AR, Plott AE, Hicklin MD, et al: Retrospective evaluation of gynecologic cytodiagnosis. II. Interlaboratory reproducibility as shown in rescreening large consecutive samples of reported cases. Acta Cytologica 1987;31:900.

44. Young NA, Naryshkin S, Atkinson BF, et al: Interobserver variability of cervical smears with squamous-cell abnormalities: A Philadelphia study. Diagn Cytopathol 1994;11:352.

45. Woodhouse SL, Stastny JF, Styer PE, et al: Interobserver variability in subclassification of squamous intraepithelial lesions: Results of the College of American Pathologists Interlaboratory Comparison Program in Cervicovaginal Cytology. Arch Pathol Lab Med 1999; 123:1079.

46. Sherman ME, Schiffman MH, Lorincz AT, et al: Toward objective quality assurance in cervical cytopathology. Correlation of cytopathologic diagnoses with detection of high-risk human papillomavirus types. Am J Clin Pathol 1994;102:182.

47. Ferris DG, Cox JT, Burke L, et al: Colposcopy quality control: Establishing colposcopy criterion standards for the ALTS trial using cervigrams. J Lower Genital Tract Dis 1998;2:195.

48. Ferris DG, Wright TC Jr, Litaker MS, et al: Triage of women with ASCUS and LSIL on Pap smear reports: Management by repeat Pap smear, HPV DNA testing, or colposcopy? J Fam Pract 1998;46:125.

49. Hopman EH, Voorhorst FJ, Kenemans P, et al: Observer agreement on interpreting colposcopic images of CIN. Gynecol Oncol 1995;58:206.

50. Ferris DG, Wright TC Jr, Litaker MS, et al: Comparison of two tests for detecting carcinogenic HPV in women with Papanicolaou smear reports of ASCUS and LSIL. J Fam Pract 1998;46:136.

51. Stoler MH, Schiffman M: Inter-observer reproducibility of cervical cytologic and histologic interpretations: Realistic estimates from the ASCUS-LSIL triage study (ALTS). JAMA 2001;285(11):1500.

52. Koutsky L: Epidemiology of genital human papillomavirus infection. Am J Med 1997;102:3.

53. Kjaer SK, van den Brule AJ, Bock JE, et al: Human papillomavirus—the most significant risk determinant of cervical intraepithelial neoplasia. Int J Cancer 1996;65:601.

54. Bosch FX, Manos MM, Munoz N, et al: Prevalence of human papillomavirus in cervical cancer: A worldwide perspective. International biological study on cervical cancer (IBSCC) study group. J Natl Cancer Inst 1995;87:796.

55. Walboomers JM, Jacobs MV, Manos MM, et al: Human papillomavirus is a necessary cause of invasive cervical cancer worldwide. J Pathol 1999;189:12.

56. Hatem F, Wilbur DC: High grade squamous cervical lesions following negative Papanicolaou smears: False-negative cervical cytology or rapid progression. Diagn Cytopathol 1995;12:135.

57. Kinney WK, Manos MM, Hurley LB, Ransley JE: Where's the high-grade cervical neoplasia? The importance of minimally abnormal Papanicolaou diagnoses. Obstet Gynecol 1998;91:973.

58. Ostor AG: Natural history of cervical intraepithelial neoplasia: A critical review. Int J Gynecol Pathol 1993;12:186.

59. Kiviat NB, Critchlow CW, Kurman RJ: Reassessment of the morphological continuum of cervical intraepithelial lesions: Does it reflect different stages in the progression to cervical carcinoma? IARC Sci Publ 1992;119:59.

60. Schiffman MH, Bauer HM, Hoover RN, et al: Epidemiologic evidence showing that human papillomavirus infection causes most cervical intraepithelial neoplasia. J Natl Cancer Inst 1993;85:958.

61. Jovanovic AS, McLachlin CM, Shen L, et al: Postmenopausal squamous atypia: A spectrum including "pseudo-koilocytosis." Mod Pathol 1995;8:408.

62. Cuzick J, Beverley E, Ho L, et al: HPV testing in primary screening of older women. Br J Cancer 1999;81:554.

63. Genest DR, Dean B, Lee KR, et al: Qualifying the cytologic diagnosis of "atypical squamous cells of undetermined significance" affects the predictive value of a squamous intraepithelial lesion on subsequent biopsy. Arch Pathol Lab Med 1998;122:338.

64. Crum CP, Genest DR, Krane JF, et al: Subclassifying atypical squamous cells in Thin-Prep cervical cytology correlates with detection of high-risk human papillomavirus DNA. Am J Clin Pathol 1999;112:384.

65. Lorincz AT, Schiffman MH, Jaffurs WJ, et al: Temporal associations of human papillomavirus infection with cervical cytologic abnormalities. Am J Obstet Gynecol 1990;162:645.

66. Liaw KL, Hildesheim A, Burk RD, et al: A prospective study of human papillomavirus (HPV) type 16 DNA detection by polymerase chain reaction and its association with acquisition and persistence of other HPV types. J Infect Dis 2001;183:8.

67. Schiffman MH, Brinton LA: The epidemiology of cervical carcinogenesis. Cancer 1995;76:1888.

68. Ferris DG, Kriegel D, Cote L, et al: Women's triage and management preferences for cervical cytologic reports demonstrating atypical squamous cells of undetermined significance and low-grade squamous intraepithelial lesions. Arch Fam Med 1997;6:348.

69. Wright TC Jr, Lorincz A, Ferris DG, et al: Reflex human papillomavirus deoxyribonucleic acid testing in women with abnormal Papanicolaou smears. Am J Obstet Gynecol 1998;178:962.

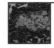

B

• Mark Spitzer

Guidelines for the Management of Colposcopic Findings

In developing evidence-based guidelines for the management of cervical cytologic abnormalities, it is important to understand the types of histologic findings that are associated with each cytologic abnormality. Once a histologic diagnosis is made, it is important to know the risk associated with that diagnosis and with the management strategies being considered. Only then can a rational and safe plan be developed that properly balances the true risk to the patient with the expected benefits of treatment. This chapter will address only squamous abnormalities of the cervix. Glandular disease is addressed in Chapter 13.

Cervical abnormalities can be divided into four categories: benign and inflammatory cervical abnormalities, productive viral infections with limited malignant potential (including cervical intraepithelial neoplasia [CIN] 1 and cervical condyloma), true premalignant disease (CIN 2 and, especially, CIN 3), and invasive cancer. The primary goal of colposcopy is to exclude cancer and to prevent it by identifying its true premalignant precursors. Consequently, it is essential that, before management guidelines are developed, the true premalignant potential for each of these categories is known. Similarly, each of these categories is found in certain proportions within each of the cervical cytologic abnormalities. For example, the cytologic diagnosis of atypical squamous cells of undetermined significance (ASCUS) is associated with some benign cervical changes, some productive viral infections, some true premalignant disease, and some invasive cancer. The more severe the cytologic abnormality, the higher the risk of true premalignant disease and invasive cancer and the lower the risk of benign cervical changes and productive viral infections. To develop a rational plan of management for women with cervical cytologic abnormalities, one must know the proportion of women with true premalignant disease and invasive cancer within each cytologic category. If the risk of true premalignant disease and cancer is high, the management approach must be more aggressive, whereas if the risk of premalignant disease and cancer is low, a more conservative approach can be taken.

ASCUS CYTOLOGY

It has always been recognized that the cytologic category ASCUS is predominantly made up of benign and inflammatory cervical changes and productive viral infections (condyloma and CIN 1). However, in this group, there is also a small number of women with true premalignant disease (CIN 2, 3) and a very small number of women with invasive cancers.[1-3] As is discussed later, there is little reason to treat CIN 1 because its premalignant potential is quite limited. Therefore, the challenge has always been to distinguish true premalignant disease (CIN 2, 3) and cancer within this group of patients. The College of American Pathology Q-Probes survey of close to 350 cytopathology laboratories and more than 1.7 million smears showed that the median rate of ASCUS reports in all pathology laboratories was 4.4% and that 13.4% of ASCUS cytology was associated with CIN 2, 3.[1] By extrapolation, this means that there are more than 2 million ASCUS smears reported annually in the United States and that almost half of all CIN 2, 3 is preceded by an ASCUS cytologic diagnosis. The ASCUS/LSIC Triage Study (ALTS) also found that 15% of 2324 women with ASCUS cytology had CIN 2, 3.[4] These findings underscore the importance of evaluating women with an ASCUS cytologic diagnosis and highlight the difficulty associated with the evaluation of such a large number of women.

Separating the true cancer precursors from the other lesions associated with ASCUS cytology has been a longstanding problem for clinicians. Because there is an inverse relationship between the sensitivity and the specificity of any test, the challenge has always been to balance the cost of any triage tool, the number of patients subsequently referred to colposcopy, and the percentage of these women who actually have high-grade disease (the positive predictive value) with how many of the women with high-grade disease are actually detected (sensitivity) and the test's ability to correctly reassure those patients with a negative result that they are really free of high-grade disease (negative predictive value). Immediate colposcopy, cervicography, repeat cytology, and human papillomavirus (HPV) testing are all triage tools that have been proposed for that role. Each of these tools is covered in greater detail in other chapters. However, in comparing repeat cytology with reflex testing for oncogenic HPV DNA types (testing the residual fluid from a liquid-based cytology specimen), the ALTS found that reflex HPV DNA testing was the most sensitive test for the identification of women at risk for CIN 2, 3 (96% sensitivity) while referring 56% of the patients for colposcopy.[4]

The negative predictive value of HPV DNA testing was 99%. In contrast, repeat cytology at an ASCUS threshold (all patients with a Papanicolaou [Pap] smear showing ASCUS or greater were referred for colposcopy) had a sensitivity of 85% while referring 59% to colposcopy and had a negative predictive value of 96%. With respect to the prevalence of CIN 2, 3, women with ASCUS cytology who are positive for oncogenic HPV types are equated to women with low-grade squamous intraepithelial lesion (LSIL) cytology and should be managed as such. Women whose HPV DNA test is negative can be managed similarly to women with negative Pap smears.

A special note should be made of the new category created in the Bethesda 2001 classification called *atypical squamous cells favoring high-grade CIN* (ASC-H). In published series,[5-8] 24% to 94% of women with ASC-H have biopsy-confirmed CIN 2, 3 compared with 5% to 10% for ASCUS smears.[4, 9-12] This is sufficient justification to recommend colposcopy for all women with ASC-H smears without the need for an intermediate triage test. However, an ASC-H report indicates that there was insufficient evidence found on the smear to call it high-grade squamous intraepithelial lesion (HSIL), and the experience with this category is still quite limited outside academic centers. Therefore, a conization for cytology-histology discrepancy is not indicated in women with an ASC-H diagnosis in whom colposcopy failed to reveal a high-grade lesion.

LSIL AND CIN 1

The cytologic category of LSIL is predominantly made up of productive viral infections (condyloma and CIN 1). However, in this group there are also some benign and inflammatory cervical changes, some true premalignant disease (CIN 2, 3), and a very small number of invasive cancers. The College of American Pathology Q-Probes survey[1] reported that the median rate of LSIL reports was 1.6% and that 13.5% of LSIL cytology is associated with benign cervical changes, 85% with CIN (68% CIN 1 and 18% CIN 2, 3), and 0.2% with invasive cancer. By extrapolation, this means that about a quarter of all high-grade disease is preceded by an LSIL cytologic diagnosis. Other studies have also shown a variable rate of biopsy-confirmed CIN 2, 3 identified in women with LSIL ranging from 10% to 70%.[13-20] In part, this reflects the high intra- and interobserver variability associated with the cytologic interpretation of LSIL. In the ALTS, only 68% of the index Pap tests interpreted as LSIL were classified as LSIL by the quality control pathology group; 26% were downgraded to ASCUS or to negative, and 6% were upgraded to HSIL.[21] The variability in the prevalence of CIN 2 and CIN 3 among series also reflects differences in the patient populations of these studies. Studies reporting a very high prevalence of CIN 2 and CIN 3 (30% or higher) often comprise women undergoing excisional procedures for persistent LSIL or conizations for CIN 1.[18, 19] These findings underscore the importance of colposcopy for all women with LSIL cytology. With respect to HPV DNA testing of women with LSIL cytology, the ALTS found HPV DNA in cervical samples from 532 (82.9%) of 642 women.[22] Because so many women require referral for colposcopy using this triage tool, there is only limited potential for HPV DNA testing to guide decisions about the clinical management of women with LSIL.

Two important details in developing a management plan for women with CIN 1 are the reliability of the histologic diagnosis of CIN 1 and the natural history of the disease. Despite the "gold standard" reputation afforded to histologic diagnoses, numerous studies have documented that there is a high level of intra- and interobserver variability in the histologic diagnosis of CIN 1. In the ALTS, only 43% of the cervical biopsies initially diagnosed as CIN 1 by the pathologists at the clinical sites were sustained by the quality control pathology group; 41% were downgraded to normal, and 13% were upgraded to CIN 2 or CIN 3.[20] The high level of uncertainty as to the accuracy of a diagnosis of CIN 1 makes the management of such patients highly problematic.

The natural history of untreated CIN 1 seems less controversial; however, in the context of the just-cited information about the reliability of its histologic diagnosis, even this information is suspect. Ostor[2] performed a comprehensive literature review of 17 studies comprising 4504 patients. He found that, in the absence of therapy, 57% of CIN 1 regressed spontaneously, 32% persisted as CIN 1, and 11% progressed to CIN 2, CIN 3, or cancer. Overall, the rate of progression to invasive cervical cancer was 0.3%. However, in the three largest reports,[23-25] 13 of the 14 cases of women who progressed to invasive cancer were lost to follow-up, appeared to have invasive squamous carcinoma at initial presentation but did not undergo colposcopy and cervical biopsy, or had CIN 2 or CIN 3 that was not treated. Only 1 in 2604 patients (0.04%) actually progressed to invasive cancer. A meta-analysis of the natural history of CIN 1 that looked at many of the same papers arrived at similar conclusions.[3] By 24 months of follow-up, 47% of lesions appeared to have spontaneously regressed, 21% had progressed to CIN 2 or CIN 3, and 0.15% had progressed to invasive carcinoma.

HSIL AND CIN 2, 3

The cytologic category of HSIL is predominantly made up of true premalignant disease (CIN 2, 3) and a few invasive cancers. However, in this group there are also some productive viral infections (condyloma and CIN 1) and a few benign and inflammatory cervical changes. The College of American Pathology Q-Probes survey reported that the median rate of HSIL reports was 0.5% and that 91.3% of HSIL cytology is associated with CIN (16.3% CIN 1 and 75% CIN 2, 3), 6.5% with benign cervical changes, and 1.7% with invasive cancer.[1] By extrapolation, this means that only about a quarter of all high-grade disease is preceded by an HSIL cytologic diagnosis. Although the positive predictive value of HSIL cytology is assumed to be very high, in the ALTS, only 47% of the cytology interpreted as HSIL was classified as HSIL by the quality control pathology group; 27% was downgraded to LSIL, 23% to ASCUS, and 3% to negative.[21] In part, this may be due to the combining of CIN 2 and CIN 3 into one category (HSIL). A similar problem is found in reporting the histologic diagnosis and natural history of high-grade CIN. Although, in each case, CIN 2 is closer in its natural history to CIN 3 than to CIN 1, CIN 2 represents an intermediary diagnosis, and so any management decision based on the positive predictive value of an HSIL Pap smear or the natural history of a high-grade CIN lesion must be viewed in that context. Consequently, whenever a discrepancy exists among the cytology, colposcopy, and histology of a high-grade lesion, each element of the data contributing to the decision to treat should be reviewed.

The natural history of untreated high-grade CIN is more difficult to study because the risk of progression to invasive cancer makes such studies unethical today. Nevertheless, Ostor[2] performed a comprehensive literature review of 21 studies comprising 767 patients. He found that, in the absence of therapy, 32% of CIN 3 regressed spontaneously, 56% persisted as CIN 3, and 12% progressed to invasive cancer. However, Ostor did note that the rate of progression of CIN 3 to invasive cancer might be higher than stated because most studies titrated to an end point of CIN 3, and longer follow-up might have yielded a higher rate of progression. The overall rate of progression of CIN 2 was 22% to CIN 3 and 5% to invasive cancer. Even patients with HSIL cytology who did not have a visible lesion had a high prevalence of CIN 2, 3 and a 1% to 5% risk of invasive cancer. Thus, observations with serial cytology or adjunctive tests short of colposcopy are unacceptable.[26-28]

FOLLOW-UP

The final concern in developing management guidelines for women with cervical cytologic and histologic abnormalities is the identification of the most appropriate tools for follow-up. Colposcopy with directed biopsy is a very sensitive tool for the detection of persistent or recurrent high-grade CIN and cancer,[29] but it is very expensive, and colposcopic resources are limited in some areas. Cervicography is also sensitive, but not specific, and its sensitivity in detecting high-grade disease is uncertain.[9, 11, 30]

A single repeat cytology is also not very sensitive. The sensitivity of a single repeat Pap smear for the detection of CIN 2, 3 when the threshold for a positive Pap was set at ASCUS or worse has been reported as 67% to 76%.[21, 31-34] To compensate for its poor sensitivity, clinicians have traditionally used serial repeat cytology. They reason that if 70% of the high-grade CIN would be detected with the first repeat smear, 21% (70% of the remaining 30%) would be detected with the second repeat smear, and 6% (70% of the remaining 9%) with the third repeat smear for a total of 97% sensitivity. This was the genesis of the practice of requiring three negative repeat smears in the follow-up of a cytologic abnormality.[12, 26, 35] However, in a well-screened population such as that of the United States, the likelihood of missing a high-grade lesion with cytology is smaller because the patient was likely screened many times before the original abnormal Pap. Therefore, in a patient with a low-grade cytologic or histologic abnormality who never had evidence of a high-grade lesion, two consecutive negative Pap smears with

an ASCUS or worse threshold are probably sufficient reassurance that a high-grade lesion is not present. This is especially true when liquid-based cytology is used.[8] However, in someone who is being followed up after treatment for a high-grade lesion, it is probably prudent to require three consecutive negative smears before releasing the patient to routine follow-up.

Data derived in part from the study of populations with ASCUS show that the sensitivity of a single HPV DNA test for oncogenic HPV types is probably comparable to multiple repeat cytology.[4] Data on patients after excisional therapy are limited but are similar to studies of patients with ASCUS smears in that the negative predictive value of HPV testing for residual disease after treatment is very high.[36] The negative predictive value of HPV testing approached 100% in two studies during post-treatment surveillance,[37, 38] and only those patients with persistent high-risk HPV DNA (screening repeated 6 months apart) were at higher risk of progressing.[27] However, the specificity of HPV DNA testing is lower in this setting.[37, 38] This means that HPV infection may persist post treatment without cytologic or histologic evidence of disease. Also, HPV positivity seems to diminish over time. It was noted at 6 to 12 months after cone biopsy or laser vaporization that 27 of 30 women were HPV negative.[39] Because the sensitivity of cytologic follow-up is so high, the overall risk of invasive cancer is so low, and the HPV DNA testing cannot distinguish patients with high-grade disease from others with HPV positivity, the value of HPV testing in post-treatment follow-up is uncertain. However, if the practitioner wants to take advantage of the high sensitivity of follow-up with HPV DNA testing while avoiding the very high rate of referral to colposcopy, the test should not be done until at least 1 year after the original diagnosis or treatment of the abnormality being followed up.

TRIAGE GUIDELINES

The central goal of colposcopy is to rule out cancer by combining cytologic and histologic diagnoses with the colposcopic impression. Colposcopy allows the clinician to localize the most abnormal areas for histologic sampling. Colposcopically directed biopsies, rather than random or four-quadrant biopsies, are performed to establish the diagnosis. If the diagnosis can be established, and invasive disease is excluded, the patient can be managed conservatively, thereby obviating the need for more aggressive treatment such as conization. Treatments for preinvasive disease include transformation zone ablation and excision.

Adherence to established triage rules during the colposcopic examination helps avoid a delay in the diagnosis of preinvasive or invasive disease and prevents inadequate treatment. The guidelines are based on the risk of premalignant disease and invasive cancer as noted previously and the risk and benefit of the management approach. One of the principles involved in managing cervical disease is whether the entire area at risk has been evaluated. When that is the case, the colposcopy is deemed *satisfactory*. Guidelines have been established to define a satisfactory colposcopy. Whenever there is a significant risk of invasive cancer, conservative management is appropriate only after a satisfactory colposcopic examination is achieved. To be certain that the colposcopic examination is satisfactory, the entire transformation zone must be visualized along with the proximal and distal limits of any lesions. To avoid inadvertent ablation of microinvasive or invasive disease in the endocervical canal, whenever an endocervical curettage is done, it should reveal no evidence of neoplasia. Any discrepancy among cytology, histology, and colposcopic impression must be reconciled before developing a management plan. This is especially true if the biopsy findings are significantly less severe than the cytologic and colposcopic findings. Because the positive predictive value of HSIL cytology is so high (discussed previously), such a wide discrepancy may indicate that a more severe lesion is present but was not sampled. If cancer cannot be definitively excluded, the patient must undergo a cone biopsy. A cone biopsy should remove the entire transformation zone, and the histologic evaluation should conclusively exclude invasive cancer. In many cases, the cone serves both a diagnostic and a therapeutic function, obviating the need for further treatment.

Lack of correlation among cytology, histology, and colposcopic impression presents a challenge for the colposcopist. Communication with the pathologist is one of the most important steps in addressing and resolving the noncorrelation issue. The colposcopist can assist the pathologist by providing a pertinent clinical history and description of the colposcopic findings. The pathologist can assist the clinician by providing clear descriptions of the pathologic findings and commenting on the adequacy of the specimen submitted (noting failure to sample the transformation zone, epithelium detached from underlying stroma, scant tissue, obscuring blood and inflammation on a cytologic specimen, etc.). Both the colposcopist and the pathologist should strive to use standard terminology to ensure that the diagnosis is meaningful to both parties and to other practitioners. One of the principal contributions of the Bethesda System was the formulation of a standardized classification and terminology system.[26] The pathologist can also review all the cytologic and histologic results to help confirm the original diagnosis and to determine whether cellular findings on the Pap smear can be explained by histologic interpretation.

SUMMARY

CIN 2, 3 (high-grade CIN) is a lesion with true premalignant potential, and some women with CIN 2, 3 have occult cancer even when it is not suspected. For this reason, it is important to identify high-grade CIN and to treat it. Because women with CIN 2, 3 are at risk for occult invasive cancer, whenever cancer cannot confidently be excluded (as when the transformation zone or the lesion cannot be viewed in its entirety), a cervical conization must be done. Women with HSIL cytology must undergo colposcopic evaluation. Because such a high percentage of these women have high-grade CIN, they should undergo cervical conization even if no lesion

is identified (once the HSIL cytology is confirmed on review). Women with LSIL cytology and those with ASCUS cytology who are HPV DNA positive for oncogenic HPV types are also at risk for having high-grade CIN, but their risk is smaller. However, there are so many women with this cytologic report that, despite the smaller risk, almost two thirds of all high-grade CIN is found in women with these cytologic abnormalities. Consequently, all women with LSIL and HPV DNA positive ASCUS cytology should undergo colposcopic evaluation. But many of these diagnoses represent cytologic overcall, and, after evaluation with colposcopy, the true risk of high-grade CIN is small and the risk of occult invasive cancer is almost nil. Therefore, conization is not indicated when a lesion cannot be identified or when the transformation zone is not fully visualized. Also, even if a CIN 1 lesion is identified, treatment is not necessary because the risk of occult invasive cancer is almost nil, and the risk of progression to invasive cancer over the next 24 months is very small.

TREATMENT DECISIONS

Women with biopsy-confirmed HSIL (CIN 2, 3; moderate-to-severe dysplasia; carcinoma in situ) and no cytologic, colposcopic, or histologic suspicion of invasive disease have a significant risk of disease progression to invasive cancer and should be treated. Those women with satisfactory colposcopy and negative endocervical curettage may be treated by ablative techniques, such as cryotherapy or laser vaporization, or by an excisional procedure such as loop electrosurgical excision. All these modalities are effective options for treatment, although cryosurgery may be slightly less effective for the treatment of CIN 3 with crypt involvement and of lesions involving more than two quadrants of the cervix (discussed earlier). With unsatisfactory colposcopy and HSIL cytology, a cone biopsy should be performed because the positive predictive value of HSIL cytology is very high and these women have a small but significant risk of invasive cancer. The cone biopsy can be performed in the office using an excisional procedure such as a laser excisional cone or loop electrosurgical cone, either of which can simultaneously accomplish both diagnosis and treatment (discussed previously).

Management of LSIL (condyloma, CIN 1, mild dysplasia) includes several options. Because the risk of invasive cancer is extremely low, the progressive potential of CIN 1 is low, the regression rate is high, and the cure rate of CIN 1 is the same as the cure rate of CIN 2, 3 using the same modalities, little is gained by treating CIN 1. Treatment is unnecessary in many of these patients because their lesion will regress without treatment. Therefore, when the colposcopy is satisfactory, the preferred treatment is observation without treatment. However, if, after consultation between the woman and her physician, a decision is made to treat the lesion, any ablative treatment modality is acceptable, including cryotherapy, laser vaporization, and loop excision (discussed earlier). Among the factors that should be considered when deciding on the most appropriate management route are patient compliance, extent and persistence of disease, prior treatment, age and parity, immune status, and patient preference for treatment. Many low-grade lesions regress spontaneously,[2, 3] and close observation with cytologic and possibly colposcopic follow-up without active therapy is the preferred management option. Although there is no evidence that cryotherapy, laser vaporization, or loop excision negatively affect future fertility or pregnancy outcomes,[40] observation or the most conservative therapy is favored in young, nulliparous women. In addition, patients with a history of in utero diethylstilbestrol exposure should be observed whenever possible because they incur a high risk of cervical stenosis after active treatment. Also, in a young, nulliparous women with no cytologic, colposcopic, or histologic evidence of high-grade disease, the risk of an unsuspected invasive cancer is exceedingly small even with unsatisfactory colposcopy.[41] Follow-up without treatment may be appropriate even with unsatisfactory colposcopy. If conization is being considered in a young, nulliparous woman, it would be prudent to seek the opinion of an expert colposcopist before a decision is made. Because of the relative unreliability of cervical cytology, whenever a high-grade cervical lesion cannot be identified, cervical smears should be reviewed before any treatment is undertaken. If large lesions or persistent lesions are present or if the patient is at risk for being lost to follow-up, active treatment may be favored.

The goal of treating intraepithelial disease of the cervix is to prevent the progression to invasion cancer, not to eradicate the HPV infection. There is no specific therapy that eradicates HPV from the lower genital tract. Patients should be made aware of the fact that HPV may persist despite effective treatment and that flat condylomata may reappear on the mature squamous epithelium of the cervix or the vagina after treatment. This does not necessarily represent treatment failure, but rather reactivation of latent HPV infection. Once the transformation zone has been destroyed, reappearance of flat condylomata on the cervix does not necessarily imply that additional treatment is necessary. Because many of these lesions regress spontaneously, the patients can be managed by careful cytologic and possibly colposcopic follow-up. Recurrence of HSIL mandates retreatment, preferably using an excisional technique to ensure that the margins are negative and that the lesion has been completely excised. This is especially true if the previous method of treatment was ablation.

ALGORITHMS

Algorithms have been developed for the management of women who have already undergone colposcopy (and/or biopsy) for evaluation of an abnormal Pap smear. Factors that were considered in development of these recommendations include

1. The results of the sentinel Pap smear(s) that led to the performance of colposcopy and directed biopsies
2. The results of the colposcopy and biopsy if performed
3. The results of HPV testing for high-risk (oncogenic) HPV types, in the case of ASCUS smears when no lesion was found on colposcopy

▼ Table 25–1

Criteria for Satisfactory Colposcopy

The entire transformation zone must be visualized.
The entire lesion must be visualized.
An endocervical curettage, if done, should not demonstrate any evidence of neoplastic disease.
The biopsy findings should not be significantly less severe than the cytologic and colposcopic findings.

4. Whether the colposcopy was satisfactory (as defined in Table 25–1)
5. The age of the patient and her desire for future fertility

A final variable is the issue of compliance or the probability that the patient will be lost to follow-up should a less than definitive treatment approach be taken. In certain communities, this last variable is remarkably pertinent. However, the algorithms that are proposed are idealized and do not incorporate modifications for the patient who is at high risk for failure to comply with follow-up recommendations.

SCENARIO 1

Sentinel Pap: ASCUS
Colposcopic findings or histologic cell type if a biopsy was done: No squamous intraepithelial lesion (SIL) found
HPV testing for high-risk (oncogenic) HPV types: Negative
Satisfactory colposcopy: Yes or no
Fertility desires: Not applicable (N/A)

The results of the ALTS indicated that the negative predictive value of HPV testing for high-risk (oncogenic) HPV types is 99% in women with ASCUS smears. These women are extremely unlikely to have high-grade disease, and their risk for occult, unrecognized cancer is virtually nil.[4] These women can be reassured that their cytologic abnormality is not clinically significant, and they may be returned to routine screening protocols.

Conization in this setting is *not* an acceptable treatment alternative.

SCENARIO 2

Sentinel Pap: ASCUS
Colposcopic findings or histologic cell type if a biopsy was done: No SIL found
HPV testing for high-risk (oncogenic) HPV types: Positive
Satisfactory colposcopy: Yes or no
Fertility desires: N/A

The risk of high-grade CIN in a patient with ASCUS cytology who tests positive for oncogenic HPV types is comparable to that in a woman with LSIL cytology.[4] This case represents a woman with latent HPV infection without any clinical lesion, a woman with a lesion at the time of the Pap smear that has now regressed, a woman who was evaluated with colposcopy when a very small and possibly growing lesion (early in its natural history) was present that may have been missed on examination, or a woman with a lesion that should have been detected on colposcopy but was not. Alternatively, the cytologic abnormality may be due to a vaginal or vulvar lesion that was missed on colposcopic assessment, or it may represent cytologic overcall. This woman should be re-evaluated in 6 months with cytology and referred for colposcopy if ASCUS or a more severe abnormality is reported on that Pap smear. Colposcopic follow-up is an option if it is available. At this visit, special attention should be paid to examination of the vagina and vulva.

Conization in this setting is *not* an acceptable treatment alternative.

SCENARIO 3

Sentinel Pap: LSIL
Colposcopic findings or histologic cell type if a biopsy was done: No SIL found
HPV testing for high-risk (oncogenic) HPV types: Positive (women with LSIL on their Pap smear are very likely to test positive for high-risk HPV types[22])
Satisfactory colposcopy: No (either because the transformation zone was not fully visualized or because there is a discrepancy between cytology and the colposcopic findings)
Fertility desires: Yes or no

This case is similar to Scenario 2 in which the woman has a latent HPV infection, a regressed lesion, a lesion early in its natural history, a lesion that was missed on examination, or cytologic overcall. Data have shown that these women have a small risk of unrecognized high-grade disease, but their risk of occult, unrecognized cancer is virtually nil. Consequently, treatment is not recommend for these women. Because conization is of value only to discover a high-grade lesion or an occult invasive cancer in a patient who can be relied on to return for follow-up, rather than proceeding to conization, it is preferable to repeat the cytology in 6 months and refer for colposcopy if ASCUS or a more severe abnormality is reported on that Pap smear. Colposcopic follow-up is an option if it is available. This approach is especially appropriate when the woman is young and desires future fertility. Treating a woman with an unsatisfactory colposcopy using an ablative modality is *not* an acceptable treatment alternative. If the repeat evaluation is negative, cytology should be repeated at 6-month intervals until the patient has two consecutive negative Pap smears. However, even after two consecutive negative Pap smears, these women should be considered at high risk and should be evaluated annually with cytology. If the repeat evaluation continues to show evidence of unrecognized low-grade disease for 24 months, consideration should be given to a diagnostic conization. It is not inappropriate to perform a conization on an older woman with this clinical picture or one who is likely to be lost to follow-up, but it is probably not necessary.

SCENARIO 4

Sentinel Pap: ASCUS or LSIL
Colposcopic findings or histologic cell type if a biopsy was done: LSIL
HPV testing for high-risk (oncogenic) HPV types: Positive (women with LSIL on their Pap smear and biopsy are very likely to test positive for high-risk [oncogenic] HPV types[22])
Satisfactory colposcopy: Yes
Fertility desires: See discussion

This case represents a woman with known low-grade disease. The risk for progression of these lesions to invasive cancer is extremely small, and, if it does occur, it does so over a period of years (at least 24 months). Data have shown that the risk of unrecognized high-grade disease is about 15%, but the risk for occult, unrecognized cancer is virtually nil.[2,3] Although these women meet the traditional criteria for ablative treatment, the preferred management of women with low-grade disease is observation without treatment. This is especially appropriate when the woman is young and desires future fertility. Follow-up should be with repeat cytology. Anyone in whom ASCUS or a more severe abnormality is reported should be referred for colposcopy. Colposcopic follow-up is an option if it is available. If the repeat evaluation is negative, cytology should be repeated at 6-month intervals until the patient has had two consecutive negative Pap smears. However, even after two consecutive negative Pap smears, these women should be considered at high risk and should be evaluated annually with cytology. If the repeat evaluation continues to show evidence of persistent low-grade disease, consideration should be given to ablative therapy. It is not inappropriate to treat an older woman with this clinical picture or one who is likely to be lost to follow-up, but it is probably not necessary.

SCENARIO 5

Sentinel Pap: ASCUS or LSIL
Colposcopic findings or histologic cell type if a biopsy was done: LSIL
HPV testing for high-risk (oncogenic) HPV types: Positive (women with LSIL on their Pap smear and biopsy are very likely to test positive for high-risk [oncogenic] HPV types[22])
Satisfactory colposcopy: No
Fertility desires: See discussion

This case represents a woman with known low-grade disease but an unsatisfactory colposcopic examination. The case is similar to Scenario 4, with the exception that the unsatisfactory colposcopy injects an element of uncertainty about the presence of unrecognized high-grade disease or occult cancer. Data have demonstrated that the risk of unrecognized high-grade disease is very low in this situation and the risk for occult, unrecognized cancer is virtually nil.[41] Follow-up should be with repeat cytology. This is especially appropriate when the woman is young and desires future fertility. Anyone in whom ASCUS or a more severe abnormality is reported should be referred for colposcopy. Colposcopic follow-up is an option if it is available. If the repeat evaluation is negative, cytology should be repeated at 6-month intervals until the patient has had two consecutive negative Pap smears. However, even after two consecutive negative Pap smears, these women should be considered at high risk and should be evaluated annually with cytology. If the repeat evaluation continues to show evidence of persistent low-grade disease, consideration should be given to conization. It is not inappropriate to perform conization in these women, especially when they are older and no longer desire fertility or when they are at risk to be lost to follow-up, but it is probably not necessary.

SCENARIO 6

Sentinel Pap: ASCUS or LSIL or HSIL
Colposcopic findings or histologic cell type if a biopsy was done: HSIL
HPV testing for high-risk (oncogenic) HPV types: Positive (women with HSIL on biopsy are very likely to test positive for high-risk [oncogenic] HPV types)
Satisfactory colposcopy: Yes
Fertility desires: N/A

This case represents a woman with known high-grade disease and a satisfactory colposcopy. In this situation, the progressive potential of the lesions is very high, and treatment should be performed.[2, 3] Such women may be treated with ablative modalities as long as the colposcopist is completely confident that the highest-grade lesion has been sampled and that invasive cancer has been excluded. Cryotherapy does have a lower cure rate for high-grade lesions and larger lesions and should probably be avoided in these patients (discussed previously). However, studies have shown that 1% to 2% of these women have occult, unrecognized, microinvasive or invasive cancer at the time of treatment despite a satisfactory colposcopy.[19, 42] For this reason, many experts recommend that these women be treated using an excisional modality such electrosurgical loop excision, laser conization, or cold-knife cone biopsy.

SCENARIO 7

Sentinel Pap: ASCUS or LSIL or HSIL
Colposcopic findings or histologic cell type if a biopsy was done: HSIL
HPV testing for high-risk (oncogenic) HPV types: Positive (women with HSIL on biopsy are very likely to test positive for high-risk [oncogenic] HPV types)
Satisfactory colposcopy: No
Fertility desires: N/A

This case represents a woman with known high-grade disease and an unsatisfactory colposcopy. The unanswered question in such women is whether they have an unrecognized microinvasive or invasive cancer. These women must have an excisional conization such an elec-

trosurgical loop excision, laser conization, or cold-knife cone biopsy.

Ablative therapy in this setting is *not* an acceptable treatment alternative.

SUMMARY OF KEY POINTS

- *HSIL.* CIN 2, 3 is a lesion with true malignant potential, and it is important to identify and treat it. Women with HSIL cytology should undergo colposcopic evaluation. Women with a satisfactory colposcopy and a negative endocervical curettage may be treated by ablative techniques such as cryotherapy or laser vaporization or by an excisional procedure such as loop electrosurgical excision. Cryotherapy may be slightly less effective for treatment of CIN 3 with crypt involvement or if the lesion involves more than two quadrants of the cervix. If no lesion is identified or if the colposcopy is unsatisfactory, a cervical conization should be performed, because the positive predictive value of HSIL cytology is very high, and these women have a small but significant risk of having invasive cancer. Observation is not an appropriate management option for women with high-grade squamous lesions.

- *LSIL or ASCUS cytology with oncogenic HPV types—lesion identified on colposcopy.* Women with LSIL cytology or women with ASCUS cytology who are HPV DNA positive for oncogenic HPV types are at risk for having high-grade CIN, but their risk is smaller than for those women with HSIL cytology. Because the risk of high-grade CIN in a woman with ASCUS cytology who is positive for oncogenic HPV types is comparable to that in a woman with LSIL cytology, colposcopic evaluation should be performed. If a low-grade lesion is identified on colposcopy, the preferred management is observation without treatment, which includes repeat cytology at 6-month intervals until two consecutive negative Pap smears are obtained. Colposcopic follow-up is also an option. If the repeat evaluation continues to show persistent LSIL, consideration should be given to ablative therapy. If a high-grade lesion is identified on colposcopy, treatment should proceed accordingly.

- *LSIL or ASCUS cytology with oncogenic HPV types—no lesion identified on colposcopy.* If no colposcopic lesion is identified, the patient should be evaluated in 6 months with cytology. Colposcopic follow-up is also an option. If the repeat Pap smear is negative, cytology should be repeated at 6-month intervals until two consecutive negative Pap smears are obtained. However, even after two consecutive negative Pap smears, these women should be considered at high risk and should have annual cytology. The women should be referred for colposcopy if the repeat cytology indicates ASCUS or a more severe cytologic abnormality. Because the true risk of CIN 2, 3 is small in these groups and the risk of invasive cancer is nil, conization is not indicated when a lesion is not identified or the colposcopic examination is unsatisfactory. However, if the repeat evaluation continues to show evidence of LSIL for 24 months, conization might be considered.

- *ASCUS cytology and negative oncogenic HPV types.* The negative predictive value of HPV testing for oncogenic HPV types is 99% in women with ASCUS cytology. These women are unlikely to have high-grade disease, and their risk for occult, unrecognized cancer is virtually nil. These women can be reassured that their cytologic abnormality is not clinically significant, and they may be returned to routine screening protocols. Conization in these women is not an acceptable management option.

References

1. Jones BA, Davey DD: Quality management in gynecologic cytology using interlaboratory comparison. Arch Pathol Lab Med 2000;124:672.
2. Ostor AG: Natural history of cervical intraepithelial neoplasia: A critical review. Internat J Gynecol Pathol 1993;12:186.
3. Melnikow J, Nuovo J, Willan AR, et al: Natural history of cervical squamous intraepithelial lesions: A meta-analysis. Obstet Gynecol 1998;92:727.
4. Soloman D, Schiffman M, Tarone R: Comparison of three management strategies for patients with atypical squamous cells of undetermined significance: Baseline results from a randomized study. J Natl Cancer Inst 2001;93:293.
5. Crum CP, Genest DR, Krane JF, et al: Subclassifying atypical squamous in ThinPrep cervical cytology correlates with detection of high-risk human papillomavirus DNA. Am J Clin Pathol 1999;112:384.
6. Schoolland M, Sterrett GF, Knowles SA, et al: The "Inconclusive—possible high-grade epithelial abnormality" category in Papanicolaou smear reporting. Cancer 1998;84:208.
7. Malik SN, Wilkinson EJ, Drew PA, et al: Do qualifiers of ASCUS distinguish between low- and high-risk patients? Acta Cytol 1999;43:376.
8. Quddus MR, Sung CJ, Steinhoff MM, et al: Atypical squamous metaplastic cells: Reproducibility, outcome and diagnostic features on ThinPrep Pap test. Cancer 2001;93:16.
9. Spitzer M, Krumholz B, Cherynys AE, et al: Comparative utility of repeat Papanicolaou smear, cervicography, and colposcopy in the evaluation of atypical Papanicolaou smears. Obstet Gynecol 1987;69:731.
10. Slawson DC, Bennett JH, Simon LJ, Herman JM: Should all women with cervical atypia be referred for colposcopy: A HAR-NET study. Harrisburg Area Research Network. J Fam Pract 1994;38:387.
11. Eskridge C, Begneaud WP, Landwehr C: Cervicography combined with repeat Papanicolaou test as triage for low-grade cytologic abnormalities. Obstet Gynecol 1998;92:351.
12. Cox JT, Wilkinson EJ, Lonky N, et al: Management guidelines for the follow-up of atypical squamous cells of undetermined significance (ASCUS). J Lower Genital Tract Dis 2000;4:99.
13. Lonky NM, Sadeghi M, Tsadik GW, Petitti D: The clinical significance of the poor correlation of cervical dysplasia and cervical malignancy with referral cytologic results. Am J Obstet Gynecol 1999;181:560.
14. Bolger BS, Lewis BV: A prospective study of colposcopy in women with mild dyskaryosis or koilocytosis. Br J Obstet Gynaecol 1988;95:1117.
15. Kinney WK, Manos MM, Hurley LB, Ransley JE: Where's the high-grade cervical neoplasia? The importance of minimally abnormal Papanicolaou diagnoses. Obstet Gynecol 1998;91:973.
16. Law KS, Chang TC, Hsuch S, et al: High prevalence of high grade squamous intraepithelial lesions and microinvasive carcinoma in women with cytological diagnosis of low grade squamous intraepithelial lesions. J Reprod Med 2001;46:61.
17. Lee SSN, Collins RJ, Pun TC, et al: Conservative treatment of low-grade squamous intraepithelial lesions (LSIL) of the cervix. Int J Gynecology Obstet 1998;60:35.
18. Andersen ES, Nielsen K, Pedersen B: The reliability of preconization diagnostic evaluation in patients with cervical intraepithelial neoplasia and microinvasive carcinoma. Gynecol Oncol 1995;59:143.
19. Bigrigg MA, Codling BW, Pearson P, et al: Colposcopic diagnosis and treatment of cervical dysplasia at a single clinic visit: Experience of low-voltage diathermy loop in 1000 patients. Lancet 1990;336:229.
20. Wright TC, Sun XW, Koulos J: Comparison of management algorithms for the evaluation of women with low-grade cytologic abnormalities. Obstet Gynecol 1995;85:202.
21. Stoler MH, Schiffman M: Interobserver reproducibility of cervical cytologic and histologic interpretations: Realistic estimates from the ASCUS-LSIL Triage Study. JAMA 2001;285:1500.
22. ALTS Group: Human papillomavirus testing for triage of women with cytologic evidence of low-grade squamous intraepithelial lesions: Baseline data from a randomized trial. The Atypical Squamous Cells of Undetermined Significance/Low-Grade Squamous Intraepithelial Lesions Triage Study (ALTS) Group. J Natl Cancer Inst 2000;92:397.
23. Nasiell K, Roger V, Nasiell M: Behavior of mild cervical dysplasia during long-term follow-up. Obstet Gynecol 1986;67:665.
24. Robertson JH, Woodend BE, Crozier EH, Hutchinson J: Risk of cervical cancer associated with mild dyskaryosis. Br Med J 1988;297:18.
25. Luthra UK, Prabhakar AK, Seth P, et al: Natural history of precancerous and early cancerous lesions of the uterine cervix. Acta Cytol 1987;31:226.
26. Kurman RJ, Henson DE, Herbst AL, et al: Interim guidelines for management of abnormal cervical cytology. The 1992 National Cancer Institute Workshop. JAMA 1994;271:1866.
27. Nobbenhuis MA, Walboomers JM, Helmerhorst TJ, et al: Relation of human papillomavirus status to cervical lesions and consequences for cervical-cancer screening: A prospective study. Lancet. 1999;354:20.
28. Stafl A, Friedrich EG Jr, Mattingly RF: Detection of cervical neoplasia—reducing the risk of error. Clin Obstet Gynecol 1973;16:238.
29. Mitchell MF, Schottenfeld D, Tortolero-Luna G, et al: Colposcopy for the diagnosis of squamous intraepithelial lesions: A meta analysis. Obstet Gynecol 1998;91:626.
30. Schneider DL, Herrero R, Bratti C, et al: Cervicography screening for cervical cancer among 8640 women in a high-risk population. Am J Obstet Gynecol 1999;180:290.
31. Ferris DG, Wright TC, Litaker MS, et al: Triage of women with ASCUS and LSIL on Pap smear reports: Management by repeat Pap smear, HPV DNA testing or colposcopy? J Fam Pract 1998;46:125.
32. Wright TC, Lorincz AT, Ferris DG, et al: Reflex HPV testing in women with abnormal Papanicolaou smears. Am J Obstet Gynecol 1998;178:962.
33. Manos MM, Kinney WK, Hurley LB, et al: Identifying women with cervical neoplasia using human papillomavirus DNA testing for equivocal Papanicolaou results. JAMA 1999;281:1605.
34. Bergeron C, Jeannel D, Poveda JD, et al: Human papillomavirus testing in women with mild cytologic atypia. Obstet Gynecol 2000;95:821.
35. American College of Obstetricians and Gynecologists (ACOG): Cervical Cytology: Evaluation and Management of Abnormalities. ACOG Technical Bulletin No. 183 (1993).
36. Wheeler CM, Greer CE, Becker TM, et al: Short-term fluctuations in the detection of cervical human papillomavirus DNA. Obstet Gynecol 1996;88:261.
37. Lin CT, Tseng CJ, Lai CH, et al: Value of human papillomavirus deoxyribonucleic acid testing after conization in the prediction of

residual disease in the subsequent hysterectomy specimen. Am J Obstet Gynecol 2001;184:940.

38. Jain S, Tseng CJ, Horng SG, et al: Negative predictive value of human papillomavirus test following conization of the cervix uteri. Gynecol Oncol 2001;82:177.

39. Strand A, Wilander E, Zehbe I, Rylander E: High risk HPV persists after treatment of genital papillomavirus infection but not after treatment of cervical intraepithelial neoplasia. Acta Obstet Gynecol Scand 1997;76:140.

40. Spitzer M: Fertility and pregnancy outcome after treatment for cervical intraepithelial neoplasia. J Lower Genital Tract Dis 1998;2:225.

41. Spitzer M, Chernys AE, Shifrin A, Ryskin M: Indications for cone biopsy: Pathologic correlation. Am J Obstet Gynecol 1998;178:74.

42. Spitzer M, Chernys AE, Seltzer VL: The outpatient use of large loop excision of the transformation zone in an inner-city population. Obstet Gynecol 1993;82:731.

• F.J. Montz
• Robert E. Bristow
• Mark Spitzer

C

Management of Positive Margins and Positive Endocervical Curettage

The clinician must take numerous variables into consideration when deciding how best to treat a patient with lower genital tract dysplasia. One of these variables is "margin status" (i.e., whether there is dysplasia in the resection margins of a cone biopsy or an electrosurgical loop excision procedure [LEEP] or in an endocervical curettage [ECC]). The health care provider must know the status of these margins, because there are few stronger predictors of success or failure of conservative cervical dysplasia therapy.[1, 2] Most experts would agree that patients with negative resection margins and a negative ECC, regardless of sentinel Papanicolaou smear, degree of dysplasia in the specimen, or fertility desires, should be followed up with repeat cytology, initially at 6 months and continuing at a similar interval for several years. Some institutions add colposcopy periodically to their follow-up protocol.

Of course, there are exceptions to this general guideline (e.g., women with glandular dysplasias), but, in general, this degree of conservative follow-up is appropriate. In contradistinction, it can be problematic to devise an optimal treatment plan for some patients who have a positive margin, such as those patients who desire fertility maintenance. In this chapter, we will discuss the challenging topics of so-called positive margins and positive ECC, reviewing their clinical importance as well as our preferred management recommendations.

INCIDENCE

A review of the literature in the 1970s and 1980s showed eight major studies[3–10] of cervical conizations. Of the almost 4000 conizations in these studies, the recurrence/persistence rate was 2.9% among patients with clear margins and 22% among those with involved margins. Spitzer et al[11] showed that the recurrence rate is higher in the endocervical margin compared with the ectocervical margin. When determining the incidence of positive margins and making clinical decisions, it is beneficial if specific data are available categorized according to four dominant variables. These variables are (1) indication for the excisional procedure; (2) cell types and degree of dysplasia, not only in the specimen but at the margin; (3) which of the numerous excisional techniques was performed; and (4) patient age. Unfortunately, such data, stratified by multivariables, are often unavailable. In the cumulative, nonstratified literature, positive margins are found in 20% to 40% of cases. These numbers simply serve to support the authors' opinion that the practicing clinician must have adequate knowledge concerning how to manage patients with positive margins.

TECHNICAL CAUSES OF POSITIVE MARGINS AND ECCs

Although knowledge regarding what specifically leads to the occurrence of a positive margin or ECC does not necessarily lead to any modification of a proposed treatment algorithm, this knowledge may serve as an impetus for future technique selection or performance improvement. In general, the only causative variable that the health care professional controls is the selection and performance of a given resective procedure. It has been recognized for more than a decade that certain procedures (i.e., LEEPs and laser cone biopsies), particularly when performed by less experienced technicians, are more likely to have positive margins.[12-15] The popularity of LEEP has led to an increase in positive margins. Gonzalez[16] reviewed 20 articles reporting on 5309 patients undergoing LEEPs. Positive margins were found in 13% to 45%, and recurrence/persistence rates with positive margins ranged between 10% and 69%. Recurrence/persistence rates in those with negative margins were between 5% and 38%. The authors concluded that patients undergoing LEEP need careful follow-up regardless of their margin status. They further concluded that the use of a second endocervical LEEP (a so-called top hat LEEP) did not reduce recurrence rates. However, there are few data supporting the belief that these laboratory findings translate into a meaningful outcome difference (i.e., rates of dysplasia recurrence).[17] Controversy surrounding this issue does exist when the underlying pathology demonstrates either a microinvasive squamous disease or an adenocarcinoma.[18] It is important to make every effort to minimize the occurrence of false-positive ECCs by ensuring that any visible ectocervical lesion is not disrupted at the time that the ECC is done.[19] One approach to minimizing this occurrence is to document with colposcopy any evident disease, before and after the ECC. In this way, any disruption of a visible ectocervical lesion can be documented.

ALGORITHMS

It is important to take into consideration at least three variables when developing rational management algorithms for women with a positive resective margin or ECC. These variables are (1) probability that residual, underlying precancer or unappreciated invasive disease is present, (2) fertility desires of the patient, and (3) risk of other procedure-related side effects or complications. A final variable is the probability that the patient will be lost to follow-up should a less-than-definitive approach be taken. Unquestionably, this last variable is remarkably relevant in certain communities. However, the algorithms that we propose here are idealized and do not incorporate modifications for the patient who is at high risk for being lost to follow-up. Additionally, we have not developed specific algorithms that adjust for volume of disease at the positive margin beyond that implied by the use of ECC status as an algorithm modifier. However, we place great clinical import on the degree of dysplasia noted at the positive margin/ECC.

These algorithms are developed for the management of women whose cone biopsies or LEEP specimen margins are positive or whose post–cone biopsy ECC is positive. Findings considered in developing these recommendations include (1) the results of the sentinel Papanicolaou (Pap) smear(s) that led to the performance of the colposcopy and biopsies; (2) the histologic cell type at the positive margin or ECC, generally without regard (except in cases of histologic findings of invasive disease or adenodysplasias) for what degree of dysplasia was found elsewhere; (3) which margin is positive (ectocervical or endocervical); (4) ECC status; and, in certain instances, (5) the

patient's age and desire for fertility. Select references from the peer-review literature are included to support a potentially controversial recommendation or to illustrate a point.

Scenario 1

Sentinel Pap: Persistent low-grade squamous intraepithelial lesion (LSIL) or atypical squamous cells of undetermined significance (ASCUS) or a single ASCUS Pap smear in a woman older than 30 years with a positive test for high-risk (oncogenic) human papillomavirus (HPV)

Histologic cell type at the margin: Low-grade cervical intraepithelial neoplasia (CIN)

Which margin is positive: Either or both

ECC: Positive or negative

Fertility desires: Not applicable (N/A)

Age: N/A

Recommendation: Repeat Pap smear in 6 months

If *positive,* repeat colposcopy and biopsies. If *negative,* follow up as per institutional routine. Some institutions add colposcopy periodically to their follow-up protocol. Hysterectomy in this setting is *not* an acceptable treatment alternative.[20-22]

Scenario 2

Sentinel Pap: High-grade squamous intraepithelial lesion (HSIL) or persistent LSIL or ASCUS or a single ASCUS Pap smear in a woman older than 30 years with a positive test for high-risk (oncogenic) HPV types

Histologic cell type at the margin: High-grade CIN

Which margin is positive: Either or both

ECC: Negative

Fertility desires: N/A

Age: N/A

Recommendation: Repeat Pap smear in 3 months

If *positive,* repeat colposcopy and biopsies. If *negative,* follow up as per institutional routine. Some institutions add colposcopy periodically to their follow-up protocol. Some authors have empirically recommended the performance of an ECC in this setting, although few data support this opinion (see later discussion). Our opinion, that the intensity of follow-up should be increased if the positive margins demonstrate high-grade squamous dysplasia, is based on studies demonstrating an increased rate of persistence in these instances when compared with cases where margins were positive for low-grade disease.[23, 24] This scenario also demonstrates the importance of knowing the status of the endocervical sampling, because it facilitates triage.[25] If this information is not available, we triage patients based on age, as discussed in Scenarios 3 and 4. Although some would perform a repeat conization or a hysterectomy in this setting (especially if the patient did not desire future fertility), unless there is another indication, this approach should not be favored.

The finding of a positive endocervical margin in the patient who is positive for human immunodeficiency virus (HIV) may be of more concern than the same finding in the HIV-negative women.[26] Margin status is generally a poor predictor of outcome of conization.[27]

Scenario 3

Sentinel Pap: HSIL
Histologic cell type at the margin: High-grade CIN
Which margin is positive: Either or both
ECC: Positive
Fertility desires: Yes
Age: N/A
Recommendation: Repeat Pap smear in 3 months

If *positive,* repeat colposcopy and biopsies. If *negative,* follow up as per institutional routine. Some institutions add colposcopy periodically to their follow-up protocol. Select authors would add the empiric performance of an ECC in this setting, although few data support this opinion.[19, 28] The finding of both a positive endocervical margin and a positive ECC, with both demonstrating high-grade CIN, increases the probability of disease recurrence or persistence.[29] Regardless, we do not change the frequency or intensity of follow-up in the young patient. In the older patient, however, the management is changed (see Scenario 4).

Scenario 4

Sentinel Pap: HSIL
Histologic cell type at the margin: High-grade CIN
Which margin is positive: Either or both
ECC: Positive
Fertility desires: Not desired
Age: Postmenopausal or older than 50 years
Recommendation: Repeat excisional procedure, because there are excellent data demonstrating that older age positively correlates with an underlying finding of unappreciated cervical cancer.[30] If a repeat excision cannot be performed as a result of local anatomic variables, consideration should be given to performing an MD Anderson class 2 radical hysterectomy in light of the increased probability of an as-yet unappreciated, underlying cancer being extant.

If the repeat excision is complete (subsequent negative margins) and there is no malignancy present, repeat Pap smear in 3 months. If *positive,* repeat colposcopy and biopsies. If *negative,* follow up as per institutional routine. Some institutions add colposcopy periodically to their follow-up protocol.

Scenario 5

Sentinel Pap: Consistent with invasive squamous cancer
Histologic cell type at the margin: Low-grade CIN
Which margin is positive: Either or both
ECC: Positive or negative
Fertility desires: N/A
Age: N/A
Recommendation: We would recommend that a repeat excisional procedure be performed. However, before

exposing the patient to the associated risk, we would strongly encourage that the cytology be reviewed by a trusted cytopathologist. If, as noted in Scenario 4, a re-excision cannot be performed secondary to local anatomic variables, consideration should be given to performing an MD Anderson class 2 radical hysterectomy in light of the increased probability of an underlying occult cancer. If malignancy is present, treatment should be based on the final International Federation of Gynecology and Obstetrics (FIGO) stage of disease.[31]

If the repeat excision is complete (subsequent negative margins) and no malignancy is present, repeat Pap smear in 3 months. If *positive,* repeat colposcopy and biopsies. If *negative,* follow up as per institutional routine. Some institutions add colposcopy periodically to their follow-up protocol.

Scenario 6

Sentinel Pap: Any
Histologic cell type at the margin: Microinvasive squamous cancer
Which margin is positive: Either or both
ECC: Positive or negative
Fertility desires: N/A
Age: N/A
Recommendation: The diagnosis of FIGO stage 1A disease can be made only in those settings where an excisional procedure has been performed and the margins are negative. Therefore, a repeat excisional procedure must be performed.[32] A simple, extrafascial hysterectomy is *not* appropriate in this setting.

If the final FIGO stage is 1A1, complete excision by any technique is adequate and avoids the additional risk of hysterectomy.

If the final FIGO stage is 1A2, the data suggest that a simple extrafascial hysterectomy is inadequate therapy and that a more extensive resection (an MD Anderson class 2 radical hysterectomy), as well as pelvic lymph node dissection, is preferable.[31] If a re-excision cannot be performed secondary to local anatomic variables, consideration should be given to performing an MD Anderson class 2 radical hysterectomy in light of the increased probability of an underlying cancer greater than FIGO stage 1A2 being extant.

Scenario 7

Sentinel Pap: Any
Histologic cell type at the margin: Invasive squamous cancer with lesion greater than 5 by 7 mm
Which margin is positive: Either or both
ECC: Positive or negative
Fertility desires: N/A
Age: N/A
Recommendation: Knowledge of margin status from an excisional biopsy that demonstrates unequivocally invasive cancer is truly moot. These patients should be treated as per previously referenced guidelines.[31]

Scenario 8

Sentinel Pap: Any

Histologic cell type at the margin: Adenocarcinoma in situ

Which margin is positive: Endocervical margin—positive, ectocervical margin—positive or negative (uncommon that this margin is positive)

ECC: Positive or negative

Fertility desires: Desired

Age: N/A

Recommendation: In this setting, it is critical that invasive cancer be ruled out to the best of the physician's ability without eliminating the woman's potential for future childbearing. A repeat cone biopsy is needed that removes a long cylinder and includes the endocervical glands. In the hands of most clinicians, this is done preferentially using a scalpel.[33] If the repeat excision demonstrates clear margins, then, after detailed informed consent has been obtained (see data below indicating potential risks to this approach), a conservative approach of repeat Pap smears and ECC can be offered the patient. There are growing data to support that this approach is safe,[34, 35] although extensive published experience supports the opinion that negative margins are a less than accurate predictor of the absence of residual dysplasia in women with adenocarcinoma in situ when compared to squamous lesions.[33, 36, 37] If a repeat excision continues to demonstrate adenocarcinoma in situ without frank invasion, we would be remarkably concerned about the presence of an occult adenocarcinoma, particularly if the ECC were persistently positive.[38] Our recommendation for an individual who desires future childbearing is that she undergo a radical vaginal trachelectomy (MD Anderson class 2)[39, 40] with concomitant placement of a cerclage. Should, on final pathology, more than the most superficial invasion be documented (FIGO stage 1A1), we would recommend that a pelvic lymphadenectomy be performed as an additional and separate procedure[41, 42] (by laparoscopy, if possible). It should be noted that early data demonstrates that conization may be adequate therapy for stage 1A1 adenocarcinoma of the endocervix.[43] Although these data are intriguing, we consider it premature to accept cone biopsy as a standard therapy in this setting.

Scenario 9

Sentinel Pap: Any

Histologic cell type at the margin: Adenocarcinoma in situ

Which margin is positive: Endocervical margin—positive, ectocervical margin—positive or negative (uncommon that this margin is positive)

ECC: Positive or negative

Fertility desires: Not desired

Age: N/A

Recommendation: When future childbearing is not a consideration, definitive surgery is recommended.

The current treatment recommendation for endocervical adenocarcinoma in situ is an MD Anderson class 1 extrafascial hysterectomy. There is concern, however, about the probability that these women harbor an unappreciated invasive carcinoma such that the performance of an extrafascial hysterectomy would be inadequate therapy.[35, 44] Our interpretation of the literature supports the opinion that this probability is so high that further attempts to rule out invasive disease must be undertaken. Therefore, our recommendation would be a large cone biopsy, one that approaches the volume of cervix removed when performing a vaginal trachelectomy. If this does not demonstrate invasive cancer, we would then proceed to an extrafascial hysterectomy. For some women, usually postmenopausal women who have undergone repeated cervical excisional procedures and have minimal cervical tissue remaining, it may not be possible or safe to attempt an additional cone biopsy or similar excisional procedure. In this setting, we recommend that the patient undergo an MD Anderson class 2 radical hysterectomy. The published literature, as well as our institutional experience, has demonstrated that in appropriate hands, this type of radical hysterectomy can be accomplished with complication and morbidity rates comparable to class 1 hysterectomies.[45]

CONCLUSIONS

It is hoped that our discussion has illuminated the multiple key points of clinical information that must be known to rationally decide how to best manage patients with a positive margin at the time of an excisional procedure or a positive ECC. Although there are special instances in which the clinician can justify an extensive or even radical surgical operation, in the majority of settings a conservative approach can be taken if the patient is able to comply with a structured follow-up protocol.

References

1. Paterson-Brown S, Chappatte OA, Clark SK, et al: The significance of cone biopsy resection margins. Gynecol Oncol 1992;46:182.
2. Phelps JY, Ward JA, Szigeti J, et al: Cervical cone margins as a predictor for residual dysplasia in post-cone hysterectomy specimens. Obstet Gynecol 1994;84:128.
3. Vaclavinkova V, Hedman AK, Nasiell K: Follow-up studies in dysplasia and carcinoma-in-situ of the cervix uteri. Acta Obstet Gynecol Scand 1978;57:69.
4. Holdt DG, Jacobs AJ, Scott JC, Adam GM: Diagnostic significance and sequelae of cone biopsy. Am J Obstet Gynecol 1982;143:312.
5. Green GH: Cervical cytology and carcinoma in situ. J Obstet Gynaecol Br Commonw. 1965;72:13.
6. Kullander S, Sjoberg NO: Treatment of carcinoma in situ of the cervix by conization. Acta Obstet Gynecol Scand 1971;50:153.
7. Burghardt E, Holzer E: Treatment of carcinoma in situ: evaluation of 1609 cases. Obstet Gynecol 1980;55:539.
8. Ahlgren M. Ingemarsson I, Lindberg LG, Nordqvist RB: Conization as treatment of carcinoma in situ of the uterine cervix. Obstet Gynecol 1975;46:135.
9. Kolstad P, Klem V: Long-term follow-up of 1121 cases of carcinoma in situ. Obstet Gyecol 1976;48:125.
10. Bjerre B, Eliasson G, Linell F, et al: Am J Obstet Gynecol 1976; 125:143.

11. Spitzer M, Chernys AE, Seltzer VL: The use of large-loop excision of the transformation zone in an inner-city population. Obstet Gynecol 1993;82:731.

12. Kristensen GB, Jensen LK, Holund B: A randomized trial comparing two methods of cold knife conization with laser conization. Obset Gynecol 1990;76:1009.

13. Montz FJ, Holschneider CH, Thompson LD: Large-look excision of the transformation zone: Effect on the pathologic interpretation of resection margins. Obstet Gynecol 1993;81:976.

14. Girardi F, Heydarfadia M, Koroschetz F, et al: Cold-knife conization versus loop excision: Histopathologic and clinical results of a randomized trial. Gynecol Oncol 1994;55:368.

15. Mathevet P, Dargent D, Roy M, Beau G: A randomized prospective study comparing three techniques of conization: Cold knife, laser, and LEEP. Gynecol Oncol 1994;54:175.

16. Gonzalez DI, Zahn CM, Retzloff MG, et al: Recurrence of dysplasia after loop electrosurgical excision procedures with long term followup. Am J Obstet Gynecol 2001;184:315.

17. Montz FJ: Management of cervical intraepithelial neoplasm. In Nichols D, Clarke-Pearson D (eds): Gynecologic, Obstetric, and Related Surgery. St. Louis, Mosby, 2000, pp 282–298.

18. Jakus S, Edmonds P, Dunton C, King SA: Margin status and excision of cervical intraepithelial neoplasia: A review. Obstet Gynecol Surv 2000;55:520.

19. Moniak CW, Kutzner S, Adam E, et al: Endocervical curettage in evaluating abnormal cervical cytology. J Reprod Med 2000;45:285.

20. Andersen ES, Nielsen K, Larsen G: Laser conization: Follow-up in patients with cervical intraepithelial neoplasia in the cone margin. Gynecol Oncol 1990;39:328.

21. Lapaquette TK, Dinh TV, Hannigan EV, et al: Management of patients with positive margins after cervical conization. Obstet Gynecol 1993;82:440.

22. Monk A, Puskin SF, Nelson AL, Gunning JE: Conservative management options for patients with dysplasia involving endocervical margins of cervical cone biopsy specimens. Am J Obset Gynecol 1996;174:1695.

23. Livasy CA, Maygarden SJ, Rajaratnam CT, Novotny DB: Predictors of recurrent dysplasia after a cervical loop electrocautery excision procedure for CIN 3: A study of margin, endocervical gland, and quadrant involvement. Mod Path 1999;12:233.

24. Jansen FW, Trimbos JB, Hermans J, Fleuren GJ: Persistent cervical intraepithelial neoplasia after incomplete conization: Predictive value of clinical and histological parameters. Gynecol Obstet Invest 1994;37:270.

25. Felix JC, Muderspach LI, Duggan BD, Roman LD: The significance of positive margins in loop electrosurgical cone biopsies. Obstet Gynecol 1994;84:996.

26. Boardman LA, Peipert JF, Hogan JW, Cooper AS: Positive cone biopsy specimen margins in women infected with the human immunodeficiency virus. Am J Obstet Gynecol 1999;181:1395.

27. Holcomb K, Matthews RP, Chapman JE, et al: The efficacy of cervical conization in the treatment of cervical intraepithelial neoplasia in HIV-positive women. Gynecol Oncol 1999;74:428.

28. Fine BA, Feinstein GI, Sabella V: The pre- and postoperative value of endocervical curettage in the detection of cervical intraepithelial neoplasia and invasive cervical cancer. Gynecol Oncol 1998;71:46.

29. Husseinzadeh N, Shbaro I, Wesseler T: Predictive value of cone margins and post-cone endocervical curettage with residual disease in subsequent hysterectomy. Gynecol Oncol 1989;33:198.

30. Kobak WH, Roman LD, Felix JC, et al: The role of endocervical curettage at cervical conization for high-grade dysplasia. Obstet Gynecol 1995;85:197.

31. Bristow RE, Montz FJ: Cervical cancer. In Ransom SB, Dombrowski MP, McNeeley SG, et al (eds): Practical Strategies in Obstetrics and Gynecology. Philadelphia, WB Saunders, 2000, pp 458–470.

32. Roman LD, Felix JC, Muderspach LI, et al: Risk of residual invasive disease in women with microinvasive squamous cancer in a conization specimen. Obstet Gynecol 1997;90:759.

33. Azodi M, Chambers SK, Rutherford TJ, et al: Adenocarcinoma in situ of the cervix: Management and outcome. Gynecol Oncol 1999;73:348.

34. Andersen ES, Arffmann E: Adenocarcinoma in situ of the uterine cervix: A clinico-pathologic study of 36 cases. Gynecol Oncol 1989;35:1.

35. Muntz HG, Bell DA, Lage JM, et al: Adenocarcinoma in situ of the uterine cervix. Obstet Gynecol 1992;80:935.

36. Denehy TR, Gregori CA, Breen JL: Endocervical curettage, cone margins, and residual adenocarcinoma in situ of the cervix. Obstet Gynecol 1997;90:1.

37. Wolf JK, Levenback C, Malpica A, et al: Adenocarcinoma in situ of the cervix: Significance of cone biopsy margins. Obstet Gynecol 1996;88:82.

38. Goldstein NS, Mani A: The status and distance of cone biopsy margins as a predictor of excision adequacy for endocervical adenocarcinoma in situ. Am J Clin Pathol 1998;109:727.

39. Covens A, Shaw P, Murphy J, et al: Is radical trachelectomy a safe alternative to radical hysterectomy for patients with stage IA-B carcinoma of the cervix? Cancer 1999;86:2273.

40. Dargent D, Martin X, Sacchetoni A, Mathevet P: Laparoscopic radical vaginal hysterectomy: A treatment to preserve fertility in cervical carcinoma patients. Cancer 2000;88:1877.

41. Schorge JO, Lee KR, Flynn CE, et al: Stage IA1 cervical adenocarcinoma: Definition and treatment. Obstet Gynecol 1999;93:219.

42. Childers JM: The virtues and pitfalls of minimally invasive surgery for gynecologic malignancies: an update. Curr Opin Obstet Gynecol 1999;11:51.

43. Schorge JO, Lee KR, Sheets EE: Prospective management of stage IA(1) cervical adenocarcinoma by conization alone to preserve fertility: A preliminary report. Gynecol Oncol 2000;78:217.

44. Poynor EA, Barakat RR, Hoskins WJ: Management and follow-up of patients with adenocarcinoma in situ of the uterine cervix. Gynecol Oncol 1995;57:158.

45. Magrina JF, Goodrich MA, Weaver AL, Podratz KC: Modified radical hysterectomy: Morbidity and mortality. Gynecol Oncol 1995;59:277.

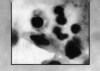

Index

Note: Page numbers followed by f indicate figures; page numbers followed by t indicate tables.